Praise from the experts for
Before Your Pregnancy

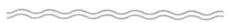

"Many people don't realize that the most important time for doing things to improve the chances for having a healthy pregnancy outcome is actually before conceiving that pregnancy. *Before Your Pregnancy* is a wonderful and invaluable resource for couples planning a pregnancy. I highly recommend this book."

—PETER BERNSTEIN, MD, MPH
Professor of Clinical Obstetrics and Gynecology and Women's Health,
Director of the Fellowship Program in Maternal Fetal Medicine,
Montefiore Medical Center/Albert Einstein College of Medicine

"Optimal preconceptional care is essential for a successful pregnancy. As Amy Ogle and Lisa Mazzullo have shown, in this beautifully executed book, there is much more to preconceptional care than folic acid supplementation. This is a comprehensive piece that synthesizes all of the important medical, dietary, and lifestyle considerations for families anticipating pregnancy. *Before Your Pregnancy* is a wonderful resource that I will be thrilled to share with my patients."

—CLARISSA BONANNO, MD
Columbia University Department of Obstetrics and Gynecology

"*Before Your Pregnancy* is a comprehensive, refreshing, and contemporary review of the complex issues that impact women and their pregnancies. With so much misinformation concerning pregnancy now available 24/7 on the Internet and other media outlets, this book should be required reading for women planning a pregnancy and their health care providers. It is well written and evidence based and is an enjoyable and educational read. I wholeheartedly recommend it!"

—LEE P. SHULMAN, MD
The Anna Ross Lapham Professor in Obstetrics and Gynecology,
Feinberg School of Medicine of Northwestern University

"*Before Your Pregnancy* will be recommended to all my fertility patients as an evidenced-based, friendly, participative guide to a successful conception and healthy pregnancy. It is by far the most complete resource I have reviewed, and I am certain it will provide a great benefit to many couples and the health of their future children!"

—JUDY SIMON, MS, RD, CD, CHES
Fertility Nutrition Specialist, Mind Body Nutrition PLLC and
University of Washington Medical Center

"I congratulate the author-clinicians for delivering this comprehensive, up-to-date, evidence-based medical guide to optimizing a couple's health in order to achieve the best possible outcome for their pregnancy. Every patient in my practice could benefit from reading this book."

—CHRISTOPHER SIPE, MD
Fertility Center of Illinois

"We strongly recommend *Before Your Pregnancy* to all of our patients. We particularly like the chapter on body weight because the focus is nourishment, nutrition, and achieving a healthy but sustainable weight. Although the information presented is current and relevant, the tone is informal and sometimes humorous, making for an enjoyable read."

—MONICA MOORE, NP, RNC
Reproductive Medicine Associates of Connecticut

"If every prospective parent took this book's advice, the future health of the American population would improve dramatically."

—KENT THORNBURG, PhD
M. Lowell Edwards Chair,
Director of the Heart Research Center and Professor of
Cardiovascular Medicine, Oregon Health & Science University

"Preconception health is so important for optimizing a woman's or man's health, and it can also optimize pregnancy outcomes. We all know that a planned pregnancy generally has better outcomes, and this book should be a great resource for women and men who want to have a baby. The information is comprehensive, current, and balanced. I applaud the authors for promoting preconception health and health care as a first step toward a healthy pregnancy."

—JANIS BIERMANN, MS
Senior Vice President, Education & Health Promotion,
March of Dimes Foundation

"Ogle, a registered dietician, exercise physiologist, and ACE-certified personal trainer, and Mazzullo, an OB-GYN, wrote the first edition of this book in 2002. Here, they present the latest information and research to help couples prepare their bodies, minds, and bank accounts for the arrival of a child. . . . An outstanding book that fills a gap in public and consumer health library collections. There are many books on pregnancy and infertility, but none addresses preparation for conception in depth as this one does."

—BARBARA M. BIBEL, Oakland P.L., CA, *Library Journal*

"What makes this book a standout is the encouraging tone. I have read many books about pregnancy and fertility, and this one feels like the advice that a caring, trusted friend would give you. Infertility is a stressful and emotional issue, and this book eases your mind at the same time that it arms you with the knowledge and information you need to prepare your body and mind for pregnancy. Whether you have struggled with infertility or not, *Before Your Pregnancy* is a valuable resource for women whose goal is to be healthy and (eventually!) pregnant."

—MARGARET G.

"Finally! A comprehensive yet easy-to-read book to help women and men prepare emotionally and physically for the joy of pregnancy! I would recommend this book to anyone who is thinking about having a baby, including my clients who have PCOS or struggle with eating disorders and body-weight issues."

—ANGELA GRASSI, MS, RD, LDN
co-author of *The PCOS Workbook:*
Your Guide to Complete Physical and Emotional Health
and author of *The Dietitian's Guide to Polycystic Ovary Syndrome*

"A comprehensive and informative book serving as a knowledge source for nurse practitioners and women of childbearing age. *Before Your Pregnancy* is something I'll share with my graduate students."

—JANIE DADDARIO, MSN, WHNP
Director of the Women's Health Nurse Practitioner Program,
Vanderbilt University School of Nursing

Before Your Pregnancy

Before Your Pregnancy

*A 90-Day Guide for Couples on
How to Prepare for a Healthy Conception*

AMY OGLE, MS, RD,

and

LISA MAZZULLO, MD

EDITED BY ALLISON KRUG, MPH

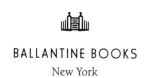

BALLANTINE BOOKS
New York

2011 Ballantine Books Trade Paperback Edition

Copyright © 2002, 2011 by Amy Ogle, MS, RD, and Lisa Mazzullo, MD
Foreword copyright © 2002, 2011 by Mary D'Alton, MD
Illustrations copyright © 2002, 2011 by Judith Soderquist Cummins

Published in the United States by Ballantine Books, an imprint of The Random House Publishing Group,
a division of Random House, Inc., New York.

BALLANTINE and colophon are registered trademarks of Random House, Inc.

Originally published in trade paperback in slightly different form in the United States by Ballantine Books,
an imprint of The Random House Publishing Group, a division of Random House, Inc., in 2002.

ISBN 978-0-345-51841-5

Printed in the United States of America

www.ballantinebooks.com

9 8 7 6 5 4 3 2

Additional illustrations by Allison Krug

Book design by Helene Berinsky

To Jamie, Sarah, and Charlie, and to my mom. —AO

To Dr. Melvin Gerbie, who has been an outstanding mentor to me and has spent his life
dedicated to improving women's health care. Without his faith and foresight,
the collaboration between Amy and me, resulting in *Before Your Pregnancy*,
would not have been possible. —LM

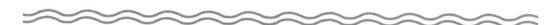

*I*n the past two decades we have witnessed enormous scientific advances in obstetrics. Sonography is used routinely to accurately date pregnancy and can provide a more precise assessment of fetal growth and well-being, important for women with medical conditions that can affect fetal growth such as diabetes, hypertension, and multiple pregnancy. Innovations in obstetric imaging technology, including the use of pulsed and color sonography, three-dimensional ultrasonography, and ultrafast magnetic resonance imaging, have allowed specialists to detect subtle problems in fetal anatomy. Genetics and prenatal diagnosis have evolved from amniocentesis for older mothers to highly sophisticated approaches to fetal diagnoses earlier and earlier in pregnancy.

Yet, against this background of scientific advances, the incidence of both structural fetal abnormalities and prematurity—the two major causes of infant death—has remained unchanged in North America. The cost of newborn intensive care is staggering; higher still is the cost of long-term care for those children who have severe handicaps. The human cost is not readily measurable.

As a practicing maternal-fetal medicine specialist, I see patients for pre-pregnancy counseling who are at risk for an adverse outcome. But targeting preconception care only to those women with risk factors results in many missed opportunities to prevent maternal and childhood disease. In this book, the authors have combined their unique backgrounds in obstetrics and gynecology, dietetics, and exercise physiology to provide an authoritative yet easy-to-read body of information to prospective families.

We health care providers must raise awareness of the importance of preconception health for women and not just women at high risk. The authors have synthesized a wealth of information into an accessible format and have a host of practical recommendations. I think they have succeeded admirably, and I am grateful to them for all of their efforts and will recommend this book to prospective parents. The material in the book attests to the extraordinary sophistication of the preconception services available today. It is my hope that the barrier separating the existing scientific knowledge from public awareness of this knowledge will be further diminished as more and more prospective parents read this book. I applaud the authors in their efforts to increase awareness of the resources available for promoting a healthy conception and birth.

—MARY D'ALTON, MD
Chair, Department of Obstetrics and Gynecology,
Director, Obstetrics and Gynecology Services,
Columbia University Medical School

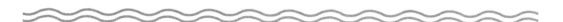

*W*hen our publisher approached us about writing a revised edition of *Before Your Pregnancy*, we recognized it as a significant milestone in how far the concept of preconception care had come. Thanks also in great part to domestic and international public health advocates such as the March of Dimes, the CDC*, and the World Health Organization, this book has had the advantage of being in the right place at the right time. The local and global effort to educate girls and women and influence public policy is working: couples are beginning to grasp the importance of preparing for the first pregnancy, and that momentum is prompting vigilance between pregnancies as well.

You may have sought information from the Internet, friends, or family, and perhaps from your doctor. Our hope is that this book can save you time and effort. We've compiled the latest research across a broad cross section of contemporary medical and lifestyle issues that many prospective parents are concerned about. Our reward is when we hear the happy endings—as one new mother put it in an email, their son was born "gloriously healthy" and mom, dad, and baby were all doing well.

This revised edition was expanded to cover the wealth of new information. Here are a few highlights:

*In 2006, the Centers for Disease Control and Prevention/Agency for Toxic Substances and Disease Registry (CDC/ATSDR) Preconception Care Work Group and the Select Panel on Preconception Care took a seminal public stand in developing ten recommendations to improve reproductive outcomes in the United States.

- Twelve steps to creating a welcoming womb by optimizing your immune health before conception
- New research on the importance of blood sugar control, and how to reduce birth defects with improved treatment of insulin resistance and diabetes
- Memorable parody ("Fatsville") to help you remember and achieve the healthiest balance of all the fatty acids (omegas, saturated, trans)
- Updates on herbs and supplements, plus new safety information on mercury and fish
- Expanded and updated medical information about depression, infectious disease prevention, vaccination recommendations, and strategies for people with physical disabilities
- New body weight guidelines, including a special section on bariatric surgery
- User-friendly preconception menu planning for men and women
- Greatly expanded gynecological and men's health sections to help you time conception more reliably and combat the most common urban legends about conception
- Reassuring guidance regarding infertility diagnosis and treatments, including specific recommendations to adjust lifestyle or health behaviors that can improve fertility before pursuing medical interventions
- Important topics for those who are between pregnancies (uncomplicated as well as more challenging pregnancy histories)

All pregnancies benefit from preconception care, but some outcomes can be dramatically improved. We hope our efforts to compile the latest information will inform and reassure you, and ultimately help you conceive the healthiest baby possible.

CONTENTS

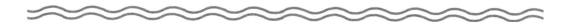

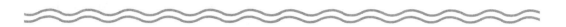

Don't Just Conceive: Preconceive!

 *I*t is every prospective parent's dream to have a child who is happy, bright, engaging, and healthy enough to experience life to its fullest. Whether you are thinking of trying to conceive for the first time or have been down this road before, we would like to help you improve your chances of making this dream come true, just as we have for countless men and women under similar circumstances. In fact, it was in the year 1995 that the idea for *Before Your Pregnancy* came into being. At the time, Amy, a registered dietitian, exercise physiologist, and personal trainer, was working with patients and private clients who were pregnant—with or without complications—or within a year or two of having had a child. She was impressed by their motivation and surprised by the number of times she heard the remark "If only I knew then what I know now, I'd have taken better care of myself before I got pregnant." It got her thinking about why there wasn't more emphasis from the medical community on health during the months before conception. After all, the scientific literature was brimming with new information on ways women and men could prepare their bodies for conception and improve the baby's health, actions that often made a difference only if begun one to three months before trying to conceive. Unfortunately, virtually none of this information was widely available to the general public.

 Determined to get the word out, Amy wrote and produced a video and accompanying booklet entitled *Before Your Pregnancy* that provided preconception nutritional and exercise advice. (Coincidentally, she became pregnant while making the video, giving her a chance to practice what she preached!) One of the professionals who edited the text, Dr. Lisa Mazzullo, a board-certified ob-gyn and assistant professor of obstetrics and gynecology at Northwestern

University Medical Center, happened to teach "Maybe Baby" classes at her hospital, covering the same topics from a medical and psychological point of view. The response to the video and preconception classes was so great that we, Amy and Lisa, ultimately decided to pool our expertise and create the book you hold in your hands, a complete resource for couples considering having a baby.

Most preconception discussions between patients and doctors—if they occur at all—are limited to "Begin taking your folic acid, and have fun!" The fact of the matter is, however, that there are many things you can do to improve your physical health and psychological readiness in the critical ninety-day period before conception. In this book we'll help you to thoroughly assess your emotional, financial, environmental, gynecologic, genetic, nutritional, and physical preparedness and provide detailed advice on how to improve in each area. If you follow our preconception guidelines, you will also improve your odds of

- Conceiving more easily
- Conceiving a healthier baby
- Giving the baby a "smooth landing" during implantation in the uterus and ensuring a strong placenta—the vascular connection between mom and baby
- Having a healthier pregnancy
- Recovering more easily in the postpartum period
- Decreasing your child's risk for certain childhood and adult health problems

You may be wondering why certain baby-friendly actions must be implemented in the months prior to conception. After all, until fertilization occurs, there isn't even a baby in the picture. Well, the egg and sperm that will eventually become that baby go through crucial genetic preparations in the weeks before conception, and you want these to occur under the best circumstances. Because genetic defects do not all occur randomly, the prospect of having some control over this risk is immensely empowering. Also, consider that most birth defects—many preventable—occur between seventeen and fifty-six days after conception, often before a woman becomes aware that she is pregnant. Preconception readiness primes the woman's body so the baby can thrive in those early weeks of development.

Here's something else that's fascinating. The maternal body directs most of its focus and energy into building and "remodeling" the placenta during the first three months of pregnancy; it's like building a solid foundation with the best materials before pouring much energy into the structural details. The placenta has always been described as the critical component that orchestrates nutrient delivery and waste disposal via the umbilical cord. It also tries to run interference, if harmful substances get into the maternal bloodstream. What you may not know is that a healthy placenta that works in sync with the maternal immune system can be key to keeping the fetus "on board" and growing well for the full forty weeks of pregnancy.

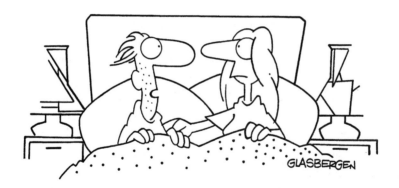

"Let's try getting up every night at 2:00 AM to feed the cat. If we enjoy doing
that, then we can talk about having a baby."
Copyright © 1997 by Randy Glasbergen. www.glasbergen.com

This is an exciting area of ongoing research, one with many potential implications for preconception and pregnancy health. You'll see more discussion about this in a new feature beginning on page 163.

Take it from us: it is also a lot easier to continue healthy habits during pregnancy and beyond if you already have them in place before you are pregnant. And eventually your children will learn the healthy habits that you, their parents, model.

We cannot emphasize enough that the preconception actions of both partners, not solely the woman, can make a difference in the health of their future child. Ultimate success comes when you both feel equally important and act synergistically as a team. You will find a lot of information in this book to help the prospective dad become healthier, better informed, and more involved in what lies ahead.

We share your enthusiasm for wanting to make your body a safe and healthy place for your baby to thrive.

HOW TO GET THE MOST OUT OF OUR BOOK

Are you planning your pregnancy several months to a year in advance, or have you already started trying? How you use this book largely depends on your personal time frame for conception. As mentioned earlier, we recommend following these guidelines for at least ninety days before trying to conceive. This time frame is ultimately best for most situations but may not be practical or necessary in all cases; we'll make a point of noting when something should be heeded earlier or later than the ninety-day timeline. Depending on what you discover from this book about your current state of preconception readiness, you may come to the conclusion that it is in your interest to postpone your plans for a few months. In the grand scheme of things, a relatively short delay is a small price to pay for improving your odds for a healthier outcome.

We've organized this book according to how you might naturally approach preparing for pregnancy. Long before you and your partner discuss preconception readiness with a health care professional, you'll determine whether you're mentally and financially ready to welcome a new being into your life. At the same time, you may start looking at your lifestyle habits (e.g., smoking, drinking) and your home and away-from-home environments with questions of wholesomeness and safety in mind. After these initial considerations, we get to the heart of preconception health, nutrition, and fitness for women and men. Finally, Chapter 17, "Romancing the Egg," can be referred to when you're both ready to start "trying"; there's now a fast-track

("zoom") and laid-back ("Zen") approach, depending on your personal needs.

It might be helpful for you to take a peek at "Romancing the Egg" (Chapter 17), just to get an idea of where you're headed and find out your "Fertility 'Personality' Profile." The profile is there to guide readers who have completed the majority of the book—and their ninety days of preconception planning—so we kept it there despite the urge to place it earlier.

Should you experience infertility, a new chapter (Chapter 18) will help reassure and guide you, including new information and specific cross-references to other parts of the book that might have initially only been skimmed. Then we delve right into ways to reassess, complement your own efforts, and get the right help to achieve your goal of having a baby.

Before Your Pregnancy is meant to be an interactive book. We encourage you to write in the blank spaces, margins, and charts. Dog-ear plenty of pages, and highlight pertinent advice with a pen or colored marker. Approach this as you would a delectable barbecue dinner: you cannot thoroughly enjoy the meal if you and your napkin remain spotless.

To further encourage you to participate in the learning process we feature exercises called Practical Applications. As the term suggests, these typically take the topic under discussion into your own specific circumstances. For example, in the section on women's medical issues, one Practical Application is to look in your medicine cabinet and write down all the medications, herbs, and supplements you find, familiarize yourself with what we recommend about them, and note which ones you should ask your physician about.

Although the information in this book is written for couples, we address the prospective mother as "you," unless stated otherwise. We're making the assumption that, for the most part, it will be women who read this book and then share pertinent portions with their partners. (Kudos to you men who ran across this book first.)

You will also notice that we use several interchangeable terms throughout the book. For example, the yet-to-be-conceived baby and the baby while in the womb both are referred to as either the fetus or the baby. Your primary health care provider is referred to most of the time as a doctor or physician but could just as easily be a nurse midwife, nurse practitioner, or physician assistant. Finally, we use the terms *partner, husband, wife, baby's mother/father, mate,* or *spouse* interchangeably.

Many of the recommendations for pre-pregnancy are also applicable later on, often for completely different reasons. When that is the case, you will see boxes titled For Future Reference with symbols indicating when the reference is to

"during pregnancy" , "after delivery" , or "family life" with children . These are for all of you information pack rats to tuck in the back of your minds for future use during the pregnancy and postpartum period. If you are the type who was driven crazy in school by a teacher who periodically went off on tangents, feel free to skim these!

This book will also help you become a more active participant in your health care. It will assist you in organizing any questions you may have for your doctor and help to clarify what he or she is telling you. That way you can make the best use of your appointment time and will be less likely to walk out of the office saying, "Oh, I wish I had asked her about x, y, and z."

SETTING A NEW PRECEDENT

As you put our guidelines into action, remember that the practice of preconception care is still relatively new in comparison to the well-established practice of prenatal (during pregnancy) care—so new, in fact, that you may periodically be faced with skepticism from your family, friends, and even some health care workers. Your partner may question the necessity of it. Don't be swayed or discouraged if people say that couples have been having healthy babies for hundreds of thousands of years and very few of them did anything to plan ahead for conception; or if they point out that there are women who abuse their bodies with drugs and an unhealthy lifestyle and then have healthy babies despite it all. It's true that women give birth to healthy babies under less than ideal circumstances—thank goodness for this general resiliency! Even so, preconception planning does improve one's overall odds for giving a baby a head start from the very moment of conception. The particulars of how and how much it helps will vary among individuals.

Occasionally we encounter a prospective parent who finds the thought of planning for pregnancy unappealing because of religious or cultural beliefs. Or you and your partner may prefer to be spontaneous and just see what happens. However, the words *planning* and *spontaneity* are not diametrically opposed. Although some couples will meticulously plan to "start trying," *true preconception readiness is a lifestyle practice in case pregnancy should occur.* Considering that almost half of all pregnancies are unplanned, this type of general pre-pregnancy readiness is a good idea for any couple of childbearing age. Following these guidelines will mean that you and your partner will be optimally ready to create a baby at any time, whether you intend to become pregnant or not.

Over the course of our careers we have counseled thousands of couples who, like you, are planning to start trying to get pregnant. Their experiences have inspired the many scenarios we have created to illustrate the information in this book. In addition, many experts outside our respective fields—psychologists, social workers, financial planners, public health advocates, geneticists, urologists/male infertility specialists, immunologists, pediatricians, and herbal researchers—have generously shared their knowledge with us to make this book as complete a resource as possible. We extend our gratitude to all who have contributed to our understanding of what it means to want a child and to selflessly act in his or her favor before conception. We thank you, too, for caring enough to learn, as we have.

Amy Ogle, MS, RD
Lisa Mazzullo, MD

Before Your Pregnancy

CHAPTER 1

So, You Want to Have a Baby

Knowing is not enough; we must apply.
Willing is not enough; we must do.
   —Goethe

For many couples, conceiving a child is one of the high points in their romantic lives. To be sure, creating another human being often represents the acme of a loving, committed relationship. Nevertheless, there are some decidedly unromantic, practical, and even mundane issues you ought to address well before you light the scented candles. Are you emotionally ready for conception? How about financially? Are your home, job, and travel environments working in your favor? Are you ready to make the kind of lifestyle changes required for responsible preconception—and future parenthood? In the first three chapters we discuss a host of topics, many of which you may not have considered relevant to preconception, and provide critical information your doctor may not have told you—or may not even know.

PSYCHED UP OR STRESSED OUT?
ARE YOU EMOTIONALLY READY?

Adam and Beth, married a few years, are driving to see their closest friends, who have just had a baby. In the car, they reminisce about all the fun they'd had as a foursome: getting together for pizza, going to jazz clubs, taking a few camping trips together. When they arrive at their friends' home they meet the baby and see all the accoutrements of new parenthood: stroller, high chair, bassinet, baby toys . . . Beth watches how naturally her friend handles the baby and how comfortably she feeds and changes him. "I could do that," Beth thinks. Adam watches his friend cradle his son ever so gently before laying him down in the bassinet. He, too, finds himself thinking, "This wouldn't be so bad." On the way home they look at each other, take a deep breath, and say, almost in unison, "Maybe we should start thinking about . . ."

Adam and Beth have just taken a huge leap toward becoming ready for parenthood. Being ready for parenthood generally means that you have taken steps, consciously or unconsciously, to adjust your physical, mental, and relational situation to create an optimal environment in which your future baby can thrive. Everything looks a little different when seen through the lens of prospective parenthood. Political issues somehow begin to seem more personally relevant. Environmental safety takes on greater importance. You start to care about the projected increase in college tuition over the next twenty years and may choose to live in an area based on the quality of the schools there. Although few of us actually manage to be fully mentally and emotionally prepared before getting pregnant, thinking about the issues that follow will give you a good head start.

It's About the Two of You

The most important thing you can do at this stage of planning is simply enjoy each other and strengthen the emotional bonds between you. Do the things you love to do together. As your friends who already have children will tell you, relish the moments of uninterrupted conversation and spontaneous outings. Once you have a baby, it will be very important to keep nurturing the person that your partner was before he or she became a parent, so that neither of you ends up losing touch with why you fell in love with each other in the first place. Dr. Arthur Segreti, a clinical psychologist, and his wife, Ramona Segreti, a social worker also in clinical practice, suggest doing "small kindnesses" for each other, such as drawing a bath, making a cup of tea, or packing a healthy lunch for your partner to take to work. They also recommend that couples keep a mutual gratitude journal, in which each person thanks the other for something that was done that day (and to do this even when you're in the midst of an argument and feeling that you have nothing to be thankful for).

You and your partner will have to make some adjustments in your relationship to accommodate the practical demands of pregnancy and of having an infant. Many couples ask us how they will know when they are ready to go from being a cozy twosome to being a sometimes frazzled threesome or foursome. "Parenthood is a natural progression in a healthy relationship," says Dr. Segreti. *Healthy* is the operative word here: there must be a solid core of love, commitment, trust, and respect between the partners for the relationship to weather the emotional storms of parenthood. Of course, by healthy we do not mean perfect. Nonetheless, when thinking about trying to get pregnant, examine your relationship closely to see what works and what needs some fine-tuning.

Think of yourselves as a team in every aspect of planning for pregnancy, especially because teamwork and mutual support will be crucial later on, when the baby's needs seem to dominate your days. Talk to your partner about what the prospect of parenthood means to you and about your hopes and fears. It's definitely easier to talk about finances and work schedules over a nice candlelit meal than it will be when you're both sleep-deprived and in the throes of adjusting to the new baby. If there are problems or tensions in your relationship, now is the time to try to work them out. Repressing or denying them won't make them go away; procrastinating will only exacerbate them. Having a child is not going to save an already troubled relationship. Rather, the added stress of caring for a newborn may be the straw that breaks the camel's back. So take as much time as you need—and seek counseling if you feel it might be useful—to make sure your relationship is on solid ground before you begin trying.

If in your discussions it becomes clear that you and your partner do not feel the same way about prospective parenthood, it is essential that you both do some soul-searching. What is driving the enthusiastic partner forward? Excitement about sharing life with a baby? Feeling that the biologicical clock is "ticking"? Hoping for unconditional love? And what is holding the reluctant partner back? Financial worries? The prospect of losing momentum in a fast-track career? Fears of repeating a difficult childhood? Many people who say they aren't ready yet do acknowledge that they want to have children eventually. Their reluctance must be respected. You may consider entering couples therapy to help sort out the issues surrounding parenthood for both of you, and to figure out if a mutually acceptable time frame can be established.

Understandably, a traumatic experience with a prior pregnancy can be enough to create fear or hesitancy in one or both partners, as can fear of having a baby with severe physical or mental challenges, especially if the parents have been down that road before. Couples who have gone through such profound experiences are going to need time and good counsel to recapture a sense of hope and optimism before trying again.

There are also other, extreme situations in which getting pregnant is just not a good idea. Spousal abuse, either physical or emotional, by one or both partners is a clear sign that the time is not right to start trying to expand your family, even if you believe that the relationship itself can be salvaged. "Domestic violence" cannot be ignored and usually escalates instead of ceasing during pregnancy and after delivery. If you are a victim, please seek help before you suffer serious harm. Look in the Yellow Pages under Domestic Violence, call your local YWCA, or ask your doctor to provide resources and references that can help you (more on this in Appendix C). Substance abuse, in either prospective parent, is a second extreme sign that now is not the time to consider pregnancy (more on this topic in Chapter 2).

There are certain life lessons that are associated with parenthood. It requires us to be patient, to set some of our own needs and desires aside, to become more aware of our community and more oriented toward the future. Studies show that parents often also experience a greater sense of purpose and meaning in their lives. The very act of loving a child deeply and unconditionally is a transforming experience. Many regard it as a superb accomplishment to be the best parent you can. We may also gain a new appreciation for the sacrifices our parents made for us, and may even arrive at new insights about our own childhood based on experi-

"I've Recently Had a Miscarriage. How Will I Know When I'm Ready to Try Again?"

Sharon and Michael experienced an early miscarriage when they were trying for their second child. Although the loss initially saddened her, Sharon now finds herself optimistic that next time will be different. Michael shares her hope that the next time they conceive, the baby will be healthy and all will proceed normally.

Sonia and Jonathan had a first-trimester miscarriage two months ago. Jonathan is eager to try again right away. Sonia is more cautious, unsure about her ability to carry a baby to term, and afraid that they will suffer another miscarriage. She admits she wakes up in the middle of the night with tears on her face from dreams about the baby that was lost. She doesn't know when she will feel ready to get pregnant again.

Sometimes the impact of a recent miscarriage can temporarily cause one partner to be more reluctant about trying to conceive. "It is important to let yourself grieve after a miscarriage," says Lois Platt, MSW, RN, who has been practicing in the Chicago area for almost twenty years and specializes in mental health issues surrounding pregnancy, parenthood, pregnancy loss, and infertility. Though everyone is different, the average grieving period after a pregnancy loss is three to six months. Some couples want to start trying to conceive immediately after a miscarriage; others need to take more time. Whether you and your spouse fall into one category or the other, keep in mind one important fact: more than 85 percent of miscarriages are random events that are unlikely to occur again.

When one partner is ready to try again but the other is not, you can often benefit from short-term counseling. Some women experience healing by visiting a counselor who is able to bear witness to their loss by listening to them and helping them process their feelings of grief, guilt, and fear. But wherever you are emotionally, be sure to use a reliable form of birth control in the meantime (even if you've had trouble conceiving in the past) and get the green light from your doctor before you start trying again.

ences with our children. All of these lessons and feelings can lead to our own emotional and spiritual development.

One question every prospective parent has is "Will I be a good parent?" You begin to think about what "mother" or "father" means to you, based on your own life experience. You consider the type of parent you would like to be, and you wonder how this ideal can be incorporated into the real, imperfect person you actually are. Comforting in this regard is the insight of psychoanalyst and author D. W. Winnicott, who asserts that our children actually need our imperfections in order to grow and mature emotionally. Imagine a child whose parents never frustrate him in any way and consistently satisfy his every need. That child will be slow to learn how to tolerate frustration, soothe himself, or take care of himself. It is adversity, great and small, that is our greatest teacher. To paraphrase Winnicott, you don't have to be a perfect parent; you only need to be good enough. If you're one who is used to perfecting most things, you'll initially be taken aback by this statement, but trust us on this one, and earmark it for when you have a child or two (it'll make better sense then).

 FOR FUTURE REFERENCE: After Delivery/Family Life

Will Life Ever Be the Same?

Most of us know that parenting is demanding and requires great sacrifice—so much so that it's hard to imagine that some of us actually volunteer for the job. It is extremely difficult to believe that the incredible power of loving a child will truly make all of the sacrifice and work worthwhile. But it does! Take it on faith if you must: you will become absolutely willing to give up everything, even your life, for your child. It goes beyond intellect: we are biologically hardwired to feel that way. You may think it will be hard to give up some of the things you love, but you will find that most of what you now think is so important will drop away quite painlessly when it's for the adorable creature you're head over heels in love with. Or you may fear the loss of your sense of self, that you somehow won't "still be you" when you have a child. But what usually happens is that the part of you that's Mommy or Daddy will eventually become part of your greater self, expanding your sense of identity. Furthermore, you will eventually find or make the time for those things that are vital to you, such as a particular sport or hobby. Although the first three months or so of a baby's life are fairly all-consuming and exhausting—and there will be times when you think that you'll never be able to take another relaxing shower again—the good news is that babies eventually develop a routine, and you'll find time to do many of the things you used to do.

Setting Yourself Up for Success

Perfection aside, it helps if you're near the top of your mental game, sharp-minded, and full of optimism and willpower to take the best possible care of yourself. Throughout this book you may run into tough choices, from dealing head-on with marital or financial issues to choosing the right foods and exercising. Building your willpower will help ensure your pre-conception period is as (wink) productive as possible. Don't despair if this seems like an impossible calling—some women actually come into their own as mothers and find that they've never been more fit or sure of themselves.

Setting goals that require self-control, focusing your attention on achieving them, and then "consciously doing" them is like exercising your willpower muscle to make it stronger. Two neuroscientists who have studied willpower, Sandra Aamodt, editor in chief of *Nature Neuroscience,* and Sam Wang, of Princeton University, caution that building willpower in one area may cause regression in another. For instance, watching finances carefully in a down economy may cause us to slip up in our healthy eating and exercise habits. Humans seem to have a finite supply of willpower, but fortunately it appears that this supply can be increased over time. Doing things that require self-control is the best mental training; do them long enough and they become a habit. Think of preconception as an opportunity to remodel your neural connections with daily learning, experience, and a healthy lifestyle.

Mary is contemplating pregnancy and wants to be at the top of her game physically, emotionally, and intellectually. She has watched her friends navigate the choppy waters of motherhood and wondered why their experiences appear to vary so widely.

Her friend Michelle is the classic übermom—after two kids, she has never felt more fit and resilient. Her productivity has increased—she knows how to cut to the chase and work quickly. She communicates in sound bytes that get attention and get things done. Her diplomacy and negotiation skills serve her well every day. Her sense of humor is unrivaled, and she's even enjoyed picking up watercolor painting again while playing with her kids on the beach. Is it possible that motherhood is a proving ground like none other?

Stacy is hang-loose and fun-loving. Though she and her husband hadn't really planned their pregnancies, they were very much wanted. Now, with her two kids in tow, she seems flustered and disorganized. She hasn't lost her baby weight and feels too pressed for time to work out. Stacy had hoped that parenthood would provide her the needed motivation to eat well and take care of her body, but the reality of parenthood has presented more challenge than momentum.

Of course Mary knows that the differences in her friends' experiences can't be entirely chalked up to preconception readiness, but being well prepared certainly can't hurt. She resolved to do what she could ahead of time to be as ready and adaptable for pregnancy as she could be.

Practical Application

Below or on a separate piece of paper, write a list of qualities you feel are key to being a "good" mother or father. Then write a list of your strengths. How do they mesh with your ideal view of parenthood? Will they help you maintain a loving relationship with your spouse? Next, write a list of your shortcomings (be as honest as you can, but don't put yourself down). Pick a couple of shortcomings to work on now, while you're preparing to become pregnant. You will feel more in control and prepared even before you see a pink or blue line on that pregnancy test.

Positive parenting qualities   Your strengths   Your shortcomings

_____

_____

_____

_____

_____

The Role Stress Plays in Your Ability to Conceive

For years, we have known that stress affects our personal relationships, work efficiency, eating habits, and sleep. You may have also heard that stress affects fertility. You may have a friend who, after months of trying, conceived as soon as she left a stressful job. Or you may have heard about the couple who immediately got pregnant when they had given up and stopped thinking about it. Catastrophic stressors such as war, natural disasters, and the loss of a child or parent have been shown to affect fertility rates in both men and women. Despite intuitive links, medical science has not conclusively proven that stress alone can cause infertility.

Studies have tied stress to reduced sperm counts and disrupted ovulation, but is the stress due to these infertility problems or is it the other way around? In May 2000, the National Institute for Occupational Safety and Health (NIOSH) was asked by Congress to examine whether mental stress in the workplace can affect fertility in men and women. More than 25 percent of employees surveyed said they were "extremely stressed out" by their jobs, yet the institute was unable to prove a link between workplace mental stress and a change in fertility or rates of conception. In contrast, studies among couples going through infertility treatments have found that those who have the highest success rates maintained lower levels of stress and a high degree of optimism and resiliency throughout treatment. Stress related to infertility or negative life events can diminish fertility by telling parts of the body (brain, pituitary, adrenals) that manage your hormones that it may not be a good time to get pregnant.[1] From an evolutionary perspective, this certainly makes sense.

One thing that has become clearer is that women and men experience stress differently and their resulting fertility challenges may also be different. Studies have shown that women who are under increased mental stress often experience changes in their sleeping and eating habits, which can lead to changes in body weight and metabolism. The body's hormones and steroids react to these changes and can often reduce a woman's ability to produce an egg. And women reporting significant marital stress were able to conceive, but they usually needed two to three times as many cycles compared to those who reported no stress.[2] Men under significant mental stress have reduced sperm counts (though not enough to change fertility rates). The good news is that sperm counts can recover within three months after the stressful period ends. (The obvious challenge to conception posed by marital stress makes it hard to isolate the independent effect of stress on fertility.)

We do know that when stress regularly overcomes your ability to meet your basic physical needs, fertility can suffer. Your overall attitude regarding the stressful situation may play a role, too. The bottom line is that every person deals with mental stress differently, and we do not fully understand all of the ramifications of unmanaged stress. Suffice it to say that reducing stress may increase your ability to conceive, and even if it doesn't, it can't hurt to lessen your

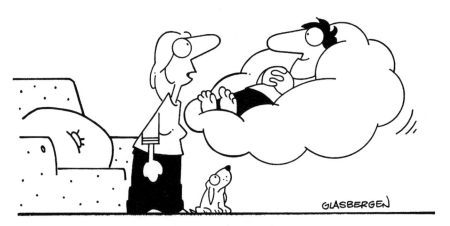

"You're getting pretty good at this stress management thing."
Copyright © 1997 by Randy Glasbergen. www.glasbergen.com

1. Nakamura, K, et al. "Stress and Reproductive Failure: Past Notions, Present Insights and Future Directions." *Journal of Assisted Reproduction and Genetics* 25 (2008): 47–82.

2. Bovin, J., and Schmidt, L. "Infertility-Related Stress in Men and Women Predicts Treatment Outcome One Year Later." *Fertility and Sterility* 83 (2005): 1745–52.

stress as you undertake the challenges of pregnancy and parenthood. Moreover, you'll have lower levels of stress hormones (e.g., cortisol) circulating in the intrauterine environment of your future baby.

Take a Load Off

Managing your stress is like eating chicken soup: it can't hurt. Here are some tips and suggestions that will help:

- **Get outside.** Researchers are now backing up what many of you already know. Spending time outdoors in nature (even in a park or tiny garden plot, for city dwellers) can help restore a sense of balance to mind and body. Feeling a connection to the earth can help make our day-to-day worries seem less significant. While looking at a nature photograph or watching nature images on a screen is enjoyable, it's no substitute for direct experience.

FOR FUTURE REFERENCE: Family Life

One of the most basic opportunities to stay positive and at ease (and fit) is fast becoming a thing of the past: time outdoors. Maintain a connection to the natural world outside for you and your family. You'll notice stress slipping away as you engage all your senses on a walk in the woods. The outdoors provides a wonderful shared learning opportunity for children of all ages, such as finding letter shapes among roots, counting points on a leaf, recognizing shapes and colors, and even learning life lessons such as perseverance and trust . . . the possibilities are endless. Even if you don't have a forest nearby, any unstructured outdoor space will do. See the world through the eyes of your child and you'll soon find an adventure (such as watching a butterfly emerge from a chrysalis or stomping in puddles after a rain). An excellent read for parents, teachers, and caregivers is *Last Child in the Woods: Saving Our Children from Nature-Deficit Disorder* by Richard Louv.

- **Get moving.** Take a walk with your dog or engage in another restorative form of exercise such as yoga, tai chi, or Pilates.
- **Reflect.** Try prayer, mindful meditation, or relaxation techniques. Set aside as little as ten or fifteen minutes a day just to be alone and quiet. Get in touch with your feelings

about the day's events. The experience of truly being focused can center and strengthen you.

- **Turn off the computer, TV, or smartphone.** Maybe not completely, but at least an hour earlier every night. Spend that hour doing something truly restorative, such as reading, journaling, meditating, taking a bath, or being with your spouse (cozying up on the couch on a cold winter's night or taking a walk under the stars on a warm summer's evening).

- **Ease the stress of commuting.** In the car, listen to enjoyable music or a podcast. Discover the world of audiobooks from your local library if you want an especially indulgent commute.

- **Cook yourself a healthy, nourishing meal for a change.** Choosing fresh, quality ingredients and making something that you love is a great way to nurture yourself and your loved ones. Conversely, if you feel you're spending too much time in the kitchen, order in and relax.

- **Treat yourself.** Buy your favorite magazine or a new outfit, or schedule a pedicure with a friend. Spa services such as facials, wraps, and massages can also be very relaxing if you can afford them. (Look for a massage school in your community—they may offer discounted rates for student massages.)

- **Get good sleep.** Try to get seven to eight hours of sleep on most nights. For pointers on how to restore healthful sleep patterns, visit the National Sleep Foundation website: www.sleepfoundation.org. Be aware that some sleep aids, particularly natural or herbal ones, may adversely affect your reproductive hormones, potentially hindering conception. For example, the popular supplement melatonin may not be advisable for jet lag during this time in your life. Later, one of the hallmarks of pregnancy and new motherhood is "mom brain"—the periodic spaciness that many women complain about. While there is some interaction between reproductive hormones and cognition, these episodes also correlate strongly with sleep disturbances during pregnancy and the early newborn weeks. Try to catch a nap—even if only twenty minutes—to restore your mind.

- **Stimulate your mind.** Experts suggest three strategies to pamper your brain, whether you're in the preconception, pregnant, or parent category:

  1. **Exercise.** Engage in a variety of physical activities to regain tone, and promote optimal blood flow and brain function (to help combat depression and stay mentally sharp, too). Exercise is the key to managing chronic conditions, such as high blood pressure, diabetes, overweight or obesity, and possibly delaying dementia. It also

FOR FUTURE REFERENCE: During Pregnancy/After Delivery

"Mom Brain"—Myth or Reality?

You may have been warned about "pregnancy brain" or "new mom brain"—periodic spacey moments—and may wonder if it's hype, stereotype, or scientifically proven. Will you be able to continue doing the things that are important to you, from work to working out? The answer is yes.

The brain is remarkably dynamic, responding to your environment, both inside and outside your body. The "pregnancy brain" phenomenon may simply be an outward manifestation of the understandably distracted state of the maternal brain, which is processing many different (and intense) stimuli at once on intellectual, physical, and emotional levels. And this isn't even counting the effect of sleep deprivation on a new mom's mental function. (For instance, we know that sleep disruptions due to shift work affect stress hormone levels, increasing the risk of cardiovascular disease.)

So, does the hormonal milieu have any impact on your mind? The evidence is overwhelming in animal models that estrogen is protective against dementia, but in humans the data is more mixed.[a] One recent study among mothers age twenty to twenty-four did not find any evidence of diminished brain power.[b] But, chances are, some spacey moments can be chalked up to fluctuating hormone levels (progesterone diminishes estrogen's effects during pregnancy, and then estrogen transiently lowers after delivery and during lactation.) But researchers remind us that these studies are limited by other factors affecting memory and cognition. And they strongly recommend against interpreting the findings with an eye to deciding how many children to have.

So take heart. Mothers across the millennia have faced these challenges, and thankfully it was an evolutionary imperative that they succeed. Mothers are well-designed beings, capable of managing the many mental distractions mentioned earlier. Regardless of your family plans or hormone levels, the tips below will help you take care of your brain by taking good care of your body.

a. Barrett-Connor, E., and G. A. Laughlin. "Endogenous and Exogenous Estrogen, Cognitive Function and Dementia in Postmenopausal Women: Evidence from Epidemiologic Studies and Clinical Trials. *Seminars in Reproductive Medicine* 27, no. 3 (May 2009): 275–82.

b. Christensen, H., et al. "Cognition in Pregnancy and Motherhood." *British Journal of Psychiatry* 196 (2010): 126–32.

confers many specific benefits, such as promoting cardioprotective levels of HDL (good) cholesterol. The benefits begin accruing as soon as you start moving.

2. **Engage.** Vary your intellectual challenges, from trying to brush your teeth with your nondominant hand to doing Sudoku puzzles. Choose one newsmagazine to

read each week to stay current on world events. Select friends who challenge you to think in new ways and can keep up with the volley of short thought bursts between interruptions.

3. **Eat.** The brain's plasticity—ability to form new connections—depends on supplying it with omega-3 fatty acids and antioxidants. Most of these vital nutrients must be obtained from our diet because they cannot be manufactured by the body. (See Chapter 10 for information.)

- **Smile plenty and laugh often.** As if we need more encouragement, there's good research to back up this recommendation. And if you need it, seek outside support from clergy or a spiritual mentor, a support group, or a mental health professional.

- **Look for the positive.** When you read about preconception and pregnancy, you'll learn about risks you never knew were there. Don't be afraid. Not only are the odds of these problems occurring very low, but the benefits that come from educating yourself are far more important.

- **Try aromatherapy.** Research has found that aromatherapy can have a beneficial effect on overall health. In one study, nonpregnant women were massaged with either scented or unscented oils. Those exposed to the aromatherapy enjoyed a reduction in heart rate, blood pressure, and anxiety, with lavender oil having the greatest relaxation and sedative effect. Although small amounts of herbal material pass into the bloodstream during massage, aromatherapy appears safe while trying to conceive (we lack such information on pregnancy). Absorption can be reduced by not preheating the oil and by using small amounts.

Practical Application

List four major stress-producing areas in your life. Then list four ways you can manage those stressors. Be realistic. And remember: the last thing you need is to be stressed out by your plan not to be stressed out!

Stress producers   Stress busters

_____

_____

_____

_____

IT'S A MATERIAL THING: FINANCES AND INSURANCE COVERAGE

Prospective parents often sense a desire to be more financially secure. Whether you have a big home or a tiny apartment, a lot of money in your bank account or not very much at all, virtually everyone experiences some stress when facing the financial prospect of bringing a child into the world. A 2009 estimate indicates that raising a child will cost $250,000 by the time the child reaches age eighteen (not including college).

Perhaps you have relatives who tell stories about growing up in a family of six or eight with only one income, two bedrooms, no extras, and everyone well fed and well provided for. Unfortunately, times have changed. The advantages of living in the twenty-first century—computers, orthodontia, and entertainment—all come at a price. The price of college alone is enough to give even the most stalwart financial planner indigestion! Plus, there are more immediate baby costs, including health care, diapers, baby food, and possibly day care.

Planning ahead not only will lessen the stress and strain but also will help ensure your smooth transition from couple to family unit. To give you a leg up, we discuss the financial issues you and your partner may encounter before, during, and after conception. Even if you and your partner are good communicators and cannot imagine being stressed by money issues, you may still find some helpful hints, suggestions, and facts in the following pages.

Getting Your Finances in Order

Often the problem is not how much money you have but how you spend it. Spending philosophies are very individualized and there is no one "right" way to spend. Kerri Sullivan-Kreiss, CFP, president of Sullivan-Kreiss Financial, recommends having at least three months of monthly expenses in reserve as a cornerstone of financial stability. This may seem like a lot to save, but as one new mother commented, "When I lost my job during the middle of my pregnancy and couldn't find another in my increasingly pregnant state, it was a relief to know we could pay all our expenses until the baby was born." Sullivan-Kreiss also suggests consolidating your debts (e.g., car payments, student loans, credit cards) to make your monthly accounting more manageable.

Other helpful financial advice includes:

- **Review and update medical, disability, and life insurance coverage.** Knowing what your medical insurance will and will not cover as it pertains to maternity coverage or infertility treatment can be very helpful before you get pregnant. Many insurance plans require that you be a member for nine months before a maternity benefit is possible. Disability and life insurance can be a source of income if something makes one spouse unable to be a financial contributor.

- **Create a budget, pay down your debt, and begin a savings plan.** Determining your monthly cash flow will allow you to fine-tune your plans for how to manage your money when you are on maternity leave (some of which is often unpaid) or when you will have extra expenses with your little one. Reducing debt will lead to extra money in your pocket for the additional expenses that accompany children, so preconception is an excellent time to start working on consolidating and eliminating debt.

- **Balance your short-term and long-term financial goals.** That is, college tuition is very important to prepare for, but remember that your retirement plans need to be continued as well. Adjusting your retirement contribution may allow more free money in the short term but will leave you at risk in the future. Evaluating your goals during the preconception period will allow more control over these issues and ultimately will reduce marital stress.

- **Seek professional expertise if needed.** Working with a certified financial planner, or CFP, will allow a trained professional to help you with the goals mentioned above.

Even if only one of you is the designated bill payer, make sure you both have a handle on where the money goes. Go over the financial worksheet in Appendix A together, or meet jointly with a certified financial planner. Alternatively, make a date to set up (or review) electronic forms of money management, such as Quicken or QuickBooks.

The Cost of Childbirth

So, exactly what does it cost to have a baby? Hospital costs and medical professional fees vary depending on the type of delivery (vaginal versus C-section), use of pain-relieving medication, your length of stay in the hospital, whether your newborn needs intensive care in the nursery, and where you live in the United States. The average delivery costs $3,500; half of all deliveries are billed to private health insurance companies, and 42 percent are paid by Medicaid (the remaining 8 percent comprise the uninsured, Medicare, and other insurance sources).[3] The amount you pay out of pocket depends on your insurance plan; it would be wise to check with your insurance company to find out how you will be billed, if at all. This information may impact your decision about where to deliver and the details of your birthing plan (such as whether or not you want anesthesia).

If you choose a midwife, costs may initially be less, but often a certified nurse midwife

---

3. Russo, C. A. (Thomson Reuters), et al. "Hospitalizations Related to Childbirth, 2006." HCUP Statistical Brief #71. April 2009. U.S. Agency for Healthcare Research and Quality, Rockville, MD. www.hcup-us.ahrq.gov/reports/statbriefs/sb71.jsp, accessed May 6, 2009.

works closely with an ob-gyn, and when that physician is called to assist in your delivery, you may be charged for both providers' services separately. People who choose to deliver in a birthing center may pay lower fees because the length of the hospital stay is usually shorter and pain medication is less widely used. Anesthesia fees can run between $1,000 and $2,000, depending on the type of anesthesia (epidural, spinal, or intravenous narcotic) and the length of your labor.

Making Sense of Health Insurance

When thinking about paying for the cost of maternity care, rule number one is that health insurance is a must! Before you conceive, it is a good idea to evaluate your health insurance policy and see what maternity provisions are available to you. If you receive insurance through your employer, you may have the option of upgrading to a more comprehensive plan. If your husband has a different insurance policy, take a look at it: his coverage for maternity care may be more comprehensive, and you might consider switching to his plan. If you think you may have trouble getting pregnant, either because of medical circumstances or your age, evaluate the provisions in your insurance policy for infertility procedures. It's also a good idea to review your health insurance plan with your insurance broker, office manager, benefits manager, human resources person, or insurance company directly.

If you receive health insurance through your employer, you have what's known as a group plan. Group plans usually encompass a few coverage options from which you can select, for example, an HMO plan or a PPO plan. The company typically decides on one as their basic plan but may allow you to choose another for an additional monthly fee. According to Ross Afsahi, vice president of employee benefits at G. S. Levine Insurance Services, if your company carries insurance through a reputable insurance company, chances are that there are no limitations on who can receive coverage. Most include prenatal and postnatal benefits as part of the basic coverage; only a few include preconception and infertility benefits in their basic plan. For new hires, there may be a thirty-day or longer probationary or waiting period before being eligible for group plan coverage, although many provide immediate coverage upon hire.

At the same time every year, businesses renew their master policies for group insurance (called "open enrollment"). Any employee who wishes to switch coverage options or add family members to the policy must do so during the month before the policy is renewed, so it is important to know when this window of opportunity opens. Here is a prime example of how this works:

Kathleen, thirty-two, and Paul, thirty-four, are engaged to be married in the fall and hope to become pregnant right away. For four years Kathleen has been self-employed and has carried an inexpensive individual health plan that offers no maternity benefits. Adding maternity benefits to

HMO, PPO, POS, and Medicaid:
Deciphering the Insurance Options

Here is a brief guide to the alphabet soup you may encounter with insurance carriers.

- **The health maintenance organization,** or HMO, is the original form of managed health care. At the time of service, there is either no fee or a small copayment. There is also no deductible (i.e., the amount you must pay for health care before your insurance will start to pay your medical bills) if you see a provider in your network. When you see a physician in your network, you see a doctor who participates with your HMO. If you desire the care of a doctor not in your network, the HMO can refuse payment or pay for only 50 to 70 percent of the fees incurred. Your primary care doctor must give you a referral to see physicians in other specialties. Depending on your HMO plan, your ob-gyn may already be your primary care provider or you may be able to visit your ob-gyn without a referral.

- **The preferred provider organization** (PPO) means your insurance company has negotiated with groups of medical providers, called preferred providers, to offer care at discounted rates; these discounted rates are passed on to your insurance company. However, if you decide that you want to see a physician who is outside of this PPO network, your insurance cannot refuse to pay. You're still covered, but in a more limited way, meaning higher out-of-pocket expenses per visit and a higher annual deductible. It is your responsibility as the consumer to ask the physician or their staff, "Are you a preferred provider for [name of your insurance]?" and "Do you contract with outside services (laboratories, sonographers) in the PPO network?" Regardless of whether you see someone in or outside of the PPO network, a small copayment for ob-gyn visits is usually required. Then, in the most typical PPO plan, an 80:20 plan, insurance pays 80 percent of anything beyond a basic office visit (e.g., lab work, medical procedures, hospitalization and delivery charges), and it is your responsibility to pay the remaining 20 percent (called a copay or coinsurance fee). A yearly deductible of $250 to $1,000 is common in PPO plans, too. This type of insurance is most often more expensive than an HMO, but allows more choice regarding which doctors you can see and may be more liberal in coverage for infertility treatment.

- **Point-of-service** (POS) plans are the most traditional type of medical insurance, allowing you to choose your own health care provider and hospital. You usually pay your own bills until a high deductible is met, after which your insurance will pay 70 to 100 percent of your charges.

- **Medicaid** is a state administered program. As such, it significantly restricts your choice of health care providers and hospitals and is available only to those families and individuals who have low income and few assets. Medicaid is also available for lower-income women who are pregnant, and those who are aged, blind, or disabled. (For more on eligibility, check www.cms.hhs.gov/medicaideligibility/02_areyoueligible.asp.)

her plan does not make economic sense. Instead, once married she will join Paul's group health in-surance plan during the annual open enrollment period in December. At the same time they will upgrade from Paul's basic plan to the slightly more expensive PPO plan that offers even more ex-tensive options for health care.

 FOR FUTURE REFERENCE: After Delivery

Sign Baby Up for Insurance Coverage

Newborns are eligible for entry into group health insurance coverage any time of the year, as long as one parent is covered at the time of the baby's birth. To qualify, the employee need only inform the employer or insurance company of the baby's name and date of birth within thirty days of the birth, and the policy will be retroactive from the moment of birth. We suggest that new parents inform their employer and insurance company even earlier—within the first few days after delivery—because if they forget and thirty days pass, the infant isn't eligible for coverage until the annual open enroll-ment period. As a reminder, put your employer or insurance company on your list of people to call from the hospital.

If you have coverage through a group insurance plan and you quit or lose your job through a layoff or firing, you (and any covered dependents) are entitled by federal law to maintain the same medical insurance coverage for up to eighteen months as long as you take over paying the monthly premiums plus a 2 percent processing fee. Check for subsidies or tax credits to help you offset the cost of premiums. Opting for COBRA (Consolidated Omnibus Budget Rec-onciliation Act) protection immediately after a job loss is recommended in case it takes a while to find a new job with new insurance. Your coverage would stay the same but the cost of your insurance under COBRA often can be double or triple what you paid while employed because your employer will not be contributing on your behalf. You must pay on time or your cover-age can be discontinued immediately. If you move to another state or city or outside the area covered by your former employer's plan, you lose the coverage.

The following is an example of how COBRA works:

Renee and Harlan have a two-and-a-half-year-old daughter and are thinking about having a sec-ond child. Renee wants to quit her job as a computer analyst to become a full-time mom before they have another baby. Because she has always been covered by her company's group insurance plan and is fond of her current ob-gyn, she decides to look into continuation or COBRA coverage. It turns out that all she has to do is advise her company's human resources manager of her desire to continue coverage when she puts in her notice; they will help her with the paperwork necessary to take over monthly payments of the premiums.

Unfortunately, COBRA laws do not apply to individual plans, which vary more than group plans in terms of whom and what they cover. Individual plans are available year-round, but generally cost more than group plans and involve more out-of-pocket expenses. You may have a high annual deductible to meet before insurance takes over some or all of the medical payments. Often certain terms of your coverage vest over a period of years—a way of sharing risk with the insurance company to prevent abuse of the system. For example, they may pay only a small portion of your bills for costly services if you have recently joined their plan, or make you wait a few years before they'll reimburse for certain preexisting conditions. Typically, the policy must be purchased before you become pregnant or the pregnancy will be classified as one of those preexisting conditions and be denied coverage.

Time Is Money

If taking unpaid time from work during or after your pregnancy is important, you may want to budget for some extra savings prior to getting pregnant. You also may want to save sick or vacation days to allow for any time you may need during your pregnancy. It is now federal law to allow a mother to have a twelve-week family leave, but this law doesn't require the hiatus from work to be at full pay, only that your job is waiting for you after maternity leave.

Child Care

This is also a good time to start thinking about the cost of child care. Does one of you want to stop working or work part-time and take care of the baby? Can you afford the reduction in income? If you both need or want to keep working, run some figures to see if the cost of child care (nanny, au pair, or day care) will be offset enough by what you earn to make the decision clear. Can you add nearby friends and family members to the day care solution? Can you and your spouse alternate shifts so the need for child care is minimized? You don't have to make a decision the minute you ask these questions, but you should start thinking about them now. Flexibility is crucial.

Your first plan for day care may not end up being as desirable once you go through the new routine for a month or so. For example, day care may cost more than you anticipated, and having you or your spouse working part-time may in fact be more cost-effective. Also, priorities may shift after you have the baby. You or your partner may find that your professional responsibilities don't compel you the way they once did. This, in turn, will affect your income if you choose to make a career change or stop working altogether.

FOR FUTURE REFERENCE: Family Life

Taking Care of Loose Ends

After you have conceived, you should write a will, consider creating a trust to provide for the care and financial needs of your future children, and evaluate your power of attorney and estate planning more closely. Does one or both of you carry life insurance or disability insurance? Planning for catastrophic events is very important when you are considering expanding your family.

TRAVEL: THE ADVENTURE IS JUST BEGINNING

The prospect of bringing a baby into your life may prompt you to plan one last carefree getaway—a weekend retreat, camping trip, or extended vacation—to escape from some of the responsibilities and stresses we've just talked about. If you're soon to be married, there may even be honeymoon plans in the works. A relaxing holiday in a developed country generally requires few, if any, preconception adjustments. Though you need not sacrifice more exotic travel when you are contemplating parenthood, there are some things you'll need to think about to ensure your preconception safety.

If you're planning far in advance for a big vacation but are going to be trying to get pregnant beforehand, you could very well be pregnant by the time you are away and should be prepared to make some concessions. Whether you plan your own vacation or employ a travel agent, consider traveler's insurance for trips involving expensive tickets, lodging, or tour fees, especially if your trip is many months away. It will allow you to cancel a trip with a small financial penalty if you do conceive and suddenly don't feel up to your plans or are concerned about travel to a place where medical care may be scarce.

The following travel recommendations are most helpful if implemented one to three months prior to conception, but some require three to six months' preparation. These recommendations can help take the strain out of business travel as well.

When You Fly

Flying is not hazardous to your fertility or to the health of a baby once conceived. The metal detectors at airport security pose no harm, and airplanes have pressurized cabins that protect you from any altitude effects. A consideration for all travelers during air travel longer than three hours is prolonged immobilization and dehydration from the climate control in the aircraft, which can increase the incidence of clots in the legs that can travel to the lungs. Once you are pregnant, these risks are even greater. When you fly, practice a few simple strategies to increase your comfort and health:

- Wear loose-fitting clothing, compression stockings being the exception.
- Drink plenty of fluids, as the pressurized cabins can cause excessive dehydration and dryness. Avoid alcoholic beverages two weeks before trying to conceive and throughout pregnancy, whether in the air or on the ground.
- Get in the habit of moving about the cabin or, while seated, stretching your legs and body every thirty to sixty minutes to relieve back tension and reduce the possibility of leg clots.

Air flight can cause significant anxiety in some travelers. If you usually take an antianxiety medication to fly, such as Valium, Ativan, or Xanax, you'll have to find an alternative way to quell your fear. Although these medicines do not reduce fertility in men or women, they can affect a developing fetus. They should be used sparingly before or during pregnancy at the discretion of your doctor. There are other ways to reduce your anxiety without having to take prescription drugs. Techniques such as meditation and visualization often work. You might try traveling with a person who calms you or traveling during low-traffic times to reduce practical factors that can trigger anxiety, such as delays and claustrophobic conditions in the airport and the airplane. Other simple strategies can work wonders.

One adventurous mother, Kayla, recently shared that she gets very nervous about flying, but doesn't want her nervousness to affect her kids' perception of flying. As she boards, she quietly tells a flight attendant that she gets very nervous in turbulence and to look out for her if it gets bumpy. Knowing in advance that an attendant will provide reassurance is comforting. If her journey involves a layover, she knows that the second flight will be easier once she gets the jitters out from the first flight. Taking care of the kids, listening to her iPod, or reading a good book distracts her enough that medication is not needed.

When You Sail

Many who suffer from seasickness, or mal de mer, control their symptoms of disorientation and extreme nausea by taking prophylactic medications such as scopolamine, an antidizziness medication, or Compazine or Dramamine, antinausea medications. However, both of these medications should probably be avoided beginning two weeks before you start trying to conceive and throughout pregnancy. Animal studies have shown no birth defects from seasickness medications, but there is little information on their effects in humans. Discuss your individual situation with your doctor.

FOR FUTURE REFERENCE: During Pregnancy

High-Altitude Travel While Pregnant

Several years ago, concerns were raised about the potential for radiation exposure when flying at altitudes over thirty-five thousand feet. This should not affect the typical business or leisure traveler, even on long international flights, but pregnant crew members are often encouraged to take desk jobs during pregnancy to avoid repeat high-altitude flights that may increase their overall exposure. One small study also intimated that flight staff who made international runs might have an increased risk of miscarriage due to time zone changes and the stress that places on the body. The low levels of cosmic radiation that occur in air flight have not been associated with early pregnancy effects and thus far have shown no link to changes in fertility in men or women.

For women with regular business trips overseas or those who are planning a vacation, it might be a good idea to consider travel insurance to cover the cost of making an unexpected change in your plans as the pregnancy progresses. (You never know whether a change in your pregnancy may alter your ability to travel.) Also, airlines and clinicians do not recommend travel after thirty-four weeks of gestation because if labor begins unexpectedly, resources are very limited onboard the aircraft and landing may not be a possibility.

Alternatives while on a boat include staying in fresh air as long as possible and keeping your eyes on the horizon. If it is an option, getting *in* the water is another tactic some people swear by. Also, pressure point wristbands, which are perfectly safe before you conceive and during pregnancy, have been shown to reduce the symptoms of seasickness in 30 to 50 percent of sufferers.

Ginger is another tried-and-true remedy for motion sickness, whether it is from seasickness or car sickness. In scientific studies, dosages of 1,000–2,000 mg/day (1–2 grams) of powdered ginger root have been more effective than placebo. This amount is deemed safe for preconception as well as pregnancy; more than this amount is not recommended. See Table 8-5 for more information on food source equivalents of ginger.

Eating and Drinking While Traveling

Most diseases contracted in foreign countries come from contaminated food or water. To keep yourself healthy while traveling, follow these safe eating habits:

Practical Application

List all the medications you may have taken during a recent trip. Check Chapter 8, "Conception-Friendly Medications and Herbs," to see if they are safe to use before you conceive.

Medications   Supplements/Herbs

_____

_____

_____

_____

- Drink only bottled or disinfected water, carbonated beverages, or fruit juices that you opened. Never accept drinks with ice unless you know that the ice was made with clean bottled water. Boiling water vigorously for one minute* is the most effective method of disinfection, according to the CDC. If this is impractical, a two-step process of filtration followed by chemical disinfection with sodium hypochlorite is recommended. Using iodine to treat water may not be advisable.
- Eat only well-cooked fish, meat, chicken, and eggs.
- Eat only fruits and vegetables that are cooked or that you peeled (but make sure your hands are clean before you eat the contents).
- At least two months prior to conception, totally avoid undercooked or raw meats, poultry, or seafood (no sushi), as well as raw eggs and eggs with runny yolks. Avoid unpasteurized cheese, yogurt, and milk, too; unpasteurized cheese that has been aged for more than sixty days may be safer but still isn't as safe as pasteurized. You should also strictly limit foods such as liver and liver products, not because of contamination concerns but because you don't want to exceed safe levels of vitamin A in your diet. See Chapters 11 and 13 for more on this.
- Heed local and national food warnings and advisories when traveling. Just to be on the safe side, pack a few good backup foods, such as nonperishable, prepackaged food items of known safety (e.g., nuts, dried fruits, granola bars).

*Three-minute boil at altitudes greater than 6,562 feet (>2,000 meters).

Traveler's Diarrhea

If you do contract traveler's diarrhea, get treated as soon as possible. You can avoid dehydration and poor nutrition by drinking fluids or by receiving intravenous fluids. You can also reduce diarrhea by using baby-friendly medicines such as Imodium A-D and Lomotil, and you can reduce fevers by using Tylenol. Avoid the use of Kaopectate if you suffer from iron-deficiency anemia and Pepto-Bismol or other bismuth products two weeks before conception. Antibiotics that can be used safely before you conceive (as long as you aren't allergic to them) include Bactrim (sulfa-based) and Keflex. Avoid antibiotics in the tetracycline family, such as doxycycline, and those in the quinolone family, such as ciprofloxacin and Levoquin, once you are pregnant, as they can affect the bones of the developing baby.

An ounce of prevention is worth a pound of cure as far as traveler's diarrhea is concerned. Frequent hand washing with potable water and the use of antibacterial gels or towelettes or antiseptic soaps can reduce your risk of becoming infected and of spreading the germs to other members of your entourage. Avoid the tap water when brushing your teeth; instead, wet the toothbrush with your travel-size oral rinse or disinfected bottled water. Unfortunately, suffering from traveler's diarrhea once doesn't confer immunity the next time you are exposed since so many different microorganisms can be culprits.

Those Pesky Bugs

Speaking of bugs, insect bites can be very uncomfortable and affect how much you enjoy your trip. More important, insect bites are the way some serious infections, such as malaria (via the mosquito) and Lyme disease (via tick bite), can be transmitted to you. By avoiding the bite of bugs that carry a potential disease, you can significantly reduce your risk of getting sick. To protect against bug bites:

- Wear long sleeves, long pants, and socks if possible. Spray repellent on your clothes as an extra measure of protection.
- If air-conditioning is available, turn it on; lower room temperatures are less bug-friendly. If not, consider sleeping under mosquito netting.
- For the most repellent power, use one that contains a low concentration of DEET (10 to 30 percent). While DEET, or N,N-diethyl-meta-toluamide, is not known to cause cancer or birth defects, the better part of prudence would suggest spraying clothing as much as possible versus directly on your skin. Be careful to avoid ingestion of DEET (so wash your hands before eating).
- Biopesticides and other DEET-free products are becoming increasingly popular, such as picaridin and natural products such as those made from oil of lemon eucalyptus or

lavender. (Use repellents in modest amounts on the skin surface, as there is scant safety data on use during pregnancy.) Vitamin B_1 (thiamin) supplements are reported to reduce your likelihood of being bitten by insects, but there is no scientific data to back up this claim. We do *not* advocate taking megadoses of vitamin B_1, but if you choose to do so, do not exceed twenty days.

Last but not least, when traveling to locales where sanitation is less than optimal or to remote places where health care systems are not the best, pack a preconception/pregnancy travel first-aid kit that includes Tylenol (known in some countries as Paracetemol), antiyeast vaginal preparations, hydrocortisone 1 percent topical cream (for skin rashes), oral rehydration packets, antidiarrheals such as Imodium A-D, sunscreen with a high SPF, and extra insect repellent.

Prevention Is the Best Cure

In addition to these precautions, when you travel to more exotic places, ensure that your routine immunizations such as measles, mumps, and rubella (MMR), tetanus, and pertussis (T dap) are up-to-date (see Table 1-1). Depending on where and when you are traveling, you may need additional shots. If you are traveling to a developing country, your doctor may recommend vaccinations against hepatitis A and B, yellow fever, or encephalitis, and medications against malaria, which need to be administered one to six months prior to your departure.

In addition to your doctor, a travel immunization center can be an excellent source of information about travel precautions. Most major hospitals have a travel advisement or immunization center. The CDC (Centers for Disease Control and Prevention) provides information about recommended vaccinations and international travel safety information. You can contact them toll free at (877) FYI-TRIP or visit www.cdc.gov/travel. A resource for world flu pandemic developments is the U.S. Department of State at www.travel.state.gov. Lastly, the World Health Organization (WHO) offers comprehensive health information for travelers at www.who.int/en. Both the CDC and the WHO have revised their websites to provide powerful interactive maps and resources that convey the latest advisories based on your intended destination(s).

Vaccinations or medications are usually thought to be safe and effective to reduce the likelihood of contracting a disease that can be at best uncomfortable (e.g., diarrhea) and at the worst, chronic or life-threatening (e.g., hepatitis B or malaria, respectively). As some vaccinations contain particles of live virus, they may lead to a reaction or sensitivity in some people (see Table 1-2). You would be advised not to receive a vaccine (during preconception or otherwise) if the following issues exist:

- If you have had a severe allergic reaction with anaphylaxis (inability to breathe) to any vaccine, a second dose or repeat dose is to be completely avoided.
- If pregnant, you should avoid all live-virus vaccines. These include vaccination against measles, mumps, and rubella; varicella (chicken pox), yellow fever, and Japanese encephalitis.
- If you have an allergy to egg products, you should avoid vaccination against influenza, yellow fever, and tetanus.

TABLE 1-1
DISEASES BY GEOGRAPHICAL AREA

Disease	*Geographical Area of Risk*
Malaria	Southeast Asia, India, Indonesia, Central Africa, Central America, South America
Japanese encephalitis	Northern and central South America, Central Africa
Yellow fever	Northern and central South America, Central Africa
Hepatitis B	Africa, India, Middle East, Southeast Asia, China, Russia, Mexico, South America, Central America, northern Canada (Australia and the United States have the lowest risk of this infection)
Meningococcal meningitis	Central Africa
Poliomyelitis	India, Pakistan, Central Africa (less prevalence compared with other areas)

Source: WHO International Travel and Health recommendations, www.who.int/ith/en/, accessed June 5, 2009.

TABLE 1-2
VACCINATION DURING THE PRECONCEPTION MONTHS

Disease	Vaccination Type	Preconception Safety
Tetanus/ diphtheria/ acellular pertussis (Tdap) (whooping cough)[a]	Toxoid/inactivated	Safe any time before or after trying to conceive (TTC)
Influenza (flu)[b,c]	Inactivated	Administer 1 month prior to flu season and preferably up to 1 month prior to TTC
Measles, mumps, rubella	Live virus	Administer 1 month prior to TTC
Hepatitis A	Inactivated	Begin series 6 months prior to travel or 1–3 months prior to TTC
Hepatitis B	Recombinant	Begin series 6 months in advance of travel (3-shot series); otherwise okay to administer any time
Varicella (chicken pox)	Live virus	Administer 3 months prior to TTC
Pneumococcal pneumonia[d]	Inactivated bacteria	Administer 1 month prior to TTC

PRIMARILY TRAVEL VACCINES

Yellow fever[e]	Live virus	Administer 3 months prior to TTC
Typhoid[e]	Inactivated bacteria, not oral live bacteria	Administer 1 month prior to TTC (safety not determined in pregnancy)
Japanese encephalitis[e]	Live virus	Administer 3 months prior to TTC
Immunoglobulins	Antibody preparations	Administer following unexpected exposure to disease (e.g., rabies)

Courtesy: CDC Health Information for International Travel, 1999–2009

a. Updated recommendations were released by CDC in May 2008 (so pay extra attention if your last tetanus shot was before then): All adults should receive one Tdap instead of the usual tetanus (Td) booster to include protection against pertussis ("whooping cough") in addition to tetanus and diphtheria. Whooping cough is life-threatening for infants and lasts for months in adults. The CDC says that it is safe to receive a Tdap *even at an interval as little as two years* since your last Td. See pages 30, 96–97, and the CDC's website for more information.

b. It is also safe for use during pregnancy, preferably after the first trimester.

c. Other late-breaking seasonal flu vaccines (such as H1N1 in 2009) that use an injectable inactivated virus may be administered 1 month prior to the flu season, or anytime before or after conception. On the other hand, please avoid the nasal version (live attenuated virus) if you could be pregnant within 1 month of administration.

d. Adults with risk factors for severe disease include those with asthma, diabetes, heart, lung, liver or kidney disease, sickle cell disease, smokers, those with a cochlear implant, HIV/AIDs or other immune suppressing condition (such as treatment for cancer or lymphoma, long-term use of steroids). Ask your doctor if this vaccine is one you should get.

e. Avoid unless traveling to a high-risk area (see Table 1-1).

Special Consideration

Men and women who are of reproductive age and are also health care providers should be aware that their risk of exposure to potential disease is greater than that of the average person. Vaccination regimens should be up-to-date before conception, and should include Tdap, varicella (if there is no history of chicken pox), MMR, annual influenza, and hepatitis A and B (see Table 1-2 for guidelines related to conception timing).

Malaria

Infection with malaria can have an extremely serious clinical impact on you and your prospective fetus. The majority of malaria cases are preventable with prophylactic medications or can be treated promptly to reduce recurrent symptoms. Once you are infected with malaria (and if you survive), it can lead to an increase in spontaneous miscarriage, stillbirth, and reduced fetal growth. Prospective mothers can suffer from fever, kidney failure, and central nervous system effects. There is no vaccine for malaria, but if you are traveling to a country during its malaria season, particularly to parts of Central and South America, Africa, and Southeast Asia, you should start malaria prophylaxis one to two weeks before you depart and continue taking the medication weekly during the trip and for two weeks after you return. Chloroquine has been used in pregnant women for decades without any reported fetal birth defects from the medication. If you are traveling to an area with chloroquine-resistant malaria, the alternative medical therapies have not been proven safe in early pregnancy. Avoid these areas of travel until your second trimester or after your pregnancy.

FOR FUTURE REFERENCE: During Pregnancy/After Delivery

Traveling with Child (in the Womb or Out): To Vaccinate or Not to Vaccinate?

Before administering anything to their child, such as medication or vaccines, most parents carefully consider the pros and cons in a discussion with their child's doctor. Pregnancy can complicate this already interesting discussion because the benefit/risk equation includes the "passenger" in the womb as well as any children who may be traveling with you. We recognize that some of our readers may feel the jury is still out regarding vaccine safety. However, as far as the medical and scientific community is concerned, three juries are in: NIH, CDC, and WHO say vaccines are a safe choice. We strongly support preconception vaccination, and we'll try to shed some light on the issue here as well as in Chapter 4, "The Preconception Visit." Please, continue the dialogue with your physician after you've delved into valid, scientific information on the topic to your satisfaction.[a]

As the incidence of autism has risen, various causes have been investigated, from genetic predisposition to environmental exposures. One small study published in the

Lancet in 1998 triggered an onslaught of concern about thimerosal, a preservative that had been used in pediatric vaccinations since the 1930s. Thimerosal was removed from vaccines in 2001 based on the theoretical risk raised (trace amounts are still used in some flu shots). Three years later, the Institute of Medicine (IOM) released a report stating that thimerosal does *not* cause autism.[b] Yet the number of children diagnosed with autism continues to rise. The original *Lancet* study was retracted in February 2010 by the journal because the authors used unethical and unscientific methods, which invalidated the findings. (Of note, in 2004, ten of the thirteen authors backed away from interpretations of the study due to concerns over unscientific and unethical practices, concerns that were confirmed by a medical review board in January 2010.) Since the original publication, more than a decade of large, rigorous studies have not been able to establish a link between vaccines and autism.

While no vaccine is 100 percent effective or 100 percent safe (adverse side effects do occur, such as high fever accompanied by seizures), the American Academy of Pediatrics, the CDC, and the WHO all strongly support routine childhood vaccination to prevent the risk of long-term health problems and death due to vaccine-preventable illness. For instance, vaccines have eradicated smallpox and nearly eliminated polio and measles in the United States, diseases that were once considered rites of passage. And before the chicken pox vaccine was licensed, more than one hundred children died in the United States each year due to complications of this "childhood disease."

You may wonder, "If these diseases have declined so much, why can't I just enjoy 'herd immunity'?" While many diseases have been reduced dramatically by vaccination, it is still important to immunize yourself and your children because modern travel makes it very easy for disease to be "imported" to your area, exposing those who were unvaccinated or not eligible for vaccination (such as newborns or those with a weakened immune system). You may even have had a measles outbreak in your area triggered by an imported case—a person who was unvaccinated and became exposed while traveling overseas where vaccination rates are lower. Also, whooping cough (pertussis) is on the rise again among adults whose immunity waned (remember to check your Tdap status).

Children are vaccinated at a very young age to prevent serious disease before exposure is likely, and to take advantage of a time when the immune system is most vigorous. There are a few exceptions to this general rule (such as a compromised immune system), and we recommend that you discuss vaccination with your physician if you plan to travel. Bottom line: what is safe in pregnancy is believed to be safe during preconception.

a. See http://necam.nih.gov/health/webresources.

b. Immunization Review Committee, National Academy of Sciences. *Immunization Safety Review: Vaccines and Autism.* National Academy press, 2004. www.iom.edu/CMS/3793/4705/20155.aspx, accessed July 1, 2009.

Practical Application

Make a list of vaccinations you received in the past, with the dates they were administered. Keeping an up-to-date list is helpful, as it will alert your health care provider to when you need a booster before your next trip. (An adult immunization schedule and detailed guidance can be found and printed at www.cdc.gov/vaccines/recs/schedules/adult-schedule.htm.)

Vaccination   Date(s)

_____

_____

_____

_____

_____

If You Want an Active Vacation

If you and your spouse enjoy active adventure vacations such as a cycling tour or a hike into the Grand Canyon, go right ahead and book your trip as long as you are physically prepared for it in advance. Exercise is something all health professionals encourage. Just be aware that fatigue is a very common side effect in your first trimester and may make a more active vacation less enjoyable.

Vacations that involve scuba diving, skiing, horseback riding, or any other sport that could involve a fall, a direct abdominal blow, or rapid changes in atmospheric pressure are best taken before you start trying to conceive. (Snorkeling is fine during preconception and in pregnancy.) Keep in mind that if you do injure yourself, treatment of your injury must take your pregnancy into consideration. For example, if you break bones, X-rays will probably be required. If you think you may be pregnant, tell the technicians so they can take the appropriate precautions to shield your pelvis and abdomen. If your injuries require surgery, general anesthesia will likely be required. While these medications do not affect your fertility, they can increase the risk of miscarriage once pregnant.

Take a Romantic Vacation for Two

Heidi and Brian, both in their mid-thirties, had been trying to conceive for several months, but to no avail. Part of the problem was that they were rarely in the same city for more than two nights in a row! Brian's consulting job had him flying around the country from Monday to Friday. "I'm beginning to forget what you look like," Heidi joked one Saturday morning. "Let's use some of your zillion frequent flyer miles and go somewhere romantic." Brian wasn't hard to persuade, and they soon found themselves soaking up the sights of Rome. Two weeks after they returned home, Heidi took a pregnancy test. It was positive. They've begun a scrapbook for their future baby with mementos of their trip.

As you and your partner prepare to conceive, feel free to plan a great, once-in-a-lifetime trip to celebrate. Then, when your adventure is over, or soon thereafter, prepare to embrace the greatest adventure of your life—that of becoming parents of a new baby.

CHAPTER 2

Lifestyle Habits: Smoking, Drinking, Drugs . . . and Caffeine?

*W*ithin the first five to ten minutes of any preconception consultation, we always ask our patients about the big four: tobacco, alcohol, illicit drugs, and caffeine. Why? Because each of these substances has the potential to affect fertility and, later on, harm a fetus. "But my mother smoked and drank through four pregnancies and we all turned out fine," one patient said, and she proceeded to do the same thing her mother did, conceiving and giving birth to a healthy first child. After that, she had one miscarriage and got pregnant again. The next child was born four weeks early and, despite overcoming the challenges of premature delivery, the baby remained smaller and more sickly than the first child, even though the patient's habits were no different from the first time around. This is just one example of how the odds play out, and they vary according to individual tolerance and genetics. Our feeling is that as far as smoking, drinking, and doing drugs is concerned, indulging is like playing Russian roulette. It's wiser not to take the risk, however small. With caffeine, you'll have some leeway with what is and what is not considered risky.

There is a considerable benefit, for both of you, to making the lifestyle changes discussed in this chapter *before* you are pregnant. While you might have heard you were born with all the eggs your ovaries will ever have, this is only part of the story. They're all there, but incompletely developed. One or more eggs resume development (meiosis I) when they are chosen for ovulation, and the final developmental stage is completed at fertilization (meiosis II). The rest stay dormant until it's their turn. Thus, unless otherwise specified, the ninety-day time frame in our book's subtitle allows the woman to make lifestyle changes that protect those final stages of egg development—reducing the risk of some genetic defects—as well as optimizing the womb environment for implantation. For men, ninety days is barely enough time for a fresh batch of sperm to develop, so we recommend three to six months lead time. You *do* have a choice in the matter. Fertility and fetal development depend on both genetics and environmental factors, and the main thing you can change is the latter.

TOBACCO: FIRST- AND SECONDHAND EXPOSURE

If you are a smoker, you probably saw this heading and thought, "Here we go again!" We know many of you may have tried to stop smoking before and that you may even have been successful, if only for a short time. You are not alone. Tobacco use is an addiction, both mental and physical, and is the largest preventable cause of death and disease among women worldwide. There are twenty-two million reproductive-age women in the United States alone who smoke. Of these, 12 to 20 percent continue to smoke throughout their pregnancies, increasing their risk of having preterm labor and infants with lower birth weight, birth defects, and developmental delays.

Why is it so important to quit smoking altogether (or, at a minimum, curtail the habit) *before* you conceive? Because nicotine decreases fertility and affects the fetus, which begins organ development on the seventeenth day after conception—potentially before you even know you're pregnant. (During the first sixteen days, the cells are dividing in preparation for the job of growing a fetus.) Between seventeen and fifty-six days after conception, the brain, central nervous system, and all of the other major organ systems begin to form. So, if you wait to stop smoking until after you know you are pregnant, you have already exposed the fetus to potential risk. Changing your smoking habits before you conceive will ensure a faster, more successful conception and healthier pregnancy. Therefore, we recommend that prospective moms quit smoking three months prior to conception, given how difficult it may be to quit smoking. This will give *you* more time to mentally ease into tobacco cessation and your body more time to heal from tobacco-related vascular changes.

Exactly How Does Tobacco Affect Your Fertility and the Baby's Health?

Tobacco smoke contains more than 2,500 different chemicals, of which carbon monoxide and nicotine are the most deleterious. Carbon monoxide is a colorless gas that constricts blood vessels, which reduces blood flow and oxygen delivery to your reproductive organs. Women who smoked took twice as long as nonsmokers to conceive. If a smoker does become pregnant, this reduced blood flow and exposure to carcinogens affects the baby, too.

Recent studies among women who smoked during preconception and pregnancy have underscored the dose-response relationship between tobacco and pregnancy complications: before pregnancy and during the first trimester, the more you smoke, the greater the risk. Smoking during pregnancy slows the baby's growth, increasing the risk of premature delivery and low birth weight (smaller than 5½ pounds and an increase in fetal cardiac defects). Smoking during pregnancy has longer-term effects, too. It doubles or triples the risk of sudden infant death syndrome (SIDS) and asthma.

If you are a nonsmoker, share the information in this section with your spouse, friends, and family members who do smoke. They are exposing you to secondhand smoke, which has been shown to have effects on you as a prospective mother that can be similar to those you would experience as a smoker yourself. Repetitive exposure to secondhand smoke at home, versus exposure at work or in a public place, has been linked to lower birth weight. This is probably due to the decreased ventilation, smaller spaces, and increased exposure time in the home.

Tip on Deterring Secondhand Smoke Exposure

When you ask people not to smoke around you, if you don't want to say that you are trying to get pregnant, claim you have (or have developed) a sinus sensitivity or an allergy to smoke.

Nicotine also decreases female fertility by constricting blood vessels and reducing blood flow to the ovaries, thereby making them less likely to produce an egg for fertilization. Nicotine is also believed to artificially increase metabolism, which can cause an increase in blood pressure, poor weight gain, and sleeplessness. Nicotine can reduce appetite, too, which can negatively affect your nutritional intake. Finally, it can change how your body uses a number of minerals and vitamins. For example, nicotine robs the body of vitamin C and leaches calcium from bones, making them more brittle as you get older.

In addition to affecting your fertility and your baby's health, smoking just a few cigarettes a day has been shown to affect your long-term health, increasing the risk of heart disease, respiratory disorders, and cancer. The type of cigarette you smoke also has an impact. A filtered cigarette exposes you to less tar than does an unfiltered cigarette, although the levels of nicotine, carbon monoxide, and other harmful chemicals often remain unchanged.

 FOR FUTURE REFERENCE: During Pregnancy

Tobacco Use During Pregnancy
The changes in a smoker's blood vessels can also affect the placenta, which is the nutritional pipeline for the fetus. When placental function is impaired by smoking, it becomes a less efficient source of oxygen and nutrients to the baby, which in turn can retard fetal growth. A number of excellent studies have also shown that when a mother's age, pregnancy weight gain, and socioeconomic status are accounted for, *tobacco is the sole culprit in increased fetal and infant death.* The bottom line is: *the more a mother smokes, the greater the reduction in the fetus's growth and birth weight.* Tobacco use resulting in poor

fetal growth, in turn, increases the risk of stillbirth and neonatal death. If you can stop smoking before you conceive or early in your pregnancy, you will have an impressive positive impact on fetal growth and long-term infant health. So even though completely eliminating tobacco from your life would be the healthiest thing to do, just cutting down the number of cigarettes you smoke a day can really help.

 FOR FUTURE REFERENCE: After Delivery

Nicotine—the Culprit

Nicotine is passed to a newborn through breastmilk, with nicotine poisoning possible if the mother smokes more than one to two packs of cigarettes per day. If you continue to smoke heavily throughout your pregnancy, at least try to cut back once your baby is born. Long-term studies have also shown an increased incidence of childhood respiratory infections and lung diseases such as asthma in infants born to women who smoke. And as noted in the sidebar earlier, smoking in the household is a major risk factor for sudden infant death syndrome or "crib death," doubling or tripling the risk.

What About the Prospective Dad Who Smokes?

Research has not been able to show the impact of tobacco on fertility in men as clearly as it has in women. In some studies, male smokers had lower sperm counts, impaired motility of sperm, and an increased number of abnormally shaped sperm. Other studies showed no effect from tobacco on sperm activity. Nevertheless, men's health risks from smoking are similar to those for women: an increased rate of heart disease, respiratory disease, and cancer. By creating secondhand smoke, prospective fathers put their future sons or daughters at risk for preterm birth, low fetal birth weight, sudden infant death syndrome (SIDS), and childhood respiratory illnesses. One report linked paternal smoking, in the absence of maternal smoking, to various childhood brain cancers. Ideally, men should cease or significantly reduce their smoking three to six months prior to trying to conceive.

Yes, You Can Quit Smoking

It's not easy to stop smoking, and it probably won't happen overnight. But as soon as you do, positive changes will occur in your lungs and blood vessels. And if you've been having trouble conceiving, your fertility problems may resolve spontaneously. An extremely slim patient who came to me complaining that she wasn't able to get pregnant confessed that she'd been smoking since she was a teenager to keep her weight under control. Her husband and medical staff joined forces and eventually persuaded her to stop. She put on about ten pounds, which to my mind she sorely needed, and—lo and behold—conceived without any further intervention.

Try making a date to stop smoking. Involve your friends and family in supporting you. But be sure to give them some advance warning, because it is not uncommon to become irritable, anxious, and unable to concentrate when you're trying to quit. You may also find educational materials from the American Lung Association, American Cancer Society, and Smoke-enders helpful.

If you wish to use nicotine replacement, such as patches or gum, or Zyban, a mild, low-dose antidepressant that can reduce the mood changes that accompany smoking cessation, you should know that there is little information on the safety of these substances for the fetus. Chantrix, the newest in medical tobacco cessation assistance, is also not recommended for one to three months prior to conception or in pregnancy because there are no safety data available. Try to quit smoking without medications first. If this proves too difficult, talk with your doctor about the best course of action. Remember, you are doing this not only for yourself but also for the health of your future child.

Practical Application

If you smoke:

How many cigarettes did you smoke today? _____

How many cigarettes did you smoke this time last year? _____

What will be your first step toward permanently quitting smoking?

_____

How do your plans for quitting compare to our preconception recommendations?

_____

If you do not smoke:

Where do you most come in contact with smokers? _____

List two or three ways to change your environment to reduce your exposure to secondhand smoke:

_____

_____

_____

If your partner smokes, ask him to take a close look at his smoking behaviors, too, and develop a plan to quit.

Acupuncture, hypnosis, and group therapy have all been ways couples have reduced or eliminated tobacco use before, during, and after pregnancy. Moderate exercise helps ease the symptoms of nicotine withdrawal and cravings and also has the potential to limit weight gain. More information is available about tobacco cessation at www.smokefree.gov, or call (800) QUIT-NOW (784-8669).

ALCOHOL

There is a great deal of evidence that women who consume a large amount of alcohol in the month or two prior to conception have a more difficult time conceiving. There is also evidence that women who keep that consumption low do not. The question of whether moderate drinking delays time to conception is still a gray area. Basically, consuming alcohol at higher volumes could change the levels of sex hormones available to the body, but ovulation may or may not be impaired. Because of this, we advise our female patients that one to three months prior to trying they should cut back to no more than one drink per day, and preferably not every day. (See Table 2-1 for what constitutes one drink.)

In case you ovulate and get pregnant a little earlier than you anticipate, *it's imperative to quit drinking alcohol altogether two weeks prior to trying to conceive* (see Table 2-2). It is also very important to ensure optimal intake of nutrients such as choline and folate, particularly if you are accustomed to having more than one or two drinks when you enjoy an alcoholic beverage. Continued abstinence is recommended for as long as you are trying and through your entire pregnancy.

By observing this rule, you will avoid one of the most common scenarios we encounter: when a woman using no birth control lets her hair down and has a few drinks because she recently got her period, but it turns out that her "period" was just implantation spotting and she is actually pregnant.(When the little embryo burrows into the uterine lining some spotting may occur.) This creates worry for her during the whole pregnancy. Although the baby will almost surely be fine, the mother's stress and anxiety could have been prevented.

Back to the question of impact on fertility, most studies find delays in conception at high levels of alcohol intake, typically more than ten drinks per week. Among couples who drink infrequently, the evidence is mixed. In one study, women with very low to modest alcohol consumption prior to conception needed fewer cycles to conceive than women who never drank. However, researchers postulated that this is due not to enhanced fertility but rather to greater relaxation accompanied by more frequent sex (in other words, the odds of conception may have increased purely because of a higher frequency of intercourse). In contrast, a study of 430 Danish couples twenty to thirty-five years old trying to get pregnant for the first time revealed that women who continued to drink between one and five alcoholic beverages per week were 39 percent less likely to conceive within six months than women who consumed no alcohol. Those who con-

TABLE 2-1
ALCOHOLIC BEVERAGES EQUIVALENT TO ONE DRINK

Beverage	*Amount Equal To One Drink[a]*
Ale, beer[b]	12 fluid ounces
Strong beer, malt liquor	8 fluid ounces
Wine: red, white, or rosé	5 fluid ounces
Wine cooler	12 fluid ounces
Distilled spirits (gin, scotch, bourbon, rum, vodka), 80 proof	1.5 fluid ounces (one jigger or small shot glass)
Liqueurs (e.g., coffee liqueurs)	1.5 fluid ounces
Sherry or port	3 fluid ounces
Other (mixed drinks)	Varies greatly: a small serving (e.g., one made with an airline miniature plus juice) counts as 1½ drinks; many others (e.g., Manhattan, martini) count as 1 to 2½ drinks, depending on serving size

a. For comparison, recall that 12 fluid ounces = 1½ cups, 8 fluid ounces = 1 cup, 4 fluid ounces = ½ cup, and 2 fluid ounces = ¼ cup.
b. Light beer contains fewer calories than regular beer, but the difference in alcohol content is negligible.

Sources: Industry data; Agriculture Handbook no. 8-14; National Consumers League, 1701 K Street, NW, Suite 1200, Washington, D.C. 20006; Distilled Spirits Council of the United States, Inc., 1250 I Street, NW, Suite 400, Washington, D.C. 20005

sumed six to ten drinks per week were 45 percent less likely to conceive, and women who had more than ten drinks per week were 66 percent less likely to conceive. Note that a limitation of these studies is the use of average consumption over seven days: Having one drink with a meal may be different than having five to ten on a weekend night or two, we just can't tell. The wisest choice if you're actively trying to conceive is to begin zeroing out your intake now.

Those who are either considering or undergoing infertility treatments may wonder if different recommendations apply to them since medicine is intervening to help fertility along. Research is limited in this area, but one prospective study in June 2009 among 221 California couples going through infertility treatment found that drinking does negatively affect fertility and the likelihood of conception. Specifically, the researchers found a dose-response relationship—the more alcohol consumed, the fewer eggs retrieved each cycle. In addition, a higher risk of miscarriage persisted among these women, even after adjusting for other lifestyle factors that adversely affect fertility, such as smoking and age. For men, the biological plausibility certainly exists that drinking adversely affects hormone levels and sperm quality, but the evidence is less solid regarding how much is too much. A recent study by Harvard University scientists of the spouses of women undergoing IVF found reduced rates of conception and fewer live births when the male consumed at least one beer daily, and even moderate alcohol consumption by the woman had a negative impact too. This is why, despite the call for more research, many doctors are recommending alcohol abstinence for both partners approximately ninety days or more prior to any ART procedures. If fertility is a concern for you, please see Chapter 18 for information about diagnostic work-ups and reassurance about the incredible advances in assisted reproduction technology (ART) available to couples today.

Did You Know?

Certain hot after-dinner drinks contain substantial amounts of alcohol. Just because they are hot doesn't mean that the alcohol evaporates!

Practical Application

Take a close look at your typical daily, weekly, and monthly alcohol intake, if any. Now ask your husband or partner to take a close look at his typical daily, weekly, and monthly alcohol intake. How do your respective habits compare to our preconception recommendations for prospective moms and dads? Is there a need for modification? While you are thinking about this, keep one eye on the present and another on the future. There are, or will be, times in your lives when, for health reasons, one of you will need to follow dietary restrictions (e.g., a low-sodium diet, a weight reduction diet, possibly a diabetic diet). It's no picnic being the one on the receiving end of these restrictions, but usually you make the best of it. Preconception and pregnancy are one such example, mostly for the female. So think about how you can support each other and be considerate of each other's positions. If you both feel a sense of solidarity by zeroing out alcohol together, then fine. But talk this through before handing down any ultimatums or directives.

TABLE 2-2
MINOR SOURCES OF ALCOHOL THAT CAN BE CONSIDERED SAFE

- Cooking with small amounts of alcohol (e.g., a little wine in a batch of spaghetti sauce) is okay if the food being prepared simmers for a good thirty minutes to allow the majority of the alcohol to cook out. After thirty minutes of cooking, 35 percent of the alcohol remains. After sixty minutes, only 25 percent of the alcohol remains. The amount of remaining alcohol per serving poses no danger.

- Desserts such as tiramisu and chocolates made with liqueurs are also alcohol sources, albeit fairly modest ones, unless you have an aunt who really goes overboard on the rum in the rum cake. In most cases, a few bites of these (e.g., sharing a dessert with friends) is fine, but we don't advise eating full portions on a regular basis.
- The alcohol found in certain medications such as prescription cough syrup is considered negligible, but again the smallest amount used or an alternative medication without alcohol is recommended. See Chapter 8 for a full listing of medications considered safe during preconception.

Men and Alcohol

Unless there is a fertility concern, men have it a little easier than women during the months prior to conception. In a handful of animal and human studies, low to moderate alcohol intake (one to two drinks a day) had no measurable effect on semen quality or ability to successfully impregnate. Heavy drinking, however, does impair sexual performance and damages sperm quality, such as motility (movement) and shape. A number of studies from 1976 to the present have shown that heavier alcohol consumption reduces the level of circulating testosterone and lowers the sperm count and quality (specifically the shape of the sperm head, which must be capable of penetrating the egg).

Although the research to date among men is limited compared to that among women, it is convincing. Thus, we strongly recommend that men cap their alcohol consumption at two or fewer drinks per day, particularly for the three to four months leading up to conception through the thirteenth week of pregnancy (we want to make sure you're covered, should you need to try again). This recommendation protects all of the developing sperm, among which resides the one that will fertilize the egg. If there is a special occasion or celebration now and then, one extra drink over the course of several hours, accompanied by food, should not be harmful to the future father's sperm, but drinking to the point of drunkenness is not wise.

 FOR FUTURE REFERENCE: During Pregnancy

Alcohol During Pregnancy

Once conception occurs, how much alcohol is safe during pregnancy? Perhaps your friends all say, "The ladies in France drink wine with every meal!" And maybe another friend got the okay from her physician to have a small glass of wine, especially during the second half of her pregnancy—advice reminiscent of that given in good conscience decades ago, when we didn't know any better. Yet here we are recommending that you begin abstaining two weeks before you conceive. Further, there are labels on alcoholic beverages and signs posted in every restaurant in the nation stating that pregnant women should not drink any amount of alcohol because of the risk of birth defects.

The research, both here and abroad, overwhelmingly supports avoiding alcohol either when you could become pregnant or at least once you have confirmed your pregnancy. The reason is simple: we do not know how much alcohol is safe, especially in the first trimester. Recall that the bulk of organ and tissue development takes place early in pregnancy, specifically, days seventeen to fifty-six after fertilization. Each day brings critical steps in the baby's development. Alcohol consumption *does* cause birth defects. Why take the chance? You'll just feel guilty later.

Yet many women do continue to drink once pregnant—and more than our mothers did a generation ago. The CDC reports that women are becoming less inhibited about drinking in general, and more specifically during pregnancy, resulting in higher rates of moderate to high prenatal alcohol exposure. At the same time, rates of the most severe type of fetal alcohol spectrum disorder, fetal alcohol syndrome (FAS), have increased sixfold in the past fifteen years. Some women who continue to drink during pregnancy may believe there are risks only with very heavy "alcoholic-type" drinking. Others may be under the impression that the recommendation to avoid even moderate amounts of alcohol stems from societal oppression of women instead of hard facts. Neither is true.

Moderate amounts of alcohol not only can increase the risk of miscarriage but also can contribute to learning disabilities such as attention deficit disorder with or without hyperactivity; lower birth weight; and low IQ, aggressiveness, and delinquent behavior often related to poor impulse control. These traits are called fetal alcohol effects and are not well publicized, nor are they often blatantly obvious at birth. In medical circles, the term *fetal alcohol effects* has been replaced by two terms, *alcohol-related birth defect* (ARBD) and *alcohol-related neurodevelopmental disorder* (ARND). These terms more accurately reflect the isolated effects of prenatal alcohol exposure, because in all but the most extreme cases, only a few of the problems emerge, if any. For example, a study of more than five hundred women and their offspring at Wayne State University (published in the journal *Pediatrics* in 2001) demonstrated that women who drank on average as little as one alcoholic beverage per week throughout pregnancy had children who were more than three times as likely to display aggressive and delinquent behaviors at age six or seven, independent of other contributing factors. Remember, most women do not vary their alcohol intake too greatly from week to week. Right now, these traits may just be benign words on a page, but when you're the parent of a child or teen who is struggling with these problems, they become heartbreakingly real.

If there is heavy drinking during pregnancy, it may result in full-blown fetal alcohol syndrome. This is characterized by lifelong brain damage (central nervous system dysfunction such as mental retardation), growth retardation, small head circumference, and abnormalities of the eyes, face, heart, joints, and genitals. The severity of these birth defects is directly related to the amount of alcohol consumed by the mother as well as the stage of pregnancy in which drinking occurs. (A woman's ethnicity also seems to play a role. For example, although black women tend to abstain from alcohol during pregnancy more often than do white women, their babies appear to be more genetically vulnerable to maternal alcohol consumption.) *The most common preventable cause of mental retardation is maternal alcohol abuse.*

ALCOHOL-FREE BEVERAGE IDEAS

Do you have a special event coming up when you might want to enjoy a few drinks—wedding, romantic weekend getaway, long vacation, special party or other celebration? Have a plan in mind, such as bringing along nonalcoholic beer or wine or a festive sparkling apple cider. Holding a wine glass filled with cranberry juice or sparkling cider prevents most people from noticing you're not drinking and may make for a more enjoyable time. Many of our patients tell us they'd like to try an alcohol-free beer or wine but don't know whether they can trust the label. Alcohol-free beverages must contain less than 0.5 percent alcohol to be labeled alcohol-free. Here is a sampling of reputable alcohol-free beers, wines, and sparkling ciders:

Alcohol-free Beers
O'Doul's Premium Amber, made by Anheuser-Busch
Kaliber, made by Guinness
Buckler, made by Heineken
Sharp's, made by Miller
St. Pauli N.A., made by St. Pauli Girl

Alcohol-free Wines
Alcohol-free versions of merlot, cabernet sauvignon, chardonnay, white zinfandel,
    and others, all made by Ariel Vineyards
Alcohol-free cabernet sauvignon and champagne, made by Inglenook St. Regis
Alcohol-free versions of white zinfandel, chardonnay, merlot, sparkling wine, and others,
    made by Sutter Home Fre

Alcohol-free Sparkling Ciders
Martinelli's sparkling cider (apple, apple-cranberry, apple-grape)
Welch's sparkling juices (white grape, red grape, cranberry)
Others (Lucky Leaf Sparkling Cider, Musselman's Sparkling Cider; certain store brands are
    available, too)

One patient, a wine broker, asked how she could possibly avoid alcohol when tasting wine was integral to her job. We suggested she opt for swishing it around in her mouth and then spitting it out, as many wine connoisseurs do, rather than taking an actual sip. And if you find yourself resenting having to give up your favorite glass or two of wine at night, or drinks at a social gathering, don't feel guilty. It's not always easy to give up something that you enjoy even though you know it's the best thing to do. You might try not drinking for a month. If you have trouble and just *can't* do it or find yourself constantly rationalizing a drink or two, consider delaying conception while you enlist additional support from family and friends, and seek counseling or help from a program such as Alcoholics Anonymous. Obviously, we are distinguishing between a natural wish that you could drink versus not being able to stop drinking.

PAINKILLERS AND RECREATIONAL DRUGS

Experimenting with or using prescribed drugs such as painkillers and illicit drugs such as marijuana, cocaine, amphetamines, and heroin peaks between the ages of twenty-four and forty-nine, right when we are at our most reproductive. Whether you use recreational drugs rarely or regularly, they can have a negative impact on your ability to conceive and on fetal development. Twenty-six percent of women surveyed who had used drugs before continued to use these potentially dangerous substances while pregnant, often because they didn't realize they had conceived. In those first few weeks after conception, your baby's genes and cells are being organized. Can you imagine how difficult it is for those building blocks to be put in order if you are stoned? We strongly recommend stopping all drug use at least three months prior to conception for women and three to six months for men. If you can quit using drugs before you conceive, often the risks to the fetus are completely eliminated. Think of your baby's health and his or her future the next time you feel the need to partake.

Marijuana

Marijuana, the most common of the illicit drugs used today, is an extract from the cannabis plant that acts as a stimulant to your brain. Marijuana today is five times stronger than what was available in the 1960s and 1970s. The main active ingredient in marijuana is tetrahydrocannabinol (THC), which is responsible for the accelerated heart rate, reddened eyes, and general euphoria noted by most people who smoke it. It can take days or even a month to clear THC from your system, which means there can be an effect on your sperm or egg one month after you last had a toke.

Not surprisingly, people who smoke dope are also more likely to smoke cigarettes and drink alcohol. This makes it harder to distinguish the effects of marijuana alone on a couple's ability to conceive. However, similar to tobacco use, the more you smoke marijuana, the greater the effect. Also, the secondhand smoke from marijuana may expose your nonsmoking spouse to its negative effects, and vice versa if your partner is the smoker. With only one exception in the literature, research has found that the chemical changes due to smoking marijuana in women reduce ovulation, which in turn makes it harder to conceive. When men smoke, less testosterone circulates in their body. This makes men less interested in sex and also reduces the quality of their sperm. So, even if they are able to conceive, it may be with damaged sperm, which significantly increases the chance of a miscarriage.

FOR FUTURE REFERENCE: During Pregnancy

If You Are Planning to Use Marijuana in Pregnancy
We don't know yet how much marijuana is too much or too little to affect your fetus, so smoking even a couple of joints while trying to conceive may have a significant impact on the health of your future baby. Babies born to women who smoke marijuana weigh ½ to 1 pound less on average than those born to women who don't. It also appears that the more marijuana you smoke, the greater the effect on your baby's growth. Children of marijuana smokers have been noted to have more frequent respiratory infections and failure to thrive or grow over time.

Amphetamines

Amphetamines, also known as speed, uppers, or weight-loss pills, act as a stimulant, making the user more alert or awake and causing the release of adrenaline. Amphetamine abuse commonly starts in high school, college, or graduate school, when body image problems peak and when studying for exams and writing papers late into the night is the norm. Amphetamines rev your internal engine, increasing your blood pressure, heart rate, and breathing rate. This puts great strain on your blood vessels, which consequently are unable to let blood flow normally to vital organs, such as the brain, ovaries, and testicles. Reproduction becomes more difficult if the egg and sperm are not being released properly because less blood flow is getting to these organs.

Amphetamines can also reduce your appetite and speed up your metabolism. This may sound appealing if you are trying to lose weight, but it is highly risky, especially when you are trying to conceive and require important nutrients to prevent birth defects and provide a nurturing environment for your future fetus.

Cocaine

Cocaine is derived from the leaves of the coca plant and, like amphetamines, acts as a stimulant. Cocaine narrows your blood vessels, raising your blood pressure and straining your heart. It also reduces the oxygen that is carried to all the parts of your body, including your ovaries and uterus, making it harder to conceive and easier to miscarry. Because blood vessels take time to heal, and because the altered consciousness of drug use means you may not even realize you're pregnant, stopping cocaine use at least three months before you conceive is hugely important for the health of your baby.

 FOR FUTURE REFERENCE: During Pregnancy

Cocaine's Toxic Effects During Pregnancy

Cocaine can cause a number of birth defects and pregnancy complications. The use of cocaine can affect the blood vessels supplying the placenta, which can cause fetal growth restriction, and placental separation or abruption, which requires immediate delivery, often preterm. Pregnant mothers who use cocaine also have a much greater risk of high blood pressure, known as preeclampsia, which can affect the maternal liver, kidneys, and blood-clotting system. In addition, the effects of cocaine on the development of fetal cardiac, gastrointestinal, and kidney systems are extremely toxic. Infants born to mothers who were cocaine users are more likely to be premature, have lower birth weights, and suffer more neonatal seizures and bleeding in the brain than babies born to non-drug-users. They also have a higher risk of dying from SIDS.

Cocaine can lead to a greater number of strokes and heart attacks in otherwise healthy men. Men who use cocaine are also more likely to smoke cigarettes or marijuana or drink alcohol. These can all affect a man's ability to have an erection and ejaculate and may reduce his libido, which obviously makes it difficult to conceive. Further, an association between poorer nutritional intake has been noted in both sexes using cocaine, which can in turn increase the risk for certain birth defects in their offspring. We recommend that men stop cocaine use three to six months prior to conception.

The Opioids

Opioids are a large group of chemical substances derived from the sap of the *Papaver somniferum* poppy or chemically synthesized. They are in the prescription painkillers (or narcotics)

Practical Application

List the medications you have taken for pain in the past week:

_____

_____

_____

In the past month:

_____

_____

_____

If you take prescription painkillers and are a "clock watcher" (you watch the clock to see how soon you can take your next dose), this is a warning sign that you could be more vulnerable to addiction. Under a doctor's supervision, make sure you're taking the lowest possible dosage and wean yourself as soon as medically responsible.

morphine, codeine, and hydrocodone, and in nonprescription narcotics (street drugs) such as heroin. Methadone is a prescription drug that is often used to help eliminate heroin addiction. Both heroin and methadone are highly addictive both psychologically and physically. This isn't to say you should avoid all pain medication when it is needed. Short courses of low-dose painkillers, used after surgery or delivery, are usually fairly safe. People who suffer from chronic pain such as arthritis, recurrent migraines, or back pain, however, may use more narcotics more often and have to be careful not to get hooked. Review your medications with your physician if you are planning to conceive.

The nonprescription opioids can reduce your appetite and deplete your nutritional stores, reducing your ability to ovulate. Women who use these drugs often have a higher number of pelvic infections, which can make it more difficult to conceive. Women who abuse narcotics during pregnancy have an increased risk of first-trimester miscarriage, preterm labor, placental abnormalities, fetal growth retardation, and fetal withdrawal syndromes.

Limited data are available about the impact of opioids on the fertility of men. It appears that men who use heroin or morphine suffer no reduction in fertility or increase in children with birth defects. However, some studies suggest that there may be an increased risk of miscarriage due to damaged sperm DNA. Other studies have tried to link paternal drug use with children's future behavioral problems, although the facts available are limited. Still, the paternal effects of drug use raise enough significant questions to encourage the cessation of drug use before you conceive.

Both male and female intravenous drug users have an increased incidence of contracting hepatitis and HIV, potentially lethal diseases that can then be transmitted to the unborn baby. If you are shooting opioids or have done so in the past, it is essential that you get an HIV test before you try to conceive.

FOR FUTURE REFERENCE: After Delivery

Opioid Use in Pregnancy
Pain medications such as codeine, hydrocodone, Demerol, and Dilaudid are often recommended after delivery. These, as well as methadone, are considered safe to use while breastfeeding if taken in doses of less than 20 mg per day. The American Academy of Pediatrics recommends that heroin users be discouraged from breastfeeding. Newborns can be exposed through the breastmilk to the same environment they encountered in utero, which can affect their growth and development. Unfortunately, HIV infection can also be passed through breastmilk.

Stopping a drug habit is most successful when done in a supportive environment. Substance abuse support groups can be contacted through your personal physician, your local hospital, or Narcotics Anonymous.

CAFFEINE
Women and Caffeine

In the early days of research on the effects of caffeine on female reproductive function, many studies neglected to separate the effects of caffeine from those of smoking and alcohol—two things known to have a negative impact on fertility and fetal health. As a result of being lumped together with smoking and alcohol, caffeine's rap may be worse than it deserves. Recent research indicates that although it is prudent for women to keep caffeine intake low before and during pregnancy, it need not be eliminated from your diet altogether.

Exactly how low you need to keep your caffeine intake remains controversial, and there is even evidence to suggest that women may vary in the way caffeine affects them. Most studies show a safety threshold of 200 to 300 mg of caffeine per day in women with no known fertility problems, so if you are new to thinking about TTC (trying to conceive), keep your caffeine intake below 200 mg per day one month prior to and all during pregnancy. But if you have any health risks such as tubal (fallopian) disease or endometriosis, further limit intake to below 100 mg of caffeine per day. And despite scant data to support benefit, if you are having difficulty conceiving, you may wish to follow the 100 mg cap on caffeine intake too. That level is so low that even if you had any increased susceptibility to caffeine's effects while you pursue pregnancy, a cup or two of soothing black or green tea could be enjoyed if desired. (See Table 2-3 to find out how much caffeine is in your favorite beverages.) This very conservative guideline leaves an ample cushion for the variations in caffeine content that inevitably occur when serving size and preparation method differ from café to café and kitchen to kitchen. Such a low intake will also not dehydrate you at a time when good hydration is very important and will have no impact on your miscarriage risk or fetal development. Finally, cutting down on caffeine may decrease the breast tenderness many women experience premenstrually and in early pregnancy.

FOR FUTURE REFERENCE: During Pregnancy

How Does Caffeine Affect the Mother and Her Fetus?

Caffeine is a stimulant and constricts blood vessels. If you consume too much, or don't clear it (metabolize it) from your system before the next dose comes along, it's a concern for you and your baby. If your blood vessels are chronically tensed up, it's a strain on your heart. Furthermore, when caffeine and its metabolites are circulating in your system, they can pass through the placenta, which can affect blood flow to the developing fetus and restrict growth. Really dilute levels of caffeine in the mother's circulation don't carry the same punch. Even if you clear caffeine more slowly than most people, 100 to 200 mg of caffeine or less per day is low enough to keep you in the safe zone. Oxygen and nutrient delivery to the baby continues unimpeded.

If you currently consume more than 100 to 200 mg of caffeine per day from beverages, reduce your intake gradually to avoid the unpleasant headache or flulike symptoms of caffeine withdrawal. We also advise preferential substitution of beverages such as water, milk, and 100 percent fruit juice according to the recommendations in later nutrition chapters. Of course, decaffeinated black and green teas, herbal teas approved in Chapter 8, and decaffeinated coffee can fill in the few remaining gaps. Just be aware that other components of teas and coffees partially bind important minerals (iron and calcium) if consumed with meals in high quantities; for people who overaccumulate iron, this can be used to their advantage. Soft drinks have a similar effect on select nutrients.

Here's something else to ponder about soft drinks. A recently published study by Harvard researchers using data from the large-scale Nurse's Health Study II showed that a diet pattern including more than two soft drinks per day was associated with reduced fertility from impaired ovulation. The findings remained the same regardless of whether the soft drinks were caffeinated, decaf, regular, or sugar-free. This finding needs to be more rigorously studied to prove or disprove, and either way, there's no research to suggest complete avoidance of soft drinks. There are, however, other reasons to reserve soft drinks for occasional use. For one, soft drink consumers tend to consume more calories and drink less milk. They may also increase the risk of type 2 diabetes among people who consume more than two soft drinks per day.

Sarah recognized that she needed to cut back on her soft drink and coffee intake, but really resisted finding an alternative. However, when a friend gave her some jasmine tea as a gift, they tried it out together. Otherwise, Sarah would have never opened the box! She wouldn't have known to be careful to get the best flavor by using water that hadn't quite come to a boil and letting it steep no longer than a minute or two. Much to Sarah's surprise, she liked both the taste and the soothing aroma. Over a short period of time, she realized that she preferred the ritual of tea drinking to that of the other two. She later regarded the occasional coffee or soft drink as a nice change of pace, but was content to mainly stick with her lower caffeine intake as a tea drinker.

After trying to cut back on caffeine before her first pregnancy, Megan came up with a solution. "Cutting back on caffeine is easier than I thought," she said. "I made my own half-caff mix and stored it in an airtight canister. I measured out an appropriate serving size and kept that spoon in the container to use. The smell and feel of drinking a hot cup of coffee cued my senses without the jitteriness I used to feel with a full-strength dose of caffeine. Now this is what I drink once or twice a day. I prefer the less-edgy me who doesn't fumble around in a mad dash, running into things on the way out to the car!"

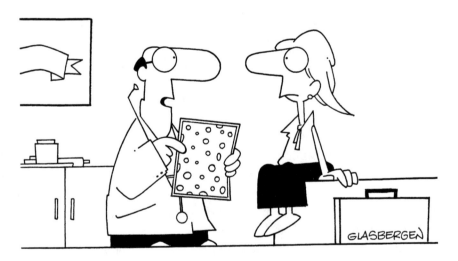

"The red blobs are your red blood cells. The white blobs are your white blood cells. The brown blobs are coffee. We need to talk."

Copyright © 1996 by Randy Glasbergen. www. glasbergen.com

TABLE 2-3

CAFFEINE CONTENT OF BEVERAGES, FOODS, AND NONPRESCRIPTION DRUGS

Beverages/Foods	*Caffeine (mg)*
Coffee, brewed, 8 fl oz	130 (up to 200)
Coffee, instant, from 1 rounded tsp	~57
Starbucks frappuccino blended coffee, avg. 9.5 fl oz	115
Espresso coffee (single shot, 1 fl oz)	40–90
Decaf coffee, 8 fl oz	3–6
Tea, 6 fl oz, green or black, brewed 3 min.	20–36
Tea, instant powder, 1 tsp	31
Tea, maté, 6 fl oz	34
Soft drinks, diet and regular, 12 fl oz[a]	35–50
Caffeine-free soft drinks, 12 fl oz	0
Energy drinks, 1 container[a]	80–295
Hot cocoa mix, 1 oz pkt.	3–8
Energy gum, mints, candies, per piece[a]	~10–150
Häagen-Dazs coffee ice cream, 8 oz	58
Milk chocolate, 1 oz	6–15
Dark, sweet chocolate, 1 oz	20
Over-the-Counter Drugs	
Midol Menstrual Complete, 2 pills[b]	120
Anacin Regular Strength, 2 pills[b]	64
Excedrin Extra Strength, 2 pills[b]	130
NoDoz Maximum Strength, Vivarin, 1 pill[b]	200

a. Watch the serving sizes and multiply the caffeine milligrams accordingly, if you're going to drink or eat the whole thing. Watch for additional herbal sources of caffeine and other stimulants as well.

b. Do not take any prescription or nonprescription drugs while you are trying to conceive unless approved by your physician.

Sources: Industry data; Agriculture Handbook No. 8 series; Starbucks Customer Relations Dept; www.energy fiend.com; Santos, I. S., A. Matijasevich, and N. C. J. Valle. "Maté Drinking During Pregnancy and Risk of Preterm and Small for Gestational Age Birth." *Journal of Nutrition* 135 (2005): 1120–23.

HERBAL SOURCES OF CAFFEINE

As long as you stay near the daily limit of 100 to 200 mg of caffeine per day, feel free to mix and match a variety of caffeine sources, or be a tea purist. The choice is up to you!

- **Tea (green, black, white, oolong).** Can be enjoyed during preconception and pregnancy up to 100 to 200 mg of caffeine per day. The upper limit for caffeine may have more of a cushion if it comes from tea than from coffee; keep in mind that tea—green more so than black—contains compounds that act as antioxidants and potentially reduce inflammation and discourage bacterial and viral infection, though more research is needed. Decaffeinated green and black teas are viable alternatives to the caffeinated versions, in relatively moderate amounts, and to our knowledge, the decaffeination process doesn't reduce the healthful polyphenolic compounds. See separate listings for naturally decaffeinated herbal teas in Chapter 8 that may be consumed in addition to their caffeinated relatives.

- **Coffee.** Can be enjoyed during preconception and pregnancy up to 100 to 200 mg of caffeine per day. Decaffeinated coffee is a viable alternative but only in modest amounts, because caffeine may not be the only compound to warrant caution. It's impossible to completely tease out the effects of the greater tendency toward smoking and less healthy lifestyles among coffee drinkers than tea drinkers, so if those habits describe you, this may be the time to clean house. There are no official preconception/pregnancy recommendations for restricting decaf coffee, but in our opinion, decaf coffee could be limited to a couple of servings per day until as much is known about it as its fully caffeinated version. Beyond that, switch to tea as the closest alternative.

- **Maté.** Very popular Latin-American caffeinated beverage that, in the few studies available, has been shown safe during pregnancy in moderate amounts; stick to the overall 100 to 200 mg of caffeine per day limit. In South American countries, maté is customarily sipped through a shared straw, a practice discouraged during preconception and pregnancy due to the threat of sharing periodontal and other infections. Maté is now commonly available in tea shops in the United States and Europe.

- **Guarana.** Strictly limit or avoid. This is a concentrated form of caffeine found in many designer drinks, weight-loss supplements, and herbal energy boosters. An 800 mg tablet of guarana contains 30 mg of caffeine (roughly equal to the amount found in a cup of tea). Guarana is frequently found in weight-loss supplements in combination with substances that should be completely avoided during preconception and pregnancy. Fans of energy drinks should be very careful to look at how many servings a container of their favorite energy drink holds.

- **Cola Nut (kola nut).** Generally recognized as safe (GRAS) when used as a flavoring ingredient and okay in small amounts. However, keep in mind that cola nut is a source of caffeine and is often found in products that contain other caffeine-containing ingredients such as guarana and herbs for weight-loss or sports performance (dietary supplements that may be unsafe altogether).

> • **Cocoa (theobromine).** Fairly negligible in terms of caffeine content, as seen in Table 2-3. See Chapter 8 for more detail.

Men and Caffeine

There is a paucity of research on the impact of caffeine intake on male fertility and the health of future offspring. Therefore, no standard recommendations exist. From the limited research that exists, it appears that prospective dads can consume caffeine in moderate doses—defined as below 300 mg per day—without fear of conception consequences. (See Table 2-3 to see how many milligrams of caffeine are in your favorite beverages.) Although some studies have shown a higher intake to be inconsequential, it is best to be prudent until more is known. Herbal or decaffeinated coffee, tea, or the occasional soft drink can always be substituted for their caffeinated counterparts, but quench most of your thirst with water.

As with most things, the larger the dosage, the more detrimental caffeine can become. The time it takes to successfully conceive may increase with paternal caffeine intake above 700 mg per day. (That's about five 8 fl oz cups of brewed coffee.) More serious problems have been observed in animal studies at the human equivalent of ten to twelve cups of brewed coffee per day: that is, a very definite negative impact on the health and survival rate of offspring was seen. However, the rates of actual conception were *not* lowered. Amazingly, these effects were perpetuated into the second generation as well. Even though these studies were done with animals, it's best to err on the side of caution and not consume inordinately large amounts of coffee, cola, and other forms of caffeine.

Practical Application

Refer to Table 2-3 and figure out your daily consumption of caffeine from beverages, foods, and medications. Make sure to compare your portion sizes to those on the chart. For example, a Starbucks single-shot espresso beverage contains 95 mg of caffeine. (Obviously, double-shot drinks have double that amount.) Their smallest serving, "short," of brewed coffee is 8 fl oz and contains 180 mg of caffeine. (Starbucks caffeine values for brewed coffee are higher than those of most brands. Be aware of how brands differ.) If either of you consistently exceeds your daily upper limit (100 to 200 mg of caffeine per day for women; 300 mg for men), slowly taper your intake by substituting alternative beverages and good old-fashioned water. Remember that at most cafés you can order "half-caff" to reduce the caffeine content but continue to drink your favorite beverage. (In Seattle, be hip and order a "split shot"!)

CHAPTER 3

Your Environment at Home and at Work

*N*ow that you understand how important it is to keep your internal environment free of such toxins as tobacco, alcohol, and recreational drugs, let's discuss how both you and your spouse can help keep your external environment, your workplace and home, free of toxins that can be damaging to your ability to conceive or your future pregnancy.

Today, men and women share many of the same hobbies and professions, so they're exposed to similar environmental risks, both at home and on the job. Exposure to potential reproductive hazards affects each gender differently, however. Because women are born with all the eggs that they will ever release, if they are overexposed to a toxin or to radiation, the genetically altered eggs may not be viable. If fertilization is able to occur, a higher risk of miscarriage and birth defects exists.

Men, by contrast, manufacture new sperm twenty-four hours a day, seven days a week. This gives sperm a chance to be rejuvenated within three to six months if exposed to a toxin in their environment. (Replacing a batch of sperm will often take at least ninety days, as this is the length of time it takes to develop one fully functioning, mature sperm. More about this in Chapter 9.) Reproductive hazards affect male fertility by reducing overall sperm numbers, changing the way the sperm move, or damaging the DNA (the genetic material) carried in the sperm. Genetic mutations can lead to male infertility as well as an increased risk of early pregnancy loss.

From experience with our patients, we know that in all likelihood your environment is quite safe. It is *very rare* to be exposed to the high levels of radiation, lead and other heavy metals, biological agents, and chemical solvents that can potentially have a toxic effect on your future fertility and offspring. Most overexposures occur through carelessness, negligence, improper handling, and accidental spills. Adequate protection at home and at work, which we will review in detail throughout this chapter, can protect you against overexposure from most chemicals.

THE SAFETY OF YOUR HOME

Maureen has gorgeous highlighted hair and enjoys the monthly "upkeep" because it forces her to take a few minutes for herself to just sit and relax. But her friends have asked, "Now that you're trying to conceive, can you continue your salon visits or should you start growing out your highlights?" She'd like to have an informed response ready the next time.

Newlyweds and pet lovers, Deanna and Jason have two cute dogs and three fat cats. Deanna recently inquired of her obstetrician whether she could contract a serious illness from caring for her cat and wondered about the routine flea and tick treatments she is giving her dogs.

With the media coverage of BPA in plastics, it's hard not to wonder whether it's safe to microwave the organic, whole-grain frozen dinner you just switched to for hurried nights. What plastics are of concern? What about sports bottles? Baby bottles? The lining of tin cans? A few simple guidelines would be helpful.

Americans on average spend 66 percent of their lifetimes in the home. Our homes are not just places where we sleep, eat, and relax. We may also engage in a number of home crafts or hobbies that involve chemicals, machinery, or metals that can have a negative impact on fertility. Even everyday household products contain toxic chemicals. Sometimes prospective parents want to enlarge or redecorate their "nest," which can involve painting, wallpapering, carpentry, and construction that may expose a soon-to-be-expectant mother or father to a variety of chemicals and toxins. Others work from home in farming or in arts or crafts and have to police themselves regarding safe disposal of chemicals, good hand-washing techniques, and laundering potentially contaminated clothing separately from other garments.

The amount of the household substance in question must be very large to qualify as an overexposure that can possibly have an impact on your fertility. Common sense is usually the key to safe use. If a substance causes you to have a headache, nausea, skin rash, or dizziness, then either avoid it or use protective devices such as masks or gloves. Make sure the area you are working in is well ventilated. Careful disposal of the waste involved will automatically increase the safe use of these substances. But try to relax and remember that even if a household chemical gives you a headache, it is unlikely that it will harm your ability to conceive or your future baby's health.

Pesticides in the Home

Whether you live in a house or an apartment, you may occasionally find yourself dealing with ants, roaches, rodent infestations, or other vermin. While trying to conceive, or if you are already pregnant, there are ways to safely use insecticides. There are also nonchemical tactics to make your home less inviting to pests. If you need professional extermination, consult with a reputable pest-control expert and ask about the least invasive treatment for your problem. If you have an indoor treatment, remain outside of the treated area for the recommended time (usually at least four hours). If your kitchen or dining room is part of the pest control zone, make sure you wash the countertops before preparing any food. Also, ventilate the living area with open windows and fans. If you prefer to do your own pest elimination, consult your physician first and, of course, follow label instructions.

The pesticides of greater concern are those sprayed on produce in an agricultural setting. Minimize exposure by using good food handling and washing techniques (see pages 413–414 for details).

Many prospective mothers ask about the safety of household products such as bleach and detergents. They feel that if it can cause their eyes to tear, it must affect their reproductive organs or potentially their early pregnancy. Indeed, the Illinois Teratogen Service receives more than two hundred calls per month about the potential reproductive hazard of household products people encounter daily in their home. As much as we would love to give women an excuse to do fewer of the household chores, most household chemicals are perfectly safe during preconception and in early pregnancy (as long as you are not drinking them).

PLASTICS IN EVERYDAY LIFE

Food and drink packaging, as well as the containers used in transport to keep food fresh, have evolved over the last decade to improve their safe use for consumers. Plastics that travel with food and beverages from refrigerator to oven to table to dishwasher are very commonly used in the home and the workplace. Though plastic containers are convenient, questions have been raised about whether certain types of plastic in these containers can be damaging to people before, during, and after conception. Here are some helpful facts:

- The majority of disposable plastic beverage containers are for single usage and contain polyethylene terephthalate (PET), which is lightweight, shatterproof, and considered safe.
- If you reuse these plastic bottles for beverages, there is an increased risk of bacterial infections unless the bottles are conscientiously cleaned. Most experts discourage reuse for this reason.

- The United States Environmental Protection Agency (EPA) states that beverage containers with PET are safe (for their intended uses) before, during, and after pregnancy.
- Freezing liquids in a PET bottle doesn't increase the risk of exposure to dioxins and other chemicals for the drinker.

Household and Personal Care

Almost half of all hand soaps and body washes (as well as a growing number of household products) purchased today include an antibacterial active ingredient such as triclosan or triclocarban. These soaps are used in hospitals to prevent infection among vulnerable patients, but their daily use in the household warrants some caution on at least two counts:

1. **Drug resistance.** Using antibacterial soap kills the weakest bugs, leaving the strongest around to reproduce. The average person's too-quick hand washing doesn't kill these hardy guys.
2. **Possible effects on the endocrine system.** Early research shows antibacterial ingredients are absorbed systemically and, in animal studies, can affect reproductive tissues.

Bottom line: whether you use these antibacterial products on your hands only or do a full-body lather in the shower, the multiple daily exposures don't offer any advantage. Regular soap contains surfactants that remove germs just fine if you lather for twenty seconds. The next best thing to ordinary soap and warm water is an alcohol-based gel—a fine substitute if soap or clean water is not available.

Another chemical in plastic food and beverage containers that has been in the news is bisphenol A, or BPA. This common component in plastic containers and resin linings in cans has raised concerns about safety for infants exposed to liquids in BPA-laden bottles. In animal studies, when BPA-laden containers were used, there were changes in uterine structure and reductions in available reproductive hormones, resulting in fewer fertile cycles, so this raises concerns about BPA's effect on human fertility and fetal development. Women with a higher concentration of BPA in the bloodstream may have a higher risk of polycystic ovary syndrome (PCOS), endometrial hyperplasia (thickening that can lead to uterine cancer), and recurrent miscarriages (discussed in Chapter 5), but more conclusive research is needed.

The Food and Drug Administration (FDA) is reviewing research conducted by the National Toxicology Program (NTP, part of the National Institutes of Health) as well as data from other countries regarding the safety of plastic products containing this chemical. The FDA concluded that it has "some" concern about the potential effect of BPA on the brain, behavior, and prostate gland in fetuses, infants, and young children.[1] Until there is a clear consensus, the NTP recommends making a few simple changes in the products we use for food and beverage storage to minimize the risk of BPA exposure among women before and during pregnancy and among infants and children:

- Use glass, stainless steel, porcelain, or ceramic containers for hot foods.
- Reduce the use of canned foods. Use fresh foods preferentially.
- Microwave in nonplastic containers such as glass or porcelain designated for microwave usage.
- Choose glass or BPA-free baby bottles.

Now for the trickier tips . . . discerning which plastic containers are BPA-free:[2]

- Try to avoid using plastics with the numbers 3, 6, and 7 in the recycling symbol (triangle) at the bottom of the container or bottle because these may contain BPA. (The number 7 symbol is a catch-all for newer plastics that don't fit into the other categories, so some may be safe. To identify the safe number 7 containers, look for "BPA-free" or the symbol "PP" for polypropylene at the bottom.)
- If you are unsure if the plastic has BPA, then avoid heating foods or beverages in it and toss it when you are through. Avoid using or reusing containers because this increases the likelihood of a small amount of the chemical leaching into your food or beverage.

A LEVELHEADED APPROACH TO WATER AND FOOD SAFETY

The human body has developed many strategies to combat environmental contaminants, and your healthy food and beverage choices can aid these natural defenses. In the latter half of the book we discuss these topics more thoroughly in the context of your best preconception nutrition. For instance, Chapter 10 covers water and Chapter 13 addresses food safety concerns. Before we move on, though, we'll specifically address one environmental contaminant that has, most notably, found its way into the water supply—perchlorates.

The industrial chemical perchlorate is a topic of growing interest because it affects the thyroid gland and blocks iodine uptake (in fact, years ago it was used as a medication to treat an overactive thyroid). Small amounts of perchlorate are found naturally, but most enters the environment from rocket fuel, batteries, chlorine-based cleaners, and drying agents, to name

1. www.fda.gov/NewsEvents/publichealthfocus/ucm064437.htm, accessed January 15, 2010.
2. http://www.hhs.gov/safety/bpa, accessed April 2, 2010. A good fact sheet on plastic safety is available from the Institute for Agriculture and Trade Policy's consumer news website (http://www.healthobservatory.org/library.cfm?refid=102202).

only a few. A CDC study found perchlorate in every person tested, indicating that the general public experiences widespread exposure to low levels of perchlorates (i.e., <35 mg/day) from some sources of drinking water and foods. Humans can safely tolerate this low level of perchlorate exposure, and it is passed through the body quickly. The biggest concern is for people with low dietary iodine *or* prolonged exposure to higher perchlorate levels, and in particular pre-pregnant and pregnant women (especially those with hypothyroidism), infants, and children.

Eating a balanced diet to meet the recommended iodine intake (see pages 348–349) is your best defense against perchlorate known to date. Do take a look at the *Annual Drinking Water Quality Report* for your local tap water supplier, especially if your water is sourced from well water or near rocket testing sites; investigate further if perchlorate made it to the list entitled "Detected Contaminants."[3] You may need to invest in a water treatment system certified for perchlorate removal (NSF International has good recommendations). Most bottled waters contain no detectable perchlorates, and if there's any question, check with the manufacturer.

WHAT'S LEAD GOT TO DO WITH IT?

Lead does not have any redeeming qualities when it comes to the human body. It not only contributes to miscarriages, stillbirths, and infertility but also causes high blood pressure, kidney dysfunction, and brain damage. Infants and children are most vulnerable to lead's often irreversible toxic effects because they are smaller and still developing. Since size matters with this issue, it's easy to see that the fetus in your womb may be even more seriously affected if you have too much lead in your system prior to or after conception. Lead can interfere with proper early development of the fetus's central nervous system, including brain function. So, for couples of childbearing age and their offspring, it is simple wisdom to minimize exposure to lead.

Overexposure to lead is relatively uncommon today unless you work in pottery making, battery manufacturing, shipbuilding, printing, or settings that expose you to a large amount of exhaust fumes (such as a garage or toll booth). Clearly, if you think you encounter lead in your workplace with regularity, you should discuss it with your employer and work out a job location change or have your blood lead level tested to determine your previous exposure. Exposure to lead in the home is more common and therefore of greater concern before and during pregnancy. Table 3-1 will help you identify potential household sources of lead, and explain how to problem-solve if you are concerned about personal exposure.

---

3. While researching this topic, we most often found perchlorates listed in a section entitled "Non-Detectable Contaminants," available only online in a link titled "Additional Tables." Current water collection data from the EPA indicates that this good news applies to most public water systems.

TABLE 3-1
SOURCES OF LEAD

Lead Source	Ways to Minimize Exposure
Exposed Soils. Primarily in cities near high-traffic areas, soils may be contaminated with lead from leaded gasoline emissions (and paint particles from older buildings to a much smaller degree). Although lead is no longer in gasoline, it remains in soil and dust.	• Cover soil with foliage or grass • Cover with a wooden deck • Professionally clear topsoil and replace with uncontaminated soil • Keep soil moist during gardening • Wear gloves and wash hands well after working with soil
Paint. In dwellings painted before 1978, but particularly those from the 1950s and earlier, there may be paint flakes or dust particles. Remodeling, demolition, scraping, or sanding of painted surfaces can increase paint flakes in your home. Also, look out for painted areas that are peeling or where there is friction or an impact surface (for example, opening and closing windows). Old peeling playground equipment, refinishing of old painted furniture, and burning of lead-based painted wood can release lead into the environment.	• Put wallpaper over paint • If paint is not flaking, consider painting over[a] • Have paint chips tested for lead content • Have professional paint stripping • Use respirators, vacuums, and masks with high-efficiency particulate air (HEPA) filters when working with paint on walls or furniture • Carefully clean off counters where food preparation will occur
Drinking water. Your water may contain lead if you have lead pipes or if lead solder was used in the water pipes. Lead content is greatest if water is obtained from the hot tap or if it has been sitting in the pipes for longer than six hours (e.g., overnight or after a workday).	• Drink from cold tap only • Run tap for at least two minutes when water has not been run in more than six hours
Imported canned goods. Some cans packaged overseas have seams that are soldered with lead.	• Don't purchase these products
Lead-glazed ceramics. Lead may occur in the glazes of some ceramics, especially those imported from or bought in foreign countries, that are used in your home for cooking and serving foods.	• Minimize cooking and serving hot foods in these containers; avoid buying food sold in these containers, such as tamarind candy
Leaded glass or *leaded crystal.* It is most problematic if these containers hold acidic beverages or alcohol or are used for storage.	• Use decoratively, not for storage • Avoid repetitive beverage use in these containers

Lead Source	Ways to Minimize Exposure
Imported home remedies. Some imported over-the-counter or home remedies may contain lead, such as azarcon and greta (e.g., Hispanic remedies for indigestion) or pay-loo-ah (an Asian remedy for rash).	• Don't purchase these products
Imported cosmetics. Kohl, a dark eyeliner, may contain traces of lead if it is imported from the Middle East. The "kohl" eyeliner you buy at drugstores or cosmetic counters in the United States does not contain lead, however.	• Use alternative cosmetics
Older venetian blinds or miniblinds. Blinds manufactured prior to the 1970s may contain lead.	• Replace older blinds with newer versions or check the date of original purchase
Shooting, fishing. Poorly ventilated indoor shooting ranges, retrieved cartridge cases and/or nonjacketed lead bullets, or home-cast lead bullets and fishing sinkers.	• Take target practice in well-ventilated facilities, and wash hands after handling retrieved cases or bullets • Use proper safety precautions with hobbies requiring casting of your own lead (bullets, fishing sinkers, etc.) or buy premade items
Domestic and imported natural/herbal remedies that may contain heavy-metal contaminants. Herbal remedies are not required to undergo FDA safety testing before being sold to the public.	• See Chapter 8's "Herbs" section.

a. Professional lead removal from your home surfaces can be very costly. Painting over nonflaking surfaces may be very cost-effective and safe.

If you suspect you have any of the aforementioned sources of lead present in your environment, there are tests to verify or disprove your suspicions. If you want to test for lead on the surface of an imported ceramic cooking dish or on a miniblind, you can purchase an inexpensive lead test kit at a local hardware or paint store. These test swabs are going to tell you only if lead is present on the surface, but give you no indication of what is underneath (as would be necessary on a painted surface that was going to be renovated). For testing paint chips, dirt, water, or imported edible goods, a laboratory analysis is recommended. For large jobs such as home remodeling lead assessments, you can have a certified professional come out to your home, collect samples, and do a full risk assessment. However, you can save money by collecting samples yourself and taking them to a qualified lab for analysis, and from there you can decide whether further action is necessary. If you choose to renovate lead-based painted walls while preparing to conceive (as well as after conception), it may be best to stay away from the work site until it is cleaned by professionals. Also, always keep your floor and counter surfaces clean, especially those counters where food is being prepared.

Dietary Defense Against Lead

You and your partner can take simple steps to protect yourselves from lead. Both iron and calcium protect the body from lead's toxic effects by partially blocking lead absorption and minimizing retention of whatever does get absorbed. Zinc may also confer a protective role. Those people who are deficient in either iron or calcium, and possibly zinc, will benefit from improving their dietary intake of these minerals, or using supplementation to fill in for dietary shortcomings, to reduce the likelihood of retaining lead in the body. Avoidance of prolonged fasting also helps because fasting prompts your bones to release nutrients such as calcium to fill the nutrient void, causing lead to leach as well.

Actual lead poisoning is much more prevalent in children, so testing is fairly common for kids, but routine lead screening in adults is seldom done, and typically is not warranted unless you live or work in a high-risk environment. Talk to your physician if you have concerns after reading this section.

HOBBIES AT HOME

Are you one of those people who like to work with their hands after a long day in the office or watching the kids? Many hobbies, such as furniture restoration, carpentry, pottery making, and auto mechanics, involve chemicals that can affect your fertility and the health of a future pregnancy if proper precautions are not taken. Arts and crafts performed in the home may involve solvents, photo-developing chemicals, and paints. Unlike the workplace, the privacy of your own home is not regulated by government safeguards for the use of chemicals, so it's essential that you take responsibility for yourself. Overexposure to the chemicals you may use in the home is rare, but with the following precautions you can safely enjoy your hobbies.

When You Need to Warm Up Your Bed

Speculation has been rampant on the safety of electric blankets prior to conception and during pregnancy. No definitive information is available, but limited studies do illustrate a link between prolonged electric blanket use and spontaneous miscarriage, as well as childhood brain cancers. An electric blanket rests directly on your body, bringing the electromagnetic waves very close to your reproductive organs. Fortunately, electric blankets produce only 15 volts/meter, whereas significant exposures are usually in the 50–100 volts/meter range. Most household electric blankets have careful temperature controls that prevent overexposure to the magnetic or electrical effects. Although a damaging effect on your fertility or pregnancy is unlikely, if you want to be on the safe side, use another source of warmth for your bed, such as a down comforter or a spouse.

General precautions that can help limit overexposure to chemicals used during recreational pursuits include:

- Storing chemicals in leakproof containers away from heat.
- Wearing protective gear, which can include filter masks, goggles, and gloves.
- Carefully disposing of chemicals after you are done using them.
- Working in well-ventilated areas to avoid inhalation.
- Avoiding direct skin contact with chemicals. If skin contact occurs, wash the area thoroughly.

Remember, most chemicals you use for home projects can be very safely handled before and after conception to ensure your reproductive health and the health of the future fetus.

Painting

Whether you paint on canvas or on walls, the paints you use contain chemicals and metals that can have an effect on your reproductive health. If you are an artist and like to mix your own paints, you can decrease your reproductive risks by using natural, vegetable-based pigments, since synthetic pigments can contain metals such as lead, cadmium, cobalt, mercury, and nickel. We know that overexposure to these metals can cause a reduction in male fertility. If you must use synthetics, consider purchasing premixed paints for your projects.

We recommend latex paints for any renovation and redecorating you may do while trying to conceive and after you are pregnant. Spray paints often contain toluene (see Table 3-2); paint thinners and cleaners also contain a number of chemical solvents proven to increase the

Making Stained Glass

For those of you who enjoy making stained glass, the greatest reproductive hazard is the lead that is present in the casement for the glass. Sanding or molding this casement can release lead dust into the air. Soldering strips of lead can also produce toxic lead fumes. Furthermore, the colors that lend stained glass its beauty can contain a number of solvents. Making stained glass involving lead-based products is *not* recommended during the time you are trying to conceive, are pregnant, or are breastfeeding. Lead-free products are available, although experts say they are more difficult to use.

rates of miscarriage and birth defects when you are exposed to them in high doses. Safe house painting suggestions include:

- Avoid using oil-based paints or paint products that contain ethylene glycols or hydrocarbon solvents. Again, latex paints are very safe to use.
- Use acetone products and shellac with caution.
- Use AP-certified (ACMI "approved product") nontoxic paints.[4]

Pottery

A variety of metallic substances such as silica, chromium, copper, lead, and cadmium may be found in pottery materials. Most modern glaze products use ground glass, which eliminates the risk of lead vapors and dusts. Firing the clay after the pottery is shaped can release carbon monoxide, as well as gases containing sulfur, chlorine, nitrogen, and fluorine. The effects of these gases on fertility are not entirely clear, but overexposure may be harmful to you, so why not reduce exposure as best you can?

In addition to the general recommendations mentioned earlier, you can improve your reproductive safety during pottery-making if you:

- Choose prepared glazes that are free of toxic metals. (Making glaze from scratch increases your exposure to the elements.)
- Make sure your kiln has exhaust ventilation.
- Clean up after a pottery project with a wet mop to prevent dust particles from lingering in the environment.

4. Art and Creative Materials Institute (ACMI) has a team of scientists review paints and determine whether they earn this AP seal (commonly seen on kids' paint labels).

Photography

Photography is an extremely common hobby. Given the advent of digital cameras, which don't use film, the following information may not be relevant to you. If you are a photography purist and still like to develop your own film, you'll be handling a variety of chemicals and preservatives, including acetic acid, bromide, and dichromate salt solutions. Color film requires even more chemicals to develop than black and white. No studies at the present time link photography to a reduction in fertility or birth defects in a prospective fetus. In the workplace, however, large exposures to solvents similar to the ones used in photography have been shown to have a detrimental effect on the developing fetus. Therefore, we suggest that you minimize your exposure to chemicals used in photography by:

- Using premixed solutions
- Avoiding direct skin contact
- Covering any chemical processing baths when not in use
- Avoiding color film processing or using strict personal protection and excellent ventilation

Cars and Carbon Monoxide

Many people like to perform their own auto engine maintenance and repair, which may involve using certain solvents. As with all chemicals, avoid inhalation of solvents, practice safe waste disposal, and protect your skin to significantly reduce the risk of overexposure. Of greater concern than solvent exposure when working with engines is carbon monoxide exposure. Carbon monoxide is a colorless, odorless gas produced by gasoline engines and other devices that burn fuel. The carbon monoxide replaces oxygen in your red blood cells, making it harder to provide oxygen to the tissues that need it. Extreme exposure can lead to neurological damage and death. Newer vehicles with hybrid engines that have gas and ion battery power can also produce carbon monoxide.

The effect of carbon monoxide on fertility is unclear. In the fetus, carbon monoxide will replace oxygen in the fetal cells, potentially damaging development of vital organ systems. The National Institute of Occupational Safety and Health (NIOSH) and the Environmental Protection Agency (EPA) have created strict guidelines to limit the amount of carbon monoxide that can be present in the home—less than 15 ppm (parts per million) over eight hours is the upper limit of safe exposure. Most carbon monoxide poisoning is accidental, usually from a malfunctioning oven or furnace or from forest and domestic fires.

In many areas of the United States, carbon monoxide detectors are required in the home. A number of appliances, such as generators, lawn mowers, and snow blowers, can release carbon monoxide into the air. Examine equipment with engines for warning labels about carbon monoxide and use such equipment outside or in well-ventilated areas. Symptoms are usually not seen until the carbon monoxide level in your blood exceeds 80 ppm. Neurological changes do not occur until the level is greater than 200 ppm.

If you think you may be exposed to extreme amounts of the gas, a blood test can determine if you are in danger. People who are toll collectors, bus drivers, and cabdrivers may be at greater risk for occupational exposure. If you are in one of these lines of work, you can reduce your exposure by keeping the windows of your booth or vehicle closed and having a fan running nearby. Most people who follow precautions will be in no danger from overexposure. If you have headaches, persistent nausea, or visual changes, you should see your doctor for a blood test. Treatment is possible with pure or hyperbaric oxygen.

Practical Application

Make a list of the chemicals you have used in the last month to conduct your recreational hobbies. Make a list of ways to increase safety within your home when you plan to try to conceive. For example, change the storage site of chemicals to be disposed of or purchase gloves or goggles to improve your protection.

_____

_____

_____

HAIR, NAILS, AND FUR BALLS (PET CARE)

If you are a cat lover, you may already know that your cat's feces may carry the parasite *Toxoplasma gondii*, which causes toxoplasmosis, which can cause miscarriages and significant birth defects if you are exposed to it for the first time immediately before or during pregnancy. Cats are more likely to carry toxoplasmosis if they are outdoor cats or are often catching mice, which can also carry the parasite. Because cats are passive carriers of this infection, they will not be ill.

Beginning three months prior to trying to conceive and continuing throughout your pregnancy, we recommend that you not take in any feral cats or adopt any kittens. If you own a cat, have a family member clean the cat box and dispose of the kitty litter. If you may have already been exposed to toxoplasmosis earlier in your life, a simple blood test, costing $75 to $100, can be done. The test will identify antibodies in your blood that, if present, mean you are immune to a new infection with toxoplasmosis. If you are found immune, you can con-

Hair and Nail Care (in the Home or Salon)

Hair and nail products can also contain chemicals that, in large doses, have been shown to affect the reproductive system. The information available about the effects of these products is still scant. When it comes to dyeing your hair, a good rule of thumb is to avoid the use of permanent hair dyes one month prior to conception and through the first three months of pregnancy. Safer options include highlighting and using vegetable-based or nonpermanent hair products. Also, try to stretch the interval between treatments. Peroxide is not considered potentially harmful. Many practitioners discourage pregnant patients from hair coloring, straightening, and permanents until the second trimester. However, since most of these chemicals are washed from your skin soon after they are applied, we feel that it is reasonable to continue these treatments until you *know* you are pregnant.

Women who work in salons or who perform manicures, pedicures, and facials can be exposed to these chemicals eight hours a day, multiple days per week. These women should work in well-ventilated areas and wear gloves to minimize skin contact from the chemicals used daily. However, if you just like regular manicures, pedicures, and other salon services, there is no reason to discontinue, because exposure to these chemicals for short intervals seems to have no long-lasting effect on a woman's fertility or fetal health. If you like to have facials done on a regular basis, inform your esthetician that you may be pregnant and she will avoid the use of high-frequency wands that heal broken capillaries. All other masks and products that do not include retinoic acid are perfectly safe for fertility and maternal-fetal health.

tinue to care for your cat's kitty litter. If you are not immune and your partner is unavailableor unable to assist in this chore, then use a mask and gloves and wash your hands thoroughly after every contact with the litter. Use similar precautions when gardening in areas cats frequent, and dampen the soil to reduce dust. (See Chapter 12 for foodborne sources.)

Other pets are safe when it comes to conception. Dogs carry no diseases communicable to you before you try to conceive. In fact, it can be helpful to have a dog at this time because having to exercise the dog means you get exercised, too! Fish, birds, hamsters, and lizards do not pose a risk to your future fertility, but late-breaking studies reveal a risk to your future fetus once you have conceived if you have direct contact with mice and hamsters. These small mammals can carry lymphocytic choriomeningitis virus (LCMV). If infected while pregnant, women can bear children who suffer from a higher likelihood of mental retardation, blindness, and seizures. Similar to toxoplasmosis, LCMV can be passed from the animal to the caretaker via breathing in dust from the feces of affected animals. If you can, have a family member or friend care for any pet mice and hamsters. If you work in a laboratory setting, wear gloves and a protective mask to avoid infection with LCMV. Careful hand washing after handling animals and when cleaning their cages is always recommended.

RADIATION AND REPRODUCTION: X-RAYS, COMPUTERS, RADON, AND MORE

Exposure to radiation is a remarkably common concern among prospective parents. Indeed, non-ob-gyn medical personnel express a similar concern when the use of radiation may be required to evaluate a mother-to-be (e.g., a chest X-ray after a motor vehicle accident; however, this is perfectly safe due to low radiation exposure to the pelvic organs). As with most of the potential exposures found at home or in the workplace, the effects of radiation on your fertility and your future fetus depend on the type, length, and frequency of exposure.

The two types of radiation that you can be exposed to are non-ionizing and ionizing. Non-ionizing radiation—radiation from microwaves, cellular phones, computer screens, radar, magnetic resonance imaging machines, and low-level electromagnetic fields such as those caused by overhead power lines—is not associated with a reduction in fertility or an increased risk of miscarriage or birth defects. Still, you may be interested to know that the majority of emissions from your microwave occur at the rear of the machinery, so putting the back of the machine near a wall or standing at least ten to twelve inches from the back of the microwave will ensure your safety at all times, not just during your preconception. Industrial microwave exposure is another story; in men, the heat from this can cause testicular injury leading to reduced sperm counts and sperm motility.

There are few prospective parents who do not use a computer either at work, at home, or in both settings. Recent studies have shown that the emissions from computer screens, which emit very low levels of electromagnetic waves, have absolutely no effect on fertility rates. Nor have these studies shown an increase in miscarriage rates or birth defects in the fetus. Antiglare computer screens can further reduce the levels of electromagnetic waves (as well as relieve eye strain). For women in the workplace, it is especially crucial to have good lighting and appropriate chair height to ensure that the middle of your screen is at eye level in order to reduce back tension and muscular strain that may be accentuated when you become pregnant.

Living near overhead power lines is often considered risky, but a number of recent studies have shown no fetal or fertility effects. Another source of non-ionizing radiation is food treatment or processing. The gamma rays that are used to irradiate food or parcels are thought to be safe during the preconception period; more about this on page 421.

Exposure to ionizing radiation—from X-rays, the atomic energy industry, and radon found in the soil and home—does pose some risk to unborn offspring (see Figure 3-1). If you are an X-ray technician or a dental or health care worker, your occupational exposure can be kept to a minimum. As you probably already know, you should shield yourself when taking X-rays or stand six to eight feet from the person undergoing an X-ray. If you are actually getting an X-ray, minimal radiation exposure to your pelvic organs occurs unless the X-ray is directed exactly at that area. Additional pelvic organ protection will be provided by shielding that area with a lead drape or apron. Even so, low-dose diagnostic radiation (less than 5 millirems) has never

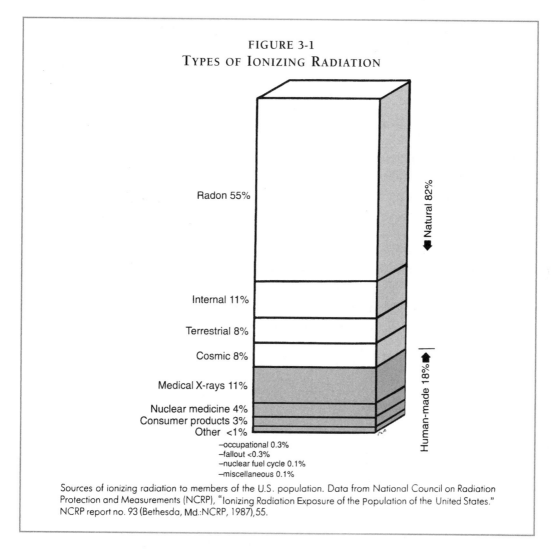

FIGURE 3-1
TYPES OF IONIZING RADIATION

Radon 55%

Internal 11%

Terrestrial 8%

Cosmic 8%

Medical X-rays 11%

Nuclear medicine 4%
Consumer products 3%
Other <1%
 –occupational 0.3%
 –fallout <0.3%
 –nuclear fuel cycle 0.1%
 –miscellaneous 0.1%

Natural 82%

Human-made 18%

Sources of ionizing radiation to members of the U.S. population. Data from National Council on Radiation Protection and Measurements (NCRP), "Ionizing Radiation Exposure of the Population of the United States." NCRP report no. 93 (Bethesda, Md.:NCRP, 1987),55.

been linked to changes in female fertility or problems with the developing fetus.In addition, you can be shielded over the pelvic organs when X-rays are being taken to further reduce any exposure that can occur. Direct radiation therapy to the reproductive organs in men and women will reduce the ability to conceive, but this type of exposure is less common and only done in the setting of undeniable need, such as if a cancer must be treated.

Let's put these radiation exposure numbers in perspective:

- 1 rem = 1,000 millirems
- Naturally occurring background radiation during pregnancy = 300 millirems

- A typical two-view chest X-ray is equivalent to being exposed to 8 millirems.
- An intravenous pyelogram (which evaluates the kidneys and their draining systems to the bladder) delivers 407 millirems.
- Nuclear Regulatory Commission (NRC) occupational exposure limit: 5,000 millirems per year. For more information check www.NRC.gov.
- NRC guideline for pregnant workers: 500 millirems per pregnancy. See page 78.

Although minimal radiation exposure is expected in dental and chest X-rays, if you might be pregnant, tell the technician, and he or she will place appropriate shielding over your belly to be extra cautious. Extreme levels of radiation exposure can lead to increased birth defects and childhood cancers, but limited changes in fertility have been seen. Such exposure is highly unlikely. In fact, the average exposure for those living near Three Mile Island was estimated at only 1 millirem and the maximum exposure for someone at the site boundary would have been less than 100 millirems.

If you have recently bought or sold a house, you may have been asked to check for radon emissions in that home. Radon, found in soil, water, and natural gas, is another source of ionizing radiation present in the work and home environment (see Figure 3-2). Although it is un-

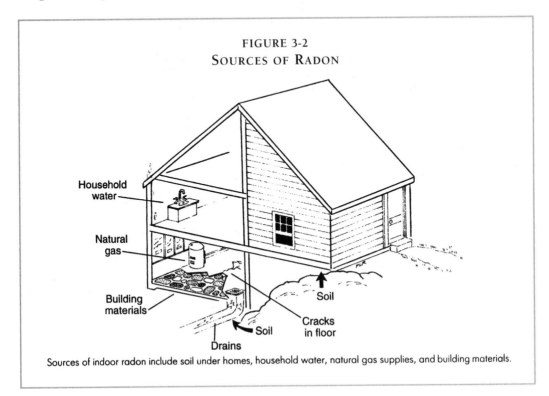

FIGURE 3-2
SOURCES OF RADON

Household water

Natural gas

Building materials

Drains

Soil

Soil

Cracks in floor

Sources of indoor radon include soil under homes, household water, natural gas supplies, and building materials.

likely to have a negative impact on your fertility, precautions are still recommended due to the potential lung problems that can result in prospective parents if exposure is not minimized. The Environmental Protection Agency (EPA) recommends that indoor radon levels should be less than 4pCi/liter of air. Your local governmental agency can test the air in your home or local firms can provide homeowners with radon detectors. Blocking points of radon entry by having good ventilation systems around your boiler equipment, house foundations, and soil sites are suggested.

OCCUPATIONAL REPRODUCTIVE HAZARDS

Kathy and Marc, a couple in their early thirties who have been married for two years, are more than ready to have their first child. Kathy has not been using protection for over a year and is concerned that she hasn't conceived yet. At her annual gynecology visit, Kathy questioned her doctor about whether the chemicals that she and her husband were exposed to in their jobs could be contributing to their difficulty in conceiving. Kathy is an industrial architect and Marc is a laboratory technician, and although they do encounter potentially toxic chemicals on a regular basis, they have been well trained to avoid overexposure.

As their doctor continued a thorough review of the chemicals used in their lives it appeared that their hobbies at home may have exposed them to some interesting substances that could affect their fertility. Kathy paints watercolors and Marc's hobby is film photography—he has his own darkroom in their home and there was concern that Marc was exposed to a number of organic solvents while developing his photos. A semen analysis revealed a reduction in Marc's sperm count. It became clear that while Marc used good safety precautions in his workplace, he was more lax in his darkroom above the garage. Marc changed his practices so that he was equally careful at home and on the job, his sperm count returned to normal after four months, and he and Kathy conceived three months later.

Like Kathy and Marc, you and your partner may have questions about how the environment you work in can affect your ability to conceive. Although the medical community is just starting to understand how various workplace hazards can affect fertility in men and women, more than a thousand chemicals can be common to your workplaces; these may have been shown to have an impact on the fertility of animals. Because the studies that show chemical effects in animals are performed on small mammals (such as rodents) in a laboratory setting where large amounts of the chosen toxin are repeatedly introduced into the animal's environment, it is hard to compare them to the effect of the same chemical or toxin in humans in a typical workplace situation. In U.S. workplaces, there are a number of safeguards against overexposure to chemicals and heavy metals that can affect male or female fertility. Government guidelines require good ventilation systems, careful handling techniques, and employee education about safety measures. This significantly reduces your potential overexposure to any concerning substances.

How to Protect Yourself from Occupational Hazards

Guidelines for your workplace safety are commonly provided by government agencies such as OSHA (Occupational Safety and Health Administration) and NIOSH (National Institute for Occupational Safety and Health). Here are their key recommendations for protecting yourself if you work with potentially hazardous materials:

- First, know the potential hazards that are present in your environment.
- Always store chemicals in tightly sealed containers when they are not in use.
- Try to avoid skin contact with chemicals. If contact with your skin is made, promptly and thoroughly wash the area.
- Use protective gear such as gloves and eye goggles.
- Always wash your hands before eating or drinking.
- Always wash potentially contaminated clothes used at work by you or your partner separately from the other household laundry.
- Participate in safety training and education programs at your workplace. If you think there is a risk or a violation, don't hesitate to speak to the person in your workplace in charge of safety training.
- Use universal precautions when dealing with human and animal body fluids, such as protective eye gear, gloves, and safe techniques for sharp object disposal (e.g., hypodermic needles).
- Make sure any work with biological agents, viruses, and chemicals is done under inhalation hoods.
- If you work with children or in health care, update your vaccinations. Exposure to viruses such as hepatitis B, rubella, and chicken pox (varicella) may be toxic to your fertility and early pregnancy. (More about this in Chapter 4.)

If You Are Being Exposed

If you take great care and use the precautions mentioned above, you are unlikely to be overexposed to a toxin that can affect your fertility. Once you get into the habit of using safe handling techniques, they will become second nature and you will perform them without conscious effort. For example, in any emergency room you will notice the entire staff, from the nurses to the doctors to the lab technicians to the custodial staff, automatically reaching for gloves and eye gear whenever coming into contact with body fluids. Nonetheless, accidents can happen and you should be prepared to minimize the risks to your fertility and general health by dealing expertly with an exposure.

- **Identify your exposure.** Find out exactly what toxin and how much of it you are exposed to. Accurate information should be available from your employer about the types of chemical agents that could possibly be in your workplace. Information about your work environment also can be obtained from a computer database that is called TERIS (Teratogen Information Service). Teratogens are substances that cause birth defects. Material safety data sheets (MSDS) for each potential teratogen on site will be listed. Remember, just because a toxin is present in your workplace doesn't mean you have had a damaging exposure.

- **Identify the timing of your exposure with respect to your reproductive cycle.** Extreme exposure at ovulation will affect the health of a possible conception. Also, you may not know that you are pregnant when you are exposed. For example, low-level radiation may not have an effect on a fetus that has been recently conceived, but extreme radiation exposure could be lethal.

- **Professionally evaluate the protective measures in your environment.** Occupational experts may be available at your workplace already, or you can find one to come to your site by:

  - Calling a poison control center in your community to get in touch with local toxicology staff.
  - Calling the occupational health division at your local major university or community hospital environmental health department.
  - Contacting OSHA for staff in your community who can assist with a workplace evaluation.

- **Avoid skin and eye contact.** If your skin or eyes become irritated, contact your workplace safety team or call a poison control center to check which solvents or liquids are best used to neutralize the effects of the contact.

- **Follow your exposure effects, if possible.** For example, if you have been exposed to lead, have your doctor check your blood levels until they return to normal. Wait until then to attempt conception to ensure a healthier fetus. Serial semen analysis may also be helpful to follow the progress of a chemical exposure that has significantly reduced sperm count.

What Are the Reproductive Hazards in the Workplace?

A link between fertility and workplace exposures in men and women was noted as far back as the 1850s, when women who worked with lead in battery production factories were noted to have miscarriages and stillbirths more often than women their age who did not work in the same setting. More recently, men who were farmers in the 1970s in southern California started to question why fewer children were produced in their families when compared to their friends who were construction workers. After testing, the farmers were found to have lower sperm counts attributed to their daily exposure to a pesticide called dibromochloropropane (DBCP), resulting in their reduced fertility. That pesticide is no longer used today.

In women, other studies revealed that overexposure from workplace chemicals or heavy metals can reduce the levels of female hormones that, in turn, control the monthly release of a mature egg. And if eggs are released less often, conception will take longer to occur. Extreme exposure to radiation or chemical solvents damages the egg and, with it, half of the genetic blueprint for the fetus. This can lead to a higher incidence of spontaneous miscarriages and birth defects. Some heavy metals and chemicals can also reduce production of the male hormone testosterone, resulting in sexual dysfunction. The following table summarizes the most common toxins that you can come into contact with in the workplace and their effects on men, women, and fetuses.

TABLE 3-2

EFFECTS OF OVEREXPOSURE TO REPRODUCTIVE HAZARDS IN MEN AND WOMEN

Toxin	Persons Exposed	Effects of Toxin		
		Men	Women	Offspring
ORGANIC SOLVENTS				
Toluene (most common)	Textile workers Printers Shoemakers	↓sperm counts[a]	↑miscarriages ↑menstrual irregularity	↓birth weight ↑birth defects
Xylene (second most common)	Painters Health care workers	none known	↑miscarriages	none known
Benzene	Health care workers	none known	? ↑miscarriages[b]	↓birth weight ↑stillbirths
Tetrachloro- ethylene	Dry cleaners	↓sperm counts	↑miscarriages	↓birth weight
Ethylene glycol	Mechanics Dry cleaners	↓sperm counts	↑miscarriages	↑birth defects

Toxin	Persons Exposed	Effects of Toxin		
		Men	*Women*	*Offspring*
HEAVY METALS				
Lead	Ceramic or pottery workers Painters Furniture refinishers	↓ sperm counts ↓ sperm motility	↑ miscarriages ↑ menstrual irregularity	↓ birth weight ↑ birth defects
	Toll collectors (car exhaust)	↓ sperm counts ↓ sperm motility	↑ miscarriages	↑ birth defects
	Factory workers (electronics)	↓ sperm motility ↓ sperm counts	↑ miscarriages	none known
Cadmium	Glassmakers Smelters	↓ testosterone ↓ sperm motility	↑ ovarian injury^c	↓ birth weight
Mercury	Shipbuilders	↓ seminal fluid nutrients	↑ miscarriages	↑ birth defects
	Dental workers	none known	? ↑ miscarriages	↑ birth defects
PLASTICS				
Polymers	Factory workers	↓ sperm motility	? ↑ miscarriages	none known
Vinyl chloride	Military	↓ testosterone	none known	none known
Synthetic rubber	Packaging staff	↓ sperm motility	? ↑ miscarriages	none known
PESTICIDES				
DDT	Farmers	↓ sperm counts	↑ miscarriages ↑ menstrual irregularity	↑ birth defects
Dieldrin (weed killer)	Gardeners	? ↓ sperm counts	? ↑ miscarriages	none known
Organochlorides	Exterminators Chemical manufacturers	↓ sperm counts	none known	↓ birth weight

Toxin	Persons Exposed	Effects of Toxin		
		Men	*Women*	*Offspring*
CARBON MONOXIDE				
Carbon monoxide	Mechanics	? ↓ libido	none known	↑ birth defects
	Firefighters	none known	none known	↑ stillbirths
	Furnace repairers			↓ birth weight
RADIATION				
Ionizing radiation	Health care workers	↓ sperm counts	↑ miscarriages	↑ birth defects
	Nuclear plant workers	none known	↑ menstrual irregularity	↓ birth weight
	Flight crews	↓ sperm motility	↑ ovarian injury	↓ birth weight
Radon	People living in affected houses	↓ seminal fluid	↑ miscarriages	none known
PHARMACEUTICALS				
Chemotherapy drugs	Health care workers	↓ sperm counts	↑ miscarriages ↑ menstrual irregularity	↑ birth defects
Hormonal preparations	Chemical factory workers	↓ sperm counts ↓ sperm motility	↑ ovarian injury	none known
COSMETICS				
Hair dyes	Hair stylists	none known	none known	rare birth defects (only with ingestion early in pregnancy)
Nail polish/ removers (acetone, formaldehydes)	Salon workers	none known	? ↑ miscarriage	? ↑ birth defects

a. ↑, increased incidence; ↓, reduction in incidence.
b. A question mark (?) before an up or down arrow implies it is a possible effect not absolutely proven yet.
c. Ovarian injury implies fewer eggs released and a reduction in the health of the eggs in the ovary, with more potential DNA damage to them.

More About Mercury

Mercury comes in three forms: elemental (vapor), inorganic, and organic. Mercury is naturally found in our environment from volcanic and geothermal activity, and is mined for industrial uses such as coal-fired power plants. Exposures to mercury can be environmental or occupational, such as proximity to waste incinerators, mining operations (or downstream of mercury-tainted wastewater), and during dental work. Regulations are in place to guide the capture and proper disposal of human-generated mercury emissions, especially near contaminated sites. Mercury is safely incorporated into some thermometers and blood pressure devices, but if damaged, these require special handling (Poison Control can provide safe instruction). Mercury-containing dental amalgam restorations have the potential to expose dental personnel and patients to mercury. Though most studies demonstrate largely inconsequential health impacts, others are more cautious not to dismiss possible risk, especially as it pertains to prospective mothers. In otherwise healthy people, any risk associated with mercury-containing amalgam restorations is quite low (according to the FDA and CDC), but alternatives are available (talk to your dentist about options and insurance coverage).

The most common form of organic mercury, known as methylmercury, is formed when mercury comes in contact with bacteria in bodies of water (oceans, lakes). Methylmercury tends to accumulate in plant and animal tissue. The safest option is to avoid eating certain varieties of fish and sea mammals, while including foods—even specific ocean fish—that are naturally protective against the harmful effects of methylmercury consumption (see Chapter 13 for an intriguing discussion of food safety and fish). Studies done in the Seychelles and Faroe islands allowed researchers to observe the traditional eating habits, specifically the fish eaten by the women in each population. They found (much to their surprise and relief) that the women's natural fish consumption was actually protecting them and their offspring from more harmful forms of mercury by ingesting the other minerals found in fish, specifically selenium. Also, omega-3s and iodine may play a positive role in reducing mercury effects from fish intake.

Remember, being able to smell a chemical solvent or insecticide or herbicide doesn't mean a damaging exposure has occurred, and in most cases it is *repetitive* and *excessive* exposure to the substance that causes the effect listed in Table 3-2.

NOISE AND VIBRATION

Noise in the workplace has not been shown to affect male or female fertility or to cause hearing deficits in the developing fetus. Reassuringly, vibrations from equipment or from driving a truck, bus, car, or tractor have not been shown to have a negative effect on fertility, either, although prolonged exposure to hand tools, such as in construction work, may have a high vibratory activity that is associated with vascular spasm. If, after you conceive, you use any of these tools in your workplace, you should review with your doctor the safety precautions to take.

FOR FUTURE REFERENCE: During Pregnancy

Safe Levels of Radiation Exposure During Pregnancy
During pregnancy, decisions regarding acceptable therapeutic radiation exposure should be made on a case-by-case basis, balancing the theoretical risks to the fetus against the benefit to the mother. Your doctor or radiologist can answer any remaining questions you might have. The IAEA offers an excellent overview of pregnancy and radiation (see http://rpop.iaea.org/RPOP/RPoP/Content/SpecialGroups/1_PregnantWomen/Pregnancyandradiology.htm).

Accidental exposure to a high level of radiation (over 10,000 millirems) will usually trigger one of nature's protective mechanisms—to miscarry, because the pregnancy is no longer viable.

PHYSICAL PROFESSIONS: FIREFIGHTING, CONSTRUCTION, ELITE ATHLETES

Angela is a thirty-four-year-old firefighter who has recently married Daniel, a thirty-six-year-old police officer. Angela's mother has repeatedly told her that if she wants a baby she must stop working, thinking that the physical exertion and danger of the job are going to prevent conception. Frazzled, Angela calls her health care providers with her concerns. Could her mother be right?

When women started taking jobs previously held exclusively by men, such as firefighting, law enforcement, and construction work, concerns about the effects on their fertility were studied. Firefighters were a particularly complicated group to evaluate because they are regularly exposed to different chemicals, such as carbon monoxide and hydrocarbons; undergo demanding physical effort; and are often exposed to high temperatures. All of this makes it hard to isolate any particular source as a potential problem. One study revealed an increased risk of spontaneous miscarriages in women firefighters compared to women in the general population who did not undertake similar physical strains. Other studies suggested that, in general, longer work shifts, along with longer hours of standing and increased repetitive bending or lifting, may affect the health of a pregnancy. This led the American Medical Association's Council on Scientific Affairs to release guidelines for work activity in pregnancy that recommend safe parameters for climbing, lifting, and standing in a workday. None of the data suggests that workplace physical exertion has any negative impact on the ability to conceive.

Some women in physically demanding professions, such as athletes, dancers, and construction workers, may experience a reduction in menstrual regularity, reflecting a reduction in ovulation. However, many women who perform extreme physical exertion during preconception show no change in their menstrual cycles. The source of this menstrual irregularity may not be due to physical exertion alone. It could also be attributed to an energy imbalance—not enough food to supply the activity level—which can significantly affect hormone levels released by the brain, which in turn can diminish the likelihood of triggering ovulation or sustaining a pregnancy.

So, as long as Angela is eating healthfully, her fertility shouldn't be affected by her job. However, she should consider modifying her work activity to reduce her exposure to excessive heat, exertion, and chemicals before conception in order to prepare for changes that will be recommended during pregnancy.

FOR FUTURE REFERENCE: During Pregnancy

What About Your Baby's First Environment? Exposure to High Blood Sugar in the Womb
As much as you don't want lead in your paint or radon in your basement, we want to be sure you view environmental toxins in proper perspective. Once you've implemented proper safety precautions and common sense, let go of very hypothetical concerns. However, don't overlook what can make the biggest difference of all: prolonged high blood sugar.

According to Adolfo Correa, MD, MPH, PhD,[a] an expert in birth defects at the CDC, uncontrolled diabetes early in pregnancy is a well-known cause of birth defects, and probably one of the most important modifiable risk factors today. Due to the increasing number of Americans who are overweight or obese, diabetes may become more common among women of childbearing age. People with diabetes do not metabolize blood sugar fully, leaving too much circulating in the bloodstream (more on this in Chapter 7).

Prolonged exposure to high blood sugar levels in pregnant women with diabetes damages tissues (the mother's and the baby's). This damage can happen early—in the first eight weeks of pregnancy, when you may not even know you're pregnant. In fact, high blood sugar levels early in pregnancy may be just as detrimental to developing tissue as most environmental health risks and the "big three" lifestyle-related choices (smoking, alcohol, and recreational drugs) discussed in the previous chapter. For example, birth defects and infant deaths are two to four times more frequent among infants born to pregnant women with uncontrolled diabetes (poor blood sugar control) than among infants born to pregnant women without diabetes.

We are equally concerned about the millions of women who are overweight or obese. They may be prediabetic, meaning their blood sugar is too high, and they are at risk for developing diabetes. These women may become diabetic at any time, even while they are trying to conceive.

"It is important that women with diabetes, or those who are overweight or obese and at risk of developing diabetes, plan their pregnancies in consultation with their doctor, and participate in preconception care," says Dr. Correa. "How well pregnant women with diabetes manage their blood sugar before and during pregnancy will influence the course and outcome of the pregnancy. Keeping excellent blood sugar control is good for all parties involved—the prospective mother, and baby."

a. Adolfo Correa, MD, MPH, PhD, is a medical officer at the National Center on Birth Defects and Developmental Disabilities, a unit of the Centers for Disease Control and Prevention.

HEALTH CARE WORKERS AND FERTILITY

During her routine gynecology visit, Julia, a twenty-nine-year-old nurse who worked in the local hospital's intensive care unit, voiced concerns about how the risks she faces as a health care professional may affect her future plans to have a child. Recently a nurse she works with had a miscarriage after taking care of a very sick patient, and now Julia is anxious that something in the ICU will make it harder for her to conceive and have a healthy pregnancy.

Health care, dental, and veterinary workers are all exposed to special risks that include infections, chemotherapeutic agents, and radiation. You can protect yourself against the latter two risks by handling medications with standard precautions and by using the safety measures mentioned earlier for radiation exposure. There are also universal precautions (precautions to be used with all patients, not just those thought to be at high risk of carrying an infection) for protecting against infections—using gloves, masks, and eye gear to prevent contamination from others' body fluids. Also, vaccination against possible infection with pertussis, hepatitis B, chicken pox (if you have never had it in the past), seasonal flus, and rubella can reduce your chances of getting an infection from patients before and after you are pregnant. Your doctor can evaluate you to determine if you already have natural immunity due to previous exposure or vaccinate if you do not have immunity. Remember, most healthy people have well-functioning immune systems and rarely contract the majority of infections a patient may have. Strict and thorough hand washing goes a long way toward protecting yourself from communicable diseases. Julia was reassured by her doctor that if she uses standard safety procedures, she has nothing to worry about.

Your home and workplace should be safe havens for you and your loved ones. By increasing your awareness of the chemicals in these environments, you can maximize your reproductive safety and produce a healthier child. Resources for more specific information are in Appendix C. In the next chapter, we will offer some helpful ways to find a health care provider who fits your medical needs. Hints and facts on how to utilize your chosen health care team will in turn allow you to optimize the health of you and your future baby.

CHAPTER 4

The Preconception Visit

*A*fter giving your relationship, your finances, your lifestyle, and your environment a good hard look, you're probably fairly well prepared mentally for conception. But what about physically? The next step is to make a pre-pregnancy medical appointment. How is a pre-pregnancy medical appointment different from a regular visit? Many elements are similar, but when your doctor knows that pregnancy is in your future, he or she will consider certain medical issues that normally might not be discussed. Even if you're in perfect health, it's still a good idea to schedule a preconception visit, as it helps you and your doctor prepare for any special needs you may have as your body undergoes the physical changes of pregnancy.

You probably already have a gynecologist or other practitioner whom you see for your yearly gynecological exams. If, however, you're not happy with your current practitioner or you're not under the care of an obstetrician or other women's health specialist, now is the time to start looking for one who will see you through preconception and pregnancy. If you have a preexisting medical condition, preconception is also the best time to add a medical doctor who specializes in your condition as well as in obstetrics; for example, a woman with diabetes or chronic hypertension may want to add a maternal-fetal medicine (MFM) specialist to her health care team if one is available. This chapter covers how to choose a practitioner who's right for you and what should happen on your first office visit and consultation.

CHOOSING A DOCTOR OR MIDWIFE

When choosing a doctor or midwife, you of course want someone who is intelligent, well trained, and well informed. But you also want someone with whom you feel comfortable discussing medical issues. The choice that you ultimately make depends on your medical needs, personal preferences and philosophy, and insurance provider network. Ask for a referral from family members and friends, especially those who share your preferences and priorities concerning medical care. Your general practitioner or internist, if you have one, is also a good source for a referral. If there's a particular hospital at which you know you want to deliver, that hospital probably has a physician referral service. Many hospitals have these lists posted on their websites, where you can search for a doctor by specialty, office location, credentials, and insurance carrier. You can also get information from your insurance company's physician directory, your local or state medical society, the American College of Obstetricians and Gynecologists (ACOG), or the American College of Nurse Midwives (ACNM). Try not to limit your options by excluding one or the other gender from your search—there are competent, sensitive, and well-respected doctors of both sexes.

Most preconception patients and expectant mothers today are cared for by an obstetrician-gynecologist (ob-gyn). However, there are other professionals who are also trained and licensed to provide obstetric care, such as family practice physicians, certified nurse midwives (CNMs), certified nurse practitioners (CNPs), and physician assistants (PAs). (See Table 4-1.) (For women choosing to see a CNM, CNP, or PA for prenatal care, an ob-gyn will oversee your care and often supervise your delivery.) If you currently have an underlying medical condition such as high blood pressure, diabetes, severe asthma, or an autoimmune disorder (such as multiple sclerosis or lupus), you may also need to begin seeing an MFM specialist as early as three to six months prior to trying, sometimes earlier. If you know in advance that you want a less medically involved birthing experience, discuss this with your health care provider to see whether he or she is comfortable with your birth preferences. If you feel that your provider is not interested in or willing to participate in a more natural birth experience, a CNM might be the right choice for you; they are particularly adept at supporting women who prefer a low-intervention, natural, drug-free delivery though they are not opposed to additional intervention for pain during labor, either. Also, if you are among the estimated 15 percent of women who need assistance conceiving, you will probably have an infertility specialist, known as a reproductive endocrinologist, on your team.

Remember, you should always check with your health insurance company to make sure that your policy covers your chosen practitioner's services or, if they are not covered, what your financial obligation will be.

TABLE 4-1
WHO'S WHO IN OBSTETRICAL CARE

Title	Degree	Training	Can perform deliveries?
Obstetrician-gynecologist	MD	4 years of medical school plus a 4-year residency in obstetrics and gynecology[b]	Yes[a]
Doctor of osteopathy	DO	5 years of osteopathic school, plus the same residency in obstetrics and gynecology as an MD[b]	Yes
Family practice physician	MD	4 years of medical school, plus a 3-year residency with 1 or more rotations in obstetrics[b]	Yes[a]
Certified nurse midwife or Certified midwife	CNM/CM (CNMs are also RNs)	Bachelor's degree plus post-baccalaureate training and certification in midwifery	Yes, when supervised by an ob-gyn
Certified nurse practitioner	CNP	Bachelor's degree in nursing plus graduate-level training (master's or PhD) and advanced clinical training	No
Physician assistant	PA	Admission requirements vary, but almost all programs require at least two years of college and some health care experience, followed by 2 years of training; all states require the PA to complete an accredited program and pass a national exam to obtain a license	No

a. Typically only an obstetrician-gynecologist or family practice MD can perform an operative vaginal delivery or Cesarean section.
b. Some MDs and DOs further their training in high-risk obstetrics and are called maternal-fetal medicine (MFM) specialists; those who further their training in reproductive endocrinology (infertility) are called reproductive endocrinologists.

By choosing your medical practitioner before you conceive, you allow yourself the luxury of time to make a thoughtful choice. One of the best ways to make that choice is to interview potential caregivers in person rather than over the phone (if their schedule and your insurance plan permit). Meeting office staff who are efficient, friendly, and cooperative regarding billing and scheduling issues will help make frequent prenatal visits more pleasant. Also, once you conceive, it's more comfortable to go for your first prenatal visit having already met the person who will be caring for you.

Some practitioners permit short, informational interviews at no cost to you, but preconception counseling cannot be conducted at these. If you want a formal interview and preconception consultation, you'll need to call for an appointment at least four to six weeks (for some busy practitioners it could be four to six months) in advance. This may seem like a lot of time, but popular doctors often are not available for a new consultation sooner than that. Also, ask about the fee for the consultation, as many insurance companies do not cover what they term a "family planning visit" or "preconception visit" and require that it be paid for out of pocket. If you will be planning your pregnancy less than a year after your last annual gynecologic exam, you can request preconception counseling then; the insurance company recognizes this as a standard well-woman annual exam and will reimburse for it accordingly.

Once you're at the consultation, here are some initial questions that may help you make a good choice:

- **What are the doctor's credentials and how long has he or she been in practice?** If the doctor is board certified, it means that he or she has been endorsed by the American Board of Obstetrics and Gynecology (or other relevant board for family practitioners and doctors of osteopathy) and has fulfilled a number of criteria that predict safe medical practice. Nurse midwives who are certified similarly have undergone training with quality control and extensive supervision. Length of practice shouldn't be the only basis by which you judge a doctor's skills, however. Young physicians who have recently graduated are usually adept at using the latest technology, and you might find it easier to communicate with someone closer to you in age. Still, more mature physicians have the benefit of years of practical experience and are also required to periodically update their clinical and technical knowledge. If you're interviewing a nurse midwife, it's important to know how many deliveries she has attended and who would be assisting and supervising her during your labor and delivery experience.

- **What is the doctor's (and/or the group's) labor and delivery philosophy?** Find out what your doctor's Cesarean section rate is (according to the CDC, the national average is approximately 31 percent). If the rate is substantially higher, ask why. He or she may specialize in high-risk pregnancies, such as multiples, which more often require surgical delivery. Is anesthesia an option, and are episiotomies typically performed? (ACOG recommends against them.) Ask if you'll be seeing the same doctor throughout your pregnancy, or perhaps you'll rotate through the staff, allowing you to meet all of the doctors—one of whom may end up being on duty for your delivery. For nurse midwives, if you're delivering at a birthing center, find out under what circumstances he or she would transfer you to the affiliated hospital.

- **What facilities are available at the hospital where the doctor delivers?** An important factor to consider is the type of nursery present at the hospital. A Level 1 nursery can care only for babies born after thirty-four weeks. Level 2 nurseries can accommodate babies born at thirty-two weeks or later, and Level 3 nurseries can care for very premature and low-birth-weight babies as well as full-term babies with medical problems. This means if you have preterm labor during your pregnancy, both you and the baby may need to be transferred to a hospital with a special or intensive care nursery, either before or after delivery. Unless your doctor has privileges at the new facility, you'd be assigned a new doctor. You may also want to know whether the hospital is a teaching facility and if medical students and residents will participate in your care. Finally, you might be interested in the amenities available at the hospital. Many maternity units now have hotel-style private rooms, whirlpool baths, and special meals. If you're interviewing a certified nurse midwife who delivers at a birthing center, find out if the center is freestanding or hospital-affiliated.

Adding Other Professionals to Your Team

Although it might be nice, not everyone can just go out and hire a personal nutritionist, trainer, or therapist to work out the minor kinks in her preconception readiness. Nor is it necessary. In these areas, this book should meet most prospective parents' needs. However, there are special situations in which adding the services of professionals outside of reproductive medicine may be helpful or even absolutely necessary to your preconception health. When this is the case, you'll usually need a physician referral. Personal recommendations can be reliable, too, if you do your homework assessing each professional's credentials. Here's what to look for:

- **A registered dietitian (RD)** is recommended if you have a preexisting medical condition such as diabetes, polycystic ovary syndrome (PCOS), anemia, an eating disorder, or a disease of the digestive system, such as Crohn's. Be aware of the distinction between the terms *registered dietitian* and *nutritionist*. The RD credential is awarded through the credentialing agency of the American Dietetic Association to those who complete an accredited bachelor's degree program followed by a dietetic internship (or coordinated program equivalent) involving more than one thousand supervised practice hours. Once these requirements are met, an RD can take a national exam, which, upon passing, leads to the RD credential and state certification and licensure. Continuing education is required to maintain this status. In contrast, *nutritionist* is a general term describing a field of interest but does not necessarily signify specific training or licensure.

- **A psychiatrist (MD), psychologist (PhD), or clinical social worker (LICSW/LCSW)** can help you deal with emotional issues that may arise as the result of a psychiatric condition, the stress of living with a chronic medical condition or eating disorder, or the aftermath of a traumatic event. If you're currently taking any medication (yes, even for trouble sleeping, depression, or ADHD, such as Xanax, Lexapro, Zoloft, or Ritalin), it's vital that you let your psychiatrist know about your plans to conceive. It may be necessary to change or temporarily discontinue the medication before conception and during pregnancy.

- **A physical therapist (PT), exercise physiologist, or certified personal trainer** may be helpful if you have chronic back problems, pelvic instability, urinary incontinence, or dyspareunia (pain with intercourse). Physical therapists who specialize in pelvic physical therapy can be very helpful with these issues. Preconception physical conditioning will help you strengthen the areas most affected by the weight gain and center of gravity shift that will occur when your pregnancy advances. They can also help keep your weight at a healthy level, both before and after conception. Recent research has also shown that core strengthening and regular exercise shorten the second stage of labor and improve postpartum recovery (regardless of whether the delivery is vaginal or by C-section).

- **A lactation consultant (specifically with an IBCLC credential)** is usually most helpful shortly before or after you give birth and start to breastfeed. However, if you have a variation in nipple structure such as a flattened or inverted nipple, have undergone breast reduction or augmentation surgery, or have had a traumatic experience that causes you extreme anxiety or discomfort around the issue of breastfeeding, you might want to consider having a preconception evaluation with a lactation consultant.

WHAT TO EXPECT AT YOUR PRECONCEPTION EVALUATION

Preconception exams generally consist of a weigh-in, medical and family history, physical exam, gynecological exam, and possibly blood tests. Lifestyle habits and environmental safety issues, such as those discussed in Chapters 1, 2, and 3, are usually broached, too. All of these are evaluated to make sure there are no medical issues that could negatively affect conception

FOR FUTURE REFERENCE: During Pregnancy and After Delivery

Is a Birth Attendant or Doula for You?

Though birth is one of the most amazing events of your life, the truth is, it's messy. This beautiful event fills many first-time parents with anxiety. A labor support person, such as a doula (the word comes from the Greek meaning "woman who serves"), who is not your spouse or significant other may be helpful as you approach the "opening ceremonies" of parenthood: birth and the postpartum period. This is especially so if your usually supportive partner is uncertain about how to handle the reality of the delivery room, where blood and other body fluids are compounded by fatigue and uncertainty about the process in general. (In busy hospital settings, many nurses will have responsibility for more than one patient until you are in active labor.) A good doula can help relax you during labor and can help your partner be a better coach. Further, for couples who deliver far from relatives or those with a deployed spouse, a doula can act as a wise "auntie" who can help with postpartum and infant care.

A doula or labor coach can cost from $350 to $1,000, depending on where you live, how many deliveries she has attended in the past, and the time she will spend with you, which may include all or some of the following: at home with you when you are in early labor, at your side in the medical setting during labor and delivery, and postpartum help with breastfeeding and your personal care. Doulas undergo certification over three to seven months, attend a birthing class and two deliveries as a labor support person, and pass a written exam, but they have no formal medical training.

It is essential when choosing a doula that you share your philosophy about pain medication usage in labor and feel that the doula will work well with both you and your partner. A doula who advocates is helpful, but one who is obstructive to your care will not be greeted happily by medical staff. To find a doula, ask friends who have had a good experience with one, your health care provider, your childbirth instructor, or your hospital referral service, or check certification websites, such as Doulas of North America (dona.org), the Association of Labor Assistants and Childbirth Educators (alace.org), or the Childbirth and Postpartum Professional Association (cappa.net). Insurance coverage is unlikely, but you can always ask. And definitely check references.

or pregnancy. If there are, you and your health care practitioner will come up with a management plan. Because it will be helpful for you to have certain information about your health at your fingertips, we've created a Women's Preconception Medical Checklist to fill out and take with you to your initial consultation (see Figure 4-1). To limit this checklist to one page, we

Dental Health and Hygiene

You may be surprised to learn that poor maternal dental health can adversely affect pregnancy outcome. Gingivitis and other oral infections may lead to pregnancy complications such as poor fetal weight gain and too early labor and delivery. Therefore, we urge you to tell your dentist about your plans to get pregnant. By identifying and treating any existing dental problems before trying to conceive, you will reap the potential systemic benefits from the moment the baby implants in your womb and placenta formation begins. Discuss preventive oral hygiene practices, too. For the record, according to the American Dental Association, routine dental hygiene and urgent oral care can be safely performed during pregnancy, should the need arise.

During preconception and then later in pregnancy, drink fluoridated water whenever possible (bottled water and well water usually aren't, but many water companies can offer fluoridated water on request). Your dentist can assess whether you're getting enough fluoride and can prescribe an oral rinse if necessary. Fluoridated toothpaste is also an excellent source of fluoride, so be sure to brush your teeth at least twice a day and floss at least once a day. These practices reduce the chances that you'll have to be treated for cavities or gum disease during your pregnancy.

had to make the type small, so you may want to enlarge it on a copier to spare your ob-gyn from reaching for his or her reading glasses!

Let's go through each step of the visit more closely now.

Before you see your doctor in the examination room, the nurse or medical assistant will ask for your height and have you step on the scale. Weight offers insight into your hormonal milieu but should always be viewed within the context of your dietary and exercise habits as well as your natural (inherited) build. Your pre-pregnancy weight is also used to determine the healthiest amount of weight you should gain after you conceive. If the thought of pregnancy weight gain is a source of stress for you (or your partner), this is the time to talk it over to ensure a healthy mind-set once you conceive. Being extremely underweight or overweight can have an impact on ovulation and, more important, may be a strain on the baby's and your health after you conceive. But there's good news—modest improvements toward a healthy body weight can dramatically improve your odds of a successful conception. When your weight is measured, your provider will probably calculate your body mass index (BMI) (you can read more about body weight and BMI in Chapter 14).

The nurse or assistant will also note some basic information (age, date of last menstrual period) and take your blood pressure. If your blood pressure is elevated, the doctor will monitor it closely, and you and your doctor will need to work to get it in excellent control prior to conception through methods discussed in Chapter 7.

The vital statistic of age won't be addressed any further during your appointment unless you'll be over thirty-five by the time you deliver your child(ren). Although many women in their thirties are anxious about their fertility, in truth, they are likely to conceive and can safely bear children into their early forties. In addition, a woman's consistency in making good lifestyle choices can ward off age-related increases in weight, blood pressure, or insulin resistance that would potentially complicate a pregnancy. However, as a woman ages, so do her eggs—largely independent of her health status. The eggs become more fragile and the genetic blueprint they carry becomes more susceptible to damage. Although there's no way to test for risks of random (noninherited) genetic problems, age-related or not, genetic testing is possible in the first and second trimesters. In terms of preconception, older eggs can mean a slightly higher rate of miscarriage and infertility for women between the ages of thirty-five and thirty-nine, and an even higher rate for women in their early forties. So getting pregnant may take a little longer than you expect, and there is a slightly greater chance that you'll need to pursue reproductive assistance. (See Chapter 18 for more information about diagnosing and treating infertility.) Do not be discouraged by these facts, as healthy pregnancies in mature moms are a regular occurrence. The education that you and your partner get before conception about the risks of being a more mature parent will empower you to examine the genetic issues ahead in pregnancy. You will both also be able to work through any ethical differences or strong opinions regarding genetic testing and choices that you and your partner may need to make during pregnancy. (See Chapter 6 for a more detailed discussion of advanced maternal age.)

Once the nurse has obtained your preliminary information, your doctor will begin the checkup by taking a comprehensive medical and family history, including information you can offer on prior pregnancies, if applicable. Using the Women's Preconception Medical Checklist, give your doctor as much information about yourself and your family as you can.

After he or she takes your history, your doctor will then perform the following:

- **The physical exam.** Your doctor will listen to your heart and lungs and check your thyroid to rule out any problems in these areas. All physicals, regardless of the woman's age, also include a breast and abdominal exam, which will look for any detectable masses. (Note: If you are nearing forty, or are over thirty-five and have a family history of breast cancer, you're nearing the time when your doctor might suggest getting a baseline mammogram if you haven't already had one. It's a good idea to get a mammogram before you conceive, because your breasts will undergo changes during pregnancy that make it difficult to read a mammogram. Also, if a lump is found, you can undergo treatment without worrying about the effect of treatment on a developing fetus.)

- **The gynecological exam.** Your doctor will now visually inspect your vulva, vagina, and cervix, do a Pap smear, and swab your vagina/cervix to check for common infections such as yeast, chlamydia, and gonorrhea. Finally, he or she will perform a bimanual

FIGURE 4-1
WHAT TO TALK ABOUT AT THE DOCTOR'S OFFICE:
THE WOMEN'S PRECONCEPTION MEDICAL CHECKLIST

Fill this out now and bring it with you to your scheduled appointment.

Your Name: _____
Age: _____ Height: _____ Weight: _____

1. My last pap smear was (date): _____;
my last complete physical exam was _____;
last menstrual period was: _____.
Any irregularities with menstrual cycle? Yes / No

2. Here is my past medical history. (Put an X by
anything you have **now** or had **in the past**.)
___ Anemia or "low iron"; or "high iron"
___ Asthma
___ Cancer (type of: _____)
___ Chicken pox (at what age? ___)
___ Crohn's disease
___ Deep venous thrombosis
___ Depression
___ Diabetes
___ Eating disorder (anorexia or bulimia)
___ Epilepsy
___ High blood pressure or heart disease
___ HIV/AIDS
___ Kidney disease
___ Lupus
___ Phenylketonuria (PKU)
___ Polycystic ovarian syndrome (PCOS)
___ Sexually transmitted disease
___ Thyroid problems

3. Some inherited diseases are more common among
certain ethnicities. My ethnic origin is: _____
The father's ethnic origin is: _____

4. I do / do not know my blood type. _____

5. I have a blood relative who has or had (put X):
___ Bleeding disorder (e.g., hemophilia)
___ Birth defects
___ Mental retardation
___ Sickle-cell disease
___ Tay-Sachs
___ Muscular dystrophy
___ Cystic fibrosis
___ Huntington's chorea

6. I've had these immunizations or shots (put X &
date):
___ Rubella (German measles) _____
___ Hepatitis _____
___ Tetanus _____
___ Td _____
___ Tdap _____
___ Pneumovax _____
___ Flu shot _____

7. I currently take the following (oral or topical)
prescription medications, over-the-counter
medications, vitamins, or herbs (include anything
within the past 6 months):

_____
_____
_____

8. *(Ask)* Do I need a prescription for a vitamin and/or
mineral supplement? _____
(Circle all that apply) I live in a northern climate > 37°
latitude; routinely wear sunscreen; have dark pigmented
skin (all pose risk for vitamin D deficiency).

9. I do / do not know whether my mother took DES
(diethylstilbestrol) while she was pregnant with me.

10. *(Ask)* Is it OK for me to continue/begin a regular,
healthy exercise program? _____

11. We now practice _____ method of
birth control (if any). Between now and the time to
start trying, we plan to use _____
method of contraception.

12. (Circle one)
Yes / No I work around chemicals, solvents, lead, or
          other potential hazards.
Yes / No I am able to take proper precautions around
          environmental hazards at home and work.
          (if not, may need to temporarily transfer to a
          different position)
Yes / No I own a cat who uses a litter box in our
          home. Who cleans it? _____
Yes / No I garden in areas where cats frequent.
Yes / No I smoke cigarettes (other _____).
Yes / No I use one or more recreational drugs like
          marijuana, cocaine, "meth," IV drugs, etc.
Yes / No I may find it difficult to cut out alcoholic
          beverages completely (including beer, wine,
          hard alcohol).

13. If pertinent, please inform your health care
provider about any previous pregnancies, miscarriages,
stillbirths, and/or abortions.

_____

14. If you have had a baby before, was he/she born
early or small, or was he/she ever in the neonatal
intensive care unit? _____

exam to make sure that your cervix, uterus, and ovaries feel normal (see Figure 4-2). If there are any concerns raised by the bimanual exam, your doctor may recommend a pelvic ultrasound, which is a painless, noninvasive procedure that allows the doctor to "see" the shape and size of your uterus and ovaries, as well as the width of your uterine lining. A rectal exam may be added to your assessment at the discretion of your doctor.

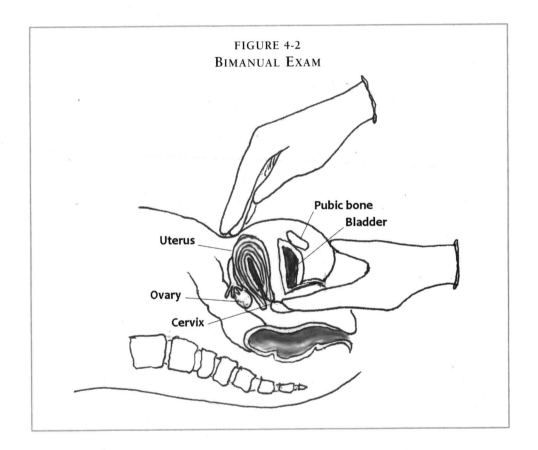

FIGURE 4-2
BIMANUAL EXAM

- **Blood tests.** Your doctor may want to check your blood sugar, the level of your electrolytes (these reflect kidney function and metabolic balance), and your thyroid-stimulating hormone (TSH) level if you haven't had it screened for two or three years.If you have been pregnant in the past and have had gestational diabetes or thyroid hormone imbalances, these lab tests will be strongly recommended. An over- or underactive thyroid is a fairly common problem in women of reproductive age and, if not corrected, can affect your fertility, menstrual cycle, miscarriage risk, and potentially the neurological development of your fetus.

The Pap Test

A Papanicolaou, or Pap, smear examines the cells of your cervix for precancerous abnormalities, which, if they are found and treated, reduces the incidence of cervical cancer by about 90 percent. Early detection of cervical abnormalities can allow treatment that prevents the cancerous cells from growing. The ideal time for obtaining a Pap smear is after your menstrual cycle is over and at least forty-eight hours after you've last had intercourse. One type of Pap smear, called Thinprep, improves the quality of the smear by providing a cleaner specimen for the technician to read, which has increased the early detection of cancer by 5 to 10 percent. Another test, human papillomavirus (HPV) typing, can also be done to see if you carry one of eighty-five strains of HPV, ten of which are associated with an increased risk for cervical cancer. If you have one of these HPV strains, your doctor will want to closely monitor you in the future to ensure any precancerous cells are caught early. (Note that only two of the known eighty-five HPV strains manifest as genital warts.)

If you have a normal Pap smear history, have negative HPV testing, and are over thirty years old, the newest guidelines suggest your Pap smear only needs to be done every three years. However, a thorough gynecologic and breast exam should still be performed yearly.

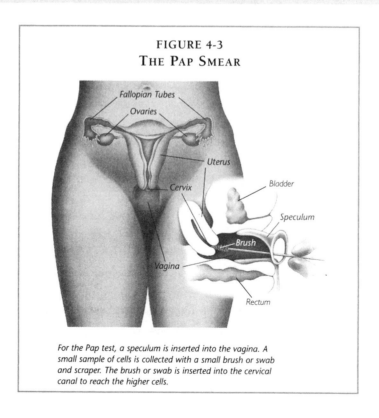

FIGURE 4-3
THE PAP SMEAR

For the Pap test, a speculum is inserted into the vagina. A small sample of cells is collected with a small brush or swab and scraper. The brush or swab is inserted into the cervical canal to reach the higher cells.

Other labs that might be ordered at your doctor's discretion include inflammatory markers (see Chapter 7), a storage form of iron called ferritin (to distinguish iron-deficiency anemia from an anemia of underlying infection or disease), and your vitamin D level. Also, let your doctor know if you eat very undercooked meat or are regularly exposed to cat feces (e.g., while gardening or changing the litter box), as he or she might want to test your blood for exposure to the parasite that causes toxoplasmosis (see Chapters 3 and 13). Your doctor may also want to confirm your immunity to diseases such as chicken pox and rubella, so that you can be vaccinated, if necessary, to protect you from illness before and during pregnancy. If you are a health care worker, it may also be helpful to do parvovirus B19 (commonly known as fifth disease) and cytomegalovirus (CMV) titers to check if you have been exposed to these diseases in the past. If you have immunity to these, then you have nothing to worry about. If you have not been exposed, conscientious use of universal precautions will allow you to reduce your exposure to these diseases, which can lead to health issues in your newborn if contracted during pregnancy. While you're checking your immunization records, ask if you've received a Tdap shot (tetanus booster with pertussis) as an adult. More on that in the next section.

You're now done with the examination part of your preconception evaluation. Let's further explore the topics of immunization and contraceptive methods as they pertain to your time line for getting pregnant.

VACCINATIONS

Margaret is a twenty-eight-year-old kindergarten teacher who has never had chicken pox. Now she and her husband are planning to start trying to conceive. At her annual gynecology exam, her doctor recommends that she get a blood test to see if she has immunity against rubella and chicken pox. Her doctor tells her that getting either disease while pregnant can have a significant effect on the developing fetus. The test found no immunity to either, so she is getting vaccines for both and is told she should not get pregnant for at least a month after the second chicken pox dose is given. She plans to continue her birth control until then.

Many patients are concerned about germs and their potential effects on their baby-to-be. They may be teachers of young children, staff members at facilities for the aged, public health workers, or retail saleswomen who must smilingly take handfuls of bills from customers who have just sneezed all over them. One woman who had worked for years in a preschool began lovingly referring to her classroom as the "germ factory" and her students as "viruses on legs."

Immunization—administered *before* you conceive—against a variety of infectious diseases, including the common flu virus, can protect you and your baby, and is important not only for teachers and health care workers but for everyone. As you have noted in media coverage about whooping cough and measles outbreaks, and new flu strains, disease outbreaks are only a plane flight away. This is also true for childhood diseases such as rubella or German measles, which may require a booster as an adult to maintain your childhood protection against these illnesses. (In fact, virtually all U.S. measles cases today are linked to imported cases contracted in countries where vaccination rates are not as high as they are here in the United States.) Risks associated with receiving vaccinations do exist, but they are rare. And the benefit of avoiding illness and potentially serious complications for both you and your baby far outweigh the risk of vaccination. A number of vaccines are routinely available as part of preconception, and the last dose (for those requiring a series of two or more) should be given at least a month before trying to conceive. We review the most common adult vaccines below, and a list is provided in Table 1-2.

- **Measles, mumps, and rubella (MMR).** Most men and women born before 1957 probably had these diseases. If you were born after 1957 you should have received at least one MMR vaccine, which supplies lifelong immunity 90 to 95 percent of the time. Your doctor can check if you are still immune to rubella with a simple blood test; if you are not immune, it's vital that you be vaccinated with a single-dose booster. If you receive a rubella booster, the CDC recommends that you wait at least twenty-eight days after vaccination before trying to conceive. The risk to the fetus if it is exposed to the vaccine in the first trimester is less than 1 percent. There is serious risk to the fetus as well as an increased risk of miscarriage if rubella is contracted during the first trimester of pregnancy. The bottom line: you can be vaccinated against MMR without concern up to one month prior to trying to conceive. If you are not vaccinated or immune prior to pregnancy, it is common practice to vaccinate you at the hospital after giving birth. (It is perfectly safe for your other children to be vaccinated with MMR if you are trying to conceive or are already pregnant.) About one in four women report joint pain after the MMR vaccination, which can persist for up to three weeks after the vaccination.

(Note: If you inadvertently conceive during the four-week postvaccination waiting period, be reassured that the theoretical risk of vaccine-associated disease in the fetus appears to be extremely low or zero [Source: http://www.cdc.gov/vaccines/pubs/preg-guide.htm]. Use good birth control after vaccination for the recommended time to avoid this concern.)

- **Chicken pox (varicella).** If you missed getting chicken pox in childhood or early adulthood, you should be vaccinated prior to conception because contracting chicken pox in pregnancy can lead to significant maternal and fetal complications. You may have been exposed to someone with chicken pox in the past and have immunity but aren't aware of it; a simple blood test can determine if you are immune to this virus or not. The chicken pox vaccine is a weakened form of the live virus that can grow in the body and produce immunity without causing illness. It is given in two doses four to eight weeks apart. You'll need to wait at least a month to conceive after the *second* dose, so use careful birth control beginning with the first dose. If you do contract chicken pox during pregnancy, you can receive VZIG (varicella zoster immunoglobulin) therapy, which is very expensive but effective if a new infection is caught early enough.

- **Hepatitis B.** If you or your spouse is at high risk for exposure, you should be tested for immunity and vaccinated long before conception. The hepatitis B vaccination schedule is a three-dose regimen; the first two doses are given six weeks apart and the third six months after the first dose. We recommend waiting one month after the last dose before trying to get pregnant (in other words, a delay in conception of seven months from the first dose of the hepatitis B vaccine is advised). Situations of high risk for infection with hepatitis B include:

  - Working in health care
  - Having multiple sex partners
  - Caring for someone infected with hepatitis B
  - Maternal infection (the disease can be transmitted from a mother to her newborn; this is why babies are vaccinated in the hospital after delivery)
  - Receiving clotting factors or blood transfusions
  - Injecting street or illicit drugs (or having a partner who does)

- **Hepatitis A.** This form of hepatitis is usually passed through a contaminated water supply, unsanitary food preparation, or general poor hygiene. The two-dose vaccination is recommended for those who plan to travel to foreign countries where outbreaks occur. As with hepatitis B, starting the vaccination series seven months before conception is best. The first dose of hepatitis A vaccine is followed by a booster six months later for lifelong immunity. If you are not vaccinated and contract hepatitis A in early pregnancy, it can lead to miscarriage and premature birth.

  A newer vaccinate, Twinrix, can combine protection against hepatitis A and B at the same time. The three-dose series is typically completed in six months (follow-up doses are administered one month and six months after the first dose). An alternate four-dose schedule confers immunity within three to four weeks and is attractive for those planning travel in the short term. In this alternate schedule, follow-up doses are administered seven days and twenty-one to thirty days after the first dose, followed by a booster at twelve months. Twinrix is a recombinant vaccine with inactivated virus and is safe to take before pregnancy; complete the series before conception (again, you'll need about seven months to get all three doses).

- **Tetanus.** Most of us have had tetanus shots in childhood, and received tetanus (Td) booster shots every ten years. Check to see if your most recent tetanus booster included pertussis, or whooping cough. You will know it did if the shot was a "Tdap" (which stands for tetanus, diphtheria, and acellular pertussis). If it was a "Td," it did not contain the pertussis component, and you should ask your doctor about being vaccinated with Tdap (pronounced "tee-dap") now. Several states have recently reported a rise in whooping cough cases. The CDC recommends all adults be vaccinated once with Tdap. The CDC says vaccination is *safe at an interval as little as two years since your last Td*, or if you can't remember your last Td (see our note about caregivers on page 98 as well). Being vaccinated not only protects you, it protects your newborn during the first six months of life, when he or she has no innate or acquired immunity yet. If your newborn is infected with whooping cough, he or she is at significant risk for pneumonia, sepsis, and death. Vaccination one month prior to conception is recommended, though it can also be safely administered anytime during pregnancy. If you contract tetanus in pregnancy, fetal death is the result about 60 percent of the time.

- **Pneumococcal pneumonia.** This vaccine is a one-dose regimen and can be given one month prior to conception. It is highly recommended for individuals at high risk for complications of pneumonia, such as those who have had a splenectomy or have lower immunity (due to illness or medication such as chemotherapy). Immunization during the first trimester is not recommended because the effects of the vaccine on the fetus are not yet known.

- **Seasonal flu (influenza).** As you may have already learned, thanks to the H1N1 flu outbreaks, the flu can make people seriously ill. The "regular" or seasonal flu is responsible for an estimated 36,000 deaths each year in the United States. The dehydration that's associated with the illness is especially harmful to pregnant women. Seasonal flu vaccine is best received between September and November, prior to flu season. In a recent *New England Journal of Medicine* study, pregnant women who received injectable flu vaccination in the third trimester not only improved their protection against two of the most prevalent flu types but also passed immunity on to their babies for three to six months after birth. More important, they did not become a source of infection for the newborn. Because the flu vaccine is created specifically for the most aggressive strains from the previous season, it must be given each fall. If you become pregnant before you are vaccinated for the season, it is safe to receive your flu shot anytime during pregnancy. Avoid the nasal mist vaccine once pregnant, as these are live virus versions of the flu vaccine.

- **H1N1.** Also commonly known as the swine flu, it was the newest aggressive seasonal flu of 2009. It contains strains of human, avian, and swine flu. Symptoms of H1N1 are similar to seasonal flu with an additional gastric component that results in nausea, vomiting, and diarrhea. H1N1 in 2009 was particularly virulent to pregnant women and newborns up to the age of six months. Since these two populations are particularly susceptible to H1N1, leading to respiratory compromise, dehydration, hospitalization, and death, vaccinating against it before infection is strongly recommended. We expect a combined flu vaccine in future years that will include the seasonal and H1N1 protection. If you are unable to obtain a vaccine, you can reduce your risk of exposure to these viruses by practicing careful hygiene in public places: thorough hand washing, use of disinfectant gels, and avoidance of sick friends and coworkers.

- **Human Papilloma Virus (HPV).** HPV vaccination is given in a three-dose regimen with two vaccines: Gardasil and Cervarix in the United States. Immunization is provided against the four strains of HPV that cause 70 percent of cervical cancers and 90 percent of warts in North America. The vaccine is given once, then one to two months later, and again six months from the first dose and is not recommended during pregnancy. If you receive the HPV vaccination when, unbeknownst to you pregnancy has already been achieved, you should not be concerned but you should wait to finish the vaccine course until after delivery. To date, no known fetal birth defects have been associated with its use. We recommend that you wait one month from the last dose before conception is attempted.

When it comes to vaccination before pregnancy, an ounce of prevention really is worth a pound of cure! For information on what vaccines your partner may need, see Chapter 9.

 FOR FUTURE REFERENCE: During Pregnancy/After Delivery

Vaccine Updates for All Caregivers of Children

Your partner and anyone else who will stay with you in the early weeks and months after your delivery should check on their vaccination status long before your due date as well. They may need Tdap, seasonal influenza, and H1N1 vaccines. They might benefit from a pneumococcal pneumonia shot or other vaccines they may not have heard about yet (such as a shingles vaccine). Because your baby is not fully vaccinated against most diseases until at least one year of age, you can help protect your baby by ensuring that those in close contact are immune.

CONTRACEPTION

At your preconception visit your doctor may give you the go-ahead to start trying. But he or she also may suggest that you wait a few months to get yourself in prime physical condition. You may need to quit smoking, lose weight, reduce your blood pressure, get a thyroid condition under control, or receive certain vaccinations. This is also the perfect time to determine whether any medication you currently take should be switched to a preconception/pregnancy-

A Word on Pregnancy Spacing

If you already have a child or children and are not racing against your biological clock to get pregnant again, keep in mind that it's best to allow at least eighteen to twenty-four months between pregnancies. This time lets you recover your strength and your best health, return to your normal weight, reduce the risk of anemia, and mentally prepare for the arrival of another little bundle of joy.

If an eighteen-month wait is out of the question for you, use the time between pregnancies to embrace preconception wellness. And, of course, if you happen to be breastfeeding a baby during this interpregnancy interval, it's triply helpful! In a study among women who waited only an average of eleven months to conceive again, those who actively incorporated healthy foods in their diet made a positive impact on both maternal health and fetal growth in their next pregnancy. These women were 50 percent less likely to reenter pregnancy overweight and had better iron stores. The babies from the second pregnancy benefited, too, as they were a little taller and bigger (also less likely to be low-birth-weight) than babies born to moms who didn't have a formal between-pregnancy nutrition plan.

friendly choice or gradually phased out altogether (see Chapter 8 for more detail on this topic). During this time you'll need to use a reliable form of birth control. Contraception is also important if you've recently miscarried and have been told to wait a few months for the green light to start trying again. If you need to hold off becoming pregnant for any reason, remember these rules of thumb:

- Don't automatically assume that the method you're using now is the best. It may be that you'll need to stop using one type and switch to another. For example, if you're currently on the Pill, we advise you to go off it two to three months before trying to conceive, so you can have at least one spontaneous menstrual cycle before conception. Since oral contraceptives increase a woman's need for the vitamin folate (as well as B_6, B_{12}, and the mineral zinc), this offers time to optimize nutrient stores, just in case.

- If you've been on Depo-Provera or recently had Implanon or Norplant removed, you probably won't spontaneously get your period for a few months, but never assume that your fertility won't return sooner than the three-to-six-month waiting period. In the interim for either scenario, use a condom and/or diaphragm (combined with natural family planning if you feel you can determine when you are ovulating) until immediately before trying.

- Even if you've had fertility troubles and haven't used birth control for years, use a reliable contraceptive method until your body is prepared to handle pregnancy. You never know . . .

Of course, any contraception is effective only if it's used correctly. See Table 4-2 for a thorough roundup of contraception methods, effectiveness, and contraindications.

TABLE 4-2
TYPES OF CONTRACEPTION

Hormonal Contraceptives ("The Pill, Patch, and Vaginal Ring")	Methods	Effectiveness (When Used Properly)	Contraindications
Estrogen + progestins	Oral pill daily	98%	Do not use if you have or had: • deep vein thrombosis (DVT) • stroke • high blood pressure • pregnancy • breast cancer • unexplained uterine bleeding
	Vaginal ring or skin patch (use 3 weeks/ off 1 week)		
Progestin only[a]	Oral pill daily		

Notes:

• Taking some medications, particularly those to treat migraines and seizure disorders, can affect your liver, which, in turn, can reduce the effectiveness of oral contraceptives.
• Studies have shown reduced effectiveness among women >198 pounds.
• Stop using 2–3 months before trying to conceive (TTC).

Hormonal Implants	Methods	Effectiveness (When Used Properly)	Contraindications
Norplant (stays in for 5 years)	Progesterone-laden rods implanted under the skin	99%	Do not use if you have or could be: • pregnant • abnormal uterine bleeding
Implanon (stays in for 3 years)			

Notes:

• Remove 3–6 months before TTC.
• Common side effects include irregular bleeding and weight gain (<10 pounds).
• May be less effective among women >200 pounds.
• Rods are sometimes tricky to remove.

a. Progestin-only pills can be used during breastfeeding and for those with medical problems that preclude estrogen use.

Intrauterine Device (IUD)	Methods	Effectiveness (When Used Properly)	Contraindications
Paraguard (copper-coated IUD, lasts 10 years) Mirena (progestin-coated IUD, lasts 5 years)		99%	Do not use if you have or had: • multiple sexual partners • recent uterine or cervical infection • pelvic inflammatory disease • a current pregnancy • abnormal uterine bleeding

Notes:

• Reduced menstrual flow. Normal menses should begin within 1–3 months of removal.
• Effectiveness not limited by weight or medications.
• May pop out in the first year of use (approximately 4%); much more likely if you have had a baby; in fact, the more children you have had, the more likely you are to have an IUD pop out.
• Recommend removal 1–3 months prior to TTC.

Barrier Methods	Methods	Effectiveness (When Used Properly)	Contraindications
Male diaphragm/ condom		85–87%	Do not use if you have or had: • Allergy to latex (use latex-free alternatives)
Female condom		75%	• You have tried this method before unsuccessfully (i.e.,
Diaphragm (fit by health care provider[b])		85%	you had an unplanned pregnancy)
Sponge/cervical cap		75–80%	

Notes:

• Can stop using immediately before TTC.
• Frequent vaginal infections and urinary tract infections are possible with use of the diaphragm, cervical cap, and sponges.

b. Must be refit if between pregnancies, or with weight loss or gain more than 15–20 pounds.

Natural Family Planning	Methods	Effectiveness (When Used Properly)	Contraindications
Standard days method	Women with cycles 26–32 days in length should avoid unprotected intercourse on days 8–19.	30–98%[c]	Discuss this method with your doctor if: • you lack commitment to carefully observing signs of fertility • pregnancy is inadvisable due to a medical condition
Symptothermal method	Use three fertility signs: basal body temperature, cervical mucus secretions, and position/feel of cervix.		

Notes:

• Can immediately TTC.
• Tools to help monitor the ovulatory cycle include basal body temperature thermometers, charts, and saliva-testing microscopes (to look for a "ferning" pattern due to peak estrogen levels at time of ovulation), and electrolyte detectors that predict ovulation based on changes in electrolyte levels in the saliva.

c. Success varies widely based on the woman's ability to predict ovulation and the couple's willingness to abstain during the fertile window. The upper end of the effectiveness range reflects those couples adhering perfectly to a method that works for them. For more information, see http://www.irh.org/nfp.htm.

Review with your doctor the best type of contraception for your needs until you begin trying to conceive. In the meantime, you may want to know more about how the reproductive system works. You'll find this in the next chapter!

CHAPTER 5

Gynecologic and Obstetrical Factors That Influence Conception and Delivery

*W*hen patients voice concerns about their fertility, it's often surprising how little information—or how much misinformation—even the most educated women have about the hows and whys of their reproductive system.

> *Danielle, age thirty-two, phoned her ob-gyn: "I know this is TMI (too much information), but for a few days every month I get this clear, slippery discharge when I use the bathroom. I've even seen a long "string" of it stretching down into the bowl (whoah!). I want to make sure I don't have a recurring infection."*

> *Martha, a twenty-eight-year-old teacher whose husband travels frequently for business, told me she was concerned about conceiving because "I can get pregnant on only one day of the month, right?"*

> *During a recent annual checkup Anna, a thirty-year-old advertising executive, told me, "I get a period every month at the same time. I know I must be ovulating."*

In this chapter we dispel the myths of how reproduction works and uncover the mystery (and wonder) of the female body. We'll also discuss some of the most common obstetrical and gynecological problems that can have a negative impact on your fertility.

Your reproductive system is in the baby-making business. From puberty until menopause, your body is responding to an elaborate concert of hormones, trying to prepare for conception every month. Ultimately, conception is fairly simple: if you can be a little patient, engage in intercourse at the right times, and let nature take its course, you will usually become pregnant with no more intervention than some candlelight and romantic music.

THE PLAYERS IN YOUR REPRODUCTIVE SYSTEM

Unlike male anatomy, which is in plain sight, the female reproductive organs are hidden from view, perhaps adding to the mystery. So let's briefly review the basics (see Figure 5-1).

- The **vulva, or external genitalia,** protects the entrance to the vagina and also houses the clitoris, a source of sexual stimulation. Although not yet irrefutably proven, studies suggest that the uterine contractions during orgasm can help propel sperm toward the egg, which may improve the odds of conceiving.

- The **vagina** is the muscular passageway through which sperm travel into the female reproductive system. The fluids produced in the vagina affect the pH level (acidity) of the vagina, in turn affecting the function of sperm and even your comfort. Normal vaginal pH is slightly acidic. Certain medications, such as antibiotics, can lower the vaginal pH and change the balance of natural vaginal flora (a.k.a. bacteria), making it less hospitable for the "good guys" but more so for the bacteria and yeast which are normally held in check.

- The **cervix** is located at the end of the vagina. As the entrance to the uterus, it is the gatekeeper to the whole system. It opens minimally during ovulation, to allow sperm in, and then widely nine months later, to let the baby out. The cervix also responds to monthly hormonal fluctuations by producing different types of vaginal mucus, which either assist or impede sperm travel. The clear, slippery, stretchy mucus noted by Danielle on the previous page is actually the hallmark of the fertile window, when ovulation is about to occur.

- The **uterus,** although normally the size of only a fist or a pear, stretches easily to accommodate a full-term infant. The walls are made of three layers: an outer membrane, a middle layer of muscle, and an inner layer called the endometrium. The last is what sheds monthly when you are not pregnant and provides a "nest" in which a fertilized embryo implants and grows when you are pregnant.

- The **fallopian tubes** are where fertilization actually occurs. The tubes, approximately four inches long, capture the eggs released from the ovaries each month during ovulation and then shuttle them along to the uterus. Interestingly, a woman can still conceive even following pelvic surgery that leaves her with one fallopian tube on one side and one ovary on the other. The odds are reduced, but the egg can still find its way to the opposite fallopian tube because these internal organs are in close proximity. The fringelike ends of the fallopian tubes undulate, causing the egg to travel to whichever tube is encouraging its passage.

- The **ovaries** contain all the eggs a woman will ever produce—she is born with approximately 1 million. By puberty, only 300,000 eggs remain for ovulation, and fertilization.

A woman will release approximately 400 eggs in her lifetime. The ovaries are also where the hormones estrogen and progesterone are produced; these are the major hormonal players in reproduction. The ovaries respond to two chemical signals from the brain: follicle-stimulating hormone (FSH), which tells them to get an egg ready, and luteinizing hormone (LH), which tells them to release the egg, known as ovulation. (Ovulation predictor kits measure a surge in the LH level, which precedes ovulation.)

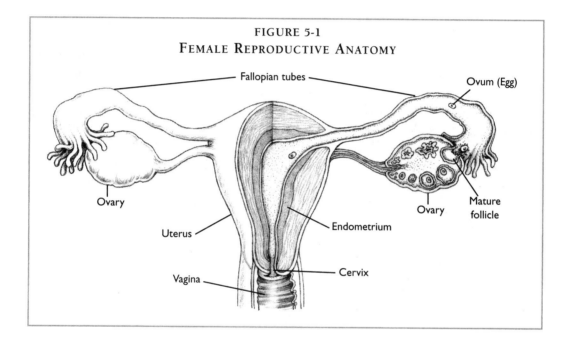

FIGURE 5-1
FEMALE REPRODUCTIVE ANATOMY

THE MENSTRUAL CYCLE

The mystery of reproduction begins with the menstrual cycle, which we can break down into two parts. The first part of the cycle, known as the *follicular phase,* begins on the day your period starts and lasts until you ovulate. The second part, known as the *luteal phase,* spans the time after ovulation until you bleed again. The length of these phases differs from woman to woman, as a normal cycle can range from twenty-four to thirty-five days. In fact, your menstrual cycle can change throughout your reproductive lifetime: the number of days between periods, the duration of each period, the heaviness of flow, and even the premenstrual symptoms may vary as you grow older, and as you have children.

Twins: The Exception to the Rule

One in 250 women will have identical twins—when one fertilized egg divides in half to create two identical embryos. While this rate has stayed relatively consistent over time and throughout the world, the likelihood of fraternal twins—two separate eggs fertilized by two different sperm—has, according to the National Center on Health Statistics, increased to about 1 in 31 (or about 3 percent). While this may seem high, remember that this average includes women of all ages, a portion of whom have had reproductive assistance. The dramatic increase in twinning is largely due to two factors: advanced maternal age at conception and the technology of assisted reproduction. Among women under thirty-five who conceive without medical intervention, 1 in 89 women will have fraternal twins.

Women in their late thirties and forties are more likely to conceive twins (the rate is approximately 4 to 5 percent), perhaps because older follicles release eggs more readily. The odds of triplets and higher-order multiples has increased dramatically in the last two decades, although these cases are on the decline due to advances in reproductive technology that mean fewer embryos need to be transferred. It is estimated that fewer than 20 percent of all triplets were spontaneously conceived.

Twinning doesn't skip generations, as people used to think, although twins do run in families. If you are a twin, your chance of having twins is about 1 in 54. If your partner is a twin, your chance of conceiving twins is 1 in 125. African Americans are slightly more likely to have twins than Caucasians, and Asians are the least likely to conceive twins.

The First Half of the Cycle: Follicular Phase

From the first day of your period, every month in your reproductive life, a simple message is sent from the brain to the ovaries: "Let's get that egg ready so it can get out there and be fertilized!" The ovaries don't always hear this message, but we'll get back to that later. In the first days of this phase, your brain produces FSH to instruct your ovaries to prepare an egg for release. Upon receiving this message, your ovaries produce estrogen, which stimulates the eggs within them to mature. The FSH also triggers changes in your cervical mucus a few days prior to ovulation, making it clear, slippery, and stretchy—similar to uncooked egg whites—so that it is easier for sperm to travel through it to meet (or wait for) the newly released egg.

Eggs form within a follicle, a small fluid-filled sac in the ovary. Each month, several follicles are prepared to release an egg, but only one follicle is ultimately "chosen" to release its egg (or occasionally two eggs) that cycle. This egg contains half of your genetic blueprint and, if it is lucky, will encounter a "chosen" sperm that contains the other half of the blueprint to make a baby. The "chosen" egg is released from its follicle, that is, ovulation occurs, after your brain produces a surge in LH—usually twelve to sixteen days, sometimes longer, after the beginning of your menstrual cycle (see Figure 5-2).

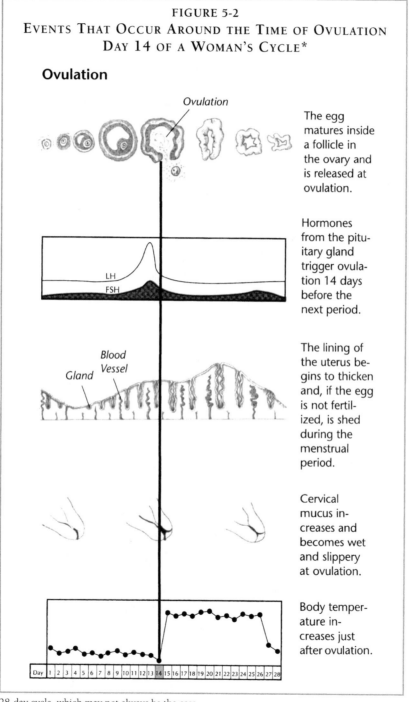

FIGURE 5-2
EVENTS THAT OCCUR AROUND THE TIME OF OVULATION
DAY 14 OF A WOMAN'S CYCLE*

Ovulation

Ovulation

The egg matures inside a follicle in the ovary and is released at ovulation.

LH
FSH

Hormones from the pituitary gland trigger ovulation 14 days before the next period.

Gland *Blood Vessel*

The lining of the uterus begins to thicken and, if the egg is not fertilized, is shed during the menstrual period.

Cervical mucus increases and becomes wet and slippery at ovulation.

Body temperature increases just after ovulation.

Day 1 2 3 4 5 6 7 8 9 10 11 12 13 14 15 16 17 18 19 20 21 22 23 24 25 26 27 28

*Assuming a 28-day cycle, which may not always be the case.

The Second Half of the Cycle: Luteal Phase

As the egg travels through your fallopian tubes, the follicle from which the egg was released becomes a corpus luteum (an ovarian cyst that is left over after the egg is released) and produces progesterone. This rise in progesterone increases your basal body temperature—one of the important cues that you have likely ovulated. Progesterone stimulates growth and blood vessel migration in the uterine lining to provide a safe haven for the fertilized egg to implant. The corpus luteum will continue to produce progesterone until the placenta takes over at eight to ten weeks of pregnancy.

If you don't conceive, the system starts to break down in order for a new cycle to start. The lining of the uterus sheds, taking the unfertilized egg with it. Your menstrual cycle begins again with the first day of bleeding (usually fourteen days after ovulation). Undaunted, your reproductive system just tells your brain that the last cycle was a no-go for conception and initiates the whole cycle again to prepare a new egg for the promise of fertilization.

PREMENSTRUAL SYNDROME (PMS)

Symptoms of PMS usually include some or all of the following, in mild to severe form, during the late luteal phase before your period starts:

- Abdominal bloating
- Breast tenderness
- Headaches
- Changes in appetite or food cravings
- Irritability and moodiness, anxiety, or depression

Tanya, age twenty-nine, had been on birth control pills ever since college to manage severe PMS and for contraception. She recently discontinued the Pill in order to start a family. Now she is experiencing the full force of her PMS symptoms again. She is comfortable taking an analgesic for a few days out of the month, but wants to try natural methods as well—foods, supplements, or herbs.

Ava, age thirty-eight, has a four-year-old son who was conceived after about seven months of trying. She recently went off birth control pills so she and her husband could try for a second child. Ava was surprised by the increased severity of her PMS symptoms. She dreads the thought of going through this every month if it takes them a while to conceive again.

Whether you have always battled PMS or are now unfortunately all too familiar with the symptoms, you may wonder if there is anything to the natural remedies you've heard about.

Though we don't have much conclusive research on nonpharmacologic approaches, some solid lifestyle and dietary improvements should make a difference. While most of natural remedies show conflicting results, demonstrate no effect at all, or have yet to be put to the test, we offer the latest information (below). We recommend that you try to meet nutritional recommendations primarily from eating a well-balanced diet, but a multivitamin-mineral supplement and omega-3s will help close any gaps. You can find more detail regarding herbs and supplements in Chapter 8 and nutritional recommendations in Chapters 10 to 14.

The following suggestions to reduce the severity of PMS symptoms are useful if implemented daily, but most effective for PMS if incorporated into your lifestyle daily from day of cycle (DOC) 14 through the first day of menses.

Lifestyle Adjustments

- **Moderate physical activity and balanced, regular meals**—don't skip breakfast, in particular! These fundamentals of a healthy lifestyle do improve symptoms, but better studies are needed to quantify their impact.

- **Stress management**—techniques to reduce stress complement dietary and lifestyle changes. These include time management, adequate sleep, and cognitive behavioral therapy in severe cases (either with the support of a therapist or learning self-help techniques such as visualization, self-talk, and biofeedback).

Dietary Recommendations—Nutrients That Stand Out in Their Effectiveness Against PMS Symptoms

- **Calcium**—1,000–1,200 mg per day, mostly from food sources, will meet and modestly exceed ordinary preconception requirements.

- **Vitamin D**—about 400–1,000 IU is recommended for women of childbearing potential, and you're encouraged to be screened and treated for this common deficiency (see Chapter 11 for risk factors). It's not easy to get all of your vitamin D from foods alone, so meeting this preconception requirement will likely involve some degree of supplementation.

- **Magnesium**—310–320 mg per day, mostly from food sources, will meet the preconception recommendation and perhaps reduce PMS-related headaches.

- **Omega-3 fats**—natural sources of omega-3 fats are highly recommended, and a small but promising area of research supports modest supplementation with fish oil (or possibly krill oil, though additional studies are needed to confirm this).

- **Vitamin B₆**—1.9 mg per day. Despite many claims of efficacy, evidence for supplementation above preconception requirements is too conflicting; aim for the current recommendation. If you still choose to supplement, keep in mind that the upper limit of safety is 100 mg B₆ per day from foods and supplements combined.

Herbal Supplements to Reduce PMS Symptoms

- **Chasteberry (*Vitex agnus-castus*)**—of all the herbal remedies touted for aiding PMS sufferers, this is the only one to date that stands up under scientific scrutiny. However, it may dampen your interest in sex and is only loosely regulated as a supplement. If taken at all, it should be stopped two to four weeks before trying to conceive.

- **Evening primrose oil**—the little research available on this supplement suggests that it is only helpful for reducing cyclical breast tenderness and is ineffective in reducing other PMS symptoms.

WHEN YOUR CYCLE DOESN'T FOLLOW THE RULES

There are a number of ways that women's menstrual cycles can vary from the norm: they may be longer or shorter, heavier or lighter, or absent altogether. Figuring out why these variations occur can help us diagnose and try to correct a fertility problem. Here are some of the most common menstrual irregularities and a discussion of what they may mean.

Amenorrhea: When the Menstrual Cycle Is Absent

In most but not all cases, a lack of bleeding signals a lack of ovulation. However, just because you get a period doesn't mean you ovulate (this phenomenon is explained in the shadow box on the next page). The most common reasons for the lack of a menstrual cycle include:

- Pregnancy
- Rapid loss of weight (with or without extreme exercise activity)
- Polycystic ovary syndrome (PCOS)
- Significant psychological stress
- Cessation of contraceptive hormones, such as birth control pills or shots
- Breastfeeding

How Is It Possible to Have a Period and Not Ovulate?

In medical terms, having a period without prior ovulation is called breakthrough bleeding or dysfunctional uterine bleeding (DUB). To recap the basics, estrogen prepares an egg follicle for release and the uterine lining for implantation. Progesterone is produced by the corpus luteum to sustain the lining for implantation. However, if ovulation does not occur, progesterone is not released. The uterine lining continues to build under the presence of declining estrogen levels until it can't sustain itself any longer and sheds, seen by you as bleeding.

Distinguishing between a "real" period and DUB is tricky. The hallmarks of DUB are irregular cycle lengths and bleeding, sometimes preceded by spotting or brownish blood. So, if Anna (from the first page of this chapter) had trouble conceiving, knowing these details about her cycle might help pinpoint a subtle issue like this.

Less common causes for the lack of menses include:

- Dramatic increases in exercise load; chronic over-exercising
- Extremes of reproductive age
- Disturbances in the levels of thyroid hormone and/or prolactin hormone
- Premature ovarian failure (early menopause)
- Asherman's syndrome (uterine cavity scarring after surgical procedures)
- Travel, accompanied by time changes

If you miss two periods (and you are not on medication with this goal in mind, such as an oral contraceptive), or if you have two consecutive cycles that are forty or more days long, you should seek medical consultation. The first thing your practitioner will recommend is a urine pregnancy test. If this is negative, the workup moves on to hormones that control your menstrual cycle, specifically those that come from the brain.

Hormones produced in the *pituitary gland,* which rests behind the eyes, include *thyroid-stimulating hormone (TSH),* which controls your metabolism, and *prolactin,* which regulates breastmilk production and can cause uterine contractions. Both thyroid hormone and prolactin levels are easily checked by a blood test anytime during the menstrual cycle.

Changes in your thyroid hormones can control how you ovulate, how you gain or lose weight, and your general feeling of well-being. Symptoms of low thyroid hormone, known as hypothyroidism, include fatigue, constipation, and constantly feeling cold. Thyroid hormone can be replaced with oral medication that is safe to take before, during, and after pregnancy. Treatment of an underactive thyroid is generally lifelong, as you need to maintain a normal metabolic rate regardless of your fertility plans.

If your thyroid produces too much hormone, a condition known as hyperthyroidism, you may be jittery, overly energetic, and unusually warm, and you may have heart palpitations. Hyperthyroidism is also associated with changes in the eyes that make people look "bug-eyed" and the formation of a goiter (swelling of the thyroid) in the throat. In this situation, medical therapy and restoration of normal thyroid function are essential to restore fertility and ensure maternal and fetal health. Correcting hyperthyroidism (see Chapter 7 for details about thyroid disease) will help restore normal menstrual cycles with more predictable ovulation and reduce the incidence of early pregnancy miscarriage. Thyroid imbalances (both elevations and reductions in the thyroid hormone) should be corrected and monitored for several months to be sure they are normal before you try to conceive.

If blood tests show that your prolactin level is high, you may also notice nipple discharge (usually milky), headaches, or visual changes. These changes may or may not mean there is a benign mass on the pituitary gland called a *prolactinoma*. This mass, if present, can be detected through blood tests and imaging with X-ray, CAT scan, or MRI. Overproduction of prolactin can be reversed with the medication Parlodel (bromocriptine), which restores normal menstrual cycles and ovulation 85 to 90 percent of the time. Parlodel may be continued until you conceive (pregnancy is naturally a high-prolactin state). Surgical intervention to remove a prolactinoma is rarely recommended.

The next step is a progesterone withdrawal, or challenge, test, which gives your doctor a chance to see how your body responds to a decline of progesterone during the second half of your menstrual cycle. The typical challenge is a seven- to ten-day course of a progesterone-containing prescription product, such as Provera 10 mg or Prometrium 200 mg (a "natural" progesterone alternative made in the laboratory from an inedible variety of wild yam; see the herbal section in Chapter 8). The choice of progesterone products for this challenge will depend on a combination of your doctor's preferences and how you have responded to using progesterone-containing products in the past.

If you have a period after completing a course of Provera or Prometrium, it suggests that your reproductive hormonal system is intact and can be restarted. More precisely, you are likely producing sufficient estrogen to build up the uterine lining, but you are probably not ovulating on your own. However, if you do not have a period up to seven days after you have stopped the oral progesterone agents, it means you are not producing sufficient estrogen to build up your uterine lining enough to cause bleeding upon progesterone withdrawal. Blood tests for FSH may be recommended to rule out early menopause (more about this later).

Asherman's Syndrome

A rare complication of surgical procedures such as a dilation and curettage (D&C) of the uterus can cause *scarring in the uterus,* leading to absent or scanty periods. Known as Asherman's syndrome, this condition can be diagnosed with a hysterosalpingogram (an X-ray using a dye for contrast). The X-ray image helps identify blockage in the fallopian tubes or irregularities in the uterus. (For those with an iodine allergy, a sonohysterogram ultrasound with saline injected into the uterus can be used instead.) Another test, called hysteroscopy, uses a telescope to visually inspect the uterine cavity under local or general anesthesia. This latter option also provides an opportunity for treatment at the time of diagnosis. Removing any uterine adhesions should be done by an experienced hysteroscopist, who is often a reproductive endocrinologist or infertility specialist.

Polycystic Ovary Syndrome (PCOS)

Polycystic ovary syndrome (PCOS) is a chronic lack of ovulation that affects 5 to 10 percent of reproductive-age women. It is the most common cause of ovulatory dysfunction in the United States. This condition is caused by an imbalance of hormones, including the male hormone testosterone (which is an important hormone for females, too) as well as estrogen and progesterone. Women with PCOS usually form small ovarian cysts, which make your ovaries on an ultrasound look like they are surrounded by a "pearl necklace" of small, benign, fluid-filled sacs. These can clear up spontaneously, but if they grow they can be painful.

You may suspect PCOS if you (or your mother, aunt, or grandmother) have these symptoms:

- Menstrual cycles that are irregular, very heavy, or scant, and fewer than eight periods per year
- Acne
- Unwanted hair growth on the face, chest, and abdomen
- Difficulty losing weight or carrying extra weight primarily around the waist
- Patchy skin discoloration, hair thinning, or baldness
- Medical problems, such as high blood pressure and diabetes, occurring at a younger age than usual
- Unexplained infertility

Reaching a diagnosis of PCOS can be challenging for the clinician, as a woman may have no symptoms or all the symptoms but no obvious shift in hormone levels. Other women may have irregularities in FSH and LH ratios. While this ratio was once thought to be diagnostic of PCOS, it doesn't detect half of all cases. Alternatives for diagnosis include a blood test to see if you have any increase in testosterone, which may explain why a woman is not ovulating or is ovulating only sporadically. Another androgen called dehydroepiandrosterone sulfate (DHEAS) may be measured as well, to see if there are adrenal gland issues to address. Your doctor will

Weight Loss and PCOS

A word of caution about sensible weight loss and PCOS: a high-protein/low-carb/calorie-restricted diet can throw the body into a state of ketosis (incomplete fat breakdown). This condition is dangerous, especially in the early weeks of fetal brain development. Instead, we encourage gradual weight loss; it's best to cut no more than roughly 250 to 500 calories per day (and expend another few hundred through exercise) before you conceive.

To achieve a healthy, balanced diet, we advocate consuming about 40 to 50 percent of calories as carbohydrates, with unprocessed carb sources and those with a low glycemic index preferable to refined starches and sugars. Such foods have the most modest impact on after-meal glucose levels and may help ease carb cravings, making weight management easier.[a] (For more information, see the "Carbohydrates" section of Chapter 10.) For the rest of your calorie intake, 20 to 25 percent should be protein[b] and the remainder should be fat, primarily unsaturated types, including ready sources of omega-3 fats. A registered dietitian's help is also recommended.

a. Choosing low-glycemic-index carbohydrates is a hot topic in PCOS research. Though consensus has not been reached, the bulk of anecdotal and scientific evidence is supportive and worthy of further research.

b. Make sure to include plenty of proteins of plant origin and fewer red meats.

recommend the best time during your cycle to do hormonal testing, usually a few days after your period has started (whether on its own or as the result of a progesterone withdrawal).

A diagnosis of PCOS can also be very challenging from a fertility perspective. Women with this condition often do not ovulate independently, and when ovulation does occur they may still have trouble getting or staying pregnant. Invasive (not to mention expensive) fertility choices such as IVF often fail unless fitness and nutrition (a.k.a. lifestyle) changes are implemented first. Regular physical activity (four or more hours of exercise per week, spread out over several days) accompanied by sensible eating has been shown to improve the hormonal profile of women with PCOS. Research has found that this improvement persists regardless of whether the woman's weight is considered normal or high. Very little weight loss may be sufficient to see an improvement. What may be most important is a decrease in the amount of fat around the belly. Slight reductions in girth may improve insulin sensitivity and restore normal menstrual function. It's prudent to delay pharmaceutical intervention to aid fertility until lifestyle changes have been aggressively pursued for a few months because this may be all it takes.

Encouraging new research has shed light on the link between PCOS and *insulin resistance,* a known culprit of ovulatory problems and pregnancy complications. This is when tissue cells

Now, About That Waistline...

You may hope that sit-ups will spot-reduce around the middle. They won't. To really get at the visceral fat deep in the abdominal area, experts suggest including vigorous activity for several of your workouts, based on your individual capability. This means if you're usually a brisk walker, incorporate intervals of jogging several days a week. Though larger studies are needed, this one may be particularly relevant because it included reproductive-age overweight women who shared some of the symptoms of PCOS.

For some women with PCOS, increased appetite and carbohydrate cravings may lead to binge eating and difficulty with weight control. Higher levels of testosterone mean that extra fat is carried in the abdominal area instead of around the hips and thighs. Obese women with PCOS and abnormal periods respond beautifully to a six-month gradual weight-loss program, including nutrition counseling, exercise, and behavior modification. Most who seriously embrace this route are able to resume normal periods in four to five months. They typically are able to conceive (spontaneously or with interventions that previously failed) and carry a healthy baby to term.

become less responsive to insulin's message to let glucose in, and the glucose builds up in the bloodstream. Correcting the insulin resistance greatly improves fertility. Lab testing to identify insulin resistance includes oral glucose tolerance tests, insulin levels, and glycosylated hemoglobin (A1C). This has led to new trends in therapy for women with PCOS, starting with nutrition and exercise interventions, two things that cannot be ignored even if time is of the essence (see the "Weight Loss and PCOS" shadow box if weight reduction is recommended). If the conservative measures of diet and regular physical activity do not work, the drug metformin may be added to reduce insulin resistance and restore a more normal hormonal milieu, and Clomid may also be prescribed to encourage ovulation. A synergy between these approaches may expedite restoration of fertility. When metformin is taken for an extended duration of time (over two years) or at a daily dosage above 1,000 mg, vitamin B_{12} levels should be monitored.

Women with PCOS who have hirsutism (abnormal hair growth) often take a diuretic known as spironolactone. This medication is not recommended in pregnancy because the hormone changes it triggers may affect male offspring by reducing the effectiveness of their testosterone during development. With this in mind, spironolactone should be discontinued when attempts to conceive start.

FOR FUTURE REFERENCE:
During Pregnancy/After Delivery/Family Life

What Is the Impact of PCOS on Pregnancy, Breastfeeding, and Later Health?

When you have a history of PCOS and you are pregnant, your risks of gestational diabetes and pregnancy-induced hypertension are greater than for a woman without the same history. Maintaining the good exercise and dietary habits from preconception will help reduce your risks during pregnancy. You may be asked to gain less weight than average to assist in reducing health risks. Also, you may undergo closer surveillance, such as earlier blood sugar testing and more frequent blood pressure checks, resulting in more appointments for prenatal care.

When your baby is born, make sure to seek out the assistance and advice of a certified lactation consultant. They are usually on staff at the hospital or in your pediatrician's office and can help ensure that your breastfeeding goes smoothly in the early weeks. A history of PCOS may pose easily correctable difficulties, such as a slight decrease in milk supply. Regular checkups for your baby will determine whether your baby is gaining weight and can confirm that your milk supply is adequate. Then resume your healthy lifestyle so you can keep up with the kids, get back into your favorite jeans, and, perhaps most important, maintain your fertility and well-being.

Less Common Causes of Menstrual Irregularity

Sue, forty-two, came in for an annual visit, complaining, "My cycle was always twenty-eight days, like clockwork, and now it's been forty-six days and a urine pregnancy test was negative. This has never happened before. Am I menopausal? Will I still be able to get pregnant?"

Many women in their early to mid-forties experience changes in their cycle. This is the unpredictable world of perimenopause: a time before menopause when cycle irregularity may begin. In other words, you're still ovulating, but not predictably or necessarily every month. You may experience a missed period and then make up for it by bleeding twice the following month. If you're considering conception during this time, missed or irregular periods can be prohibitive and frustrating. These irregularities are often perfectly in keeping with what Mother Nature plans for all women, but we recommend that you seek medical attention to confirm your good gynecological health.

Sara, an extremely active thirty-four-year-old mother of two, was trying to conceive her third child when her menstrual cycle just stopped. Three urine pregnancy tests were negative. She reduced her workout intensity and gained six pounds, but after ninety days without a period and increasing hot flashes she went to her doctor to discuss the problem. Blood tests indicated she was in early menopause.

Premature ovarian failure, better known as *early menopause,* occurs when ovulation and the menstrual cycle completely stop prior to age thirty-five. This is a rare phenomenon, diagnosed by testing your blood FSH levels twice, at least a few weeks apart. The causes of premature ovarian failure are poorly understood, though occasionally it follows an inherited pattern (e.g., mother and daughter both suffer from the problem). If you want to consider conception under these conditions, consult a reproductive endocrinologist right away. Egg donation is your best chance, although it is fraught with ethical and legal dilemmas and can be emotionally stressful and financially challenging.

Another unusual cause of menstrual irregularity or cessation is fluctuations in steroid levels—either too little or too much. These conditions are known as *Addison's disease* or *Cushing's disease,* respectively. Steroids are the building blocks for most hormones in our body. An imbalance of steroids can be diagnosed by blood tests and treated with medication. Normal menstrual cycles should resume within three months of treatment.

If Your Periods Are Too Frequent or Too Heavy

For some women it is not a lack of periods that concerns them but a too frequent or too heavy menstrual cycle. Though hormonal imbalances can be the culprit, the majority of these cases are caused by abnormal (though primarily benign) growths in the reproductive tract. Some of these growths, such as *uterine fibroids* (see Figure 5-3), are actually fairly common and go unnoticed unless they cause symptoms.

Irene, a thirty-one-year-old married woman, came in after trying to conceive for three years. She had a history of heavy menstrual cycles, and on the worst day she changed a sanitary napkin every two hours. For the past six months she had been experiencing worsening cramping with her cycle. An examination revealed that her uterus was two and a half times normal size. The ultrasound scan showed two uterine fibroids, one potentially blocking the entrance of the right fallopian tube into the uterus.

Common reasons for heavy menstrual periods include:

- **Fibroids.** Smooth muscle masses that grow on the surface of the uterus, in the uterine wall, or into the uterine cavity (see Figure 5-3), fibroids are usually discovered during a routine pelvic exam or ultrasound. They are benign the majority of the time and are thought to be dependent on estrogen, which is why they often grow during pregnancy, when estrogen is at its highest level. Up to 20 percent of women have fibroids that produce symptoms such as heavier bleeding or a fullness in the abdomen. Black women are more likely to have symptomatic fibroids, for reasons that remain unclear. (See pages 119–121 for more information.)

- **Endometriosis.** This condition occurs when endometrial tissue that implants outside the uterus responds to the hormonal stimulation of ovulation and menstrual cycling, causing cyclic pain that can occur at midcycle or before the menstrual period. Over time, the bleeding and scarring from endometriosis can cause fallopian tube blockage and continuous pelvic pain, particularly during intercourse. Read "Complementary Care of Endometriosis (below) and see Chapter 18 for more detailed information on this condition.

Complementary Care and Endometriosis

The chronic pain that accompanies endometriosis can affect your whole life, and your general sense of well-being may be almost nonexistent. A healthy lifestyle that includes physical activity combined with healthy food can go a long way toward helping endometriosis sufferers feel better. You'll benefit most from regular moderate-to-high-intensity activities. Mind-body exercise such as yoga is very helpful for women dealing with endometriosis. Although formal study is scant, it is believed that deep breathing and balance exercises, such as yoga or Pilates, stimulate the release of natural painkillers (known as endorphins) and modify the brain's pain pathways.

Women with endometriosis are no different from other women planning for conception. They need a balanced diet, emphasizing vegetables and fruits as well as keeping protein sources varied (thereby limiting red meat), according to the USDA's MyPyramid (more on this in Chapter 12). What makes these women unique, though, is their tendency to be more sensitive to abdominal discomfort if their intake of carbohydrates lacks variety or is not evenly spread out over the day. A balanced approach is even more important for comfort's sake. The health of the endometrium is also bolstered by ensuring you consume the following nutrients: omega-3 dietary fats and dietary fiber (discussed in Chapter 10), vitamins C, E, and A (or beta-carotene), and the minerals calcium, selenium, and zinc (detailed in Chapter 11).

If you are considering taking an herbal remedy to alleviate gynecological pain, your top priority is to assess whether the product is safe for preconception and, equally important, whether it is effective. Although there are no known herbal cures for endometriosis, warm soothing decaffeinated herbal teas are what we recommend most often. Please refer to our herb safety tables in Chapter 8 before trying any herbal tea or remedy.

- **Polyps.** These are finger-like projections that emerge from the endometrial lining and are almost always benign. Some fertility experts believe that polyps can interfere with fertility by blocking the fallopian tubes or increasing the risk of miscarriage. They can be diagnosed with ultrasound or hysteroscopy and can be left untreated if they are not growing or blocking the fallopian tube openings. If you are trying to conceive and polyps are present, most reproductive endocrinologists will recommend removing the polyps to create a more hospitable uterine lining for the embryo to implant. The hysteroscopy procedure used to remove endometrial polyps is minimally invasive.

- **Endometrial hyperplasia.** This is an overgrowth of the uterine lining caused by too much estrogen exposure, either from medication or from high levels caused by PCOS and obesity. Symptoms include irregular vaginal bleeding between cycles and excessive bleeding during menses. Endometrial hyperplasia is more prevalent in women over the age of forty. It can be diagnosed by in-office endometrial biopsy, dilation and curettage (D&C), or hysteroscopy, and can be treated with medication if there is no evidence of atypical or abnormal cells.

- **Infection in the endometrial lining (endometritis).** Infection can occur after any surgical procedure that involves the cervix or uterus such as endometrial biopsy, D&C, or cervical cone biopsy. Cramping and an odorous vaginal discharge are the most common symptoms. Treatment with antibiotics should restore normal periods and reduce the incidence of scarring in the uterus and tubes, which could prohibit conception.

A Little More Information About Fibroids

Fibroids are the most common source of abnormal uterine bleeding in reproductive-age women. The medical community still does not know for sure why some women develop fibroids and others who experience the same shifting hormonal patterns do not. Often found incidentally during your pelvic exam, it is the size or position of the fibroids that determines whether they pose problems for fertility or future pregnancies (see Figure 5-3). Treatment is individualized, depending on the severity of symptoms, the woman's desire for conception, and how quickly the fibroids are growing. If a woman has no symptoms prior to pregnancy and the fibroids are not pressing on other organs, observation without additional intervention is often the norm. Fibroids are almost always benign, but if there is rapid growth, a tumor called a sarcoma may be the reason. Regular physical exams by your doctor and/or regular ultrasound evaluation will help determine if there is any concern. When fibroids are suspected and there are no other fertility issues, the physician will likely recommend a hysterosalpingogram or sonohysterogram. These diagnostic techniques can help determine if fibroids are blocking the fallopian tubes, which could make it difficult to get or stay pregnant. Fibroids are rarely the sole source of infertility problems. However, if a complete infertility evaluation determines that fibroids are preventing you from conceiving, you may want to undergo surgery for fibroid removal, known as myomectomy. Unfortunately, myomectomy can lead to significant blood loss and postoperative scarring, which itself may block your tubes and prevent conception. The chance of fibroid recurrence can be as high as 20 percent after surgery. As with all surgery, you and your physician will want to assess the risks and benefits of the procedure to determine if it is in your best interest. If you choose to have surgery, you can usually begin trying to conceive three to six months afterward, but do discuss this with your doctor.

FIGURE 5-3
POSSIBLE FIBROID LOCATIONS IN THE UTERUS

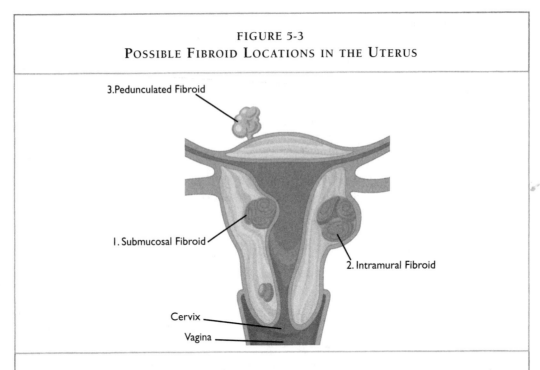

1 Fibroids pressing into the uterine cavity may distort it and increase the risk for miscarriage. These are submucosal fibroids.

2 Fibroids present in the middle layer of the uterus may increase the size or bulk of the uterus but may not affect the cavity or impinge on the fallopian tubes. These are known as intramural fibroids.

3 Fibroids that are protruding outside the bulk of the uterus are rarely a problem during pregnancy (except for discomfort to the mother). They are called pedunculated or subserosal fibroids.

FOR FUTURE REFERENCE: Before Delivery

How Prior Fibroid Surgery (Myomectomy) Factors into Your Delivery Plan

If you had a myomectomy before pregnancy, it is vital to know whether the uterine cavity was entered or not during the procedure. If the uterine cavity or a significant amount of uterine muscle was disturbed during the myomectomy, a Cesarean delivery is strongly recommended. After a myomectomy, changes to the thickness of the uterine wall may lead to uterine rupture during labor contractions. A uterine rupture would endanger both mother and baby and require an emergency delivery via C-section.

Even if the uterine wall was not disturbed during myomectomy, you remain at greater risk for adhesions or scarring around the fallopian tubes, which can increase the risk for ectopic pregnancy. If you miss a period after myomectomy is performed, please do a urine pregnancy test. If it is positive, see your doctor for blood tests (specifically serial beta human gonadotropin or bHCG pregnancy levels) to show normal increases consistent with an intrauterine pregnancy, not an ectopic pregnancy, until a pelvic ultrasound would be helpful to confirm an intrauterine pregnancy at around six weeks gestation.

One of the few nonsurgical options to treat fibroids is Lupron, an injectable medication that can shrink the fibroid by inducing temporary menopause. Lupron, a GnRH agonist, can temporarily reduce the bulk of the fibroid by up to 25 percent and is usually used before surgery to reduce the significant risks of bleeding that can occur with fibroid removal. It is not recommended as medical therapy alone. Another nonsurgical treatment, developed in the 1990s, that can reduce the size and symptoms of fibroids, is a radiology technique known as uterine artery embolization (UAE). This procedure deprives the uterine fibroid of its nourishment by clotting off the blood vessels that supply it. The long-term risks of menopause, possible fertility difficulty, and regrowth rates of the treated fibroid after embolization are still not known.

Until researchers better understand the impact that UAE has on fetal growth during pregnancy and uterine muscle performance during labor, the procedure is not recommended to treat fibroids if pregnancy is desired. While there have been a number of documented pregnancies after UAE, these women seem to have a higher incidence of growth restriction in their baby-to-be when compared to age-matched controls. To date, there have been no long-term studies on fetal safety after UAE, to answer these concerns. However, for some patients embolization may be desirable over surgery, and a decision to pursue this option must be considered on a case-by-case basis in consultation with the physician.

SEXUALLY TRANSMITTED DISEASES

While it may be uncomfortable to talk about having had a sexually transmitted disease, it is important that you do so with your doctor and your partner. And if you want to have a baby, it is absolutely essential.

Sexually transmitted diseases (STDs) can be either bacterial or viral, and seeking medical attention if you or your partner has symptoms is very, very important. While STDs have been officially renamed sexually transmitted infections (STIs), the former acronym remains more widely used and recognized by the public, so we will stick with STD. An STD that is treated promptly will usually not impair your fertility. People who are at higher risk for STDs are those who started sexual activity early in life, particularly those with multiple sexual partners.

- **Chlamydia** is the most common bacterial STD. Women who are infected may have no symptoms or have a copious amount of vaginal discharge with pelvic discomfort. Men can experience penile irritation, urethral soreness, or redness of the penis, or they may have no signs at all. Chlamydia is diagnosed by swabbing the cervical or penile opening. The disease can cause cervicitis (inflammation of the cervix), salpingitis (tubal inflammation), or urethritis (inflammation of the bladder opening or urethra). Prompt treatment with antibiotics reduces the long-term occurrence of pelvic inflammatory disease (PID), chronic pelvic pain, and tubal blockage. If chlamydia is suspected, your clinician will most probably err on the side of caution and treat both you and your partner.

- **Gonorrhea** is the second most common bacterial STD. Usually this is an infection in the cervix, although it can also affect the oral cavity, urethra, and rectum in both men and women. Symptoms appear two to three weeks after contact with the affected partner: vaginal discharge or burning or pelvic pain in women and penile discharge and pain with urination in men. The diagnosis is made by swabbing the cervical opening in women and the penile opening in men. Treatment is often by antibiotics that cover both gonorrhea and chlamydia because they tend to travel together. This will help prevent the chronic pelvic pain and infertility often caused by these diseases.

- **Human papillomavirus (HPV)** is another common STD that is not itself a deterrent to conception, but treating precancerous lesions caused by HPV may affect the strength of the cervix. This virus is present in seven out of ten sexually active men and women. Among the infected women, almost 30 percent will have an abnormal Pap smear at least once in her lifetime. Thirty percent may also have warts, known as condylomata, that typically appear on the vulva and perineum. The real concern with HPV is not infertility but cervical cancer: studies have revealed that more than 95 percent of cervical cancers contain strains of HPV. If abnormal Pap smears persist and the changes in them become more abnormal looking, the risk of cervical cancer may increase. However, the majority of abnormal Paps can persist for years and spontaneously resolve to normal, never leading to cervical cancer. Your cervix can be evaluated with the aid of a colposcopic exam and directed biopsies before, during, or after pregnancy. The more severe cervical changes associated with HPV are treated with the removal of a dome-shaped piece of the cervix (loop electrosurgical excision procedure, or LEEP). Treatment can cause the opening of the cervix to be tighter than usual (stenotic) or looser than usual (incompetent, or compromised and more likely to open during pregnancy). The likelihood of cervical incompetence increases with the number of cervical procedures.

• **Syphilis** is caused by the bacterium *Treponema pallidum* and used to be the most common of the STDs. With the advent of penicillin it became less and less common until its resurgence in the 1990s. Syphilis can affect the growth and development of the fetus, particularly if the mother is exposed to it during the first trimester. It is therefore vitally important to treat syphilis prior to pregnancy and to avoid exposure to this disease while you are pregnant. Syphilis can present as a hard painless lesion on the penis or vulva, joint pain, fever, and rash, or with no symptoms at all.

Andrea, a twenty-six-year-old virgin, is engaged to be married three months from now. She noticed a sore on her vagina and was shocked to learn she has herpes because she has had only oral sex.

At her annual visit, Lita, thirty-three, expressed concern about her history of herpes, contracted during college. She has had no outbreaks in two years. Does she have to be concerned about her ability to conceive?

Valerie, a thirty-four-year-old banker, has a long history of herpes and is getting an outbreak every month. How can she get pregnant if she can't have sex on a regular basis?

• **Herpes,** also known as herpes simplex virus (HSV), can be transmitted through oral-genital, genital-genital, or genital-anal contact. If oral contact is the source, the herpes virus involved is often HSV type 1, which tends to be less aggressive; HSV type 2 is usually contracted via genital-genital contact. Both types are extremely contagious and you should avoid all intimate relations during an outbreak. Most initial outbreaks occur ten to thirty days after contact, and it's important not to ignore the signs, however subtle. But the first HSV genital infection is usually the most obvious and most painful, heralded by ulcerated sores and discomfort during urination. Subsequent HSV outbreaks tend to happen in a similar location but with a decreased intensity of symptoms, and can occur on any mucous membrane surface including the eyes or mouth. The best way to avoid active transmission to others is to avoid skin contact of your affected mucous membranes and those of your partner and loved ones for seven days after the lesions first appear. While HSV itself does not affect fertility, genital outbreaks demand that you refrain from lovemaking, possibly lengthening the time it takes you to conceive. Baby-friendly medications, such as Valtrex and Zovirax, taken orally, can be used daily to suppress recurrent outbreaks before and after conception.

New research is changing the traditional belief that the most contagious period is just before or during an outbreak. Instead, the viral load seems to rise and fall indiscriminately. Thus, to be safe one must use condoms and antiviral medications to prevent the spread of the virus. At the present time, there is no cure or vaccine to prevent the herpes virus. With this in mind, you might want to consider viral suppression whether you get frequent outbreaks or not.

FOR FUTURE REFERENCE: During Pregnancy

Managing Herpes While Pregnant

If you have herpes lesions while you're pregnant, you can be treated with a pregnancy-safe medications to reduce your discomfort. If you've had one or a number of outbreaks during pregnancy, you may be asked by your health care provider to take an antiviral medication daily, beginning at thirty-six weeks gestational age, to reduce the risk of an HSV outbreak during delivery and to avoid exposing your infant. If you have been infected with herpes prior to conception, when you get an outbreak during pregnancy there will be no risk to the fetus of contracting herpes as well. However, if you have a herpes outbreak during labor, a Cesarean delivery will be recommended to help the infant avoid direct exposure to the herpes virus. Suppression with Valtrex or similar baby-friendly medications in the last month of pregnancy will reduce the likelihood of an outbreak and allow you to pursue a vaginal delivery.

Unless you have an active genital lesion, vaginal birth is a safe option for delivery. When you are asymptomatic, the chance of giving your newborn herpes as it travels through the vaginal canal is rare. Only HSV outbreaks in the genital and anal areas will increase infant risk of transmission. If oral or ocular sores occur at or before delivery, a vaginal trial of labor is strongly recommended.

- **Human immunodeficiency virus (HIV)** can cause acquired immunodeficiency syndrome (AIDS) and is transmitted through the exchange of blood and body fluids such as semen. The virus can be sexually transmitted through genital-genital or genital-anal contact. There have been no reported cases to date of HIV infection solely attributed to oral-genital contact. Safe sex practices are helping to slow the spread of HIV and AIDS. While HIV can be diagnosed from one month to six months after contact with an infected partner, it is possible to contract HIV but not actually develop AIDS for two to twenty years. If a prospective mother is HIV-positive, she can pass the virus to her fetus up to 35 percent of the time. If someone who is HIV-positive conceives, we can reduce the risk of transmission to the fetus by about a third using a variety of medications to strengthen the maternal immune system. A healthy diet, adequate rest, and exercise also help. Getting diagnosed prior to pregnancy is crucial because HIV affects not just your life and the life of your prospective child but also your ability to care for your child in the years ahead.

IF YOU'VE MISCARRIED

Charlie and Pam just had their first pregnancy miscarry at eight weeks. They want to know what their chances are of having that happen again. Can they do anything to reduce the risks?

Charlie and Pam, like many couples, were happily anticipating their first child, only to be disappointed by a miscarriage. This devastating, but likely random, event is more common than most women realize, occurring in 15 percent of all pregnancies when the woman is under the age of thirty-five, increasing to 20 to 25 percent of all pregnancies among women age thirty-five and over, and rising to 30 to 40 percent among women over forty. Because very sensitive tests can detect pregnancy up to five days before your period is due, you may be aware you are pregnant before the embryo successfully implants. In fact, *half of all fertilized eggs are lost spontaneously,* usually before the woman knows she is pregnant.

A spontaneous miscarriage in the first trimester (usually between weeks seven and twelve) is often nature's way of telling us this would not have been a healthy pregnancy. A nonviable fetus actually sends a signal to the body that the pregnancy should not be maintained. After waiting at least one and preferably two menstrual cycles, couples are encouraged to start trying again. (Note: The first cycle after miscarriage is independent of the bleeding immediately after the miscarriage, which may be seven to fourteen days long.) The chance of miscarriage the second time around is no higher than that of the general population.

Whether you've had one miscarriage or more than one, conscientious preconception planning, beginning at least ninety days in advance, may help reduce your risk of experiencing another one. Why?

More than 80 percent of miscarriages are due to random genetic problems, hormonal imbalances, obesity, or uncontrolled diabetes, and less commonly caused by exposure to teratogens (substances known to cause birth defects) or environmental toxins. Reducing your environmental exposures and fine-tuning your body weight and medical conditions (see chapters 3 and 7 for details) may make your womb more hospitable to a baby. Keep in mind, random genetic mismatches, the most common reason for miscarriage, occur more frequently with advancing maternal and paternal age. There is only so much you can do to limit potential exposures. Try not to feel guilty, and take control of what you can—just live as healthfully as you can, for you and for your baby.

After a miscarriage, a woman's body will often be somewhat confused and may not revert immediately to the pre-pregnancy hormonal norm. A little patience is required to allow the normal menstrual cycle to occur. If it doesn't return within six to eight weeks after a miscarriage, consult your health care provider.

Fewer than 1 percent of women experience more than two spontaneous losses in the first trimester. If you are one of them, your doctor may recommend further evaluation and/or a referral to a reproductive endocrinologist to rule out causes other than random misfortune. While no medical cause can be identified for 15 to 50 percent of recurrent losses, others can be attributed to hormonal imbalances, immunological issues, anatomical issues, or genetic abnormalities. The workup for recurrent miscarriage includes a number of studies to assess your immune and endocrine systems, the shape of your uterine cavity, and the genetic makeup of both you and your partner. Here are some of the more common conditions identified in these evaluations:

- **Endocrine (hormone) imbalances** such as corpus luteal defect cause a deficiency in progesterone to support the fetus prior to the placenta's development at eight to ten weeks. While experts are still not certain that low progesterone has a significant impact in causing a miscarriage, many doctors provide supplemental progesterone because it is not harmful to the fetus and may even help. If a nonviable pregnancy exists and you take progesterone, it will just delay the spontaneous loss begun by nature. Other endocrine conditions that can have a significant impact on the risk of miscarriage involve disturbances in thyroid and glucose metabolism. Glucose fluctuations are most common if you have insulin resistance, diabetes, or polycystic ovary syndrome.

- **Autoimmune diseases,** such as anticardiolipin and antiphospholipid syndromes, can cause changes in the blood vessels serving the placenta. In extreme cases clots can form, leading to reduced blood flow between mother and fetus. Celiac disease (intolerance to wheat gluten) can also contribute to unexplained infertility or recurrent pregnancy loss.

- **Uterine anomalies** are abnormal uterine shapes and/or structures that may make implantation of the fetus difficult. These uterine changes can vary from a septum that divides the uterus down the center to unicornuate or bicornuate (heart-shaped). Usually these changes are linked to second-trimester miscarriages (thirteen to twenty-three weeks gestation), as opposed to those in the first trimester.

- **Genetic problems** are variations from the norm that are carried by one or both spouses; random genetic mutations can also occur during egg or sperm development or just after conception. Other genetic issues that may increase the risk of recurrent pregnancy loss are inherited blood clotting disorders (thrombophilias) in the prospective mother. These disorders may affect how well blood flows to the placenta, meaning the blood may clot too easily and the placenta may not receive enough nourishment. A blood test can identify the following mutations: MTHFR (variant in folate metabolism), factor V Leiden, and protein S and C deficiencies. Once a diagnosis is made, the physician can recommend targeted vitamin supplements and/or medications to promote normal clotting.

Other genetic mutations occur when a parent carries an extra copy of a chromosome, which means the embryo will have three copies (trisomy) instead of just two. One such trisomy is Down syndrome (trisomy 21); other trisomies of the 13, 15, and 18 chromosomes can be lethal to the embryo. A trisomy can also happen at different times during egg or sperm development, known as meiosis (a type of cell division unique to eggs and sperm). Human cells have twenty-three pairs of chromosomes, for a total of forty-six. When the egg and sperm combine, they must have only half of each pair in order to create an embryo with the right number of chromosomes. Meiosis ensures that only one half of each pair of chromosomes is present, in the mature egg and sperm. If an extra copy of one chromosome is present it will be passed on to the embryo and result in trisomy. This extra chromosome will often lead to miscarriage. While age increases the general risk of trisomy, the overall risk is much lower than if a parent already carries an extra copy. This is why parental karyotyping (remember those "photographs" of the chromosomes early in this chapter?) to identify extra chromosomes may be in order for those who have suffered three or more fetal losses.

Kathleen and Michael want very much to have a baby, but they had a miscarriage at sixteen weeks gestation. They are beginning to lose hope. Kathleen asked her physician if he thought she and Michael could ever have a healthy baby. Was there anything they could do to improve their chances of having a full-term pregnancy?

Kathleen and Michael represent a rarer group of couples who have a miscarriage after they reach the twelve-week mark and are convinced that their pregnancy is normal and viable. The reasons for their second-trimester loss are very different from the likely random genetic events that happen before twelve weeks gestation. Second-trimester losses are instead due to uterine anomalies, cervical weakness (when the cervix opens without labor), the separation of the placenta from the uterine wall (known as an abruption), and birth defects that are structural (not genetic), such as severe heart abnormalities or neurological defects. A genetic cause also can be the reason for this heartbreaking loss. Before you try to conceive a second time, a thorough workup for all of these possible causes of second-trimester loss will be recommended.

For couples like Kathleen and Michael, it is very difficult for them to believe that the usual reassurances offered throughout the first trimester can really apply to them. If a reason for the second-trimester loss is found, often an intervention can eliminate the issue, making the next pregnancy safer. Although a loss between thirteen and twenty-three weeks may remain unexplained even after a thorough evaluation, the very absence of a concrete problem makes a recurrent episode less likely. If you have had a second-trimester loss in the past, a second opinion with a maternal-fetal medicine specialist to review future risk may be a good idea before you conceive again.

FOR FUTURE REFERENCE: During Pregnancy

Previous Gynecology Surgery and the Risk of Miscarriage

If you have had three or more procedures that opened or cut into your cervix, such as a D&C, cervical freezing (cryosurgery), cervical cone biopsy, or LEEP (recall page 123) for cervical dysplasia, you may have a slightly higher risk of cervical problems associated with second-trimester miscarriage. If you have a cervix that is too loose (cervical incompetence or cervical weakness), your doctor may recommend placing a stitch in your cervix, known as a cerclage. This is done between the twelfth and fourteenth weeks of pregnancy to hold your cervix together until thirty-six weeks gestation or when labor begins. Anticipating a problem with the cervix and intervening early significantly improves your chances of having a healthy baby.

Third-Trimester Loss: Stillbirth

A stillbirth—loss of a pregnancy after twenty weeks—is rare and the overwhelming majority remain unexplained even after careful medical review. Causes include a knot in the umbilical cord, which compromises blood flow to the fetus; a problem with the placenta; or genetic or physical birth defects. Understandably, women who have gone through a stillbirth are extremely anxious during subsequent pregnancies. If you have experienced this, try to reduce your anxiety by seeking evaluation with a maternal-fetal medicine specialist to confirm that the right testing has been done to rule out any issues that may cause another stillbirth. The specialist will propose a close surveillance plan for your pregnancy that can reduce fetal risk and increase the likelihood of catching any problems before they happen. The good news is that the overwhelming majority of stillbirths occur without medical explanation and many couples go on to have normal full-term births after such a loss.

IF YOU'VE HAD AN ABORTION

Karen, a thirty-six-year-old architect, had an abortion ten years ago when she was single. Now she and her husband have spent six months unsuccessfully trying to conceive. Karen is consumed by guilt and is concerned that she has sabotaged her ability to have a child.

Many women struggle with profound feelings of guilt over having had an elective abortion. Often this decision occurred at a time in life when raising a child seemed unimaginable. Now if they experience difficulty conceiving or carrying a child, they beat themselves up with "if onlys" and self-recrimination. The fact is that if an elective abortion is uncomplicated by infection or hemorrhage, it's unlikely to impact future fertility. However, if you have had more than three elective abortions, your cervix may be weakened and you may be less likely to carry a child to term. Let your doctor know so that he or she can examine your cervix to decide whether a cerclage (stitch) should be placed to secure your cervix after twelve or thirteen weeks gestation.

IF YOU'VE HAD A PRIOR ECTOPIC PREGNANCY

Jan and her husband, Peter, had one son three years ago in an uncomplicated pregnancy. But the second time around, Jan experienced vaginal spotting beginning at six weeks. Her doctor did a blood test and sonogram, then diagnosed a right tubal pregnancy. He prescribed methotrexate, an injectable medication that can dissolve the tubal pregnancy about 85 percent of the time. Six months later, Jan finally feels ready to start trying again, but she is worried about having another ectopic pregnancy.

Ectopic pregnancy is when a fetus grows outside the uterus, most commonly in one of the fallopian tubes. The incidence of ectopic pregnancy has been rising in the past twenty years, possibly due to the use of assisted reproduction technology and the increased incidence of sexually transmitted infections. Approximately 1 to 2.5 percent of all pregnancies are ectopic. In the past, ectopic pregnancies often went undetected until the tube ruptured, putting the mother's life at risk. Fortunately, more sensitive blood markers (beta-human chorionic gonadotropin, or bHCG) and early ultrasound have improved so dramatically that an ectopic pregnancy is usually diagnosed long before the fallopian tube can rupture. It can, however, take one to two weeks to follow the trend in the bHCG levels to confirm the diagnosis of an ectopic pregnancy. During this time, you and your doctor will be closely monitoring your clinical symptoms as well to detect any sign that a possible ectopic pregnancy is beginning to rupture. An ectopic or tubal pregnancy diagnosed in the first five to eight weeks of pregnancy allows time for prompt treatment, avoidance of emergency surgery, and reduced likelihood of a poor outcome for the mother.

The risk of an ectopic pregnancy is increased with IVF, previous ectopic pregnancy, ovarian or uterine surgery, previous Cesarean section, or a history of pelvic inflammatory disease. The incidence of recurrent ectopic pregnancy is increased by a history of previous ectopic pregnancies, surgery, or pelvic inflammatory disease. Heterotopic pregnancies—where one fetus is in the uterus and the other is outside—are extremely rare, occurring in one in ten thousand pregnancies. The incidence of these has increased as well since IVF has become more common.

If you've had an ectopic pregnancy in the past, there is a 15 to 20 percent chance of having one again, regardless of whether you had surgery to remove it from the tube or took medication to treat it. So, once you start trying again and miss a period, you need to seek immediate medical attention to confirm the placement of your pregnancy in the uterus.

The most common symptoms of an ectopic pregnancy are pelvic pain, from bleeding into the abdomen, and vaginal bleeding. If you experience any of these signs early in your pregnancy, your doctor will first check your blood level of bHCG, which usually rises 50 to 60 percent every forty-eight hours in a healthy pregnancy. If the bHCG is not rising adequately, ultrasound will detect whether the embryo is implanted inside or outside the uterus. Progesterone levels can also be helpful as levels greater than 15 to 20 mg/mL imply that an intrauterine pregnancy exists.

INTRAUTERINE GROWTH RESTRICTION

Another issue you should mention to your ob-gyn is any history of an infant delivered at less than the tenth percentile of weight for gestational age (for instance, babies weighing less than six pounds after thirty-seven weeks of pregnancy—the normal range for the weight of a full-term infant is 6 pounds 6 ounces to 8 pounds 14 ounces). Infants with low birth weight have an increased lifetime risk for heart disease, diabetes, high blood pressure, and obesity. Because the chance of recurrence can be as high as 20 percent, it is important to understand the risk factors and try to reduce as many of them as possible.

Risk factors for intrauterine growth restriction are related to maternal health, fetal health, and placental anatomy. Maternal risk factors include being less than sixteen or more than thirty-five years old, low BMI, poor pregnancy weight gain, tobacco and recreational drug use, and medical conditions such as diabetes, high blood pressure, collagen vascular disease (such as lupus), and heart disease. Fetuses are at risk for growth restriction if they have been exposed to certain viral infections or have a genetic abnormality. Placental factors, such as inflammation or abruption (detachment from the uterine wall), are the hardest to predict before they affect the fetus. Placental abruption can restrict the flow of nutrients through the placenta and deprive the fetus of enough nutrients for adequate growth.

The following may help reduce the likelihood of delivering a low-birth-weight infant:

- Excellent dental care within the six months before trying to conceive (TTC)
- Good control of chronic conditions, such as controlling blood sugar levels and blood pressure with baby-friendly medications, beginning three months before TTC
- Elimination of tobacco and drug use at least three months before TTC
- Elimination of alcohol use beginning two weeks before TTC
- Being at a healthy weight before conception, followed by careful and consistent weight gain (no loss) throughout the pregnancy. (Note: If being under- or overweight has been an issue for you, pay particular attention to Chapter 14.)
- Early ultrasound dating—due date confirmation in the first trimester of pregnancy with ultrasound can eliminate the question of smaller fetal size due to gestational age miscalculation

PRETERM LABOR AND/OR DELIVERY

Michelle and Dan were expecting their first baby in May, but in March of the same year Michelle started having severe back pain and didn't realize she was in early labor at thirty weeks gestation. Within forty-eight hours of the diagnosis of preterm labor she went on to have a vaginal delivery of a 2-pound 12-ounce baby boy who spent eight weeks in the special care nursery. Their son, Matthew, is now a healthy two-year-old (though still requiring occupational therapy for a few developmental delays), but Michelle is very stressed thinking that the same thing could happen with their next pregnancy.

Preterm labor and delivery can be an extremely stressful experience for both mother and infant. Delivery before thirty-seven weeks gestation (or three weeks early) is considered preterm, but infants born between thirty-five and thirty-seven weeks rarely need intensive interventions to assist with breathing, eating, and temperature regulation, issues that are more common among infants born before thirty-five weeks. However, the premature delivery of an infant is the number one reason why newborns have severe health problems or die, so your health care team will make every effort to understand any risk factors you may have and take every precaution to avoid this happening again. While a preterm delivery is often unexpected the first time, having a history of preterm delivery increases the odds that it may happen again. For example:

- With one preterm delivery (before thirty-seven weeks), the risk of recurrence is 16 percent.
- With two preterm deliveries, the risk of recurrence increases to 41 percent.

Note that if a preterm delivery happened in a prior twin or triplet pregnancy, the next pregnancy with a single baby should not pose an increased risk of preterm delivery.

Studies have identified several known risk factors for premature delivery, including African American and Hispanic ethnicity, tobacco use, body weight that is too low, gaining too little or too much weight *during* pregnancy, underlying inflammation or infection, and pregnancy less than a year following a preterm delivery. There have also been a few studies in the dental literature suggesting that poor periodontal hygiene or gingivitis increases the risk for preterm labor and delivery. Most of these risk factors can be best addressed between pregnancies, at least ninety days before trying to conceive. Prospective mothers are encouraged to try to wait at least eighteen months between pregnancies, unless age is an issue. They should eliminate tobacco and recreational drug use, get a preconception dental checkup and maintain good dental hygiene habits, attain a more optimal weight, and improve their overall medical health during preconception to decrease the risk of preterm labor. Daily folic acid supplementation has been long recommended during preconception to reduce the incidence of neural tube defects in the baby-to-be. But a recent cohort study revealed that taking a folic acid supplement for *one year prior to conception* was also associated with a dramatically reduced (by 50 to 70 percent) incidence of preterm birth prior to thirty-two weeks of pregnancy when a baby would be at greatest risk for long-term medical, mental, and developmental difficulties. Fortunately, research like this has noted specific steps we can take to help ensure the baby gets as close to a full forty weeks as possible.

As you work on reducing any risk factors under your control, your health care team will monitor you closely throughout your pregnancy. For instance, your cervical length may be measured at eighteen to twenty weeks with ultrasound. While this increased surveillance does not necessarily reduce the likelihood of another preterm delivery, it certainly increases the likelihood of early intervention if there are any signs of trouble.

Maureen, thirty-six, and Scott, thirty-eight, were first-time parents who had conceived after three years and three trials of IVF. They were almost twenty-four weeks pregnant when Maureen's water broke. Medical interventions were begun immediately to stop labor and help the infant optimize lung capacity (by giving Maureen steroids forty-eight hours before delivery). Little Brian was born two days after admission to the hospital at 1 pound 8 ounces. He underwent resuscitative measures but, tragically, died three days after birth. About eight months later, when Maureen and Scott spontaneously conceived, Maureen received weekly intramuscular injections of 17-hydroxyprogesterone and was able to deliver their daughter, Ava, at thirty-two weeks, a 3½-pound infant who is now a precocious sixteen-month-old.

Several medical interventions introduced in recent years have shown a significant improvement in gestational age for a subsequent delivery among women with a history of preterm delivery. For women who have had an extreme preterm delivery (less than twenty-six to twenty-eight weeks) accompanied by cervical incompetence (premature cervical dilation), a cerclage (stitch) can be placed in the cervix at the end of the first trimester to keep it closed tightly until term. If there was no evidence of cervical compromise, progesterone therapy (17-hydroxyprogesterone caproate) can be given weekly between twenty and thirty-six weeks of pregnancy to reduce the incidence of preterm delivery. Progesterone therapy also reduces complications in the premature newborn such as intracranial bleeding, severe gastric problems, and respiratory distress. There are very few side effects to this treatment and studies have shown a statistically significant increase in gestational age at delivery (by two to four weeks).

Careful preparation, excellent nutritional health, and a team effort between prospective parents and their health care providers can reduce the risk of these obstetrical problems in future pregnancies.

FOR FUTURE REFERENCE: During Pregnancy

Prior Medical Complications During and Between Pregnancies

Women whose past pregnancies were complicated by medical issues such as gestational diabetes (abnormal blood sugar tolerance while pregnant), pregnancy-induced high blood pressure (an isolated finding of hypertension), or preeclampsia (when high blood pressure is accompanied by protein in your urine and changes in blood tests that show kidney and liver stress) have a 15 to 20 percent risk of similar problems in the next pregnancy. In addition, the likelihood of continuing to have these issues after the baby is born is about 10 percent. Women who have had these medical issues during or after a prior pregnancy should be screened prior to or during a subsequent pregnancy.

Before a second pregnancy, you can reduce your odds of having a medical problem by losing weight gained in a previous pregnancy and achieving the healthiest weight for your body build, stopping tobacco use, and controlling high blood pressure with regular exercise and baby-friendly medications that can be continued during the pregnancy. Researchers are studying whether preconception and early pregnancy dietary measures can reduce the risk of preeclampsia. While some dietary changes may be helpful, nothing can rival the importance of simply getting to a healthy weight (see pages 426–429). Once you have achieved that goal, resolving vitamin and mineral deficiencies such as vitamin D and calcium, respectively, can help. A balanced intake of omega-3 and omega-6 fats and a daily multivitamin combined with a healthy diet full of veggies and fruits may lower the risk of preeclampsia but, contrary to widely circulated advice, aspirin or megadoses of vitamin C have not been found to reduce the risk of hypertension in your next pregnancy. We suggest you talk to your doctor about the latest research on this topic when trying to conceive. Once you do conceive, continue with close medical supervision.

IF YOU HAVE HAD A PREVIOUS CESAREAN SECTION

There is a growing concern among obstetrical health professionals about the rising C-section rate. The overall rate of first-time C-section is as high as 30 percent in some parts of the United States. The increase in C-sections is believed to be a result of increased patient desire for elective C-section, growing reluctance to try a vaginal birth after a previous C-section (VBAC), malpractice concerns (C-sections are perceived to offer a reduction in fetal risk during delivery), and increasing obesity, leading to large-for-gestational-age infants who are difficult to deliver vaginally.

If this is your first pregnancy and you think you want an elective C-section, don't be surprised if your doctor tries to talk you out of it. Today, C-sections are the most common surgical procedure performed on women in the United States. They seem to be quite convenient—a scheduled delivery (pick your baby's birthday!) that takes only one to two hours instead of the projected six to eighteen hours of labor in a vaginal delivery. The problem is that C-sections, while a safe procedure overall, put future vaginal deliveries at risk by a medical "domino effect."

After one previous C-section, there is an inherent risk of the old uterine incision rupturing in a future labor, leading to an emergency C-section and putting mom and baby at significant risk. Also, when the placenta implants in a uterus that has already been cut open, the placenta may penetrate into the uterine muscle wall, causing hemorrhage during delivery and potentially requiring a hysterectomy to correct that problem. The *New England Journal of Medicine* published a study in 2005 that reported the risk of uterine rupture in labor after a previous C-section closer to one in three hundred women (prior to this study, clinicians believed the risk was more like one in six hundred women). In 2010, ACOG somewhat relaxed its position regarding VBAC. The group encourages a vaginal trial for those women who have had up to two C-sections in the past or who may not be clear on the previous type of incision they had during their C-section. However, inherent risks remain. Careful discussion and counseling with your health care professionals before you deliver is essential.

If you have had a previous C-section and have gained more than ten pounds between pregnancies, there are new data to suggest an increased risk for a repeat C-section. This is especially true if you were also diagnosed with gestational diabetes in a prior pregnancy. This new information reinforces that a healthy weight and regular exercise between pregnancies can improve the chances of a successful vaginal birth after a previous C-section.

Common reasons for a first-time, medically necessary C-section include problems with where the placenta is located (such as placenta previa) or problems with labor progression, including failure of the fetus to progress through the birth canal while the mother is pushing, lack of progress in labor despite intervention (such as drugs, activity, or positions to move things along), and malpresentation (such as a breech position). If your previous C-section was for a non-labor-related event, you should be optimistic about a successful vaginal delivery in future pregnancies. If you had a labor progression issue, the odds of successful future vaginal deliveries are lower.

The advantage of vaginal delivery over C-section is a more rapid maternal recovery and ease of future vaginal deliveries after the first. Infants often need less respiratory support if they are squeezed in the vaginal canal. Think of the baby as a sponge—mucus and excess fluids are squeezed out during the delivery process. When you have other children at home, a two-week vaginal recovery versus a four-to-six-week C-section recovery can make a difference.

Many couples like to discuss delivery options before they conceive again to clearly understand what a safe and comfortable birthing plan might be for the next pregnancy. For instance, many physicians and midwives work in hospitals that do not have twenty-four-hour anesthesia services. If that is the case, your provider is unlikely to offer a VBAC trial because if the uterus ruptures during labor and you need an emergency C-section, the anesthesiologist may be twenty minutes away. Find out if the facility you plan to use has the capacity to deal with this type of urgent delivery so you can make informed decisions regarding the facility where you will deliver. Discussion before pregnancy will eliminate avoidable stress during the pregnancy itself. But remember, your choice regarding the mode of delivery will be revisited many times, so take your time to gather information and make a decision that is good for you and your family.

SO, WHEN CAN WE MAKE A BABY?

Now that you understand your cycle and have identified any gynecological issues you may need to consider, you're probably very excited to get going on baby making. Later chapters will enlighten you about nutrition—knowledge that will serve you well long after your baby-making career is over. Your role as the family's nutrition and health gatekeeper cannot be overstated. So take this time to invest in setting up healthy lifestyle routines. Get to know the produce section of your grocery store a bit better. Experiment with new "slow food" recipes. Find the local farmers' market. Set up walking or jogging routes that fit into your day. This way, once your baby arrives, you won't have to struggle to regain your old self. You'll already have those healthy patterns in place.

We know some of you are wondering about your fertility. In fact, many patients say they want to have their fertility tested before they even start trying to conceive. Unfortunately, there is no simple way to predict a woman's fertility. But statistics show that most women will not have fertility problems. And those who do need some extra help have many options available, some of which are neither invasive nor expensive.

The vast majority (85 percent) of women under age thirty-five will conceive within one year or twelve menstrual cycles, and 90 percent of those who don't get pregnant within the first year will be able to conceive the old-fashioned way within their next twelve menstrual cycles. If you are between thirty-five and thirty-nine, your chances of success are a little less: about 70 to 75 percent of women can conceive spontaneously after twelve cycles (though most women over the age of thirty-five are advised to seek medical assistance and evaluation after six months of trying).

After you turn forty, fertility drops another 10 to 20 percent, and it continues to decline each year. That means that approximately 50 percent of women between forty and forty-two can conceive without the assistance of reproductive technology. Unfortunately, the likelihood of miscarriage increases with age, just as fertility is fading. Women in their early forties have a 30 percent risk of miscarriage, making the likelihood of getting and staying pregnant about 35 percent.

But what about the 15 percent of women under the age of thirty-five or the 20 to 30 percent of women over thirty-five who are having trouble getting pregnant? At first the very idea of making a baby is sweetly thrilling. But as months become a year and a year turns into two, confidence can turn into despair and eagerness into blame and fear: "Is it me? Is it him? Is it our past catching up with us?" Each menstrual cycle becomes an emotional roller coaster, with soaring excitement at the promise of conception and searing defeat when your period comes and it is clear you are not pregnant that month.

If you have been there and done that, we understand your keen interest in expediting conception. Please feel free to skip to Chapters 17 and 18 to brush up on your ovulation timing and identify any fertility issues you may have. Then do come back and review the other chapters. While you're waiting for your next ovulatory "window," take this time to focus on you and your good health.

CHAPTER 6

Ancestry and Age: Your Baby's Genetic Legacy

NATURE VERSUS NURTURE: THE INFLUENCE OF YOUR GENES ON YOUR BABY-TO-BE

When people consider the prospect of becoming pregnant, they begin to fantasize about what their little one will be like: "Will he have my eye color?" "Wouldn't it be nice if she inherited my husband's musical talent?" In other words, they begin to think about genetics.

In the centuries-long discourse over nature versus nurture, genetics represents nature, the underlying blueprint, and nurture is represented by external environmental factors such as where we grew up, how we're raised, the quality of our diet, and how we interact socially. At the heart of the debate is the question of which factors have the greater influence on our overall development. Our position is that your environment and your genes combined make you the person you are. The good nutrition, exercise, and behavioral habits we recommend to foster a healthy pregnancy will stack the nurture cards in your baby-to-be's favor. But what about nature? How much do genes matter? In this chapter we answer these questions, as well as provide general guidance about whether you should explore genetic counseling and/or blood testing (which may or may not be covered by your insurance).

Each parent contributes twenty-three chromosomes that contain all the genes underlying the elaborate blueprint of how we are made. Your future baby's appearance, medical predisposition, and personality are coded within those genes. It's possible to sample cells from blood or body tissues to obtain a "photograph" of the chromosomes—called a karyotype—to make basic observations (such as change in the number or structure of the genes). Looking for a specific disease or trait requires targeted testing of a specific gene (or genes).

FIGURE 6-1
KARYOTYPE OF A FEMALE FETUS

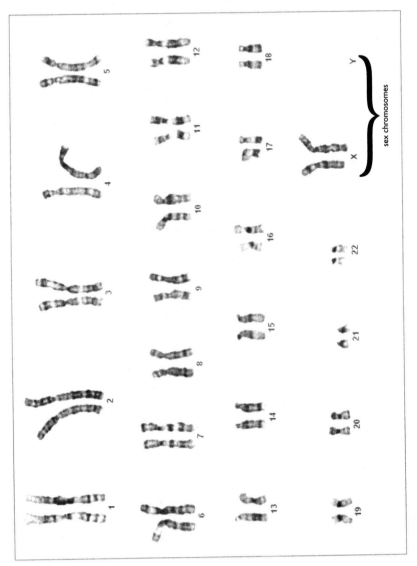

This is a normal karyotype for a little girl, hence the two X chromosomes. Each chromosome contains hundreds to thousands of genes that act as an instruction manual for how we should be built when we are just embryos. The chromosome pairs you see above are from the mother and father—an equal division of labor in building a baby. If a fertilized egg is missing a whole or partial chromosome, or if an extra chromosome appears, there can be abnormal growth or problems in the fetus.

FIGURE 6-2
TURNER SYNDROME—BABY WITH A MISSING X OR Y CHROMOSOME

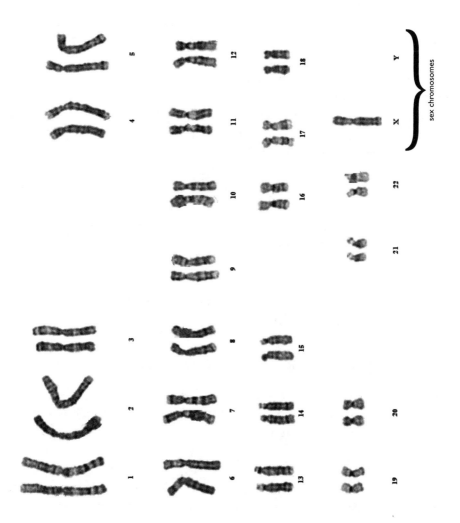

This fetus carried a random genetic mutation called Turner Syndrome, which means it lacked one of the two necessary sex chromosomes. Notice in the upper right-hand corner (by the bracket) that another X chromosome would have made this fetus a girl, whereas adding a Y would have made the gender a boy. In approximately 99 percent of Turner syndrome cases, the fetus is miscarried.

When a baby is conceived, it inherits some part of the genetic information provided by both parents' ancestry. For example, Alisa is the only one in the family with red hair, and she remembers overhearing her parents respond to the question "Where did that red hair come from?" with jokes about the milkman. Her parents actually did some research to find out from whom Alisa had inherited her beautiful hair. They went back four generations and found red hair on both sides of the family. These red hair genes are recessive, so they'd been carried for generations in the presence of dominant genes for dark hair. But when the two recessive red genes found each other in the embryo that would become Alisa, they were finally able to be expressed in her hair color.

Occasionally, genes break, get mixed up or lost, or duplicate themselves, making it more difficult to read the genetic blueprint and resulting in a baby that is unhealthy or developmentally challenged. Between 50 and 90 percent of miscarriages in the first trimester are the result of a random genetic problem that makes the fetus nonviable, and this rate varies widely by maternal age (see Figure 6-2 for an example of how the genes would look in an embryo with one of the most common random genetic mismatches, Turner syndrome). These spontaneous mutations rarely repeat themselves. In fact, in the general population, 2 to 3 percent of all fetuses conceived may be affected by a genetically influenced birth defect. Many of these are miscarried so early that the woman may not even be aware she is pregnant. There are, however, some genetic problems which are not random, and as you are preparing to conceive a child, you need to examine the factors that might place you at higher risk for producing a baby with hereditary diseases or birth defects.

ARE YOU A CANDIDATE FOR PRECONCEPTION GENETIC SCREENING?

When it comes to understanding your personal genetics, knowledge is power. While you can't control your genetic makeup, knowing the medical and genetic histories you and your partner will contribute to your future child(ren) can inform your decisions about having a family.

Your genetic makeup is only part of the story. The rest is history—your family's history, that is. Based on your family's history of birth defects, disorders, or diseases, you may be eligible for preconception genetic counseling. While this is sometimes a difficult subject to broach with extended family, it's very important to find a way to tactfully gather such information.

As you reach out to family, you might consider using humor to place your request in context. For example, you could blame it on your age: "Due to my *advanced maternal age,* ha ha, I am eligible for genetic counseling and need to have some information about our family handy for the appointment." Many insurance carriers routinely offer genetic counseling for women over thirty-five years of age. Additionally, you may offer to share any insights you gather, such as with siblings who may be carriers for a specific disease that runs in the family. They may be quite interested in finding out their odds of passing it on to their children. Consider using gentle phrases, such as "Do you know of any children in our family who were born with special needs?" to ease into the topic.

Start with capturing what you know on paper. Consider using a worksheet such as that prepared by the March of Dimes (www.marchofdimes.com/files/GYP_PrenatalQuestionnaire.pdf).

You may want to ask for prepregnancy genetic screening if you have one or more of the following risk factors:

- One or more prior pregnancies that have ended in fetal death after twenty weeks
- Recurrent first-trimester miscarriages (two or more)
- Children (your own or elsewhere in your family) with genetic issues such as hemophilia, cystic fibrosis, muscular dystrophy, dwarfism, or fragile X syndrome (see Table 6-1)
- Family history of adulthood diseases such as Huntington's disease or muscular dystrophy
- Family history of unexplained mental retardation, severe learning disabilities, or behavioral problems
- Ethnic background that implies a predisposition for a specific genetic problem—for example, sickle-cell anemia if you are black and specifically of African American descent (see Table 6-1)

There is no right or wrong choice when it comes to deciding whether to undergo genetic counseling and testing. Some people choose not to, reasoning that if anything was wrong they would have the baby anyway. Others feel more comfortable knowing as much as possible in advance so they can make plans for further tests during pregnancy and decisions based on those tests. The correct choice is the one that you and your partner find acceptable. Our philosophy is that it is usually better to be prepared before conception than to be surprised when you are pregnant and have very emotionally and ethically difficult decisions to make. To find a genetic counselor, ask your doctor, or contact:

- The genetics department of your local university hospital.
- Your local branch of the March of Dimes (www.marchofdimes.com). Ask if there are genetic counselors who concentrate on the type of genetic problem you are interested in. For example, if you have a family history of Tay-Sachs disease, the March of Dimes has local referrals for genetic counseling.
- The National Society of Genetic Counselors (www.nsgc.org) and Gene Clinics (www.geneclinics.org) offer a list of clinics searchable by state.

- Medical organizations such as the American College of Obstetrics and Gynecology, which can provide you with a list of medical doctors in your area who specialize in genetics.
- Friends who have consulted a geneticist in the past.

Most genetics counselors are well versed in all aspects of genetic illnesses related to pre-conception and pregnancy, so it is not too late to ask for a consultation after conception if you opted to skip pre-pregnancy genetic screening.

HOW DOES YOUR BABY INHERIT A GENETIC DISEASE?

There are many pieces of family health history carried in your genetic code. When you and your spouse pass your genes on to your baby-to-be, they'll include some of this medical information, and also the potential for disease.

Genetic conditions can be inherited in a number of ways. If a disease has an *autosomal dominant* inherited pattern, only one parent has to carry the gene that codes for that particular problem. When one parent has the disease, and each child has a 50-50 chance of inheriting it; if both do, up to 75 percent of all children conceived can be affected by the same disease. Examples of autosomal dominant diseases include polydactylism (extra digits on hands or feet), achondroplasia (a form of dwarfism), and Huntington's disease (a debilitating neurological condition). Huntington's doesn't develop until middle age, so you may have already had children by the time you realize you have this life-altering disease. A preconception blood test exists for this disease and should be considered absolutely essential if your parents or their siblings have Huntington's.

The second, very common way to inherit a genetic disease is in an *autosomal recessive* pattern. In this case, both parents have to carry the affected gene and the child has to inherit one copy from each in order to manifest the disease. If both parents are carriers, neither will have the disease, but each offspring will have a 25 percent chance of being affected. The most common autosomal recessive diseases are prevalent in the gene pools of specific ethnic groups, probably as a result of generations of endogamy (the practice of marrying within a social group). If you are a member of an ethnic group listed in Table 6-1, you may be a carrier of the specific genes in question and should consider having a blood test to find out for sure. If you are a carrier, your partner should also undergo genetic blood testing. If you are both carriers, you can substitute donor sperm or eggs to conceive without the carrier gene risk, and have early prenatal testing to determine if the fetus is affected so that you can mentally prepare yourself, or discontinue the pregnancy.

While on a trip to Naples, Anthony and Maureen met some of their relatives who had not immigrated to the United States. Maureen used this opportunity to ask her relatives about a type of ane-

mia that those of Mediterranean descent may develop because no one in her immediate family back home knew of a family history. Sure enough, her husband's grandmother had beta-thalessemia. When they got back to the United States their doctor ordered blood testing, which ended up being negative.

TABLE 6-1
AUTOSOMAL RECESSIVE DISEASES

Disease	Ethnic Group	Carrier Rates	Birthrates	Childhood Effects
Cystic fibrosis[a]	Caucasians, Northern Europeans, Ashkenazi Jews[b]	1:35–1:70	1:3,600	Pneumonia, inflammation of pancreas, increased mucus and sweat production, frequent hospitalizations Life expectancy in the 30s
	Hispanics	1:46		
	Asian Americans	1:94		
	blacks (of all ancestry)	1:65		
Sickle-cell disease	blacks (with highest incidence in African Americans)	1:8	1:256	Changes in blood cells that reduce oxygen to organs and may require hospitalization for pain, anemia, and infection
	Native Americans	1:560	1:354,000	
	Latinos	1:700	1:960,000	
Spinal muscular atrophy (SMA)	Caucasians	1:35	1:10,000	Severe neuromuscular weakness: difficulty walking, learning disabilities, ataxia (difficulty with directed movement and balance issues with ambulation)
	African Americans	1:66		
	Asian Americans	1:53		
	Latinos	1:117		
Tay-Sachs[b]	Ashkenazi Jews[b]	1:30	1:3,600	Mental retardation, central nervous system damage and weakness, death before age 5[c]
	French Canadians	1:150	1:90,000	
	Louisiana Cajuns	1:300	1:360,000	
Canavan disease[b]	Ashkenazi Jews[b]	1:40	1:6,400	Developmental delay, seizures, difficulty swallowing, death by age 10
Gaucher's[b]	Ashkenazi Jews[b]	1:25	1:2,500	Fetal hydrops[d]; stillbirth common

Disease	Ethnic Group	Carrier Rates[a]	Birthrates	Childhood Effects
Alpha Thalassemia	Asians, Asian Americans	1:20		Fetal hydrops[d]; poor weight gain
Beta Thalassemia	Mediterraneans (Turkish, Greek, Italian)	1:7		Fetal hydrops[d]; anemia, fatigue, poor weight gain

a. ACOG guidelines, as of May 2001, recommend cystic fibrosis testing for all Caucasians who are planning to be or are already pregnant. Both parents must be carriers before prenatal tests will be offered.

b. There are three tiers of preconception testing for couples of Ashkenazi Jewish descent that ultimately allows one to test for up to eighteen diseases in this population, as of 2010; this number has tripled in the last decade. The first is for the most common genetic diseases that could affect your offspring, including Tay-Sachs disease, cystic fibrosis, Gaucher's, and Canavan disease. The final tier is for the rarer metabolic diseases, such as Niemann-Pick disease and—in fewer than 1 in 300,000 offspring—Fanconi's anemia and Bloom's disease.

c. There is a rare form of Tay-Sachs that doesn't cause death until adolescence.

d. Fetal hydrops is a severe form of anemia that causes fluid to accumulate in the cavities of the fetal body.

MORE ABOUT AUTOSOMAL RECESSIVE GENETIC DISEASES

The genetic diseases commonly passed on to the next generation as autosomal recessive traits are also some of the easiest to test for before conception and often have the greatest impact on decision making and childhood quality of life.

Cystic fibrosis (CF), which is carried more commonly but not exclusively by Caucasians of European, North American, and Ashkenazi Jewish descent, can lead to a shortened life span and almost certainly will lead to frequent hospitalizations for pneumonia and pancreatitis. However, great strides have been made in CF treatment, and the average life span is now thirty-seven years. Preconception testing for cystic fibrosis became the standard of care after 2001. As of 2010, testing for up to 250 CF mutations was made possible in a single blood test.

For healthy prospective parents, genetic counseling with a health care provider is essential prior to making the weighty decision to undergo blood testing. Prospective parents should also have a private conversation about how each would foresee using the information gathered from genetic testing. For instance, the testing may reveal that one or both partners carry a gene that will increase the odds of their baby having an inherited disease. How would you respond? Do you know how your partner would feel? Full disclosure helps reduce the angst and tension between couples who may not be on the same page about how to handle such a situation. Of course, actually finding out some troubling information may change the equation for one or both partners, but a conversation beforehand lays the framework for how to handle such news.

The X-Factor

Maria was visiting her elderly aunt when she heard a story about a cousin who died from hemo-philia, the same disease that plagued the son of Tsar Nicholas and Empress Alexandra in early eighteenth-century Russia. Maria started to wonder if there was a chance that she could be car-rying the gene and could pass it on to any sons she might have. She decided then and there that she would seek preconception genetic counseling.

When an egg and a sperm combine to create an embryo, the mother's and father's chromosomes match up to form twenty-three pairs. All are evenly matched except in boys, where the twenty-third pair, which contains the sex chromosomes, is made up of an X chromosome from the mother and a shorter Y chromosome from the father. (Girls have two X chromosomes, one from each parent.)

Because boys carry only one copy of the X chromosome, any disease or characteristic carried on that chromosome automatically has an autosomal dominant pattern: boys need to inherit only one copy of the gene to have the condition. These conditions are called X-linked traits. Girls must inherit two copies of the affected gene, one from each parent, making these conditions much rarer among female offspring. Girls who have only one copy generally will not be affected or will be affected only slightly, but they will be carriers, meaning that their sons will have a 50 percent chance of inheriting the trait or disease. Classic examples of X-linked genetic problems are color blindness, spinal muscular atrophy, muscular dystrophy, and hemophilia A.

Hemophilia A is a deficiency in the blood-clotting system. Decades ago, those affected with hemophilia often died in their youth of internal hemorrhage, but today the missing clotting factor, most commonly factor VIII, can be replaced and significant bleeding avoided. Nowadays, the risks are more likely due to contracting disease by blood transfusion (hepatitis B and C, HIV infection) and limited availability of blood supply. You can test to see if you carry this gene before or after conception. Being prepared will reduce fetal and newborn risks of bleeding.

Another common X-linked disease is fragile X syndrome. This means that a baby boy has a 50 percent chance of being conceived with the disease if his mother is a carrier. This disease can lead to behavioral challenges and learning disabilities that can range from mild to severe mental disabilities. If you have a family history of fragile X, a child born to you with fragile X, or a relative with unexplained mental retardation or behavioral problems, you may want to request genetic screening.

Duchenne's, the more common form of muscular dystrophy, is an X-linked genetic disease that affects 1 in 3,500 male children (one-third of the cases are new mutations in the gene pool of a family) and results in muscular weakness and learning disabilities that begin at age three to five. Boys with this condition are often wheelchair-bound from early childhood. As adults, these men may be infertile, can have heart abnormalities, and may have a life expectancy limited to the second or third decade.

Spinal muscular atrophy (SMA) is a newly identified genetic disease that can be tested for in the preconception period or in early pregnancy. A severe neurological disease, SMA is an X-linked disease with three subgroups, one of which can lead to death by the age of two from muscle weakness resulting in respiratory distress. Those suffering from other types of SMA have difficulty walking or doing activities related to daily living, such as bathing or cooking. Genetic testing offers 90 percent predictive accuracy by checking for changes in the survival motor neuron (SMN) 1 and 2 genes and can determine if someone has the potential to carry SMA. Because SMA is found in all populations, predicting likelihood by ethnicity is not possible.

HOW TO MAKE A FAMILY TREE

The tool geneticists use to organize your family's genetic history is a pedigree, or family tree. Even if you don't have a genetic concern, it's a helpful way to imagine how a disease or characteristic such as blue eyes can be carried through the generations (see Figures 6-3A and B).

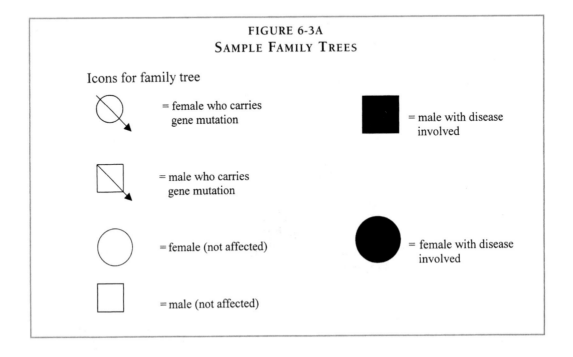

FIGURE 6-3A
SAMPLE FAMILY TREES

Icons for family tree

= female who carries gene mutation

= male who carries gene mutation

= female (not affected)

= male (not affected)

= male with disease involved

= female with disease involved

FIGURE 6-3B
EXAMPLE OF X-LINKED RECESSIVE INHERITANCE, SUCH AS HEMOPHILIA A

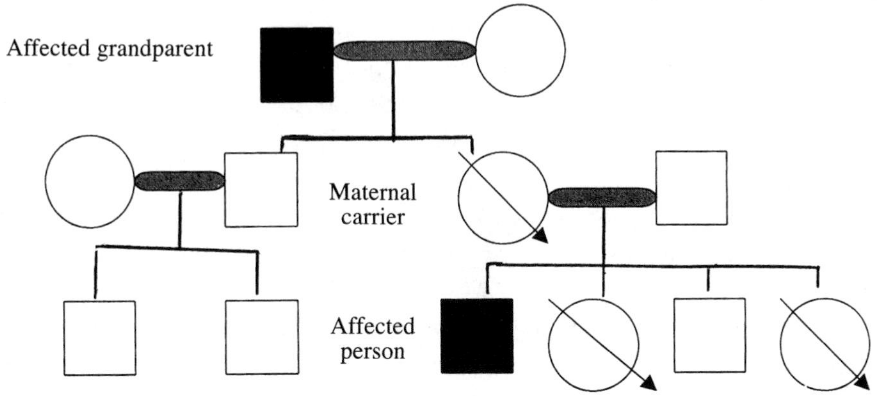

Affected grandparent

Maternal carrier

Affected person

EXAMPLE OF AUTOSOMAL RECESSIVE INHERITANCE, SUCH AS CYSTIC FIBROSIS

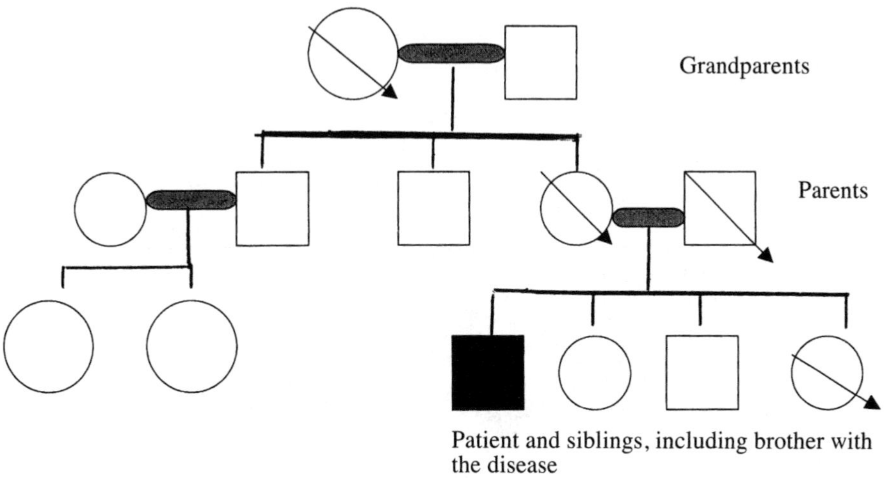

Grandparents

Parents

Patient and siblings, including brother with the disease

Practical Application

Make a family tree of your own, using both your and your spouse's family members and going back at least two generations, if possible. Make a list of the potential inheritable birth defects or diseases that may place your future baby at risk. Your families can be invaluable resources for insight into your genetic ancestry. (Also refer to Chapter 4, Figure 4-1, for the family section of the women's medical checklist, the men's medical checklist in Figure 9-4, and Table 6-1 for a list of conditions associated with ethnicity.)

Start with the two of you (bottom circle and square); then move up to your respective parents. You can also note any siblings by adding circles for sisters and squares for brothers. The top row is your grandparents.

The family tree below can also be used in an attempt to predict other traits, such as blue eyes or red hair. Have some fun and use colored pencils to "decorate" your family below and see what you think your future baby will look like. Bear in mind that eye and hair color are expressed by multiple genes but generally follow this oversimplified rule: brown is dominant over blue (for eyes) and blonde and red (for hair).

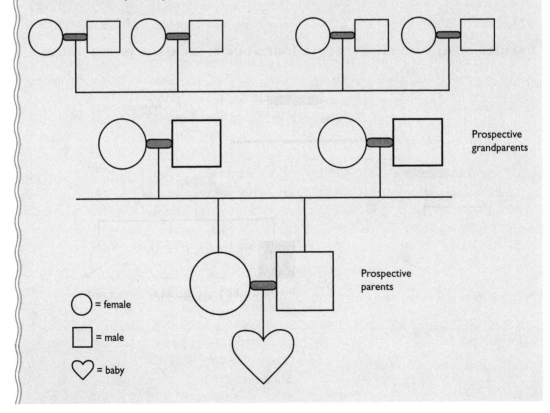

GENETIC TESTING ALONG THE CONCEPTION CONTINUUM

Anne and Daniel, both of Eastern European Jewish descent, have been married for several years and are thinking about having children. Anne's doctor recommended she be tested for the "Jewish panel" of genetic diseases: Tay-Sachs, Canavan, Gaucher's, and Niemann-Pick disease. But when Anne told Daniel that she'd made an appointment for the blood test, he hit the roof: "How could you even consider genetic testing? What are we going to do with it?"

Anne was completely taken aback. "I just want to know what our chances are of having a child with one of these dreadful diseases, so that we can decide if we want prenatal testing later on."

"Why?" Daniel retorted. "I can't imagine anything that would make me feel comfortable about getting an abortion."

"Well," Anne sighed, "if the child is going to die before the age of two, then I don't think it's fair to bring him into the world—for him or for us." Daniel and Anne have a lot to think about.

If preconception genetic screening revealed you were at risk for having a child with a serious disorder or birth defect, would you avoid pregnancy? The answer to this question is a totally personal one. Knowing your genetic risks before conception enables you and your spouse to educate yourselves about the potential challenges and, like Anne and Daniel, work through some difficult questions before a baby is even part of the equation.

As we've noted previously, it is vitally important that you and your partner open a respectful and caring dialogue about your family histories and any potential genetic disorders. If you are not in agreement about genetic evaluation and the ethical issues surrounding testing, it makes pregnancy very stressful, even before conception. Counseling and education before pregnancy will empower you to make decisions together with the best interests of your future baby at heart, and in the context of your faith if that is a factor for you. Addressing any disagreements in advance will make it possible to respond quickly to the question of genetic testing during pregnancy, if needed (such as during the first trimester).

When a genetic disease is almost a foregone conclusion, such as in the case of Huntington's disease or cystic fibrosis, you and your partner could consider alternative methods of building your family, such as adoption or donation of an egg or sperm.

Preconception Genetic Screening for Moms- and Dads-to-Be

It makes sense to consider preconception genetic testing if you have an inherited disorder, have a family history of a congenital or inherited disorder, are at high risk for certain diseases due to your ethnicity, or have had a previous child with a genetic disease or chromosomal abnormality. The blood testing is done on one partner to see if he or she is a carrier for the disorders in question. Depending on the results, the other partner may or may not need to be tested. These results may inform your decision about whether or not additional genetic testing is warranted as you progress through your journey to have a baby.

If your carrier testing was done more than five years prior to trying to conceive, ask your doctor whether additional tests have been added to the screening profiles. For example, Jewish carrier screening currently spans twenty-two different diseases, and five years ago it screened for only ten. You may be a carrier for a disease recently added to the screen, and you and your partner would not be aware of it.

Preimplantation Genetic Testing: Genetic Screening that Can Occur with IVF

Couples who have an inherited risk for disease, who have gone through repeated miscarriage (following either spontaneous conception or IVF), or where the woman is older than thirty-five may choose to consider preimplantation genetic testing, also known as preimplantation genetic diagnosis or PGD. The advanced technology used in this testing requires IVF in order to have access to the embryo in a lab setting. At an early stage of development, one or two cells are extracted from the embryo (called embryo biopsy). The DNA from these cells is analyzed for the presence of chromosomal abnormalities or specific genes that indicate that an inherited disorder has been passed on to the embryo. The PGD process is safe, and now the first six-to-eight-year-olds who were embryo-tested with PGD are doing wonderfully. A possibility for ethical abuse of PGD exists (such as for gender selection versus trying to avoid conceiving a baby with a gender-related disease like fragile X). Testing in this fashion is strictly regulated and will require extensive counseling for you and your partner. This technology is truly amazing. Parents who have watched a previous child die of an awful genetic disease can now have real hope to deliver a healthy child (at least one without the same disease) and avoid the fear of trying to conceive.

We should add a note of caution as well. While PGD was expected to increase the likelihood of implanting a healthier embryo, recent research has called this expectation into question. In a randomized, controlled trial of PGD published in the *New England Journal of Medicine,* women undergoing the procedure actually had significantly fewer pregnancies continue past twelve weeks and significantly fewer live births compared to women who did not receive PGD. Also, only one cell is extracted and examined in PGD, and if there is a mosaicism, that is, some normal and abnormal cells sharing the same embryo, PGD can be falsely reassuring if only a normal cell is checked. The IVF field is evolving rapidly, and your doctor will be able to advise you about the latest thinking. Clearly, improving the odds of successful implantation and live birth is the goal for all concerned.

FOR FUTURE REFERENCE: During Pregnancy

Prenatal (During Pregnancy) Genetic Testing

Once you and your partner are expecting your baby, you may be offered genetic screening of the fetus. If you already know that you or your partner carries the potential for a genetic disease, you have had a child in the past with a genetic abnormality, or you are at least thirty-five years of age, prenatal genetic testing will be offered to you. For everyone else who is not at higher risk, noninvasive genetic screening is possible for re-assurance about the health of your fetus (such as first-trimester nuchal fold measurements by ultrasound, hormone levels, and first- and second-trimester blood tests).

If you are at risk for having a child with a genetic abnormality such as fragile X or Down syndrome, you may wish to test your fetus while in the womb. Again, the decision to test a fetus, usually via chorionic villus sampling (CVS) or amniocentesis, is a personal one. These tests are acceptable at any maternal age, but the risks of the procedures must be outweighed by the benefits to each set of prospective parents. What you intend to do with the information obtained from the testing should determine if you do the test at all. That is, if you want the test to help you mentally and emotionally prepare by gathering information from pediatric staff or a support group, or if you will discontinue a pregnancy if a child is affected, then requesting a test is an excellent idea. Otherwise, the risks of the procedures may not be warranted (see Table 6-2). Most insurance companies will pay for part or all of the genetic screening if you or your spouse is at risk. Finding out in advance will save you from the shock of the genetic testing cost if it is not covered.

FIGURE 6-4
GENETIC TESTING DURING PREGNANCY

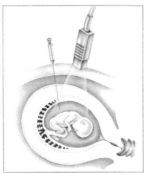

Amniocentesis is a diagnostic test. Ultrasound is used to guide a slender needle through the woman's abdomen into the amniotic sac to withdraw a small sample of the amniotic fluid. Amniotic fluid contains cells from the fetus that have the same genetic makeup as the fetus. These cells can be tested for a number of genetic disorders.

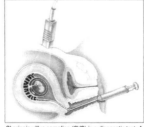

Chorionic villus sampling (CVS) is a diagnostic test. A small sample of cells is taken from the placenta where it is attached to the wall of the uterus. This is done either through a thin tube passed through the vagina and cervix or through a needle passed through the abdomen and uterus. Cells from the placenta reflect the genetic makeup of the fetus.

TABLE 6-2
PRENATAL GENETIC TESTING

Test	Timing (Weeks Pregnant)	Risks		Accuracy (Predictive)
		Fetus	Mother	
NONINVASIVE				
• Triple screen MSAFP[a] becomes a quad screen if inhibin is added	15-21	None	Emotional	Chromosomal abnormalities: Predictable: 65–75% False positives: 25% False negatives: 5–10% Neural tube defects (NTDs): Predictable: 85–90% False positives: 10%
• First-trimester[b,c] screen	11–13	None	Emotional	Chromosomal abnormalities (trisomy, especially 13, 18, 21): Predictable: 85–90% False positives: 10% False negatives: 5%
• Harmony Test (maternal blood test that detects fetal DNA fragments)	10 or more	None	Emotional	Chromosomal abnormalities (trisomy, especially 13, 18, 21): Predictable: 98–99% False negative <1% NTDs: not tested
INVASIVE				
• Amniocentesis (collects fetal cells in amniotic fluid)	15–18[d]	1:400–500[e] miscarriage; rare fetal injury	Infection	Chromosomal abnormalities: Predictable: 99% NTDs: 99%
• Chorionic villus sampling (CVS, collects chorionic villi, cells that will form placenta)	10–12	1:400[e] miscarriage; limb deformity[f]	Vaginal bleeding	Chromosomal abnormalities: Predictable: 98% NTDs: not tested

a. Tests the blood levels of bHCG, maternal serum alpha-fetoprotein (AFP), and estradiol.

b. Uses ultrasound to look at the fetal nuchal fold and a blood test to check maternal levels of PAPP-a and bHCG.

c. If first trimester screening or MSAFP raises the age-related risk for trisomy 13, 18, or 21 (Down syndrome), then another blood test called Materna 21 can be done and is predictive of these genetic abnormalities with up to 99% accuracy.

d. Genetic amniocentesis can be performed at any time during pregnancy but is optimal for safety and decision making between fifteen and eighteen weeks.

e. Rates of miscarriage from CVS and amniocentesis are dependent on the experience of your physician or institution. Check with your health care provider for the rates quoted specifically for their practice.

f. Limb deformity is more likely to occur if CVS is performed prior to ten gestational weeks.

WHAT IF I'VE BEEN ADOPTED?

Monica was reading a magazine at the hairdresser's about a family who had a child with cystic fibrosis and it started her thinking. She had been adopted and had no information about her ethnicity or family history. What about her own chances of passing on a problem to her prospective offspring? The more she thought about it, the more interested she became in genetic screening tests that could be performed before getting pregnant.

If, like Monica, you or your husband was adopted, your particular family history or ethnic background may be unknown. You need not be concerned. Autosomal recessive diseases, in which a child needs to inherit two copies of the defective gene, require only one partner to be tested. If the nonadopted partner is Italian, for example, he or she should be tested for beta thalassemia. If the test is negative, then the adopted partner does not need to be screened for beta thalassemia at all. If you and your husband are both adopted and of the same race, you can be tested for the most common genetic concerns in that population. For example, if you and your husband are Caucasian, one of you could be tested for cystic fibrosis and Tay-Sachs disease. If you are both African American, one of you should be tested to see if you carry sickle-cell disease. Armed with this information and any inklings of your own, you and your doctor can discuss whether it's necessary to probe further. It's important not to lose sight of the fact that the odds of having a favorable genetic predisposition are overwhelmingly in your favor.

Open adoptions—those that support direct contact between the child and his or her birth family—facilitate access to medical information by allowing the exchange of calls, emails, and letters between parties. If you or your partner was adopted, consider checking into the legality of obtaining information about the birth parents. The laws vary by state, but you may find that certain information can be disclosed to individuals over the age of eighteen or twenty-one.

FETAL ENVIRONMENT, FETAL GENES

Genetic problems in a fetus can occur in three ways: they can be passed on from the mother or father, they can result from damage to an egg or a sperm, or they can result from damage to the fetus itself at an early stage in the pregnancy. We've been talking about the first scenario—when nature (inherited genes) are the cause, a situation beyond your control. In the second and third cases, it's nurture that is to blame: a genetic change is caused by something in your or your partner's preconception environment or the fetus's womb environment.

The best way to minimize your risk of having this kind of problem occur is to see your respective doctors at least ninety days before trying to conceive. Discuss being proactive with every aspect of your health, starting with anything you flagged on your Preconception Medical Checklists (Figure 4-1 for women and Figure 9-4 for men). Focus on your nutrient intake and pre-pregnancy body weight, as well as taking a multivitamin that contains folic acid, which is protective against birth defects. Make certain behavioral changes such as avoiding alcohol (especially binge drinking) and recreational drugs. Avoiding exposure to certain infections (such as rubella, syphilis, and cytomegalovirus) and non-baby-friendly medications will also help prevent a large percentage of the following nonhereditary genetic concerns.

- **Neural tube defects (NTDs).** The neural tube, which develops into the brain, spinal cord, and nerves, forms by four weeks of life, often before you realize that you are pregnant. The most common NTD is spina bifida, when part of the spinal column is exposed or protrudes through an opening in the vertebrae that protect the spine. This condition is not lethal but often requires surgical correction to avoid paralysis and promote normal infant growth and development. The second most common NTD, anencephaly, is when the baby is born missing part of its brain and dies shortly after birth. Defects in the neural tube can occur in 1 out of 1,000 births, but are more likely if you have already had a child with an NTD or if you or your spouse has a personal history of an NTD the risk of NTD in your offspring can be as high as 1 to 3 in 100. In women with no prior history of an NTD-affected pregnancy, research has shown that 400 mcg of supplemental folic acid taken daily at least one month prior to conception and through the first two missed periods can reduce the incidence of NTDs by 70 percent. Recent evidence suggests that better intake of choline can further decrease the incidence of NTDs as well (see Chapter 11 for additional nutritional details).

- **Congenital heart disease.** This heart problem, usually diagnosed while the fetus is in the womb, can result from maternal infection with rubella or syphilis. Getting tested for immunity to or being vaccinated for these diseases several months prior to conception can minimize the risk of having a child with this problem (see Chapter 4). It may also be caused by random or inherited genetic issues, such as Down or Turner's syndrome, or by a poor perinatal environment, such as extreme alcohol abuse by the mother, poor nutritional status, or environmental exposures.

- **Pyloric stenosis.** This blockage between the stomach and intestines, which is usually diagnosed and surgically repaired after delivery, has been associated with maternal undernutrition.

- **Cleft palate and clubfoot.** Research has established a clear link between the incidence of these issues and excessive alcohol or drug use by the mother; vitamin inadequacies have also been implicated. Cleft palate is a gap in the lip or hard palate of the fetus. Clubfoot is a foot that is twisted inward at the ankle, making weight-bearing difficult. By reducing the intake of problematic substances before and after conception, you can reduce the risk of these abnormalities. Although these conditions are not lethal, they do require medical or surgical intervention, which carries its own risks to an infant as well as unnecessary pain.

- **Fetal alcohol spectrum disorders, the most severe being fetal alcohol syndrome.** These are characteristics caused by alcohol consumption when pregnant (most often from bingeing, but also from moderate regular drinking), especially during critical windows of fetal development. The baby can have varying degrees of sleep and feeding disturbances, growth and facial abnormalities, and later have exasperating—or worse, heartbreaking—behavior problems and learning disabilities. (It's not uncommon for patients to voice some degree of skepticism over whether moderate drinking should really pose concern. If this applies to you, please see, at a minimum, the "For Future Reference" on pages 41–43.)

Other nonhereditary medical issues that may increase the risk of having a child with a birth defect include:

- **High blood sugar** during preconception and early pregnancy in a prospective mother. This is one of the most common yet underrecognized causes of birth defects. Even if you are not diabetic, make absolutely sure that your blood sugar levels are within normal limits. (Being overweight increases the odds of being prediabetic.)

- **Exposure to certain medications** that are known teratogens (any agent that interferes with normal development of an embryo or fetus). Examples include the antibiotic doxycycline, lithium (sold under the brand names Eskolith and Lithobid), Dilantin, and isotretinoin (also known as Accutane or Clavaris). A full list of known teratogens can be found in Chapter 8.

AM I TOO OLD TO HAVE A BABY?

Judy, thirty-eight, comes in for her annual gynecologic exam with excellent news: she has finally met her soul mate. They plan to marry next spring and want to start their family shortly there-

after. She confesses that she always imagined it would be terribly romantic to conceive a baby on her honeymoon. But she is also worried: "I'll have turned thirty-nine just before our wedding, so I could be forty when the baby is born." Her friends warn her that she may be too old to have a healthy baby. She wants the facts: is she too old to be considering pregnancy?

The simple answer is no, Judy is not too old to responsibly consider pregnancy. In our parents' generation, the medical community discouraged childbearing after thirty years of age; now research supports, and we can vouch for, the success and safety of conception in women who wish to have babies in their mid-to-late thirties and early forties. Still, although you may think of yourself as a chipper thirty-five, from a medical and reproductive point of view, you are given the charming designation of being a woman of advanced maternal age. Your eggs have been with you since your mother conceived you, and they become more fragile as the years pass because they are dormant until ovulation and are not undergoing routine cellular repair. Friends and family members may be tormenting you about your biological clock, or you may be doing a fine job of fretting all by yourself, but rest assured you are not alone: overall birthrates have been on a slow, steady rise and increasing parental age has become much more common over the past thirty years.

In fact, according to the National Center for Health Statistics, births to women over age thirty are at an all-time high since the mid-1960s (the end of the postwar baby boom). Births to women ages thirty-five to thirty-nine have seen twenty-nine consecutive years of increases and the most recent data released indicate the rate is at the highest level in forty years. The birthrate is steadily increasing among women over forty years of age as well.

What societal drivers are causing advanced maternal age to become more common? There are more women in the workforce who are delaying childbearing until their professional goals have been met. Mature adults are also waiting longer before they decide to start a family in order to provide a more stable and financially secure environment. Keeping pace with our social trends, science provides assisted reproduction technologies that support the aging maternal and paternal birth trend.

What Is It About Age Thirty-five?

From early adulthood, women are told to have their children before the age of thirty-five, if possible. Why is this year of your life the magic year of fertility change and genetic concern? Actually, in the past thirty-five was simply the approximate age at which the risk of having a child with Down syndrome or other chromosomal abnormality surpassed the risk of miscarriage if you underwent a procedure to check for such genetic problems (about 1 in 350 procedures). This meant that for many women, thirty-five was the age at which it became worth the risk to have prenatal genetic testing. In 2009, new research reported an even lower risk of

Down Syndrome

Down syndrome, also known as DS or trisomy 21, occurs when the fetus has an extra copy of chromosome 21, causing varying degrees of learning disabilities, heart defects, short stature, and distinct facial features. The incidence of DS increases as the prospective mother ages, but preconception testing cannot yet predict the likelihood of DS, because the vast majority of instances are not inherited. The exception to this rule occurs with a family history of DS. One extremely rare type of DS can be screened for prior to conception. However, prenatal genetic testing can be performed for DS on pregnant women via amniocentesis or chorionic villus sampling. If DS is diagnosed during pregnancy, it's impossible to know how mild or profound the clinical effects will be. If you have had a child with DS in the past, you have a 1 percent chance of having a child with DS in a future pregnancy. If you will be over thirty-five years of age when trying to conceive, discuss your risk of DS with your doctor.

miscarriage (that is 1 in 500) as a result of undergoing invasive genetic testing with CVS or amniocentesis. This new genetic testing risk now matches the chance that DS will occur in a prospective mother who is thirty-two years old. As we incorporate this new understanding of invasive genetic test risk, women of all ages who are pregnant can be offered definitive genetic screening with CVS or amniocentesis, if prospective parents desire more exact results to allow maximum accuracy for decision making during a pregnancy.

TABLE 6-3
CHROMOSOME ABNORMALITIES IN LIVE-BORNS BY MATERNAL AGE

Maternal Age	Approximate Risk of Down Syndrome
25	1:1,250
30	1:1,000
32	1:500
35	1:350
40	1:100

Just to make sure you have an accurate picture of your odds of conceiving and carrying a baby to term when you are over thirty-five years old, here is what is known. Research has found that approximately 70 percent of women age thirty-five to thirty-nine are able to conceive within the first year and approximately 75 percent of those women will have a healthy early pregnancy, free of miscarriage. Statistics on women age forty to forty-two are less easy to come by, but approximately 50 percent conceive spontaneously in their first year of trying (happily, an additional 10 to 20 percent will conceive if you include women assisted by reproduction technology), though for women over forty the miscarriage rates rise to 30 to 40 percent.

Late Fatherhood

> *Charles, an excited new father, is a vigorous fifty-year-old with salt-and-pepper hair. He is walking down the hall of the maternity ward with his newborn son in his arms when a well-wisher passes and asks if this is his first grandchild. "No," he says. "Actually, it's my first child."*

What role does an older father's genes play when it comes to genetics and fertility? We've all heard of or perhaps known a man who remarried late in life and proudly started a new family. We know men can reproduce well into their senior years. But what are the implications of paternal age for fertility and healthy conception?

A man's sperm are not as fragile as a woman's aging eggs because new sperm are constantly being produced. But there are changes noted in the sperm of older men. One study examined men who were over fifty-five at the time of conception and had partners who were under thirty-five. In these patients, an increase in Down syndrome and birth defects was noted, unexplained by maternal age alone. Increasing paternal age also seems to increase the risk of autosomal dominant diseases such as Turner syndrome, in which all or part of a chromosome is missing.

Men over forty may also be more likely to have medical conditions such as high blood pressure that necessitate taking drugs that can sometimes affect libido, potency, and ejaculation. Obviously, decreased ability to engage in sexual activity can affect fertility rates. But it is reassuring to know that just as modern medicine offers much in the way of fertility support to women, men also have options when they need a reproduction assist. If this is pertinent for you or your partner, refer to Chapter 9 and discuss it with your health care provider.

If your man is tempted to go it alone by heading to the supplement aisle of your health food store, think about sharing this information with him: a number of male baby boomers look to "anti-aging" dietary supplements such as DHEAS, a hormone precursor, in hopes of turning back the clock or improving sexual function (mainly erectile dysfunction). However, DHEAS has a notorious record of poor quality control and insufficient proof of effectiveness. More important, he should be cautious of any supplements that alter hormone levels. Too many are tainted with legal (or illegal) contaminants, something you cannot identify from

A Y-Chromosome Link to Autism?

Researchers are also exploring the degree to which a man's age may affect the likelihood of autism among their children. Autism is a disease that results in abnormal social development, communication problems, and unusual behaviors and is associated with learning disabilities. The underlying cause of autism still baffles the medical community, and many different etiologies have been proposed, such as genetic predisposition, maternal medication usage, vaccination, and environmental exposures. Some theories have been subsequently debunked by more carefully controlled research (such as vaccinations in childhood). That said, recent studies have offered a link between more mature maternal or paternal age as an independent variable for the increased risk for autism and reduced neurological development. Other studies from 2006 reported a relation to advanced maternal age as an isolated factor that can increase the risk of autism in offspring. In a large Israeli study that controlled for maternal age, the age of prospective fathers definitely affected the incidence of autism. For men under the age of thirty, the chance of conceiving a child with autism was 1 in 1,000, but for those in their forties, the risk tripled to 3 in 1,000, and over age fifty, the risk quintupled to 5 in 1,000. While there is no way to change paternal age, it is helpful to have an increased awareness of the risks all prospective parents undertake.

reading the label. See more on individual herbs and dietary supplements in Chapters 8 and 9, and remember that the best way to naturally revitalize your man is through encouraging physical activity and good nutrition.

As Mother Nature Ages...

The main reason that miscarriage and lowered fertility rates rise steadily with age can be traced to Mother Nature, who gives each woman all the eggs available for procreation at birth. As we grow older, our eggs can become more fragile and their genetic material more likely to break, duplicate, or be lost. So the rates of genetic abnormalities or missed ovulation rise more dramatically from thirty-five to forty-two years of age than prior to thirty-five.

FOR FUTURE REFERENCE: During Pregnancy

What Is the Impact of Maternal Age on Pregnancy Health?
Pregnant women over thirty-five face higher risks of medical problems, such as pregnancy-induced hypertension (PIH) or gestational diabetes than their younger coun-

terparts. Researchers have long understood that advanced maternal age introduces risk factors for a complicated pregnancy. For instance, a study conducted in 1996 by investigators at Mount Sinai Medical Center in New York City found that women between ages thirty-five and thirty-nine had preeclampsia and gestational diabetes at twice the rate of women who conceived in their twenties. By entering pregnancy in peak physical condition you can reduce those health risks.

A large study conducted at the University of California, Davis, in January 1999 reported on the safety of women who delivered babies after the age of forty compared to women who delivered prior to the age of thirty.

- There was an increase in Cesarean sections for the women who were over forty. In fact, 47 percent of women over forty who were having a first-time pregnancy underwent C-section; by comparison, women under thirty had Cesarean sections only 22 percent of the time (the national average at the time).
- For women who were over forty but having a second or third child, the Cesarean risk was 29.6 percent: not as high as for first-time mothers, but still much higher than the 17 percent of their younger counterparts having a second or third child.

We are not absolutely certain what causes the higher rate of Cesarean deliveries in older mothers, but there are a few likely possibilities. First, the uterine muscle may not labor as effectively as that of a younger woman. Also, the baby doesn't drop into the proper position as often as it does in prospective mothers under the age of thirty, making C-section a safer mode of delivery for these infants. The study did not show any significant differences between the two age groups in terms of premature delivery, birth weight, or birth trauma to the infant, indicating that the majority of neonatal outcomes were good—reassuring information for those who wish to be moms later in their reproductive years.

When you have successfully conceived over the age of thirty-five, you will be offered several tests to evaluate the normalcy of your developing baby (see Table 6-3). New technology is evolving regularly to determine the genetic health of a prospective fetus without increasing the risk to the pregnancy itself. For now, ultrasound and laboratory testing in the first and second trimesters of a pregnancy can predict the risk of genetic abnormalities such as Down syndrome and assess congenital anomalies (birth defects that can affect your fetus's anatomy without having a genetic irregularity as the cause), respectively. A blood test called the triple screen MSAFP (maternal screen alpha-fetoprotein) can predict certain chromosomal abnormalities with a moderate level of accuracy. The most accurate way to test your fetus for genetic abnormalities is through invasive procedures such as chorionic villus sampling and amniocentesis. These technical advances have helped couples to decide if they are willing and able to embrace a future that includes a special-needs baby. Most of the time, though, these tests serve as reassurance that all appears well with the baby.

With an element of luck and some work of your own, your biological clock may reward you with an easy conception and pregnancy, especially if you've maintained good health over the years. Even if you haven't, it's never too late to make a change for the better. The middle section of this book will help guide you through nutritional and fitness changes you can make to improve your health and reproductive potential.

CHAPTER 7

To Your Health: Your Immune System and Other Medical Matters

Those that take their medicine, but neglect their diet, waste the skills of their physician.
—Old Asian aphorism

We live in extraordinary times. Women in the United States live almost two decades longer than their counterparts of only fifty years ago, and maternal mortality is at an all-time low (7 to 8 per 100,000 live births). Improvements in preventive health care, nutrition, and exercise, as well as advances in medicine and medical technology, have made women today healthier than ever. Only twenty-five years ago, women who had medical conditions such as diabetes, lupus, or heart disease were strongly advised by their doctors to avoid pregnancy to ensure their own continued good health. With today's improved preconception and prenatal care, women with these sorts of medical conditions usually can become the mothers of healthy babies. Moms-to-be whose medical history may include hypothyroidism, breast cancer, physical disabilities, or depression can successfully conceive and carry a child, too.

A Note from the Authors to *All* Readers

In this chapter, we have added new recommendations pertinent to *every* reader—how to help prepare your immune system to welcome your baby from the very start (implantation in the womb), and how you can actively decrease the risk of a too-early birth. This is a must read (see next page).

Further, though the majority of you reading this book will not have the clinically diagnosed medical problems detailed in the following pages, resist the urge to skip the rest of this chapter. At least familiarize yourself with the risk factors or warning signs listed under each medical condition. Who knows—you may be the first to detect signs of a medical problem that, if ignored, can affect your fertility, your general health, and the developmental milestones of your baby. Here's to your health!

The best time to start discussing any potential special needs is before conception has occurred. As we show, women who have their medical problems under good control, often by taking baby-friendly medications and optimizing their body weight and general health, will increase their fertility, decrease miscarriage risk, and improve their overall prenatal health.

If you do have a preexisting medical condition, our most important piece of advice is not to avoid pregnancy but rather to avoid an *unplanned* pregnancy. Knowledge is your friend when it comes to your preconception health: the more you know about your physical and mental health before your pregnancy, the better equipped you and your health care team will be to manage any medical conditions you have now or that might arise or worsen during your pregnancy.

When you have a preexisting condition you may find it useful to raise the following questions when you begin to work with your doctor or midwife:

- Is it appropriate for me to consider conceiving a baby at this time? If not, are there steps I can take to prepare for pregnancy?
- Will my medical condition change when I'm pregnant? How?
- Will my medical condition pose risks to my unborn fetus? What are those risks?
- How can my medications be managed before, during, and after pregnancy? Which medications are optimal, and which are absolutely unacceptable?

Naturally, the answers to these and other vital questions must be tailored to your individual needs. Care of a given condition begins with medical management and is enhanced by nutritional, exercise, and psychological components. If you need to manage your health for several weeks or many months before you get the go-ahead to conceive and are feeling frustrated, remember: if you don't master your own health, your future baby's health may be off to a rocky start.

MAKING YOUR BODY A WELCOMING PLACE: THE IMPORTANCE OF A HEALTHY IMMUNE SYSTEM

If you are science-minded, the first part of this section on the immune system will offer a fascinating rationale for placing this discussion front and center. However, some of you may prefer to move directly to the action steps on page 165, "12 Tips to a Welcoming Womb."

When you conceive, your immune system sets off on a uniquely maternal course of multitasking. Here's how:

- First and foremost, your immune system remains true to its purpose of protecting your body from harmful foreign substances, particularly infectious viruses or bacteria. Immune recognition of these "foreigners" triggers inflammation, then methodical elimination of the perpetrator.

- Second, during pregnancy, the immune system cannot overreact to the introduction of a baby in your womb, which is half familiar, but also half "foreign" genetic material (that of dad). Scientists used to think that the mom's immune system would automatically weaken during pregnancy, to spare the fetus from attack. Recent research suggests that the immune system, in fact, remains as strong as ever.
- Third, in order to build a healthy placenta—the lifeline between you and the fetus—a swift, efficient inflammatory response from the implantation site in the womb is required to tidy the area where the placenta will develop in the womb. If this immune system response is weak, the pregnancy struggles or doesn't continue.
- Lastly, a normal inflammatory response occurs in the placenta when delivery is imminent, preferably as close to full-term as possible. Sometimes the immune system "jumps the gun" causing preterm labor, the reasons for which are not entirely understood.

How do our bodies resolve these conflicting goals of the immune system? Studies from Dr. Gil Mor's Reproductive Immunology Unit at Yale University School of Medicine propose that amazingly, the immune system, womb lining, and building blocks of the placenta work in concert to "educate" each other once you conceive. Your immune system learns what's a real threat (viruses and bacteria) and what's not (the fetus). (More about Dr. Gil Mor's immune theory can be found on page 165.)

Luckily for us, our bodies have had a long time to perfect this art of baby making. However, it isn't a perfect system, and infection, whether viral or bacterial, is often a cause of miscarriage and preterm labor, especially if the inflammation was smoldering undetected in the body prior to conception. Such "silent" inflammation occurs with low-grade infections (e.g., dental or vaginal) as well as in chronic medical conditions (e.g., obesity, insulin resistance/metabolic syndrome, vascular disease). Entering pregnancy with an immune system already under duress is potentially risky. Sadly, the appropriate inflammatory responses to a real threat (infection) can backfire on a pregnant woman as her immune system tries to overwhelm the invaders and protect the vulnerable mother-to-be.

As mentioned later in this chapter, reproductive-age women with autoimmune diseases such as lupus and rheumatoid arthritis need to optimize their immune systems before pregnancy to improve maternal and fetal health. But what about everyone else who doesn't have an autoimmune disease? Shouldn't we all be optimizing our immune systems to prepare for pregnancy by reducing inflammation, which can irritate the reproductive system? Researchers are just starting to address these questions, and the possibilities are very interesting.

FOR FUTURE REFERENCE: During Pregnancy

The Role of Your Immune System During Pregnancy

When you become pregnant, your immune system will play a big role in making your body a welcoming place. When your baby is only sixteen cells large, called a blastocyst, it must burrow into your womb to successfully implant (a critical factor for a full-term pregnancy). Normally such an "invasion" from something that isn't 100 percent Mom's genetics sets off all sorts of alarms and triggers the immune system to attack. What happens instead? We asked Yale University's Dr. Mor, an expert in reproductive immunology whose research has overturned fifty years of conventional thinking about the maternal immune system. Here's what he has to say:

"The pregnant mother's immune system is vigorous and dynamic, engaging in a constant dialogue with the fetus to protect the health of mother and baby. When threats arise, such as inflammation or infection, the placenta coordinates the immune response. But in serious conditions, the placenta has to choose which life to spare, and it is biased to protect the mother's life. This necessary choice can lead to problems with implantation, preeclampsia, premature delivery, and, unfortunately, congenital defects. By adopting some specific health habits before and during pregnancy, you can optimize your immune system's ability to juggle competing needs, so that the placenta is not forced to make such a difficult choice. The authors of this book have pulled together a dozen recommendations based on the latest research. You can play a key role in improving reproductive outcomes by following these guidelines beginning in the preconception period."

12 Tips to a Welcoming Womb

1. **Avoid exposure to infectious microorganisms in the first place.** This prevents unnecessary activation of your immune system. Though there's no need to be compulsive, proper hygiene by you and your partner is key. For starters, hand washing and bathing with ordinary soap and warm water (no need for antibacterial soaps—though antibacterial gels are appropriate if you have no access to clean water or soap) would spare you exposure to many germs. It's important to understand that different types of bacteria live peacefully (and serve various functions) on your body and probably should not routinely be wiped out by overcleansing or vigorous scrubbing. (In fact, two active ingredients in antibacterial soaps have recently been found to disrupt hormone signaling systems; see page 57.) You've heard this before, but feminine hygiene includes properly wiping yourself when you use the restroom to avoid contamination

from your anus (wipe from front to back, never going back over the same area with the same piece of toilet paper); keep this same concept in mind during sexual intercourse (you don't want anal bacteria entering your vagina).

2. **Do not douche or aggressively wash the inside of your vagina with soap.** Douching rinses away friendly bacteria that protect you from infection, and it disrupts the balance inside the vagina. Your vulnerability to infection increases even more dramatically if you douche when you become pregnant.

3. **Don't wait until you're pregnant to see your dentist.** Pre-pregnancy is the best time to treat undiagnosed periodontitis (oral and gum infections increase the risk of preterm delivery and poor pregnancy outcome).

4. **Consider a lab workup.** This can help your doctor assess inflammatory markers such as C-reactive protein (hs-CRP) and possibly homocysteine. A test called HbA1C, or A1C, is an excellent indication of long-term blood sugar control (recall from the end of Chapter 3, chronically high blood sugars can cause inflammation in blood vessels and may cause birth defects). These labs could uncover hidden problems or at the very least identify women who need to be extra vigilant in following these anti-inflammation guidelines. This workup is mainly advised if you are overweight or have a strong personal or family history of periodontal disease, heart disease, or colon cancer. One last test, especially if you are overweight or have heavily pigmented skin, is to make sure you have healthy levels of vitamin D.

5. **Avoid smoking and being around those who do smoke.**

6. **Keep your gastrointestinal tract healthy.** Your digestive tract is prominent in the defense of your immune system, so you want it to be healthy. This means it's probably a good idea to regularly eat yogurt or kefir with live and active cultures to keep friendly strains of bacteria thriving in your intestinal tract (they are not perceived as a threat by your immune system). Research on a wider variety of probiotic strains (e.g., primarily types of lactobacilli) are promising, albeit preliminary, in protecting against urinary tract infections and some vaginal infections. Further, make sure to eat yogurt with live cultures if you ever require antibiotics, which can wipe out natural, protective bacteria and leave you vulnerable to an overgrowth of potentially harmful bacteria or yeast. (Also, please be sure to finish the course of antibiotics, because stopping early leaves the most resilient bugs alive and encourages the emergence of new drug-resistant strains.)

7. **Enjoy foods that appear to have an anti-inflammatory effect on the body.** Although scientists are still sifting through evidence that specific foods may minimize

inflammation, we do know a few things for certain. An emphasis on whole grains, nuts, legumes, a wide variety of fruits and vegetables, low-fat dairy foods, culinary herbs and spices, fatty fish, and olive or canola oil all have a welcome effect on the body. Eliminate trans fatty acids (hydrogenated fats) as best you can, and cut back on fatty meats and saturated fats, but don't make the mistake of replacing these with refined carbs or sugar. This is only the briefest overview. There's more on dietary advice in Chapter 10; for specific antioxidant and anti-inflammatory herbs, seasonings, and supplements, see Chapter 8.

8. **Take 400 mcg of folic acid in a daily supplement** (which can also contain other vitamins and minerals). Folic acid might mediate early intrauterine infections that could contribute to very early preterm birth, especially if it is taken daily for one year before conceiving.

9. **Follow safe food handling recommendations to prevent bacterial or viral contamination.** (See the end of Chapter 13, for both you and your hubby.)

10. **Eat just enough to maintain a healthy body weight.** Or if you are overweight, pore over Chapter 14 to get motivated to lose some weight prior to conception. This cannot be ignored, because obese people have higher levels of systemic inflammation and greater susceptibility to infectious insults (such as urinary and genital tract infections, poor wound healing).

11. **Make daily exercise a top priority.** Moderate physical activity lowers inflammatory markers and improves immune function. If you need any vaccinations prior to trying, moderate aerobic exercise appears to improve a vaccine's efficacy. Most research on this exercise effect has been conducted among those receiving the flu vaccine. Exercise improves the recruitment of the body's "first responders" to the injection site, thus triggering a swifter and more efficient immune response. Note that prolonged, heavy exercise (such as a marathon) does not have this helpful effect, and may even temporarily depress immunity.

12. **Manage stress.** Some stress is fine, but too much wreaks havoc. Wanting to have a baby is the best excuse in the world to slow down and take the time to de-stress your life. We talked about ways to accomplish this in Chapter 1 when contemplating emotional readiness.

That wraps up the "required reading" for all prospective mothers, independent of health status. Now it's time to segue into warning signs of potential medical conditions (we suggest that you skim over the shaded boxes before moving on to the next chapter). And if you already know you have a preexisting condition, let's move on to how you can begin refining your pre-conception plan with your medical team.

CAREFUL CONCEPTION: MANAGING YOUR MEDICAL PROBLEMS

Preparing for conception is a great opportunity to renew your commitment to good health. Now you are walking or jogging, remembering to take your meds, or saying no to those cheese fries! We'll begin our discussion of possible preexisting conditions with one of the most common medical diseases that can be positively affected by preconception fine-tuning: diabetes.

DIABETES

Diabetes mellitus is one of the most common medical conditions that can have a significant impact on women of reproductive age. When you have diabetes, your body is unable to effectively use its main fuel source: sugar, also known as *glucose*. The result is an overabundance of glucose in the system that can affect the blood vessels, kidneys, nerves, and the ability to fight infection. Approximately 5 percent of women have diagnosed cases of type 1 or type 2 diabetes at the time of conception, and another 5 to 7 percent will develop a form of diabetes during pregnancy known as *gestational diabetes*. Gestational diabetes usually subsides after delivery, but these women will be at a higher risk for either type 2 diabetes or insulin resistance after pregnancy. There are two main types of diabetes mellitus that require preconception care:

Type 1 (formerly called insulin-dependent diabetes or juvenile diabetes)
- Usually occurs before age thirty
- Has an abrupt onset
- Requires multiple daily insulin injections or an insulin pump because the body cannot produce its own insulin
- Can be more challenging to reduce fluctuations in glucose levels

Type 2 (formerly called non-insulin-dependent diabetes or adult-onset diabetes)
- Usually occurs after age forty but is becoming more common in younger, reproductive-age women as well, due to the increasing prevalence of overweight and obesity
- Has a gradual onset
- Does not generally require insulin injections because the body usually produces some of its own insulin; oral medications may be necessary to facilitate insulin production and/or uptake, but during pregnancy insulin is almost always required

"Borderline"?

Are you insulin resistant or prediabetic? Do you have borderline high blood pressure? Are you a little heavy around the waistline?

We all know that there's no such thing as being borderline pregnant. But with blood sugar levels, blood pressure, lipids, weight, and "silent" inflammation, there's a gray area of risk—although your numbers may not yet merit a true clinical diagnosis, you haven't dodged the bullet, especially once you become pregnant. Getting these issues under control now could be the tipping point that determines your pregnancy outcome.

If you're otherwise healthy but have (or suspect you have) one or more mild abnormalities involving blood glucose, blood pressure, thyroid hormone levels, or weight (especially increased abdominal girth), you should not wait until after you're pregnant to get things under control. Research tells us that it's women who begin pregnancy healthy who have the best outcomes, often because so much is determined in the early, early weeks of a pregnancy. You're protecting your baby from day one.

The blessing of having a "borderline" health condition is that the solution can usually be found in your efforts to modify personal habits (and possibly include a simple baby-friendly medication) rather than in more invasive medical treatments. It's usually a matter of making a few fundamental lifestyle changes, with increased physical activity and nutritious eating taking the lead. Take a close look at the immune system, diabetes, cardiovascular, and thyroid sections not only for lifestyle modifications but also for tests you may need to help rule out full-blown medical conditions.

- Is a less volatile condition and often goes undiagnosed in its early stages; can usually be controlled, and in some cases reversed, through diet and exercise if caught early, although medications may be needed eventually

Claudia, twenty-nine and married, has had type 2 diabetes since she was in her mid-twenties. At the time of diagnosis, she was cautioned by her doctors not to conceive unless her blood sugars were in good control for at least two to three months beforehand, to minimize the risks to her and the future baby. Last year, in anticipation of wanting to be pregnant by age thirty, she and her health care team ramped up efforts to get her hemoglobin A1C (HbA1C) (see page 172) from around 8.5 percent to the goal of below 6.5 percent. Their main focus revolved around what it would take to get her body weight into the healthier range—the verdict being a gradual weight loss of thirty-five pounds through healthy diet and increased daily activity. She set her mind to the task and, with a little guidance, set up a weight reduction and exercise program that she could track on her computer (see

Chapter 13). Claudia was thrilled to see that this was working and she became more in tune with her body. By the time she reached her goal, she was down to the lowest possible dosage of diabetes medication to control her blood sugars. She had an eye exam with her ophthalmologist, a twenty-four-hour urine collection to assess her kidney function, and an electrocardiogram to assess her heart. Each was found to be normal, and her doctor agreed that she could start trying to get pregnant. He also tested her HbA1C, which was just below 6.5 percent, and her daily blood sugars were within safe parameters. With all this good news, he happily gave Claudia the green light. Claudia was pregnant three months later.

Perhaps the greatest difficulty in managing diabetes is its constant presence in your life. The body of a person with diabetes is simply not as forgiving as the nondiabetic body when food, exercise, medication, and lifestyle do not work in harmony. Minimizing the short-term and long-term consequences of diabetes demands your diligence, but the payoff is a healthier baby and a healthier you. While you dedicate yourself to getting ready to conceive, continue to use effective birth control methods until you hear those golden words: "It's okay to begin trying!"

SHOULD YOU BE SCREENED FOR DIABETES?

If you have any of the following conditions, it's a good idea to be screened for diabetes before trying to conceive.

- If you are overweight with a BMI (body mass index) greater than 25 (see Chapter 14 to find out how to calculate your BMI).
- If you have close relatives with diabetes.
- If your ethnicity is one of the following: Native American, African American, Hispanic, Asian, or Pacific Islander (including Native Hawaiian).
- If you've had gestational diabetes in a prior pregnancy or have had a baby whose birth weight was over 9 pounds.
- If you have high blood pressure (regardless of whether it is under control with medications).
- If you have a low HDL ("good") cholesterol level (35 mg/dl or less) and/or high triglyceride level (250 mg/dl or more).
- If your blood sugars have ever been tested and you were told they were borderline or that you have impaired glucose tolerance or prediabetes.
- If you have polycystic ovary syndrome (refer to Chapter 5 for detailed information).
- If you were born prematurely or with a birth weight below 5½ pounds.
- If you have had a prior pregnancy in which your baby had a birth defect, such as a cardiac malformation or a neural tube defect.

Making Helpful Changes Prior to Conception

The demanding but rewarding job of achieving blood glucose control requires a team effort among you, your partner, and the health care professionals who are rooting for you. These usually include an endocrinologist and a maternal-fetal medicine (MFM) specialist or general obstetrician, a certified diabetes educator (CDE), and a registered dietitian (RD), in addition to your primary physician. Many hospitals offer a clinical setting where the entire team works together and sees you regularly through preconception and pregnancy. If you have not had an eye exam within a year of trying to conceive, we advise that you visit your ophthalmologist or optometrist for a comprehensive eye exam.

Your partner can be an essential part of your winning team. Women with a supportive partner maintain better blood sugar control, which leads to improved fertility and maternal health once pregnant and fewer first-trimester losses. In relationships considered nonsupportive, higher numbers of unplanned pregnancies were noted, in which poorly controlled blood sugar levels that placed mother and baby at significant health risk were observed more often than not. A supportive partner who doesn't expect you to "go it alone" may help cook healthy meals, promote exercise, and indulge his sweet tooth outside of the home to reduce temptation for you. He may also take an active interest in the disease itself so he can be informed enough to be helpful or, at a minimum, more empathetic. (But being supportive does not mean becoming the food police!)

So, Why Control Your Blood Sugar?

Your keen attention to controlling your blood sugar will help to ensure your ability to have a healthy full-term baby. Successful control of blood sugar will lead to:

- A greater likelihood of fertility, especially with a history of insulin resistance.
- A reduction in the likelihood of miscarriage, birth defects, abnormal fetal growth (too large or too small), and stillbirth.
- Slowing the advance of detrimental changes in your eyes, heart, or kidneys.
- A reduced risk of high blood pressure and stroke.

Conversely, if you have poor blood sugar control, you will be at higher risk for:

- A baby with multiple birth defects, including defects of the heart, brain, spine, upper lip, soft palate, kidneys, gastrointestinal tract, and limbs. The damage is done very early in the pregnancy, by eight weeks from your last menstrual period, and may be even more likely if you are obese prior to conception. Remember that prolonged hyperglycemia is a more common likely cause of birth defects than all of the environmental exposures covered in Chapter 3.

- Preterm labor and delivery.
- Preeclampsia, a syndrome that includes high blood pressure, hypersensitivity of reflexes, protein excreted in the urine, swelling of the hands and feet, impaired liver and kidney function, and clotting problems.
- Speeding up the progression of eye and kidney problems in yourself.

What Other Tests Should Be Done?

As part of the preconception exam, all women with preexisting diabetes should have, at a minimum, the following additional tests, according to the ADA: HbA1C, serum creatinine, thyroid function, urine testing to see if there is protein being spilled into the urine, and ferritin (iron stores). Women with type 1 diabetes (or type 2 if on metformin) should also be tested for vitamin B12 levels and if they have bowel complaints, an evaluation for celiac disease.

Colette, twenty-four, has had type 1 diabetes since she was sixteen years old, but resented having to use conspicuous vials and syringes and her glucose meter in public. She had poor blood sugar control as a result. But these reasons really masked the bigger issue: it was easier to stay thin when her blood sugars ran high, luring her to skip or cut back on insulin unnecessarily. She and her husband desperately wanted a child but didn't want to risk conception until her diabetes was better controlled. She talked to her health care team about relatively painless, discreet alternatives to syringes (e.g., insulin pens) for insulin delivery. She also worked with her CDE dietitian and a psychotherapist experienced in eating disorders to address fundamentals of food and weight attitudes. She soon felt reassured that her weight wouldn't get out of control with better blood sugar control. Within a few short months of making changes, Colette was more confident and comfortable in caring for her diabetes. It took four additional months of good blood sugar control before she got the go-ahead. She conceived surprisingly quickly and later delivered a healthy 8-pound 10-ounce baby girl.

The Importance of Blood Sugar Monitoring

Now we know what the blood sugar level is supposed to be. But how do we measure it? There are two primary ways to do this. Blood sugar control can be self-monitored at home by finger stick and a blood glucose meter, or by blood test in a medical office. Long-term blood sugar control (that of the past two to three months) can be determined by a single test, the glycated hemoglobin test (HbA1C, or simply A1C). Recent studies have shown that lower A1C levels, usually less than 6.5 percent, predict the best possible maternal and fetal health during a pregnancy.

Special Circumstances for Women with Type 1 Diabetes

In type 1 diabetes, the blood vessels of the eyes, kidneys, and heart can be damaged as a result of poor blood sugar control. Nerve endings and your fertility can also be affected. If you have one or more of these complications, work with your endocrinologist or diabetologist to identify the severity and stabilize the condition before you try to conceive. If you have any of these medical problems but don't know it, you can put yourself and your unborn baby under unnecessary strain. We suggest you get an electrocardiogram, eye exam, urinalysis, and blood pressure check. Identifying potentially problematic changes in these organs before pregnancy will allow you to minimize their effect on your pregnancy and the pregnancy's effect on you. Excellent blood sugar control for one to three months prior to trying to conceive is optimal. Usually this is accomplished through intensive insulin therapy with continuous subcutaneous insulin infusion (via an insulin pump) or multiple-injection regimens of short- and long-lasting insulins. Most doctors recommend regular A1Cs (optimally less than 6.5 percent) before and after pregnancy to keep tabs on your overall blood sugar control.

Note: Only in rare cases is it too dangerous for a woman with diabetes to try to get pregnant. If you are making every effort to control your diabetes but your doctor still advises against conception, a second medical opinion as well as counseling with an endocrinologist and maternal-fetal medicine specialist may be helpful.

Unless you use a device for continuous glucose monitoring, self-monitoring blood glucose with a fingerstick blood sugar (FSBS) test will give you the best feedback on food-to-blood-glucose relationships. Women with type 1 diabetes are experts at FSBS monitoring, and continued frequent sampling is essential once pregnancy occurs. However, if you have type 2 diabetes, you may not have been encouraged to self-monitor your glucose levels until now. To assess your sugar fluctuations you may be asked to test yourself as a woman with type 1 diabetes would, before each meal and snack, as well as do occasional spot checks one to two hours after a meal, in the middle of the night, or anytime you suspect low blood sugar. Food diaries, in which you record what you ate and your sugar levels after meals, are the best way to have an accurate understanding of the way certain foods affect your blood glucose levels and body weight. Pricking your fingers several times each day is no picnic, but keep in mind the wonderful service you are doing yourself and, by extension, your baby-to-be. In addition to your food journal, make notes of any questions you have for your dietitian, such as "Why did my blood sugar shoot up so high after I ate a bagel with nothing on it?" (You'll be amazed to discover that some bagels are the equivalent of three to five pieces of bread.)

Counseling before pregnancy will give you an opportunity to see how effectively your blood glucose and weight fluctuations can be managed. Women with preexisting diabetes will be asked to follow the same weight gain guidelines during pregnancy as do women without diabetes. This proactive approach to making the lifestyle and nutrition changes necessary for preconception health will better equip you to assess your timing for conception.

Once you are ready to conceive, you may be advised to stop taking pills—Actos, Avandia, Glucophage (metformin), acarbose, or glyburide (Diabeta)—and start giving yourself insulin shots (recall there are relatively new, pain-free devices for this). Why go from pills to injections? The side effects on the fetus from these oral glucose-lowering medications are not completely understood. Current studies suggest that metformin may be safe to take while pregnant, and it has been used in the first trimester with no reported fetal effects to date. We do know that some oral agents can pass through the placental barriers, causing excessively high levels of circulating insulin in the fetus. If you're taking medications for other conditions, such as high blood pressure, your doctor will evaluate whether any of them need to be discontinued or switched at some time.

The following are the criteria from the American Diabetes Association (ADA) for optimum blood sugar control prior to conceiving. The closer you are to these guidelines (though some physicians advocate even tighter goals), the better the outcome for you and eventually for your baby:

Goals for Pre-pregnancy Plasma Glucose Levels[1]
- 80 to 110 mg/dl before meals
- Less than 155 mg/dl two hours after the beginning of a meal

1. Laboratories separate the blood and analyze only the plasma glucose. Most of the newer meters are plasma referenced, too. See the directions that accompany your meter to see what it measures.

 FOR FUTURE REFERENCE: During Pregnancy

How to Maintain Glucose Control in Pregnancy

Once you are pregnant, the fluctuations in your blood sugar can have widespread implications. That is, if your glucose is too high on a regular basis, you will be at risk for poor weight gain, fetal birth defects, and irregular fetal growth (often too much or too little). High blood sugar (hyperglycemia) is one of the few teratogens over which we have some control. Once you are pregnant, your blood glucose control will need to be even tighter than the pre-pregnancy recommendations listed above, namely:
- Fasting glucose (first thing in the morning): 60 to 90 mg/dl; before subsequent meals, 60 to 105 mg/dl[a]

- One hour after the beginning of a meal: less than 140 mg/dl;[b] the ADA prefers tighter control of 100–120 mg/dl one hour after meals[a]
- Two hours after the start of a meal: less than 120 mg/dl
- Middle of the night (~2–3 a.m.): make sure blood glucose isn't dipping below 60 mg/dl

a. American Diabetes Association (2007).
b. American College of Obstetricians and Gynecologists (ACOG).

Avoid Hypoglycemia

When switching from oral agents to insulin injections, or adjusting your usual insulin regimen, close follow-up with your medical team is essential. If you are using insulin injections for the first time, you may find that being observed by a diabetes educator can be helpful. This is helpful to implement one month prior to trying to conceive to ensure early pregnancy health for mother and baby-to-be. Alterations in your insulin regimen are common in early pregnancy as you may be unable to eat regularly or may suffer from nausea or vomiting. Hypoglycemia is defined as a blood glucose level less than 60 mg/dl, though symptoms may occur at 70 mg/dl or less. Learn how to recognize and treat hypoglycemia, to ensure good fetal and maternal health.

SYMPTOMS OF HYPOGLYCEMIA

Common symptoms of hypoglycemia or low blood sugar are:

- Shakiness, weakness
- Light-headedness
- Quickened heart rate
- Irritability, anxiousness
- Confusion
- Extreme hunger

- Sweating
- Headache
- Blurred or double vision
- Nausea
- Numb lips or tongue
- Difficulty verbalizing, slurred speech

Studies show that women who intensively manage blood glucose levels prior to conception have fewer severe hypoglycemic episodes during pregnancy and are better at identifying and treating it when it does occur, which improves the overall health for mother and fetus. A glucagon emergency kit is essential for treating severe hypoglycemia, but sugar in the form of glucose tablets or ½ cup of juice or regular soft drink works fine for less severe episodes. Mild episodes of hypoglycemia (with low blood sugars that remain between 50 and 70 mg/dl) may even be best treated with a cup of milk. Make sure your family members are aware of emergency strategies for your treatment of hypoglycemia, as you may be unable to treat yourself.

Your Healthy Preconception Diet

In the old days, diabetics were simply handed a heartbreaking list of excluded goodies. Now we realize that there is no such thing as a one-size-fits-all diet for those with diabetes. In fact, the diabetic diet is actually one that we should all strive for! You will be happy to discover that a little knowledge in the grocery store, kitchen, and restaurant, combined with a commitment to eating healthfully for yourself and your baby-to-be, will enable you to develop a nourishing and satisfying food plan that will carry you through preconception and into your pregnancy.

What goes into developing your preconception meal plan? Individual women's needs vary, but most basic plans consist of a daily breakfast, lunch, dinner, and bedtime snack. The rationale behind this format is the need to eat every four and a half to five hours while awake (with the nighttime snack coming approximately four hours after dinner). Once you commit to a plan, meal skipping is not an option, though those on insulin pumps have a little more freedom to adjust to changes. If you have a problem with that standard plan—say, if you're not a breakfast person or prefer a very late dinner—speak with your dietitian about an alternative meal plan. Your daily calorie intake will break down roughly as follows:

- 45 to 50 percent carbohydrates (low-carb diets are not recommended)
- 15 to 20 percent protein
- 30 to 35 percent fat (with an emphasis on monounsaturated fats and omega-3 and omega-6 polyunsaturated fats, as discussed in Chapters 10 and 12)

Consult Chapter 8 before you consider any herb or supplement that's said to "naturally lower blood glucose." Be equally cautious about foods that claim therapeutic effects on blood sugars. For example, periodic meals containing a traditional vegetable in Mexican cuisine called nopal (prickly pear cactus, minus the spines) may have beneficial effects on the after-meal blood sugar level with no major downside, whereas the seeds or juice extracts from bitter melon, a common food in Indian and Asian cuisine, may similarly lower blood glucose but could cause miscarriage.

Keep That Body Moving

Women with diabetes seeking to become pregnant will enjoy the same advantages of physical fitness as women without diabetes. But there is a second fitness agenda that applies to people with diabetes: significantly reducing the risk of coronary heart disease. Studies have found that having diabetes puts you at the same risk for a heart attack as those who have already had one, but on the flip side, these studies have also confirmed that blood sugar control significantly reduces that risk. When muscles are exercised, they use a lot of glucose and become more responsive to insulin, which transports glucose into muscle cells. The result: glucose can more readily move from the bloodstream into the muscle, where it becomes fuel and reduces the amount of supplemental insulin needed.

Being overweight or obese is a relatively common challenge for some people with diabetes, so the weight control associated with exercise (combined with diet) is another of its important benefits. Plus, it is not uncommon for exercise and weight management to correct type 2 diabetes to the point where it can be controlled with little or no additional medication (whether pills or insulin). Once you become pregnant, the need for extra insulin gradually increases, so proper diet and exercise are typically not enough. You will likely need insulin in addition to or in place of pills.

The safest pre-pregnancy fitness plan is one that has been approved by your doctor, particularly for women over forty or those who have had diabetes for fifteen years or longer. Your health care team will help you design an exercise program around the following five points:

1. The exercise plan must work for your lifestyle. Don't create a plan that requires an expensive gym membership if that is going to ruin your budget.
2. Make sure you can adhere to your plan. All the best intentions in the world won't help if your plan is overly ambitious or too difficult to fit into your busy day.
3. Try to exercise at about the same time each day and expend roughly the same amount of energy for each workout. These factors will minimize your blood sugar fluctuations, making them easier to predict and manage.
4. Try to combine aerobic and resistance training for best results.
5. Make sure to monitor pre- and post-exercise blood sugar levels. Work with your medical team to identify what constitutes safe ranges for pre-exercise blood sugars, when to delay exercise, and what to target for post-exercise blood glucose levels.

Physical activity that is not accounted for in your normal plan, such as a long weekend hike, will require food and beverage adjustments as well as closer self-monitoring of blood glucose levels before, during, and afterward. A lot of unplanned or sporadic exercise is not wise in pre-pregnancy and pregnancy because it makes control of your blood sugar levels too difficult.

AT THE HEART OF THE MATTER: CARDIOVASCULAR DISEASES

> *Sabrina is a thirty-two-year-old newlywed who wants to have children. As a child, she had to be extra careful because she was born with a "tight" heart valve and her parents never wanted her to have corrective surgery. She was always the one who tired easily and couldn't run around as much as the other children on her block. Now, as an adult, she occasionally gets short of breath with vigorous activity and feels chest "flutters" or palpitations at least twice a week. She and her husband are nervous: is it safe for her to conceive?*

If, like Sabrina, you suffer from heart valve abnormalities, have other heart ailments such as high blood pressure or congenital heart disease, or have had a valve replacement, then an assessment by a cardiologist, ob-gyn, or maternal-fetal medical consultant before conception is essential to minimize problems before, during, and after pregnancy. When you become pregnant your heart normally goes into hyperdrive, pumping up to 20 percent more blood volume in the first trimester and up to 50 percent more blood volume after twenty weeks gestation. This extra effort on the part of the heart during pregnancy sends more nutrient-carrying blood to the growing baby inside of you. Many women are not diagnosed with heart disease until after they deliver because changes in the heart after delivery put particular stress on the cardiac system.

The medications that are used to treat heart disease before and during pregnancy must improve cardiac function while maintaining a good safety profile for the baby-to-be. Medications used to improve heart pumping strength and blood flow must be reviewed at least three months prior to trying to conceive because many of them are not baby-friendly and will need to be safely adjusted to a more appropriate choice by your health care team, which would comprise a cardiologist, an ob-gyn, and possibly a maternal-fetal medicine specialist. Stability on new medications before conception will improve how you tolerate pregnancy day to day and maximize fetal health and growth (see Chapter 8 for examples of baby-friendly cardiac medicine choices). When you are pregnant, continued close follow-up with your medical team is essential. Fine-tuning your heart health before conception will ensure better outcomes for you and your baby during and after the pregnancy.

FOR FUTURE REFERENCE: Between Pregnancies

Special Cardiac Concerns

If you do suffer from cardiac disease and you are a smoker, stop immediately! Tobacco not only increases complications of cardiac disease such as stroke and heart attack but also has proven to negatively affect fertility and your future fetus. Smoking is identified, along with alcohol and recreational drugs, as a risk factor in preterm labor, ADHD, and SIDS. It is not going to get any easier to stop smoking once your baby is born, and among the risks associated with infant exposure to cigarette smoke are increased colds, ear infections, and breathing problems.

If you had a cardiac problem diagnosed after your first pregnancy, you need to make sure your recovery is complete and that you wait at least twelve months from the prior delivery (and at least six months from recovery of a cardiac episode) to the next pregnancy. Optimizing body weight and exercise tolerance between pregnancies is also essential to your goal of good cardiac health in the next pregnancy.

High Blood Pressure or Hypertension

If you have high blood pressure, you are probably already under the care of an internist or cardiologist in addition to your obstetrician. If you're not sure, have your blood pressure checked; most people have no symptoms with elevated blood pressure. Headache, which is commonly thought to be the first symptom, usually occurs only in the most severe cases. If your blood pressure is elevated, you and your doctor can begin to control it with a healthy diet and an exercise regimen at least three months prior to conception. If your blood pressure remains uncontrolled, you will be at risk for:

- Stroke and heart attack
- Miscarriage and stillbirth
- Poor fetal weight gain or delays in fetal growth
- Pregnancy-induced hypertension (PIH) or preeclampsia (complication of pregnancy involving high blood pressure and protein in the urine beginning after twenty weeks gestation)

Amazingly, for more than 95 percent of adults with hypertension, the cause is unknown. In young women, the remaining 5 percent may be due to side effects of hormonal medications such as oral contraceptives, underlying kidney disease, adrenal illness, or congenital heart disease. Your internist or cardiologist will be able to rule out these causes of hypertension by taking a thorough history.

SHOULD YOU BE SCREENED FOR HIGH BLOOD PRESSURE OR
CARDIOVASCULAR DISEASE?

Even if you do not suffer from known heart disease or high blood pressure, if you have any of the following risk factors, do have a preconception evaluation:

- Family history of hypertension, heart attack, or congenital heart disease
- Personal history of preeclampsia (also known as toxemia or high blood pressure of pregnancy) in a past pregnancy
- Obesity, with a BMI greater than 30
- Personal history of high cholesterol
- Personal history of other medical problems such as lupus, kidney disease, or diabetes
- Smoking
- Race: High blood pressure is more common among black and Hispanic women.
- Age: if you are thirty-five or older (with increased risk if you are over forty)

If you have one or more of the above risk factors:

- Get a medical checkup with a blood pressure and urine analysis.
- Obtain a baseline EKG, cholesterol screening, and blood chemistries to check your kidney function.
- If you are taking high blood pressure medication, make sure it is baby-friendly (see below). If it's not, discuss alternatives with your doctor.

The safest high blood pressure medications before and after conception are beta-blockers, such as propranolol and atenolol, which are vasodilators (they cause a relaxation of the walls of the blood vessels), labetalol, and methyldopa. Diuretics, commonly used to treat high blood pressure, are thought to be safe as well but are rarely used during pregnancy because they adjust fluid levels in the blood, which fluctuates regularly when you are pregnant. Diuretics also may contribute to platelet abnormalities that can lead to excessive bleeding in infants (see Chapter 8). If you have a calcium deficiency due to diet or bowel disease, a calcium supplement may help reduce your high blood pressure.

Managing Your High Blood Pressure

What was your last blood pressure? Was the systolic pressure (top number) greater than 130? Was the diastolic pressure (the bottom number) greater than 80? New criteria have been developed that increase the scrutiny of blood pressure and hold us to a stricter normal. If your blood pressure is greater than 130/80, you may have prehypertension (classic hypertension is 140/90). One other way to measure your risk for developing heart issues can be via a blood test measuring C-reactive protein. If these tests indicate risk for high blood pressure, you will be asked to adopt changes in lifestyle to maintain a blood pressure closer to 120/80. Weight loss if appropriate, reducing unhealthy fats and high-salt foods, and regular exercise can have a very positive impact on your blood pressure and concomitant cardiac risk. If your blood pressure doesn't respond to these attempts, further evaluation may be recommended and medication offered (particularly if you have a blood pressure equal to or greater than 140/90).

Your Heart-Healthy Diet

Many of the changes you make in your lifestyle and diet for preconception heart health will continue to serve your needs throughout your pregnancy. The following suggestions will start you off in the right direction, and you and your health care team can individualize it for you as needed.

- Lose any extra pounds prior to conception to reach a healthier body mass index (BMI) that respects your genetically predisposed body weight.
- Once pregnant, put on the recommended amount of weight according to your pre-pregnancy BMI (see Chapter 14). Gaining too much or too little places extra stress on your heart and the rest of your body.
- Guidelines for alcohol and caffeine consumption are generally no different than our pre-conception guidelines for all women. A few general rules: for the one to three months prior to conception, limit your alcohol intake to no more than one drink per day and eliminate it completely two weeks prior to trying to become pregnant; limit your caffeine intake to less than 200 mg per day. (For more about alcohol and the caffeine content of beverages and foods, see Chapter 2.)
- Drink enough liquids throughout the day to remain well hydrated. Your urine should be pale yellow most of the time.
- Eat a well-rounded diet, the most common being the Dietary Approaches to Stop Hypertension (DASH) diet (almost identical to the preconception-friendly diet in this book), a copy of which can be provided by your health care professional or found online. You and your baby-to-be really are what you eat.
- Follow general preconception guidelines for vitamin, mineral, and herbal supplements. Avoid vitamin deficiencies specifically in calcium, potassium, and magnesium, to maintain optimal blood pressure. Plenty of minimally processed whole grains, low- and non-fat dairy products, vegetables, fruits, nuts, beans, and legumes, along with small servings of lean meat, poultry, and fish, provide vital nutrients. The American Heart As-

sociation recommends at least two servings of fish, preferably fatty fish, per week, which falls within our safety specifications for pre-pregnant and pregnant women.

- You may need to restrict your sodium prior to conception to help lower your blood pressure, but do not significantly restrict sodium during pregnancy unless advised to do so by your physician.

A heart-healthy diet with just under 50 percent of calories from carbohydrates is as good for you as the DASH diet (which gets almost 60 percent of calories from carbs), if not more so for some, provided the difference is made up with plant-based protein sources and unsaturated fats (many monounsaturated); you may recognize this as closer to a Mediterranean dietary approach.

Pay particular attention to the section of Chapter 10 where we discuss ways to include heart-healthy fats (poly- and monounsaturated fats) while limiting those that may harm (saturated fats and trans fats).

Keep It Moving

According to the American College of Sports Medicine, regular moderate-intensity physical activity "is the cornerstone therapy for the primary prevention, treatment, and control" of high blood pressure. It may also protect against developing high blood pressure during pregnancy. The most dramatic improvements are seen in women who go from being completely sedentary to being moderately active—doing something as simple as walking around the neighborhood. If you are already active, maintaining your regular exercise routine will continue to improve your health. Low-intensity warm-up and cool-down periods are especially important to those with high blood pressure.

Weight training can be incorporated into your physical fitness program if your doctor feels it would be appropriate. Show your doctor the fourteen-step pre-pregnancy strength training workout in Chapter 15. If you belong to a fitness club, work with a qualified trainer to develop a program that includes proper lifting and breathing techniques. Lighter weights and additional repetitions are generally the safest practice when beginning to work out or in pregnancy. If you have high blood pressure that has been chronically uncontrollable or begins during pregnancy, your doctor likely will tell you to minimize your level of activity.

When the Heart Valves Are Too Tight or Too Loose

The heart has four valves—aortic, pulmonary, tricuspid, and mitral—which control the blood flow into and out of the four chambers of the heart. Any of these valves can be too tight (stenotic) or too loose (prolapsed), thus preventing the proper flow of blood to and from the lungs and body. Either of these variations can be mild, moderate, or severe. Treating and sta-bilizing existing cardiac valve problems before conception will minimize health risks to mother and baby. Your preconception evaluation should include an EKG and an echocardio-gram in addition to a physical exam.

(Note: If you suffer from cardiomyopathy or congestive heart failure, an unplanned preg-nancy should be avoided at all costs. Be sure to see your cardiologist or ob-gyn before you start trying to conceive.)

 FOR FUTURE REFERENCE: During Pregnancy/After Delivery

If You or Your Offspring Were Born with a Heart Defect

Congenital heart disease is a physical defect of the heart that is present at birth. If you have a congenital heart condition, such as a hole in the heart (atrial septal defect) or tetralogy of Fallot, your children may be at slightly higher risk for the same condition. There is no way to reduce this hereditary risk before conception, but be sure to discuss it with your medical team once you are pregnant so that they can take particular care in evaluating the heart of your baby-to-be. If you have had a child with congenital heart disease in the past, your risk of having another similarly affected child is 1 to 2 percent. Under these circumstances, a fetal echocardiogram will be suggested at nineteen to twenty-two weeks gestation. If you have had a previous heart defect repaired, prophylac-tic use of antibiotics is recommended during labor and delivery.

If you are among the 10 percent of reproductive-age women with *mitral valve pro-lapse,* discuss this medical issue with your physicians even if you are asymptomatic. This will allow them to assess your condition and consider antibiotic use in labor to reduce the risk of inflammation and infection in the heart valve. The current thinking among cardiologists, however, is that antibiotics are not generally required during delivery to prevent heart valve infections. Also, pay careful attention to adequate hydration through-out your entire pregnancy. If you experience palpitations, shortness of breath, or chest pain, bring this to your doctor's attention immediately.

The Vitamin K Connection

Foods that are high in vitamin K, which aids blood clotting, have to be eaten in predictable amounts if you are taking Coumadin prior to pregnancy or heparin after you have conceived. Look at the list of good sources of vitamin K below and decide (along with your physician) how much you will consume every day. Consistent intake is more important than limited intake.

- Vegetables: spinach, collards, turnips, kale, and other green leafy vegetables; broccoli, cauliflower, Brussels sprouts, cabbage, asparagus; very spare use of parsley and dry seaweed
- Legumes: lentils, garbanzo beans, soybeans, tofu
- Nuts: pine nuts, cashews
- Fruits: kiwi fruit, prunes, dried figs, blackberries, blueberries, grapes, avocado
- Oils: soybean oil

Despite what you may have heard, tea as a beverage is not a source of vitamin K; the vitamin K stays in the tea leaves, which you won't be eating.

Many other foods are sources of vitamin K but in normal portion sizes do not interfere with blood thinners. Make sure your physician is aware of any herbal supplements you may be taking, as some may interfere with Coumadin or heparin therapy.

Severe stenosis of the pulmonary, aortic, or mitral valve may require surgical correction prior to pregnancy. If you have already undergone replacement of a heart valve and are currently taking anticoagulants (blood thinners), your health care team will need to review your medications before you become pregnant. Most affected women take an oral blood thinner, Coumadin, which can cause birth defects if taken during pregnancy. Coumadin can cross the placenta into the baby's environment. Even though placental tissue doesn't begin to function until weeks eight to ten of pregnancy, discontinuing Coumadin at least one to three months prior to that time is considered safest. In stopping Coumadin use you will need to change to a more baby-friendly blood thinner such as heparin or Lovenox, which do not cross the placenta and do not cause any known adverse fetal effects.

BARIATRIC SURGERY AND BEYOND

For those who have tried what seems like everything to accomplish their goal of health-promoting weight loss and are unsuccessful, bariatric surgery may be considered to aid in this endeavor. Bariatric surgery reduces the stomach capacity, forcing one to eat very small meals, significantly reducing caloric intake and resulting in more rapid weight loss, as well as nutrient loss. The two most common types of bariatric surgeries are laparoscopic banding and gastric bypass. The former wraps an inflatable band around part of the stomach to reduce caloric intake. Gastric bypass removes part of the stomach and causes weight loss via reduced calories and some malabsorption of food and vitamins normally used by the body for energy sources.

Samantha is a thirty-five-year-old mom who found herself one hundred pounds heavier after her first two pregnancies, the first of which was complicated by a preterm delivery and the next by gestational diabetes. She had gained too much during both pregnancies and never took it off. Samantha's BMI was 37 (clinically obese). She underwent laparoscopic banding and lost sixty-five pounds over eight months. She was able to maintain her new healthier BMI of 27 for eight more months before trying to conceive her third child. As a precaution against gaining too much during this pregnancy, her doctor opted not to loosen the band unless a need arose. At twenty-eight weeks gestation she complained of abdominal pain and an uncontrollable nausea and vomiting. She was briefly hospitalized for the treatment of dehydration with intravenous fluids and subsequently had her laparoscopic band deflated for the rest of her pregnancy. At thirty-nine weeks and just shy of her fifteen-pound weight-gain goal, Samantha delivered a healthy 6-pound 8-ounce son.

Recent studies among women who undergo bariatric surgery before pregnancy have found improvements in fertility, decreased miscarriage risk, and less severe medical problems during pregnancy such as preeclampsia, gestational diabetes, and very large babies that weigh more than 8 pounds 13 ounces. With fewer pregnancy complications, these women were more likely to have a safe and full-term delivery.

For Samantha and most women who undergo bariatric surgery, the greatest weight loss occurs over the first twelve to eighteen months after surgery. However, it is important to take note of the significant nutritional challenge that occurs immediately after bariatric surgery, known as "dumping syndromes." This "dumping" effect on nutrients eaten can lead to deficiencies in iron, zinc, vitamin A, B complex, vitamin K, calcium, and vitamin D—all of which are crucial to keeping mother and baby healthy. For those women who conceived within the first year of a bariatric procedure, there was an increased risk of fetal growth restriction and miscarriage. With this in mind we strongly recommend waiting at least twelve to eighteen months after bariatric surgery before trying to conceive. During pregnancy, women who have had weight loss surgery are more likely to have band migration (as Samantha did in our anecdote above), intestinal obstructions, and hernias. Chapter 14 provides specific guidance on recovering from bariatric surgery and making the most of your weight loss and good health prior to conception.

THYROID DISEASE

Andrea, twenty-eight, is overweight and occasionally misses a menstrual cycle. For more than two years, she and her husband have not used birth control. Now, however, they wish to conceive. For the past three months Andrea has complained of worsening fatigue. She finally goes to the doctor, who palpates her thyroid gland, takes a blood sample, and discovers she has a low thyroid hormone level. She receives medication to correct her hormonal imbalance and for the next three months her menstrual cycle is like clockwork. On the fourth cycle she becomes pregnant.

Beth is a thirty-two-year-old who recently delivered a healthy 7-pound 5-ounce baby boy. Three weeks after delivery she was complaining of heart palpitations and extreme fatigue. Although it isn't unusual to be more tired after a new baby joins the household, she knew something wasn't right. She saw her doctor and had thyroid testing, which revealed she had postpartum thyroiditis, which initially releases a large amount of thyroid hormone into the body and then burns the thyroid out in varying degrees, leaving very little thyroid hormone available to run the metabolism. After treatment, Beth's symptoms were completely gone within two weeks. When she wanted to conceive again she had her blood tested three months in advance to be sure her thyroid function was normal, and she had no difficulty getting and staying pregnant.

The thyroid is a gland in your neck that produces hormones that control your metabolism. Thyroid disease commonly affects women during their reproductive years, which can lead to fertility problems, lack of ovulation, and a lack of general well-being. Even borderline thyroid changes have been shown to negatively affect fertility and miscarriage rates. Reversal of a thyroid problem will restore normal menstruation and ovulation and improve the possibility and ease of conception, as well as maintain good fetal health once you are pregnant. New research has placed greater emphasis on making sure your thyroid is normal before conception and between pregnancies.

Thyroid problems can be detected with a simple blood test that measures your thyroid-stimulating hormone (TSH) level. The criteria for treatment of an underactive thyroid (hypothyroidism) are changing to encompass what used to be a borderline state of hypothyroidism. This change in thinking reflects newer research, which has noted that even small reductions in available thyroid hormone can impair normal fetal neurological development.

A Dietary Connection to Hypothyroidism

Iodine deficiency is one cause of hypothyroidism, but it is a less common cause in the United States because in the majority of households, our salt is iodized (note: the label *must* clearly say "iodized salt"). Iodine is also found in seafood (but, ironically, not sea salt, which is wildly popular among foodies), dairy products (especially milk), eggs, commercially made breads and cured products, seaweed, and kelp. (See Chapter 11's iodine section for important safety information about sea vegetables.) Most vitamin-mineral supplements do not yet contain iodine (150 mcg being a good supplemental amount), but there is a push from the global medical community as well as the American Thyroid Association to change that. Stay tuned. Women with hypothyroidism often experience constipation and will benefit from a high-fiber diet with plenty of fluid intake.

SHOULD YOU BE SCREENED FOR A THYROID CONDITION?

Even if you have never suffered from a thyroid imbalance in the past, there are factors that may place you at higher risk, such as a family history of Hashimoto's or Graves' disease or a personal history of other endocrine diseases such as diabetes or hyperprolactinemia. Some symptoms that might tip you off to a thyroid problem include:

Hypothyroidism
- Weight gain
- Slowed pulse or low blood pressure
- Unexplained fatigue, depression, or anxiety
- Long menstrual cycles
- Dry or lusterless skin and hair
- Oversensitivity to cold
- Constipation
- Difficulty conceiving

Hyperthyroidism
- Unexplained weight loss
- Faster heart rate
- Altered mood states, especially anxiety
- Irregular menstrual cycles
- Inability to sleep
- Heat intolerance
- Bowel changes
- Bulging eyes

Even if you do not have any of these risk factors or symptoms, current medical practice is to have a thyroid screening test before you conceive—borderline or early hypothyroidism without symptoms can impact maternal and fetal health. Many diseases can mimic each other, but if you recognize two or three of the symptoms listed above, talk to your doctor.

To evaluate your thyroid, he or she will perform a simple blood test to measure TSH and palpate your neck to feel for a goiter. If there are nodules, you may need imaging and biopsy of the thyroid. If your TSH is elevated, this means you are producing too little thyroid hormone. If it is too low, you are producing too much thyroid hormone. You should wait at least three months after normalized thyroid function has been restored before trying to conceive.

HYPERTHYROIDISM

Hyperthyroidism is a condition marked by sustained overproduction of thyroxine (T4), one of the hormones produced by the thyroid gland. If your thyroid is overactive, it can negatively affect your ability to conceive because you won't ovulate regularly. Further, conceiving while excess thyroid hormone is circulating in your body can affect fetal growth and development. Excess thyroid hormone can speed up all those body functions that are already fluctuating during early pregnancy, leading to maternal heart palpitations, anxiety, weight loss, and miscarriage.

Hyperprolactinemia

Of particular importance to reproductive-age women is the relationship between hypothyroidism and hyperprolactinemia. Hyperprolactinemia is an excessive secretion of prolactin, a hormone released from the pituitary gland that causes breastmilk to be produced. Prolactin levels may be elevated if you suffer from an untreated thyroid disease or if there is a benign mass, known as a prolactinoma, growing in the pituitary. The latter can be microscopic and clinically negligible, or it may be large enough press on the nerves serving the eyes. Complaints include irregular or absent menstrual cycles, galactorrhea (production of breastmilk or colostrum when not pregnant), headache, reduced libido, and visual changes.

A simple test can diagnose a prolactin disturbance. If your prolactin levels are elevated, you should have an MRI or CT scan of your pituitary gland. Treatment options often depend on the size of the mass and the severity of symptoms. If left untreated, hyperprolactinemia can affect fertility. Bromocriptine (brand name Parlodel), a medicine used to suppress the secretion of prolactin, can be used prior to conception to restore normal menses and prolactin levels. When preparing for conception, discuss with your physician how to discontinue Parlodel.

The most common reason for an overactive thyroid is the often hereditary Graves' disease. Treatment is available with propylthiouracil (PTU), which stops the thyroid from releasing and manufacturing excess thyroid hormone and is safe in the preconception period. After treatment with PTU, your thyroid may become underactive and your doctor may prescribe thyroid hormone replacement with Synthroid or Levoxyl, both of which are baby-friendly medications. If you've been treated for hyperthyroidism with either surgery or radioactive iodine, wait until your thyroid hormone levels have been normal for at least one to three months before you try to conceive. Avoid radioactive iodine during pregnancy because the fetal thyroid can become enlarged if exposed to excess iodine.

ASTHMA

Approximately 9 percent of reproductive-age women in the United States are affected by asthma (the prevalence is higher among Puerto Ricans, non-Hispanic blacks, and American Indians). Asthma restricts the air passing through the bronchi (tiny airways in the lungs) by causing spasms in the muscles that surround them. An acute flare of asthma may include coughing, wheezing, a feeling of tightness in the chest, and overall difficulty in breathing. Asthma often is triggered by an allergic reaction to an environmental factor such as dust, animal dander, cigarette smoke, exercise, or a cold. Most women who avoid the triggers or proactively treat themselves when they anticipate exposure to an irritant are able to tolerate their asthma very well.

During pregnancy, women who suffer from asthma may find it either improves or worsens, 30 and 23 percent, respectively. Researchers have not found a direct relationship between asthma attacks and fertility, but if your asthma is not controlled well and affects your sleep patterns or dampens your ability to be physically active, we think these factors may influence fertility. Steroids and other medications used to treat asthma may have an indirect effect on fertility (see Chapter 8).

Medical Therapies for Women with Asthma

"I want to start trying to get pregnant, but if I don't take my asthma meds I have attacks requiring emergency room visits. Can I take my medications and still have a healthy baby?"

Absolutely. Preconception control of asthma with medication and medical surveillance can reduce the number of asthma attacks before and after conception, improving your health and that of your prospective baby. You'll be much less likely to have complications, such as preterm delivery, if your asthma is well controlled. Consider the following tips when you and your doctor develop your preconception medical plan:

- **Single-agent therapy is best whenever possible.** Avoid the use of multiple medications, such as inhalers plus over-the-counter medication, to minimize fetal exposure.

- **Avoid medications with iodine unless approved by your doctor.** Be particularly cautious with over-the-counter expectorants, such as potassium iodide, otherwise known as SSKI, containing concentrated amounts of iodine, because they can cause fetal hyperthyroidism and goiter if taken while pregnant.

- **Inhalants** such as Proventil (albuterol), which is a bronchodilator, have shown no detrimental fetal effects.

- **Using a peak flow meter** may be helpful prior to conception to aid in decisions about medication.

When single-medication bronchodilator therapy is not sufficient to control the asthma attack, a steroid may be added. When you are trying to conceive, inhaled steroids such as Azmacort are preferable to systemic (oral or intravenous) steroids. In general, you should avoid chronic use of steroids, which can lead to glucose intolerance (symptoms like diabetes) and bone loss. If you absolutely need inhaled budesonide (a common steroid, safe to use in pregnancy) on a regular basis for maternal health, blood sugar testing should be done regularly throughout pregnancy.

SHOULD YOU BE SCREENED FOR ASTHMA?

You may need to be tested for asthma if you have some of the following risk factors or symptoms:

- Need to catch your breath during a cold-weather activity
- Chest tightness or wheezing with exertion
- Frequent cold and flu symptoms that are slow to recover
- BMI over 30 and you notice frequent mouth breathing at rest
- You are a smoker
- Other family members have asthma

To diagnose asthma you can begin with a physical exam. Breathing tests, called peak flow measurements, can be done to measure the capacity of air movement through the bronchi. Any treatment will include avoidance of your triggers or allergens in the environment and medications to reduce inflammation and open up air passages. Make sure your internist or pulmonary specialist knows you are trying to conceive; the medication choices can then be tailored to baby-friendly options.

Eating Well and Breathing Easy

If you have asthma, one of the best things you can do for yourself is to keep well hydrated at all times to minimize mucous secretions. You know your body: if certain foods aggravate your asthma, avoid them. Although it is atypical for foods to trigger asthma, the following are the most frequently noted culprits: generous servings of wine or beer (due to sulfites), milk, eggs, nuts, soy, wheat, fish, and shellfish.

Asthma researchers have taken an interest in the anti-inflammatory role that omega-3 fats might play in managing asthma and possibly reducing the risk of your offspring developing it, but results from studies are still too inconclusive to recommend supplementing with omega-3s with those goals in mind. However, what they do know is that there is no disadvantage for asthmatics who increase the amount of omega-3s in their diet to levels consistent with our preconception recommendations. (See Table 10-3 for nutrition tips.)

Exercise That Works for You

If you have received approval from your physician to participate in a regular exercise regimen, be sure to do so. Physical activity can prepare your lungs for the extra work of pregnancy. Be certain that you know how and when to use your inhaler before and after exercise. An asthmatic incident is unlikely to occur if you take the time to incorporate a long, slow warm-up and cool-down into your exercise routine. Also, avoid exercising in frigid conditions, in extreme humidity, or when the pollen count or pollution is at its highest. It may be prudent to wear a small fanny pack to accommodate your inhaler (and an emergency epi kit if advised by your doctor—injectable epinephrine can give more immediate bronchodilation if an allergic reaction occurs). That way you can be prepared to immediately treat an asthma attack should one occur while you exercise.

TUBERCULOSIS

Though less common today in the United States than it was twenty years ago, tuberculosis (TB) is a highly contagious disease caused by airborne bacteria. If you have TB and it is not diagnosed prior to trying to conceive, you may have scarring in your fallopian tubes that can lead to infertility. Testing for TB is advised for high-risk individuals.

You may be considered at risk and in need of screening if you:

- Have lived in or traveled through developing countries
- Work in a health care setting or in a long-term-care facility for the elderly or disabled
- Have close contact with persons known to have TB
- Have a medical condition that reduces your immune system's activity, such as HIV infection or an organ transplant

Testing for TB can be easily performed in your doctor's office with an under-the-skin injection of tuberculin or purified protein derivative. If a welt appears after forty-eight hours, a chest X-ray should be performed to confirm the diagnosis. Medical therapy with isoniazid (INH) for six to nine months is recommended; INH has never been shown to cause fetal side effects and is safe for use during pregnancy and breastfeeding. If a new TB infection is diagnosed before conception or in the first trimester, ethambutol is a safe option for mother and fetus; after sixteen weeks of gestation, rifampin is used.

BLOOD DISORDERS

Your blood contains red blood cells that carry oxygen to your body tissues, white blood cells that help your body fight infection, and platelets that make a clot to prevent significant bleeding. All of these elements exist in balance. When there is too much or too little of any one of them, the resulting illness can affect your health during and after conception.

Too Little of a Good Thing: Iron-Deficiency Anemia

Anemia is a condition characterized by too few red blood cells to carry oxygen to the sites that need it. The most common cause is iron deficiency. Symptoms include a general feeling of fatigue, weakness, paleness, and in some cases headaches. If you experience heavy menstrual bleeding or have had pregnancies less than one year apart, or if you have had bariatric surgery less than twelve months prior to trying to conceive, you are at increased risk for iron-deficiency anemia. The workup to figure out if you have anemia starts with a simple blood test called a complete blood count (CBC), which will also allow your health care provider to rule out other causes of anemia such as vitamin B_{12} deficiency. Another sensitive way to detect low iron is to get a separate test for serum ferritin.

Variations in hemoglobin levels, not due to iron deficiency, occur in smokers (whose hemoglobin is slightly higher than that of nonsmokers), African Americans, and those of Mediterranean or Asian descent who may have beta- or alpha-thalassemia, respectively.

When it comes to anemia, it is hard to play catch-up after conception, because your iron requirements double during pregnancy. (See Chapter 11 for more on iron-rich foods and iron supplements.) If you are anemic before and after conception, you are at greater risk for delivery of a low-birth-weight baby and preterm labor. According to researchers from Johns Hopkins University, if iron deficiency persists beyond your pregnancy, it can negatively affect the mother-child bond, probably because fatigue is more likely with anemia and it is hard to be emotionally invested in your newborn if you are exhausted. Resolving anemia can help you be a more responsive, resilient mommy. If you suffer from iron-deficiency anemia, treatment usually begins with dietary increases in iron and iron supplements.

SHOULD YOU BE SCREENED FOR ANEMIA?

You may want to pursue testing for anemia if you have noticed any of the following:

- Worsening, unexplained fatigue
- Heavy menstrual bleeding
- Cravings for red meat and other iron-rich foods (see Table 11-3)

> • Cravings for cornstarch, laundry starch, plaster, chalk, dirt, clay, ice, or freezer frost are called pica. Notify your doctor if any of these cravings apply to you.

When There Is Too Much Iron: Hemochromatosis

Hemochromatosis describes a condition in which excessive iron is absorbed through the intestines and stored in the liver, pancreas, kidneys, and pituitary. This ailment can be hereditary, especially among those of Northern European descent, or the result of acquired defects in iron absorption, commonly found among alcoholics. In women, too much iron stored in the liver can impede the processing of the reproductive hormones, leading to irregular menstrual cycles and a lack of ovulation. This is another good reason to avoid alcohol before and after conception—your liver will have enough to deal with if you have hemochromatosis. In men, hemochromatosis can lead to testicular atrophy (a reduction in testicular size), which can reduce sperm production. Further, in both men and women, hemochromatosis can cause a reduction in libido.

Anyone with hemochromatosis should avoid mineral or vitamin supplements containing iron and/or vitamin C. To de-emphasize iron absorbed from food sources, you can drink milk, tea, or coffee (decaf or small amounts of regular) with meals and snacks, particularly with foods known for their high iron content. Your diet should be rich in fiber-containing foods, including whole grains and beans. Calcium-rich foods and a daily calcium supplement of 500 mg may also help to partially bind the unwanted iron. Become a friend of the Red Cross by donating blood regularly.

 FOR FUTURE REFERENCE: During Pregnancy

Pregnancy After a History of DVT or PE

If you have had a prior deep vein thrombosis (DVT) or pulmonary embolism (PE), you may be at a higher risk for this blood abnormality when you are pregnant, perhaps because of a hereditary disposition (see more about hereditary thrombophilias in Chapter 5). The blood of a pregnant woman is sluggish and more prone to clotting, so if you have had a DVT (an inflamed vein, often in your lower extremities, that reduces blood flow, causing a clot) or PE (a clot that blocks a vein in the lungs) in the past, you have a 4 to 13 percent risk of recurrence while pregnant. You will also be at a higher risk for preeclampsia, so you should be monitored closely in pregnancy for symptoms of this as well. You are also at risk for DVT if you are obese or diabetic. Being vigilant and educated about the symptoms of a potential DVT or PE are critical to early treatment and reduced maternal morbidity. Having a high index of suspicion is the best preparation to avoid recurrent blood clots in your legs and lungs.

If you had a DVT or PE during the first three months of a past pregnancy, or in association with oral contraceptive pill use, medications will be recommended during pregnancy to prevent a DVT or PE. Prophylactic medications to reduce the likelihood of a blood clot while you are pregnant need to be individualized to your particular needs by your medical team. Prophylaxis with Lovenox or heparin must be injected (so it's not very convenient) and increases your chance of bleeding, so these medications should be used only when absolutely necessary. If you take Coumadin (mentioned earlier in the heart valve section of this chapter) on a regular basis to reduce blood clotting, you will need to stop it and get accustomed to heparin or Lovenox prior to pregnancy. Coumadin is a known teratogen and needs to be discontinued at least one to three months before you try to conceive to allow for your body to become accustomed to a new treatment.

Sickle-Cell Disease

The medical care of those with sickle-cell disease has improved dramatically over the past three decades, and as a result, more women with this condition are reaching reproductive age. Though preconception counseling can make a difference, women who have sickle-cell disease are not without pregnancy-related risks. These include:

- 2 percent risk of maternal mortality
- 18 percent increased risk of preeclampsia
- 26 percent increase in preterm delivery due to fetal or maternal reasons
- 16 percent risk of poor fetal growth due to changes in blood flow through the placenta
- Increased risk of kidney infection and sickle-cell crisis in the prospective mother

To maximize your chances of a healthy pregnancy, you should seek treatment for preexisting anemia, begin prophylactic vaccinations against infections, eat healthfully even during painful episodes, and start a multivitamin containing folic acid at least three months before conception. Hepatitis B and HIV testing, particularly if you have received blood transfusions, is vital to evaluating your health prior to conception. Also, pneumococcal pneumonia and flu vaccinations are recommended, as your immune system may not be up to fighting these infections while pregnant. Frequent urine testing after conception can identify early bladder infections that are otherwise without symptoms. If left untreated, a bladder infection can precipitate a sickle-cell crisis or become a kidney infection. To help avoid precipitating a sickle-cell crisis prior to and during pregnancy, we recommend that you maintain good hydration and get adequate rest—advice all expectant mothers should follow.

Preconception genetic testing can help you determine the chance of passing the disease to your child. Sickle-cell disease is hereditary, and if you have it or carry the trait for it, your partner should be tested to see if he carries a related mutated gene. Both parents have to carry the gene mutation to pass it on to a child. If you do not have sickle-cell disease but are of African American or Native American ancestry, you (and your partner if he is of similar ethnicity) should undergo genetic testing. Details about the odds of having sickle-cell disease are found in Table 6-1.

Thrombocytopenia

Normal platelet levels are usually greater than 200,000 per ml; thrombocytopenia or a low platelet count is suspected when the platelet count drops below 100,000 per ml. Most people who have low platelet numbers have no symptoms. Diagnosis and treatment of this problem prior to pregnancy will reduce the risk of life-threatening bleeding for you and your baby. A CBC and occasional bone marrow samplings may be required to make a definitive diagnosis. Idiopathic thrombocytopenia (ITP) is diagnosed when there is no source of bleeding to explain a reduction in platelets. Symptomatic ITP, with active bleeding or platelet counts under 50,000 per ml, can be treated safely with oral or intravenous steroids and immunoglobulin before and during pregnancy. If you have no symptoms, you'll be observed closely, but you're not likely to require treatment.

SHOULD YOU BE SCREENED FOR THROMBOCYTOPENIA?

You should be screened for thrombocytopenia if you have experienced any of the following:

- A flat rash on the arm that looks like red pin dots under the skin (a.k.a. petechiae)
- Easy bruising
- A longer time for cuts to stop bleeding
- Fatigue, related to heavy menstrual flow
- Thrombocytopenia in a previous pregnancy

FOR FUTURE REFERENCE: During Pregnancy

What Are the Implications of ITP in Pregnancy?

If you have ITP during your pregnancy, your platelet levels will be tested every trimester because these levels have important implications when it comes to choosing which type of anesthesia you can have access to in labor. For example, if your platelets are under 80,000 per ml, an epidural may not be an option, because there is too high a risk for bleeding into the spinal cavity. C-sections would be done under general anesthesia. Pain control in a trial of vaginal labor is done with narcotics that are short-acting and can be counteracted to ensure that the baby is not adversely affected. Under these circumstances, short-term narcotic use is considered baby-tolerant (instead of baby-friendly).

It is also important for your health care provider to know if your platelet counts are low because the baby may initially have low platelets as well. Since there is a higher risk of bleeding with minimal provocation, vaginal deliveries with forceps or vacuum and internal fetal monitoring (an electrode stuck to the fetal scalp to monitor the heartbeat more carefully) are generally avoided. Maternal risks in labor are lower if the baby is born via vaginal delivery because there is less bleeding compared to a Cesarean section. Often thrombocytopenia takes three to five days to show up in a newborn; therefore, pediatric follow-up a few days after birth is advised. Also, any surgery on the newborn, such as a circumcision, should not occur until normal infant platelet counts are confirmed.

IF YOU WERE BORN WITH A HEREDITARY DISORDER

Phenylketonuria

Phenylketonuria (PKU), a hereditary disease, occurs when you lack an enzyme required to break down the amino acid phenylalanine (phe); if PKU is left untreated, levels of phe can become toxic and cause mental retardation (and other birth defects for a developing fetus). Federal recommendations require that all newborns be tested for this at birth. Fortunately, the prognosis is excellent for babies born with PKU if treatment begins soon after birth, provided the mother was only a carrier or had carefully managed PKU prior to and through pregnancy.

If you were a PKU baby and are now a prospective mother with PKU, you will find a registered dietitian an excellent resource to assist you in planning a diet very low in phe, if you haven't already done so. Once you've established your food program, you'll need to follow it for at least three months prior to conception and throughout your pregnancy. Ideally, it's best to follow it for life. Foods that are naturally low in protein are the basis of this diet; however, it must be supplemented with medical foods such as specially formulated phe-restricted mixtures, usually in beverage form. The phe-free formula is high in vitamins, minerals, and calories and will ensure that you have a balanced diet that will prevent your body from breaking down your own muscle protein, which causes phe to be released into the bloodstream. This diet will make a label reader out of you. Aspartame, which we know as Nutrasweet, contains phe, too, and is found in diet soft drinks, some foods, and even medicines. Take a look the next time you're in the supermarket: these products exhibit warning labels that read, "Attention phenylketonurics: This product contains phenylalanine."

Let's be honest: this is not an easy diet to follow. It is quite restrictive, and the special phe-restricted formula has never won a blue ribbon for taste. But what you are accomplishing through your strict adherence to the program, including gaining enough pregnancy weight, will win you the best prize of all: a healthy baby. Even if your baby is born with PKU, he or she can remain healthy with careful medical attention and adherence to the PKU diet.

Cystic Fibrosis

Advances in medical care have extended the life expectancy for people born with cystic fibrosis (CF). This hereditary disease now affects reproductive-age men and women who have increased mucus production in the lungs, pancreas, and upper respiratory system. Before you conceive, a nutritional status workup to correct imbalances of micronutrients and essential fatty acids, as well as a medical evaluation to confirm good blood sugar control, is strongly recommended. It is also important to get vaccinations against the seasonal flu and pneumonia to reduce the risk of these diseases. If you have cystic fibrosis or are a carrier of CF, your spouse should be tested; if your spouse is also a carrier, there is a 25 percent chance that your offspring could inherit this disorder (see Chapter 6 for details). Men who have CF may inquire about a semen analysis before they try to conceive due to an increased risk for low sperm counts due to an absent vas deferens, which is the highway the sperm must travel to be ejaculated. In women, frequent respiratory infections must be minimized and baby-friendly medications used if you are trying to conceive.

GASTROINTESTINAL DISEASES
Inflammatory Bowel Disease: Crohn's and Ulcerative Colitis

There are two forms of inflammatory bowel disease (IBD): Crohn's disease and ulcerative colitis, both of which can have an impact on your nutritional status during pregnancy, indirectly affecting fetal growth and development. If prior to conceiving you frequently experience flare-ups of either condition, you'll probably suffer episodes during pregnancy as well. However, some sufferers find great relief during pregnancy, which naturally affects your immune system and reduces your inflammatory response.

Table for One: Nutrition for Crohn's or Ulcerative Colitis

Dietary management of IBD is very individualized. It is not unusual for two women with this condition to have very different food tolerances. During flare-ups the diet is most restricted: low fiber, with limited fat and lactose (milk sugar). When you are feeling better, introduce healthy foods you enjoy back into your diet with the assistance of your doctor. Probiotics combined with prebiotics (fiber and fiber-like compounds) are being investigated as possible adjunct therapies for IBD. To date these show promise, but they require more rigorous study before a blanket recommendation can be made; ask your gastroenterologist about the latest advances.

Nutrients that are often depleted and require particular attention are folic acid (folate), iron, vitamin B_{12}, magnesium, vitamin D, calcium, and omega-3 fats. Be careful of prenatal vitamin supplements, which can replace these nutrients—often they contain stool softeners (e.g., Colace), because the iron in them can cause constipation. If you have IBD, you may find the stool softener causes diarrhea. In that case, request a supplement without a stool softener.

A careful diet, vitamin supplementation, adequate hydration, and, often, medication will keep your IBD flare-ups to a minimum. Steroids and sulfasalazine can be used in preconception and pregnancy without any negative effects on you or your baby. Avoid therapies that involve mercaptopurine (5MP), azathioprine, and metronidazole (Flagyl) due to concerns about their potential fetal effect. The team members most likely to help with management of inflammatory bowel disease are your registered dietitian, gastroenterologist, and obstetrician, who can work with you to orchestrate a safe time for conception.

IBD should not be confused with other gastrointestinal disturbances such as irritable bowel syndrome, or IBS. Although IBS has certain symptoms in common with IBD, the person with IBS will have normal imaging studies, and little to no effect on fertility or perinatal outcome has ever been documented. Often IBS can be treated by diet alone for the comfort of the prospective mother. The other gastrointestinal problem that is often misdiagnosed as IBD is an autoimmune disease called celiac disease, which can impact fertility if left untreated. The treatment differs from that for IBD. We discuss celiac disease next.

SHOULD YOU BE SCREENED FOR CROHN'S OR ULCERATIVE COLITIS?

You should be screened for these conditions if you have:

- Bloating after meals
- Frequent bouts of diarrhea or bloody bowel movements
- Severe cramping after meals

- Family history of either disease
- Nonspecific, unexplained abdominal pain

If you and your health care provider are concerned that you may have IBD, diagnosis can be confirmed via colonoscopy or CT scan/barium enema. Blood testing for anemia is also advised before you conceive.

Celiac Disease (Gluten Intolerance)

Celiac disease is really an autoimmune condition with complex genetic roots. When people with celiac disease eat wheat, rye, or barley products (and often oat products unless they are free from traces of other grains), a natural protein called gluten in these foods causes damage to the lining of the small intestine. This damage is responsible for malabsorption of key baby-friendly nutrients from the diet and has been linked to both mild and severe problems, including lowered fertility and possibly miscarriage. Celiac disease in its full-blown form affects 1 percent of the population, but many others are gluten intolerant. Two simple, fairly inexpensive blood tests can be used to screen for this disease, and an intestinal biopsy makes the diagnosis more definitive. You and your health care team have to have a high index of suspicion to test for this disease because other bowel disease symptoms commonly overlap. Getting the actual diagnosis of celiac disease may take years, since it is not commonly tested for and symptoms are so highly variable.

Once you are diagnosed with celiac disease, lifelong adherence to a gluten-free diet is the only known way to heal your gut and rid yourself of symptoms such as abdominal pain, diarrhea, constipation, fatigue, and weight loss (though you could be overweight and still have celiac disease). If lactose intolerance has also developed, it may eventually go away as you stick to the gluten-free diet. Initially, adopting a gluten-free diet can be overwhelming as you familiarize yourself with which foods contain gluten and which ones are safe. You should definitely consult a dietitian. In addition, an excellent resource to simplify this daunting process is the book *Gluten-Free Diet* by Shelley Case, RD; she teaches you all the tricks and offers a multitude of resources (one being the Celiac Sprue Association).

Chronic Hepatitis B or C Infection

If you suffer from a severe illness related to hepatitis B or C, such as cirrhosis of the liver, you face a very possible reduction in fertility and increase in miscarriage rates. There are no treatments prior to conception that can eliminate the real risk these diseases pose to a fetus. Education by your hepatologist, internist, or ob-gyn about the risks to you and your prospective child will help you make compassionate, responsible life decisions.

When a woman knows she has a chronic hepatitis B or C infection, preconception counseling can be essential in two ways:

- **Determining the severity of the current liver disease.** The milder the disease, the less risk in pregnancy for high blood pressure, preterm labor, and fetal growth abnormalities. Asymptomatic or dormant hepatitis (i.e., no active liver disease) has been shown to have little impact on the developing fetus.

SHOULD YOU BE SCREENED FOR CELIAC DISEASE?

You should be screened for celiac disease if you have:

- Abdominal pain
- Diarrhea
- Constipation
- Chronic fatigue
- Weight loss (though overweight/obesity doesn't preclude a diagnosis)
- Unexplained dermatitis
- Herpetiformis (itchy, blistery rashes)
- Unexplained anemia
- Unexplained infertility or miscarriage
- Low bone mineral density
- A relative with celiac disease
- Rheumatoid arthritis, type 1 diabetes, or thyroiditis
- Numbness or tingling in your hands or feet

Warning! Do *not* go on a gluten-free diet until after the testing has confirmed celiac disease. (Doing so will interfere with an accurate diagnosis.)

- **Screening for other infections that can have an impact on maternal and fetal health.** Chronic hepatitis B and C are often associated with other viral infections. Identifying these additional infections before conception allows early intervention to reduce risks to mother and fetus. For example, if HIV infection is diagnosed before conception, medical therapy to reduce transmission of the infection to the fetus is available.

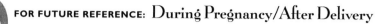

FOR FUTURE REFERENCE: During Pregnancy/After Delivery

Protecting Your Newborn Against Hepatitis B & C

Unfortunately, 70 to 90 percent of babies born to a healthy hepatitis B–positive mom will become asymptomatic carriers of the disease. Whether a baby is born via a Cesarean or vaginal route, there is no significant difference in the rate of transmission. Prophylactic vaccinations and immunoglobulins are now routinely administered at birth and can reduce a newborn's risk of contracting active hepatitis by 95 percent.

FOR FUTURE REFERENCE: After Delivery

Breastfeeding with a Maternal History of Hepatitis B or C?

There are no definitive guidelines regarding breastfeeding and hepatitis. In general, many consultants recommend breastfeeding to protect the baby against infections in general, and there is little risk for the baby if he or she is provided the hepatitis B vaccine and antibodies against hepatitis B immediately after birth. Others advise against it to limit the baby's exposure to hepatitis B and C from an affected mother's breastmilk. Careful counseling with your doctor will help you make your decision.

SHOULD YOU BE SCREENED FOR HEPATITIS B OR C?

If you have not been diagnosed as either having or carrying hepatitis B or C but have concerns about possible exposure or answer yes to any of the following questions, you should consider blood testing for hepatitis B and C.

- Have you had a blood transfusion in the past fifteen years?
- Have you had sexual intercourse with an intravenous drug user or previous user?
- Do you work in health care or mental health care?
- Have you had multiple sexual partners?
- Are you a past or current street or illicit drug user?

Blood testing for exposure to this infection is easily done. Women who are pregnant are automatically screened for hepatitis B, but it is preferable to know before you conceive. When you see your doctor for a preconception visit, consider hepatitis and HIV testing. Your doctor may even recommend it before you get a chance to bring up the subject.

AUTOIMMUNE DISEASES

An autoimmune disease occurs when cells of the immune system fail to recognize a particular cell or part of the body as "self" and attack it with antibodies. The result of this attack is seen as inflammation throughout the body. It is treatable with lifestyle modifications (such as stress reduction) and medication, and may be followed by a long period of time without any symptoms, known as remission. It is best to delay conception until you are in remission for at least three to six months to allow your body and your immune system to grow steadily stronger. Autoimmune diseases can also affect fertility, miscarriage rates, and fetal growth. Preconception evaluation with your rheumatologist or internist and obstetrician will help you modify your medications to ensure the safest internal environment for baby to grow.

Systemic Lupus Erythematosus

Lupus predominantly affects women of childbearing age and is more prevalent in women of black, Hispanic, Asian, and Native American descent. It manifests as intermittent inflammation in different joints or blood vessels throughout your body, often feeling like migrating pain. Lupus can be diagnosed with blood tests that measure antinuclear antibody (ANA) levels. Symptoms of lupus can include arthritis, facial rash, fatigue, anemia, and non-infection-related inflammation of the heart or kidneys. You may find it hard to believe while in the midst of a flare-up, but remission is a definite possibility.

If you are able to achieve remission of your symptoms for three to six months prior to trying to conceive, you will improve your fertility, reduce your miscarriage risk, and positively impact your future baby's growth and overall health. If you have not had a lupus flare-up for at least six months prior to trying to conceive, your miscarriage risk drops to the same as that of the general population: approximately 15 percent if you are under thirty-five years of age (up to 25 percent if you are between thirty-five and forty). Under these conditions, your chances of having a lupus flare-up after conception is less than 7 percent. If your lupus is not under control when you become pregnant, you have an increased risk of miscarriage (20 to 40 percent), fetal birth defects, preterm delivery, and a low-birth-weight infant.

Fortunately, lupus doesn't appear to affect fertility rates, but some of the medications used to tame lupus flare-ups can temporarily stop ovulation. Usually ovulation resumes within one to three months after the medication is discontinued. However, antimalarial medications (helpful in treating lupus arthritic symptoms) and cyclophosphamide should be discontinued at least one month prior to pregnancy. Though managing your lupus requires commitment, patience, and a team effort with your doctors, successful conception is within your reach.

Because lupus inflames the blood vessels, circulation to a prospective fetus may be impaired, because the vessels to the placenta can be compromised; this may result in a higher risk of first-trimester miscarriage. You will be at special risk for this if you also have anticardi-olipin and antiphospholipid antibodies in your system, commonly found in women with lupus. Your doctor may recommend that you take a low-dose aspirin, heparin (which thins blood), and/or steroids (which reduce inflammation) to counter these effects. Improved circulation will lead to improved blood flow to reproductive organs when you're trying to conceive, as well as improving nutrient delivery and blood flow through the placenta. These medications can also significantly reduce the risk of miscarriage and birth defects, advantages that outweigh the rare side effects of bleeding and sugar intolerance.

In addition to conventional lupus treatments, do what you can to boost your immune system health through lifestyle measures outlined at the beginning of this chapter. You'll want to add one more thing to that list: you may also find it helpful to be vigilant in limiting your sun exposure to prevent flare-ups of the butterfly-shaped facial rash so common in women with lupus.

SHOULD YOU BE SCREENED FOR LUPUS?

You may need to be screened for lupus if you experience any of the following:

- Previous babies born with heart block (causes an arrhythmia)
- Recurrent unexplained miscarriages (two or more)
- Rheumatic diseases such as arthritis or Raynaud's disease (hypersensitivity to cold in hands and feet)
- Family history of lupus
- Unexplained migrating joint pain or a butterfly-shaped facial rash

If you think you may be at risk for lupus, a complete history and physical exam, as well as simple blood tests by your doctor, can confirm this diagnosis. Medical therapy is available and options that are baby-friendly do exist, but being in remission for three to six months prior to conception is strongly recommended to reduce maternal and fetal risk.

Rheumatoid Arthritis

This autoimmune disease has no effect on fertility, miscarriage rates, fetal birth defects, or pregnancy outcome, but it can be mighty uncomfortable if you have a flare-up while pregnant. The good news is that most women find that rheumatoid arthritis (RA) symptoms improve while they are pregnant (but the symptoms return with a vengeance after delivery).

Most women who suffer from RA experience joint pain, joint swelling and stiffness, and difficulty walking. Preconception treatment usually consists of therapeutic exercise in conjunction with nonsteroidal anti-inflammatory drugs (NSAIDs) such as ibuprofen or Aleve, aspirin, steroids, Remicade, or methotrexate (MTX). Remicade is a chemotherapeutic agent that doubles as an arthritis medicine that reduces joint pain, and MTX is a selective chemo agent that is also a teratogen, particularly attracted to developing fetal tissue, and is to be completely avoided during pregnancy. If you are on MTX, please stop taking it for three to six months before pregnancy, and take special care to maximize your folic acid, B_6, B_{12}, and possibly choline intake. These B vitamins can be compromised by MTX and can lead to increased risk for neural tube defects in your prospective fetus. Remicade, also known as infliximab, is a synthetic antibody that can fight inflammation in joints and binds to tumor necrosis factor, but only in humans and chimps, so traditional animal safety studies are not helpful. Common sense should rule—if you need a medication to ensure your overall good health, then the risk is outweighed by the benefit.

Prolonged steroid usage, common in the treatment of RA, can cause diabetes and bone loss, and NSAIDs can reduce fetal amniotic fluid production and affect fetal vascular circulation, so your medical team will probably advise discontinuation before conception or as soon as possible during the first trimester. Treatment with gold (yes, real gold) and penicillamine is no longer widely used and should be avoided if you are planning to become pregnant.

Healthy body weight, adequate calorie and protein intake, optimal balance of omega-3 and omega-6 fats, and intake of calcium and antioxidant vitamins (especially vitamins C and E) deserve special attention, in addition to the lifestyle measures suggested at the beginning of this chapter to promote immune system balance, so the "troops" are ready to fight at any time. According to a recent study conducted at the University of Arizona's Department of Medicine, as long as there are no drug-nutrient interactions, it might help to consume a couple of daily servings of fresh ginger or fresh-brewed ginger tea (better than crude ginger extract) for its joint-protective effects. As mentioned earlier, physical activity actually improves mobility and reduces joint pain; exercise in warm (not hot) water is particularly soothing if you have RA. Again, happily, the majority of women who suffer from rheumatoid arthritis find it improves during pregnancy.

FOR FUTURE REFERENCE: During Pregnancy

Myasthenia Gravis
Another autoimmune disease, myasthenia gravis, causes muscle weakness; the effects can vary from drooping eyelids to severe chest muscle weakness that can lead to respiratory distress. Fortunately, this diagnosis has no impact on fertility or miscarriage, but more than 50 percent of women with myasthenia gravis experience an intensification of their symptoms during pregnancy. Severe cases may require respiratory support.

Common treatment for myasthenia gravis includes steroids and anticholinesterase medications, which have not been shown to cause fetal birth defects. Avoid therapy with azathioprine, an immunosuppressive drug, because it may be potentially harmful to the developing fetus. Medical technology has improved over the years, making pregnancy for women with myasthenia gravis safer than ever. Still, you should have a serious discussion with your neurologist and obstetrician before conception to determine your individual risk. As with other autoimmune diseases, it's better to wait until you're in remission for three to six months before trying to conceive.

CANCER SURVIVORS AND CONCEPTION

Having been treated for cancer with chemotherapy, radiation, and/or surgery adds a whole new level of anxiety when you're contemplating conception:

"How do I know my ovaries can work?"
"What if my cancer recurs when I'm pregnant?"
"Will my baby have cancer if I had cancer and was treated with chemotherapy?"

The impact of cancer-fighting drugs on your fertility depends on the chemotherapeutic agents used. Your age is also a factor: the older you are at the time of the chemotherapeutic treatment, the higher the risk for premature ovarian failure or early menopause. Chemotherapy can also affect other organs, such as the heart and kidneys. Speak with your oncologist about a time frame for becoming pregnant and any pertinent testing you should consider before you try to conceive. For example, after a diagnosis of breast cancer, some oncologists advise waiting to conceive until you've gone three to five years without evidence of recurrence of the cancer. Your doctor's recommendations will often depend on the original stage and extent of your cancer and the types of treatment you have been exposed to. For example, lymphoma and leukemia are among the more common cancers that occur in reproductive-age women and men. If you have suffered either of these cancers, be sure to review your previous medical treatments with your obstetrician and oncologist before you attempt conception.

If you are having regular menstrual cycles and have been in remission for a number of years, getting pregnant shouldn't be a problem. If your periods are absent or irregular, have your FSH level checked—it may need to be adjusted to improve your fertility. This can be a potentially challenging situation, so be prepared to work closely with your mate and your medical team.

Nobody wants to think about a diagnosis of cancer just as they are beginning to contemplate starting a family. Yet it is far better to find out before you conceive than when you are pregnant. For both men and women, detecting cancer prior to conception gives you more options to preserve fertility. Evolving reproductive technologies are improving freezing, or cryopreservation, of eggs, so women who previously might have despaired of ever using their own genetic material to conceive after a cancer diagnosis can now cure their cancers and return years later with a younger, healthier egg for conception. Freezing and thawing sperm is a technique that is already very reliably accomplished. This ability to save eggs and sperm can reduce concerns about sterility that could result from lifesaving chemotherapy, radiation, and surgical treatments. If a diagnosis of cancer is made, be sure to let your oncologist know you are hoping to have children at some future date. As hundreds of thousands of cancer-surviving moms will tell you, not only is there life after cancer; there can be new life, too.

Influence of Diet and Lifestyle Habits on Cancer

Lifestyle factors such as smoking, inactivity, and obesity contribute to cancer development (or recurrence). And though there is no way to completely protect yourself, you can cut your risks by not smoking, being physically active on a daily basis, and being lean without being underweight. Scientists are on the cusp of discovering interactions between diet and genes that will yield more targeted dietary advice, but for now, a healthy, varied diet that emphasizes plant-based, minimally processed foods and little to no alcohol is already known to lower risk. Supplementing with high amounts of single vitamins or minerals makes some cancers worse, not better. Do not use any dietary supplements in amounts exceeding our preconception guidelines.

For those battling cancer, especially breast or colon cancer, research strongly supports the role of regular moderate exercise in improving your prognosis; whether this benefit comes directly from exercise or indirectly through exercise's impact on weight control, hormone balance, or immune system readiness is not entirely clear.

SHOULD YOU BE SCREENED FOR BREAST CANCER?

Though the overall incidence of women affected by breast cancer is not rising, an increasing number of reproductive-age women are being diagnosed with this disease. This is most likely because women not only are well educated about breast self-examinations and screening mammograms but also are choosing to become mothers when they are more mature. So, who should undergo preconception breast cancer screening? Consider it if:

- You have a mother or close relative with premenopausal breast cancer.
- You have a personal history of breast cancer, in which case you will want to make sure you are disease-free prior to conception.

- You are at or beyond the age of forty. This is when an initial screening or baseline mammogram is standard practice in the United States, according to the American Cancer Society and the American College of Obstetricians and Gynecologists. If you have a strong family history of breast cancer, a mammogram may be recommended sooner (usually ten years before the youngest family member with breast cancer was diagnosed).

At her preconception visit, Danielle's doctor discovered a breast mass that was subsequently diagnosed as cancer. Before her surgical and medical therapies were complete, Danielle and her husband discovered they were pregnant. They didn't know what to do: should they continue Danielle's life-saving therapy, exposing their unborn child to risks such as significant developmental problems and childhood cancers, or discontinue the pregnancy? The dilemma was unbearable. With the help of their physician and religious leaders, they decided to continue modified chemo after twenty weeks. Danielle is now the healthy mother of a healthy three-year-old son.

FOR FUTURE REFERENCE: During Pregnancy

Can Chemotherapy Be Used in Pregnancy?

Using chemotherapy medications while pregnant is associated with considerable risk and uncertainty because a portion of whatever drugs you take will be passed on to your baby. Chemotherapy is lethal to cancer cells, but unfortunately, it also kills healthy cells. The medical community doesn't yet know exactly how exposure of chemotherapeutic agents to the fetus translates into the long-term incidence of early childhood diseases and leukemia. But it is more or less standard to recommend that chemotherapy be completely avoided during the first and second trimesters. Radiation therapy to the extremities is acceptable, as it allows the rest of the body to be protected, but radiation therapy that involves the chest or the abdomen needs to be delayed until later in the pregnancy or after childbirth.

HEADACHES AND OTHER NEUROLOGIC DISEASES

Why do some women get headaches every time they have a period? Why do some people with seizures have none for years, while others need complex medication regimens to keep seizures at bay? The workings of the brain and central nervous system are still fairly mysterious. Fortunately, however, we do have some clues as to how neurological disorders affect fertility and fetal health.

Migraines

Melanie, twenty-eight and married for two years, has had menstrual headaches since puberty. They are severe enough to put her out of commission two or three days a month. Her ob-gyn told her that these headaches resulted from fluctuations in her hormones through her menstrual cycle. What will she do when she gets pregnant and her hormones rise?

Severe, throbbing headaches often accompanied by nausea and blurred vision are known as migraines and are common in reproductive-age women during the premenstrual time of the month, as well as in early pregnancy. If you experience increasing headaches before conception, an ophthalmologic exam will help to rule out other possible causes. The majority of women who experience migraines during pregnancy find they improve after fifteen to twenty weeks of gestation.

Safe medications to use for headaches before pregnancy include Tylenol, aspirin, and NSAIDs such as Advil, Aleve, and Motrin, which are not associated with causing birth defects. Once you are pregnant, Aspirin and NSAIDs are not usually recommended because the former can make you bleed more than normal and the latter can affect the fetal heart structure if used during the third trimester. Exceptions to this precaution occur when aspirin products are used to prevent recurrent first-trimester miscarriages associated with anti-phospholipid antibody and anti-cardiolipid antibody syndromes. Another exception is the use of ibuprofen-containing medications at the discretion of your health care provider. Ibuprofen-containing medications can be essential and safe for the treatment of preterm labor before thirty-four weeks gestation. Prescription-strength painkillers such as Tylenol with codeine, Fioricet, and Vicodin can be used safely, though only if necessary, in early pregnancy. Migraine medications such as Imitrex and Maxalt have been associated with birth defects in animal studies and should not be used during the month prior to conception and throughout pregnancy. Until more information becomes available, it is best to use proven baby-friendly medications for your migraine headaches before conception.

To minimize the frequency of migraines, whether or not they are triggered by your menstrual cycle, avoid dehydration, low blood sugar, and overexhaustion. Drinking sufficient fluids (limited caffeinated beverages), not skipping meals, and getting at least six to eight hours of sleep a night will reduce the sensitivity of the nervous system and, in turn, reduce the incidence of migraines. Oftentimes, a detailed food diary that includes time of month, weather conditions, and stress level will reveal foods (e.g., chocolate, red wine, aged cheese, and lunch meats) that trigger a migraine for you; these are not the same for everyone and may act in combination more than in isolation, so take the time to find out what your triggers are. Further, you should take medication to treat your headache as soon as possible after you begin to get symptoms so as to lessen the intensity and severity of your headache.

Epilepsy and Neural Tube Defects (NTD)

Women who are treated with anti-seizure medication for epilepsy have an increased risk of having children with NTDs. Taking 1–4 mg (1,000–4,000 mcg) of folic acid has been shown to reduce the incidence of NTD in the offspring of epileptic mothers, but the American Academy of Neurology states that at least 400 mcg offers similar protection. While the precise amount of extra folic acid that is most effective is still controversial, research suggests that 400 mcg of folic acid supplementation is beneficial for *all* prospective mothers.

Epilepsy

Some women's epileptic seizures are controllable by medication, others are cured by time (the frequency of seizures drops over time without medication), and still others have continued seizure activity despite medication. Regardless of which category you fit, if you've ever suffered from epilepsy, it's a good idea to undergo preconception counseling to learn about the fetal effects of the disease and the fetal risks associated with the medications currently available. The majority of women who have epilepsy and take antiseizure medicines have healthy children. If your seizures are under control prior to conception, there's a good chance they'll remain at bay during pregnancy. Among people with epilepsy who choose to conceive, a small percentage will enjoy a reduction in their symptoms, a small percentage will suffer an increase, and approximately 45 percent will experience little change in their seizure disorder while pregnant.

Epileptic seizures can be severe (grand mal) and involve involuntary muscle movements and loss of consciousness, or very mild (petit mal), associated with an odor, visual aura, or brief feeling of forgetfulness. The initial seizure disorder can be caused by fever, infection, head injury, or even allergies. Though no specific genetic link is known for epilepsy, there is a 1 to 10 percent risk that your offspring may also have seizures. Uncontrolled seizures resulting in physical trauma or oxygen loss can injure both the mother and the growing baby. Epilepsy can be diagnosed by a complete physical and an EEG, which measures brain wave patterns.

If you have been seizure-free for three to five years prior to your interest in becoming pregnant, you may be able to go without antiseizure medication before conception and for the first trimester of pregnancy (this is something to be decided with the help of your neurologist).

Neurologists who specialize in epilepsy among women suggest that consultation occur at least one year prior to trying to conceive to maximize safe medication usage and discontinuation. The medical jury is still out on which is the best antiseizure medication to take before and during pregnancy. If you need to keep taking medication, some potentially safe alternatives include carbamazepine (Tegretol), Lamictal, and phenobarbital. Dilantin, also known as phenytoin, is associated with a high risk of birth defects and should be avoided. Valproate (also referred to as valproic acid) is another medication to avoid because it is associated with NTDs in 1 percent of exposed children. Recent research also revealed that children born to mothers who took valproate during pregnancy had impaired physical and mental development at age three. It is essential to change to more baby-friendly medications well before conception to avoid fetal risks and reduce the incidence of recurrent seizures that may come with changes in your medication regimen.

SHOULD YOU BE SCREENED FOR A SEIZURE DISORDER?

Even if you don't think you've ever had a seizure, you may still want to be evaluated by your doctor if you seem to "lose time," that is, have episodes where you are awake but don't remember portions of time. Consider testing for epilepsy if you:

- Have a family history of seizures
- Have had a recent head injury or trauma
- Use recreational drugs or excessive amounts of alcohol (see Chapter 2)

Your doctor or neurologist will make a diagnosis by carefully taking your history and by conducting an EEG. Treatment can then be initiated. You should have either no seizures or at least good control over their severity for at least three months prior to conception.

If you have epilepsy, keep in mind that lifestyle changes along with folic acid supplementation at least three months prior to conception will not affect your fertility rate but will certainly improve your fetus's health. And your own health will benefit if you reduce the stress to your neurological system by getting adequate rest and avoiding alcohol and drug use.

Multiple Sclerosis

Multiple sclerosis (MS) is a progressive disease of the nervous system that is characterized by generalized fatigue and progressive muscular weakness. Unfortunately, MS most frequently occurs in women between the ages of twenty-five and forty—in other words, reproductive prime time. On the positive side, MS often improves during pregnancy and in itself offers no risk to fetal health or fertility. Many women with MS find that their symptoms are exacerbated during the first three months of the postpartum period, limiting their ability to care for their newborn and other children. Where MS is concerned, preconception counseling should include discussion with your mate about how you will handle the care of your children, the household, and, not least important, yourself, should you be incapacitated by a flare-up of your condition. Minimizing the medications needed for the treatment of MS is advised. Complete discontinuation of immune system modulators such as cyclophosphamide and azathiopurine is recommended because they are known to cause increased risks for early miscarriage and premature birth if used during pregnancy. To maximize the baby-friendliness of your body, steroids should be discontinued as well. Conception after a remission of three to six months is considered optimal to ensure a safer pregnancy.

A comprehensive approach to MS is empowering. So in addition to conventional MS treatments and approved medications, flip back to the beginning of this chapter to see how you can strengthen your immune system through healthy lifestyle measures. We also recommend that you pay particular attention to the vitamin D section of Chapter 11. You'll especially appreciate the payoff of the nutrition interventions, which help decrease problems with gastric reflux and constipation, and of the fitness guidelines, which reduce fatigue, improve balance (which will be further compromised when you have a pregnant belly), and help fight infection.

Spinal Cord Injuries

With the advent of improved medical treatments, physical therapy, and emotional support, more young women who are challenged by a physical disability are reaching reproductive age with the desire to have children. These women may use a wheelchair or crutches and have limited use of their hands, arms, or legs, but there is no limit to the ability these women have to love and care for a potential child. Rehabilitation medicine, occupational therapy, and the determination of prospective parents have opened the door to conception for couples where one may have a physical disability. Many women and men who are affected by physical disabilities now have the ability to be independent and completely capable of self-care. Special consideration before pregnancy for these women should include:

- Strengthening your physical condition, including cardiovascular and muscular fitness
- Optimizing your body weight
- Avoiding infection in the genitourinary system by maintaining scrupulous personal hygiene (i.e., if skipping a shower is easier on some days, use a baby wipe to "sponge bathe"), and the sterility of catheter use is essential
- Assembling a medical team that can direct and support your conception plans and make you feel welcome as you pursue prenatal care

The cause of your physical disability may raise some concerns about genetic risk to your offspring. Most reproductive-age men and women with disabilities are victims of trauma, muscular dystrophy, neurological illnesses, or injuries during birth. If there is a genetic reason for your physical limitations, the chances that your children might have the same should be discussed. Risk can range from 25 to 50 percent (depending on the genetic abnormality) and can be tested for in early pregnancy to provide reproductive choice to a couple. (See Chapter 6 for more information on genetic disorders and testing options.)

Before conception, encourage a team approach among the specialists managing your care—one option might be to ask for a case manager if your health plan provides that service. A case manager can minimize the hassle factor during this busy time of your life by helping to ensure that the proper referrals are in place to cover all your specialist visits. If you have not already done so, ask for a consultation with a maternal-fetal medicine specialist. Although you are likely already well informed, we are compelled to mention a few cautions here just in case they have slipped through the cracks.

A spinal injury increases your risk for osteoporosis unless you are able to integrate physician-approved, weight-bearing exercises that place your body in a standing position. These include passive static standing machines with standing frames, continuous passive motion machines, harness-assisted treadmills, and/or parallel bars. To slow bone loss, make sure your daily diet contains 1,000–1,300 mg calcium (more than this can create a different problem—constipation). Also, ask your physician if your vitamin D level is fine—any deficiency should be treated aggressively.

Adequate birth control while you are fine-tuning your body weight, physical strength, and overall medical condition is essential. Limitations in mobility increase the inherent (albeit slight) risk of clot formation when using oral contraceptives. Reassuringly, current medical opinion is that birth control pill use is safe for those with a spinal injury. Other options include barrier methods, such as condoms, and an intrauterine device (IUD) can be considered if birth control is anticipated for at least two years (it's cost-prohibitive if used for less than two years).

KIDNEY (RENAL) DISEASE

Your kidneys, located on either side of your midback, filter your blood to remove waste products. When you become pregnant, your blood volume increases by 30 percent, making your kidneys work overtime (hence the increased frequency and amount of urination common in early pregnancy). If you suffer from an underlying kidney disease, this increased workload may exacerbate your condition significantly with each subsequent trimester of your pregnancy. Optimizing your kidney function at least three to six months before conception will improve your fertility and reduce your risk of preterm labor, preeclampsia, miscarriage, and poor fetal growth.

FOR FUTURE REFERENCE: During Pregnancy

Urinary Tract Infections in Pregnancy

During pregnancy, vaginal bacteria near the urethra can make their way up to the bladder and tend to accumulate there with little warning before progressing to a urinary tract infection (UTI). These bacteria are normal and healthy in the vagina (so don't over-cleanse inside the vagina or douche!), but they don't belong in the bladder. Sometimes a UTI is missed during pregnancy because you're already urinating more frequently, a key symptom that would otherwise trigger a test to see if you have an infection. If you are pregnant, a UTI can more easily lead to a kidney infection, a condition known as pyelonephritis, because the growing uterus compresses the ureters, the tubes that carry urine from the kidney to the bladder, disrupting the flow of urine. Kidney infection, in turn, can lead to a higher incidence of low-birth-weight infants, preterm labor, premature rupture of the membranes, and high blood pressure. If you are prone to UTIs before conception, your ob-gyn may have you take urine tests as part of your routine pregnancy exams to help diagnose UTIs earlier and prevent a kidney infection.

To help prevent a UTI you should:

- Maintain proper hydration.
- Empty your bladder shortly after intercourse.
- If you have recurrent UTIs, limited evidence supports regular consumption of cranberry juice to change the acidity of urine to discourage bacteria growth in the bladder.
- Women with recurrent UTIs after intercourse may be prescribed a prophylactic antibiotic to take after intercourse, such as nitrofurantoin, which can be used safely before and after conception. Although this may increase the resistance of bacteria in your bladder to one antibiotic, there is usually a second baby-friendly and effective choice should the need arise.

Polycystic Kidney Disease

This is an inherited disorder that appears in a woman's late thirties and early forties. Evaluation of this condition is accomplished through urinalysis, kidney ultrasound, and twenty-four-hour urine creatinine collection. The more severe a prospective mother's kidney disease, the greater her pregnancy risk of high blood pressure, preterm labor, abruption of the placenta, and premature rupture of membranes. You have a 50 percent chance of passing this on to your offspring. This disease progresses with age, so you may wish to start your family as early as you healthily and happily can.

Severe Kidney Disease and Kidney Transplants

Women with severe kidney disease (due to a condition you were born with, complications of diabetes, drug abuse, or toxic prescription medication use) are at significant risk for reduced fertility and more pregnancy complications. Although there is commonly a negative impact on fetal growth with this condition, the rate of birth defects is no higher than that in the normal population. If you have renal insufficiency or require dialysis, pregnancy may not be advised because it increases the strain on the kidneys significantly. However, there are exceptions, and vigilant preconception preparation makes the critical difference.

If you have undergone a successful kidney transplant, your probability of carrying a healthy baby to term is much greater than if your kidney disease is unresolved. If you are waiting for a transplant, remember that pregnancy can accelerate the deterioration of your kidneys. Trying to conceive may not be advisable until roughly two years after your transplant has taken place. Immune system modulators necessary after transplant to reduce your body's rejection of the new organ are not advised in pregnancy; your medication regimen should be reviewed with your transplant team and ob-gyn thoroughly before conception is attempted. Much can be accomplished in the interim. Well before you get the green light to start trying, make sure you are working with a complete multidisciplinary team of experts, including renal and obstetric doctors, and a renal dietitian.

DEPRESSION/ANXIETY/MENTAL HEALTH

Jennifer and Alan have been married three years and want to start a family. Jennifer has suffered from an anxiety disorder for years, but thanks to medication (Zoloft) and bimonthly therapy sessions, she leads a normal life. Fearful of the effects on her unborn child, Jennifer secretly took herself off her medication before they conceived. Thirteen weeks into her pregnancy she had a nervous breakdown and had to stop work, go back on heavy doses of medication, and receive intensive counseling.

Experts estimate that at least 10 to 15 percent of reproductive-age women suffer from depression? If you are one of them, you are in the company of millions of others who hold jobs, maintain relationships, and raise families while coping with anxiety or depression. Preparing to conceive can increase your stress and compound any emotional difficulties that you may already be experiencing. A preconception discussion with your partner, therapist or psychologist, and ob-gyn can help you to make the transitions from preconception to pregnancy to motherhood. Fortunately, mild depression appears to have little impact on fertility or miscarriage, and more than 30 percent of women with depression notice an improvement in their mood during the second and third trimesters of pregnancy, often to the point where they are able to reduce or discontinue their medications.

If you are struggling on a daily basis with debilitating depression or anxiety, it is very important to assess your ability to care for yourself and those around you, including a new baby. Some women decide to defer pregnancy for the time being; others go forward. If, after consultation with your partner and mental health care provider, you choose to plan for a baby, you'll need to assess the safety of your medication.

The most common medications used to treat depression, anxiety, and premenstrual syndrome mood changes are *selective serotonin reuptake inhibitors* (SSRIs), such as Prozac, Zoloft, Lexapro, Effexor, and Celexa. Though they are considered safer for pregnancy than other medications that could treat depression, concerns remain about temporary changes in your newborn related to his or her withdrawal from these medications, which have been circulating in your system. Symptoms of withdrawal in a newborn include reduced ability to suckle, failure to thrive, and an increased sensitivity to noise and light. Optimal medication management for depression and anxiety is accomplished through minimizing the dose and number of different medications used, and securing the best possible support system before, during, and after pregnancy. If this is done prior to conception, the positive impact on the health of your baby-to-be and yourself is clear.

Recent research on a common SSRI, Paxil, used for the treatment of depression and anxiety revealed increased negative effects on prospective offspring. There was no change in fertility rates in women who used Paxil, but those who took the medication in their first trimester were more likely to have infants with cardiac defects. A similar observation of women on Zoloft and Prozac did not find negative outcomes for the baby; hence, these are the preferred medications to treat depression and anxiety during pregnancy.

Treatment of depression and anxiety before, during, and after pregnancy is best done with a multidisciplinary approach:

- Establish a supportive relationship with your therapist.
- Stick to regular exercise patterns, which release endorphins that improve your mood.
- Stabilize your mood on a medication that is baby-friendly at least one to three months before conception.
- Involve your partner in the pursuit of mental health—time together concentrating on your relationship, not chore performance, can be helpful in reminding you why you plan to conceive.
- Simplify your work life and eliminate the stressors you have control over, such as saying yes to extra projects at work or at your older child's school, to allow more time for exercise, healthy meals, and quiet time.

Jennifer could have continued her meds safely and avoided her breakdown. Baby-friendly choices can be used to prevent emotional disintegration. When considering medicine for depression and anxiety before and during pregnancy, you have to make the choice that is right for you as an individual. (See "For Future Reference" on page 217.)

Other medications that treat mental illness have no effect on fertility but can pose problems for the fetus if continued through pregnancy. The drugs listed below are best avoided one month prior to trying to conceive. You may even want to transition to a more baby-friendly medication up to three months prior to conceiving to allow your system to acclimate itself.

Drugs that are not recommended for treatment of mood disorders when you may become pregnant include:

- **Tricyclic antidepressants, such as Elavil.** Although the tricyclics do not delay conception or cause birth defects, they can cause lethargy and other problems in newborns. If these medications are needed during pregnancy, stopping two weeks prior to delivery will limit the drug's neonatal effects.

- **Benzodiazepines, such as Xanax and Valium.** Valium taken during the formative weeks of the first trimester is associated with cleft palate, but it can be reinstituted after the first trimester in the lowest possible doses.

- **Monoamine oxidase inhibitors (MAO inhibitors), such as Nardil.** These can cause birth defects if used in the first trimester. These drugs also have dangerous interactions with other drugs, such as cough and cold preparations (especially those with dextromethorphan), antiasthma drugs, and foods that are pickled or smoked, leading to severe decreases in blood pressure.

SHOULD YOU BE SCREENED FOR DEPRESSION?

If you experience any of the following symptoms for more than a few weeks, speak with your doctor or get a referral to a therapist or psychologist:

- Decreased interest in daily activities, hobbies, and sex
- Disturbance in your usual sleep patterns (whether too much or too little)
- Reduction in appetite or weight loss due to lack of appetite
- Heightened irritability or moodiness
- Inability to concentrate or increased indecisiveness
- Unexplainable fatigue
- Unrelenting thoughts of death

There is no blood test to determine if you are depressed or anxious. Your instincts are your best diagnostic tool. You should also have a general checkup to rule out other medical problems, such as thyroid disease and Cushing's disease, that can affect your mood.

 FOR FUTURE REFERENCE: After Delivery

The Facts Regarding Postpartum Depression

If you have used medications to treat a mood problem in the past, have an eating disorder, or had postpartum depression (PPD) after a previous delivery, you are at a much higher risk for PPD in the current or future pregnancy. With this in mind you should strongly consider restarting your usual medications two to three weeks before your due date or immediately after delivery, whether or not you have symptoms at the time. Like many women, you were probably feeling emotionally well in the second and third trimester, but physical, emotional, neurochemical, and hormonal changes after delivery may have triggered a return of your depression or anxiety. It is even possible that your symptoms may be more severe than prior to or during pregnancy. As you already know, depression and other mood imbalances take a toll on your health and can disrupt the initial bonding with your infant, and for some women can even lead to violent outbursts with unintended, tragic consequences (e.g., shaken baby syndrome).

The upside here is that restarting medications before or just after delivery can head off these symptoms. In addition to medications that will reduce the intensity of your PPD, we recommend taking steps long before delivery to strengthen your support system. For instance, to help minimize fatigue, consider saving money to have a night nurse after delivery (even if you are breastfeeding) and stagger family help over two months if possible (instead of only the first two weeks). Finally, plan some alone time with your spouse.

If you choose to not restart antidepressants before or after delivery, we recommend close follow-up with your ob-gyn and therapist to improve your successful transition to parenting.

Breastfeeding while taking antidepressant medication appears to be safe for the baby, although taking the lowest possible effective dose is recommended to reduce even further the minute amount that can be present in breastmilk. Zoloft and Prozac are considered safe options in these circumstances.

Exercise Plus Traditional Therapies: A Key Combination for Depression

If you have a history of depression and make a point of incorporating moderate physical activity into your life, you probably know all too well how your mood can suffer when there is a lapse in routine. We're talking about aerobic exercise where you break a little sweat—moving freely and mindfully, preferably outdoors, almost every day. As long as you get a good thirty minutes, physical activity serves as a kind of therapy for your mind and body, with no downside when done responsibly. You may even find that you need less medication (with doctor approval, of course) and your sleep is sounder.

If your doctor or psychotherapist and you have not discussed how to make fitness an integral part of your treatment plan, waste no time before reading Chapters 15 and 16. Make sure he or she is aware of your intentions, begin to make gradual changes, and relish this new form of emotional resuscitation—it's like spa time for your soul.

Can Specific Nutrients Do Anything for Depression?

First and foremost, depression can impair your motivation to take good care of yourself and may dampen appetite, causing weight loss or an unbalanced food intake. Some antidepressants, notably the SSRIs, may initially result in weight loss but eventually have a side effect of weight gain and low-grade body inflammation. But body weight won't tell the whole story. Knowing this, it might be helpful to get a referral to a registered dietitian who can help you stay on track to be well nourished before conception, through pregnancy, and into the postpartum period.

With regard to individual nutrients, pay particular attention to getting an optimal supply of healthy oils (especially the omega-3s EPA and DHA), folate, vitamin B_{12}, selenium, zinc, vitamin D, and possibly magnesium and riboflavin. Your vitamin D status may also be worth adding to your preconception panel of blood tests. Since you are planning on conceiving, refer to Chapter 8 for information on the safety of natural supplements or herbal remedies that make claims about mental health.

More Situations Where Mental Health Care Professionals Can Help

Even if you do not experience symptoms of anxiety or depression, it is wise to consider a preconception psychiatric evaluation if you have any of the following:

- History of depression, anxiety, eating disorders, psychosis, or attention deficit disorder
- History of sexual abuse
- Intense fear of labor and delivery
- Past history of postpartum depression or traumatic pregnancy event, such as a stillbirth
- Current marital difficulties

Mental illness can sometimes pose challenges that make parenthood impractical and even irresponsible. If someone is psychotic or delusional, pregnancy is too overwhelming a stressor. Often, women in these conditions have difficulty caring for themselves, much less a new-born. If you suffer from a disorder such as manic-depression (bipolar disorder) or schizo-phrenia, your medical regimen will require attention, but the risks to your baby from your medication may be outweighed by the benefits to your mental well-being. Lithium or Lamic-tal is commonly prescribed for bipolar disorder but at higher doses is known to cause birth defects. Lithium levels should be lowered during pregnancy to avoid unintentional toxicity to the mother and her developing baby. Some women who are in remission from bipolar disor-der may be able to stop taking this medication entirely, but they still need to be closely moni-tored during pregnancy.

FOR FUTURE REFERENCE: During Pregnancy/After Delivery

Getting Support

Many local hospitals host support groups moderated by mental health professionals to help with the transition into motherhood and to provide assistance with postpartum depression. Day care for other children is often available in these settings, and bringing your infant with you to sessions is encouraged. Partner and family support after delivery can make a very positive difference for these new mothers.

ATTENTION DEFICIT DISORDER (ADD) OR ATTENTION DEFICIT/HYPERACTIVITY DISORDER (ADHD)

There is a growing population of reproductive-age women who suffer from ADD or ADHD. The symptoms of these disorders can often mimic other mental health disturbances and are often misdiagnosed as anxiety. Observational studies report up to 15 percent of parents of children with ADD or ADHD also suffer from the same disorder. You may be affected by ADD or ADHD if you have at least two of the following symptoms for at least six months or more:

- Inattention, as seen as a lack of detail-oriented thinking, careless mistakes made in school or work projects, failing to finish a project, being easily distracted during every-day activities
- Difficulty following through on projects at home or at work
- Trouble organizing work-related or leisure activities
- Nervous physical activity such as fidgeting or an inability to sit for needed periods of time to finish a task
- Difficulty maintaining a patient manner when engaging with others

Most women affected with ADD or ADHD recognize having had symptoms for many years prior to diagnosis, but they had been able to mask these issues to fit into their workplace or educational setting. Therapies for ADD and ADHD include behavioral techniques and medications that may reduce one's neurological chemistry. Common medications include Strattera, Adderal, and Focalin; these are contraindicated in pregnancy because negative changes in blood pressure, heart rate, and sleeping patterns are common and the potential for fetal birth defects is not well-known. Discontinuation of medications is recommended for one to three months before conception to allow you to practice functioning without them, and adjustments can be made without an affect on your fetus. A team approach to your care involving your psychiatrist and obstetrician before, during, and after pregnancy will maximize your successful transition without medication for ADD or ADHD.

WHAT'S NEXT?

Modern medicine has made it possible to not only live with a chronic condition but thrive with it, and that includes building a family. The next chapter reviews the preconception and pregnancy safety of common medications, herbs, and supplements. Your partner will be interested in checking out Chapter 9 for specific recommendations to help his sperm get into the best shape of their lives. Chapters 10–16 are chock-full of information about nutrition and fitness so *you'll* be in the best shape of your life heading into pregnancy as well!

CHAPTER 8

Conception-Friendly Medications and Herbs

MEDICATIONS

Knowing ahead of time which medications are safe during pregnancy helps you avoid the worry of realizing you used medications of questionable safety for baby prior to conception. Medications, both prescription and over-the-counter, can range from being completely safe to being absolutely unacceptable for use prior to and after conception. Perhaps the most devastating and dramatic example is thalidomide. This drug was widely used in the late 1950s and early 1960s to treat morning sickness before it was found to cause severe fetal limb deformities as well as kidney and heart defects. In the thirty-five years since the effects of thalidomide were discovered, there have been only thirty drugs proven to be teratogens, substances that can potentially cause a birth defect in an otherwise normal fetus. These teratogens have been promptly removed from the market or are clearly labeled to be avoided during preconception and pregnancy (see Table 8-1).

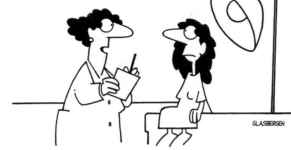

"This will help you feel less moody, stressed, and irritable. It's a prescription for chocolate."

Randy Glasbergen, www.glasbergen.com

TABLE 8-1
UNSAFE PRESCRIPTION MEDICATIONS
DURING PRECONCEPTION AND PREGNANCY

Medication	Treatment for	Fetal Effect	Alternative Therapy[a]
Accutane[b] (isotretinoin), Retin-A Claravis Roaccutane	Acne	Central nervous system (CNS) defects, bone and heart defects, ↓ fetal growth, ↑ miscarriage, mental retardation	Topical antibiotics: erythromycin or clindamycin
ACE inhibitors[b] (e.g., Captopril, Enalapril)	High blood pressure	Kidney failure, ↓ birth weight, ↓ fetal growth	Beta-blockers (e.g., Inderal), methyldopa, hydralazine
Coumadin (warfarin)[b], blood thinner	Valve replacement, prevention of blood clots	Face and eye defects, CNS defects, ↓ fetal growth	Heparin, Lovenox
Dilantin[b,c] (phenytoin)	Seizure disorder	Facial, heart defects, ↓ fetal growth, mental retardation	Tegretol, Lamictal
Imitrex	Migraine	Vascular defects	Tylenol
Lithium[b]	Manic-depression or bipolar disorder	Heart defects	Tegretol
MAO inhibitors (e.g., Nardil)	Anxiety, depression	? ↑ miscarriage risk, ? ↑ birth defect risk, newborn lethargy	Prozac, Zoloft
Methotrexate[b]	ectopic pregnancy, choriocarcinoma, rheumatoid arthritis	DNA damage, ↑ miscarriage risk, ↑ birth defects	None, specifically. Rely on MD discretion.
Paxil	Anxiety, depression	? cardiac/CNS damage	Prozac, Zoloft
Prilosec	Gastric ulcers	? ↑ miscarriage risk, ? ↑ birth defect risk	Zantac, antacids
Quinolones (e.g., ciprofloxacin)	Infections	Cartilage deposits, may weaken bones	Cephalosporins (e.g., Keflex)

Medication	Treatment for	Fetal Effect	Alternative Therapy[a]
Radioactive iodine[b]	Hyperthyroidism	Fetal goiter	Propylthiouracil
Testosterone, Danazol[b]	Decreased libido, endometriosis	Virilization of female	None
Tetracycline[b], Doxycycline	Bacterial infections	Bone, teeth changes	Penicillin, erythromycin
Valproate[b]	Seizure disorder	Neural tube defect[c] ↓ cognitive ability	Tegretol

a. Alternatives in this table represent only some of the choices that are safe. Discuss options with your health care provider.

b. These medications are either suspected or known to cause birth defects in human studies. (Pregnancy Categories D or X)

c. Most antiseizure medications have some effect on neural tube defect risk. This risk might be reduced by taking a separate folic acid supplement above the usual 400 mcg dose, but typically not exceeding 1,000 mcg/day. The American Academy of Neurologists recommends *at least* 400 mcg/day for all women of childbearing age with epilepsy.

This may be obvious, but just remember that the medications discussed in this chapter all have known safety profiles based on rigorous safety testing in nonpregnant humans and animals. Safety profiles for medication usage for the transition to pregnancy have always been difficult to formulate, though, because pregnant women are not actively enrolled in clinical trials. Data are collected retrospectively (usually in cases when the exposure took place before the woman found out she was pregnant). Unfortunately, such retrospective research is complicated by the fact that many other variables could have affected the health of a fetus. The medical community bases its perinatal advice about medicines on animal study, limited human observation, and common sense. When you're considering medication or treatment while pregnant, the potential risks to the fetus must be outweighed by the benefit to maternal health.

During the preconception phase and first trimester of pregnancy, if a medication is not absolutely necessary, it is best avoided. If changes or discontinuation of medications are planned, contact your health care provider to aid you with these transitions. Preferably, try to adopt this new medication regimen at least one to three months before you want to start trying to conceive. Preconception changes allow you to determine if additional baby-friendly medications may be needed, and the best time to determine and adjust these medications is before a fetus enters into the scene. Regardless, there are many safe and effective medications to use for a variety of ailments both before and after pregnancy (see Tables 8-2 and 8-3). All prescription medications are classified into a pregnancy category (A, B, C, D, or X) by the Food and Drug Administration (FDA). The criteria for the FDA's five categories are defined as follows:

- **Category A.** Well-controlled animal and human studies among pregnant women found no fetal risk.

- **Category B.** Animal studies found no fetal risk but no human studies have been conducted among pregnant women; *or* animal studies found risk but no adequate studies among pregnant women were able to confirm the risk.

- **Category C.** These fall into a gray area. Studies among animals have found evidence of risk to a fetus; *or* there have been no studies conducted among either pregnant humans or animals. In some cases, the benefit to the mother may outweigh the risk to the fetus.

- **Category D.** There is clear evidence of risk to a human fetus, but in some serious conditions the benefit to the mother outweighs the risk to the fetus.

- **Category X.** There is clear evidence of risk to a human fetus, and the benefit does not outweigh the risk for women who are or may become pregnant.

Many of the OTC drugs in Table 8-2 were once prescription drugs and formerly had an A, B, or C pregnancy category, but comparable classifications don't exist for OTCs. Every OTC drug should have a Drug Facts or Warnings section on the label where pregnancy safety is addressed. Medications in Table 8-2 should not impact fertility and most of them demonstrate no risk to fetal development, though some have more limited use during pregnancy (possible risks are often isolated to a specific stage of pregnancy). Read the footnotes for clarity.

Similarly, Table 8-3 lists prescription-only drugs that are safe choices for preconception and pregnancy. Most are Pregnancy Category A and B, and a few are C; we detail the explanations for you in the footnotes. What you need to know is that if your physician is writing a prescription (or recommending an OTC drug), she will balance the safety of the medications for the fetus against the benefit to your health according to the following five basic principles:

- **Weigh the benefits as well as the risks.** Potential side effects for the fetus if you take the medication must be balanced against the harmful effects to you if you don't.

- **Choose the most baby-friendly medicine possible.** This will allow you to minimize the health risk to you and the fetus. If your previous medical regimen was more effective in controlling your condition, let your doctor know your experience.

- **Use single-agent therapy, if possible.** The use of one medication rather than several to treat a problem significantly reduces fetal risk. For example, multiple medicines are typically used for the treatment of asthma or high blood pressure, but often your regimen can be safely scaled back to a single drug during preconception and pregnancy, if needed.

- **Take the lowest dose possible.** Many medications are safe at a low dose. Taking the minimal dose needed to get the desired medical benefit will significantly reduce the risks to the fetus.

- **Discontinue for a short period of time.** If a medication is preferable but not essential, consider discontinuing it during the development of the fetal organ system, which takes place between the seventeenth and fifty-sixth day after conception. Restart your medication after the first trimester, beginning at thirteen weeks.

TABLE 8-2
SAFE OVER-THE-COUNTER (OTC)/NONPRESCRIPTION DRUGS FOR COMMON AILMENTS DURING PRECONCEPTION AND PREGNANCY

Condition	Medication[a]
Allergy symptoms	Sudafed, Benadryl, saline nasal sprays
Constipation[b]	Colace, Citracal, Benefiber, Metamucil
Cough[c]	Robitussin (DM type), lozenges without licorice
Diarrhea	Imodium A-D, Kaopectate[d]
Headache[e]	Tylenol is the drug of choice; Fioricet for more severe headaches
Hemorrhoids	Tucks, Preparation H, Anusol
Heartburn/gastroesophageal reflux[f]	Antacids such as Mylanta, Maalox, Tums, and Pepcid; Zantac
Itching or skin rash	Topical steroids such as hydrocortisone cream 0.5% to 1%, zinc oxide cream, oral Benadryl
Lice	Quell shampoos and topical products
Muscle soreness	Tylenol, NSAIDs[e] (e.g., ibuprofen and Aleve); aspirin[e]
Sleeping aids	Benadryl, Tylenol PM[h]
Yeast infection (vaginal)	Monistat[g], Gyne-Lotrimin, Vagisil

a. Physician consultation is recommended as you transition from pre-pregnancy to pregnancy.

b. Avoid overtreatment with these medications, as diarrhea can lead to dehydration, which is unhealthy for prospective mother and fetus.

c. The amount of alcohol in most cough preparations is negligible. Cough drops should not contain licorice. Limited use of codeine is recommended for the treatment of persistent coughs. (See Table 8-4 for herbal ingredients.)

d. Occasional usage is considered safe in pregnancy, but repetitive dosing throughout the pregnancy can lead to restricted growth in the fetus.

e. The NSAIDs ibuprofen and naprosyn (Aleve), and aspirin are pain relievers and anti-inflammatory medications that are not known to cause birth defects. They are safe to use *before* pregnancy but should be used at the discretion of medical staff once you are pregnant. Aspirin may increase bleeding in the prospective mother and fetus but under certain clinical circumstances, such as habitual miscarriages and known immunological alterations in antiphospholipid and anticardiolipin antibodies, it can thin the blood, allowing better flow through vessels that nourish the placenta and the growing fetus. NSAIDs can be safely used in limited amounts during pregnancy for the treatment of preterm labor and fibroid pain but must be regulated carefully to avoid low amniotic fluid and changes in the fetal heart.

f. In OTC antacids, magnesium should not exceed 350 mg per day (no limit on magnesium found naturally in foods, just supplements). A limit of approximately 1,000–1,500 mg calcium per day from supplements leaves room for calcium from food too. See Chapter 11 for more details about getting enough, but not too much of, minerals.

g. Monistat is best used in the second and third trimesters. First-trimester use should be discussed first with your health care provider. It is perfectly safe to use before conception.

h. Sleeping aids can be habit-forming and should always be discussed with your health care provider before use. Alternatives such as regular exercise, relaxation techniques, light snacks, and warm baths are better first choices. If these meds are used, be careful to hydrate well after use.

TABLE 8-3
SAFE PRESCRIPTION MEDICATIONS FOR COMMON AILMENTS DURING PRECONCEPTION AND PREGNANCY

Condition	Prescription Medication[a]
Allergies with sinusitis	Zyrtec, Rhinocort, Nasocort[b]
Bacterial vaginosis	Cleocin (vaginal suppositories)
Chlamydia	Zithromax, erythromycin
Depression	Zoloft, Prozac, Ativan[c]
Diabetes	Insulin, from human or synthetic sources; metformin
Genital warts	Aldara, trichloroacetic acid
Heartburn/gastric reflux[f]	Zantac, Pepcid, Protonix
Herpes	Zovirax, Valtrex
HIV	AZT (zidovudine)
Hypertension	Aldomet, Labetalol, Inderal, hydralazine
Hyperthyroidism	Propylthiouracil (PTU)[d]
Hypothyroidism	Synthroid, Levoxyl
Kidney infection	Keflex, clindamycin, gentamicin
Migraines	Tylenol with or without codeine, Fioricet, Darvocet
Nausea/vomiting[e]	Zofran, Compazine, Reglan
Sleeping aids	Ambien[c]
Syphilis	Penicillin
Upper respiratory infections	Ampicillin, Zithromax
Urinary tract infections (UTI)	Macrodantin, Keflex, Penicillin
Yeast infection (vaginal)	Diflucan, Terazol

a. Check the package insert for the pregnancy category assigned by the FDA (e.g., A, B, or C).
b. Use only as needed because these medications can cause dehydration. Pay particular attention to getting enough fluids to avoid dehydration.
c. Used in the lowest possible doses and preferably not in the first trimester.
d. PTU should be discontinued by the twelfth week of pregnancy; after that time, a developing fetus can begin to produce its own thyroid hormone and can be affected by maternal intake of PTU, leading to hypothyroidism and a goiter.
e. The benefits of better nutrition and maternal comfort will outweigh the risk potential if medication is needed.
f. Tagamet is also a Category B medication used for gastric upset, but unlike the other medications listed, one animal study reports the occurrence of benign testicular tumors in the animals given this drug. No additional studies have raised human fetal concerns, but we recommend a conservative approach and prefer the drugs listed in Table 8–3.

Practical Application

Make a list of the over-the-counter and prescription medications you have used in the past month and bring it to your preconception appointment. Better yet, bring the containers with you.

Drug name   Using to treat . . .

_____

_____

_____

_____

_____

As we've noted, pregnancy category D and X drugs are teratogens, meaning they may cause some babies to be born with birth defects if they are exposed to these drugs. Medications are categorized into D or X according to this risk calculation: whether or not the benefit to mother and/or baby outweighs the risk of a birth defect. Drugs in category D must be used sparingly at the discretion of your health care provider—in some serious situations, a particular drug may be your only choice for treating a condition vital to your health and that of your baby. A few examples of category D medications:

- **Spironolactone** is a diuretic used for those with high blood pressure and in polycystic ovary syndrome to reduce hair growth and water retention. There have been no drug-associated birth defects, but there are concerns about the antiandrogenic effect this medication can have on the developing fetus, especially if it is male.

- **Oral hypoglycemics** such as metformin and glyburide are used to control blood sugar in nonpregnant women with type 2 diabetes.[1] Insulin has long been the drug of choice for pregnant patients with type 2 diabetes to maximize sugar control and avoid potential fetal effects. Recent studies have shown that women might gain less excess weight and have fewer hypoglycemic episodes in early pregnancy with these newer oral drugs. Although a number of structural anomalies or birth defects were noted among the babies

---

1. While metformin is not yet the standard of care for pregnant women, many women are using metformin during preconception and through their first trimester; then insulin is added to aid in blood sugar control. We may be seeing more practitioners adopt this strategy in the future, particularly when obesity or PCOS is an issue.

born to mothers in these studies, the incidence was not higher than the expected risk of birth defects among babies born to mothers who have diabetes. (The risk of birth defects can be reduced by maintaining good blood sugar control. See Chapter 7 for more on this.)

- **Antidepressants** are used by many men and women for the treatment of anxiety, depression, and premature ejaculation. Clearly, if you have tried lifestyle adjustments to balance your mood (such as good exercise, sleep, and nutrition habits) but have not experienced adequate improvement, these drugs may be essential and the benefits may offset the known and unknown disadvantages of taking these medications. The most baby-friendly choices—both during pregnancy and breastfeeding—are listed in Table 8-3: Zoloft and Prozac, which are selective serotonin reuptake inhibitors (SSRIs). Almost all of the medications in this group can cause a reduction in libido, but Zoloft and Prozac have never been associated with causing a birth defect. Recent studies have shown that Paxil (listed in Table 8-1), a different SSRI, has been associated with an increase in fetal cardiac defects and some neurological abnormalities; thus it is now considered an unacceptable choice for use before and during pregnancy.

Category X drugs may cause some babies to be born with significant problems, and the benefit to the mother never outweighs the risk (see Table 8-1). Any medication not considered safe after conception should be avoided before trying to conceive, because you cannot be certain of the moment of conception and might unknowingly expose the fetus. *If you are using a known teratogen, you need to be unwavering in your use of safe, reliable birth control to absolutely prevent birth defects in your offspring.*

FOR FUTURE REFERENCE: During Pregnancy/After Delivery

Most of the medications that are safe in pregnancy are safe during breastfeeding, but don't start or stop medications until you consult with your physician. Alternative treatments such as herbal remedies are available but may interfere with prescription medications, so make sure your physician is aware of anything you are self-prescribing. And some of the medications that are not recommended during pregnancy can be used at the lowest dose while breastfeeding because such a small portion is excreted in the breastmilk. Your potential medication needs in the postpartum period should be reviewed with your ob-gyn and pediatrician before delivery to maximize the ease of transition into new (or repeat) motherhood.

HERBS

Many women want to try natural ways to take care of themselves while preparing for conception and the marvels that occur afterward. We encourage that, but it is extremely important to be every bit as careful with herbs as you would be with over-the-counter and prescription drugs. In fact, it is prudent to be even more cautious because although most herbs are much less potent than medications, there are more unknowns about herbs. Unlike prescription drugs, the manufacturing, labeling, and marketing of herbal products is not regulated.

Even the most knowledgeable experts in herbal medicine agree that the one to three months prior to conception are not the time to be testing the safety limits of herbal preparations (and other non-nutrient "natural" supplements). Rather, now is the time to *stop* taking herbs that have an unproven track record in reproductive health. Now is also the time to strictly avoid herbal body purification or detox programs that claim to offer internal cleansing or colon purification. Such programs are cleverly marketed but can be dangerous. In contrast, much is known about the benefits and safety of foods and certain vitamin-mineral supplements; these warrant separate discussions in later chapters that focus on essential nutrients (Chapters 10 and 11).

Just because a substance is natural does not guarantee its safety. And though an active ingredient in a particular substance might be helpful (or harmless) for the mom, it may not be baby-friendly. Like medications, many herbs carry the potential for adverse side effects, which are a great concern when a vulnerable new life is on the way.

The late Varro E. Tyler, PhD, ScD, a renowned author and distinguished professor emeritus of pharmacognosy at Purdue University, offered timeless, valuable input for the first edition of *Before Your Pregnancy*. He agreed with us that even those supplements in Table 8-4 are only "probably safe." He continued: "I do not recommend the use of herbs by pregnant women or nursing mothers, not necessarily because all are potentially toxic, but because in the United States there are no enforced standards of quality for such products. One simply cannot be sure that what is listed on the label is actually in the package. If the products were approved as drugs with assured standards of quality, I would feel differently about some of them."

Unlike countries such as Germany, where herbs are classified as drugs and held to the same stringent regulations, the United States does not regulate herbs, as Dr. Tyler noted. In the United States the supplement manufacturers are the ones who determine whether their products are safe and effective. They have to submit evidence to the FDA that their product is "reasonably expected to be safe," but no formal FDA testing or approval is required before it goes to market. This is unfortunate, because many a good herb gets a bad rap in the United States solely because it gets lumped together with inferior and worthless products that are allowed into the marketplace. Very few supplement companies are willing to spend what it takes to make voluntary improvements in quality control. Consumers should be aware that not all products live up to their claims, and some may not even be of the purity or dosage stated on the label. For example, numerous natural weight-loss supplements contain undeclared pharmaceutical ingredients (including legal and illegal drugs), while some Ayurvedic and traditional Chinese herbal medicines sold in the United States have been found to contain high levels of lead, mercury, and arsenic, putting mom and future baby at risk.

To date, trained practitioners in herbal medicine have deemed only a handful of herbs "probably safe" in moderation for women who are pregnant. The same recommendations hold true for the one to three months leading up to conception, unless you've been instructed otherwise by an experienced health care professional. For your convenience, we've categorized several common herbs and dietary supplements into three tables: in Table 8-4 are those that are probably safe during preconception and pregnancy; in Table 8-5 are those that warrant caution; and in Table 8-6 are those that should be completely avoided. We have primarily limited our discussion of their safety to specific concerns affecting women's fertility and the maintenance of health during pregnancy. Your physician should be made aware of all the herbs and supplements that you are considering taking.

Practical Application

If you currently take, or want to start taking, herbal/natural supplements for any reason in any form (pill, capsule, tea, tincture, extract, drops, powder, injection, cream), please write them down on the Women's Preconception Medical Checklist in Chapter 4 (Figure 4-1) that you will be taking with you to your preconception medical visit. If you have been taking supplements to treat a medical condition, this is an ideal time to discuss traditional medical approaches as well.

We discuss how supplements affect male fertility in Chapter 9. For now, your partner should be aware of the herbs and dietary supplements in Tables 8-5 and 8-6, especially those that are toxic and potentially dangerous to organ systems. Men who take legitimate dietary supplements to enhance sports performance should also understand that many of these are intentionally (or unintentionally) mixed with illegitimate substances such as hormones, stimulants, and contaminants that won't be listed on the label but could decrease his fertility, damage the sperm's DNA, and harm overall health.

TABLE 8-4
HERBS AND DIETARY SUPPLEMENTS THAT SHOULD BE SAFE DURING PRECONCEPTION AND PREGNANCY

Following is a list of herbs that may safely be used by women prior to and during pregnancy, provided that the product is what it says it is. But understand that because product purity and dosage cannot currently be guaranteed in the United States, they are not completely without risk. Also, these guidelines hold true only when intake remains moderate, that is, no more than the suggested servings per day for each of the teas and only according to manufacturer's labels on the others (e.g., safe herbal cold aids). In some cases we note the abbreviation GRAS: this means "generally recognized as safe," a designation ascribed by the FDA based upon expert opinion.

The approved teas are our favorites, because sipping tea can be one of many soothing ways to take time for yourself. Begin with one-half or one serving per day and go higher only if you like it. Sometimes a little milk, sugar, or honey improves the taste. Many women alternate the various teas throughout the week for variety.

- **Cinnamon and cinnamon bark.** Safe to consume in amounts normally found in foods and recipes. Higher amounts of cinnamon are being investigated for possible therapeutic value in lowering blood sugar and potentially treating men for premature ejaculation; however, women who could become pregnant should avoid supplemental doses in case fetal risks are uncovered in the future.

- **Cocoa (theobromine).** Safe when consumed as a food; should be a safe component of the cocoa butter that some women use to prevent stretch marks during pregnancy (though there is no evidence to support or refute this practice); the amount of caffeine in cocoa products is low, and even a daily serving of dark chocolate or hot cocoa falls way below our daily limit of 100 to 200 mg caffeine per day.

- **Culinary herbs and spices (e.g., rosemary, oregano, thyme, parsley, horseradish, sage, curry, turmeric/curcumin).** Recommended as excellent sources of concentrated antioxidants and phytonutrients; safe when limited to moderate use for cooking or garnish; these are not intended for repeated daily use in higher medicinal quantities.

- **Jewelweed.** In cases of poison ivy skin irritation, jewelweed appears to be a safe and effective alternative treatment to drugs such as corticosteroids; it is intended only for short-term topical use.

- **Lemon balm (melissa).** Under medical supervision, lemon balm may be effective in treating cold sores (herpes simplex virus 1) with no known effects on reproduction; short-term topical use should be safe.

- **Menthol.** Menthol is safe for topical use or in cough drops when taken according to package instructions, short-term; if there are other ingredients in question, check with your physician.

- **Omega-3 fatty acids.** Chapter 10 focuses on extensively researched sources of omega-3s such as fish oils and vegetarian alternatives; there are insufficient scientific study and safety data to make recommendations about the relatively new krill oil (from the crustaceans that whales love to eat), which has a lower level of omega-3s but more mono-unsaturated fat (same healthful fat as in olive oil), but you could ask a registered dietitian about updates.

- **Peppermint.** Peppermint tea has been shown to settle heartburn, indigestion, and nausea and is safe to drink in moderation (approximately two to three cups per day) during preconception and pregnancy; however, according to *The Nursing Mother's Herbal* by Sheila Humphrey, consumption should be more limited during breastfeeding, particularly if you are having trouble with low milk supply. Peppermint can be consumed in amounts commonly found in food or garnishes; avoid peppermint extracts (please refer to "Essential Oils" later in this chapter).

- **Probiotics.** Supplements that contain probiotics (substances that support the growth of friendly bacteria in your intestinal tract) are best reviewed by your doctor before consuming. However, foods and beverages, such as yogurt, acidophilus milk, and kefir, that contain live and active cultures should be safe during preconception and during pregnancy. These can be a healthy part of your diet, especially during flu season or if you have been on antibiotic therapy; if you are currently taking antibiotics, it is prudent to take your probiotic a couple of hours before or after the antibiotic. Also of interest are lactobacillus vaginal applications that, under medical supervision, may treat vaginal infections (e.g., bacterial vaginosis); evaluation of pregnancy safety is underway. Women with a weakened immune system are strongly advised to consult their physician before taking any probiotic. A well-balanced, high-fiber diet also helps probiotics work their best.

- **Psyllium (plantago seed or husk).** Psyllium is a form of soluble fiber that acts as a bulk-producing natural laxative (not to be confused with harsher stimulant laxatives of herbal origin described in Tables 8-5 and 8-6). Psyllium is the active ingredient in prepackaged products such as Metamucil. It is also sold in bulk. Psyllium is appropriate for healthy women who already eat a high-fiber diet, maintain good hydration, and exercise, yet need constipation relief. This form of fiber may also ease symptoms of irritable bowel syndrome. See Chapter 10 for information on dietary sources of fiber.

- **Red bush tea (rooibos tea).** This herbal tea is almost completely caffeine-free and unusually low in tannins compared to most herbal and black or green teas. It is also a satisfactory source of vitamin C. All of these properties make it very appealing to prospective moms.

- **Witch hazel.** This herb, particularly the hydroalcoholic extract of the leaves, is considered a safe and effective astringent for skin irritation and to reduce the inflammation of hemorrhoids as long as it is restricted to topical use as directed.

TABLE 8-5
HERBS AND DIETARY SUPPLEMENTS THAT WARRANT CAUTION DURING PRECONCEPTION AND PREGNANCY

- **Alfalfa.** Leafy portion possibly safe in small amounts (one to two servings in tea), and may exert a mild diuretic effect. It is best to avoid alfalfa seeds and large amounts of any other alfalfa products, especially if pregnancy is possible.

- **Barley grass (barley green).** Likely safe in culinary amounts, but avoid barley sprouts. If consumed in a "green" juice, look for one that is pasteurized; also watch other ingredients that may not be approved for safety.

- **Bitter melon.** Eaten as a vegetable in India and Asia and a component of some curries. May lower blood sugar levels with short-term use. Before pregnancy, small culinary amounts of bitter melon may be safely consumed as a vegetable or as a component of curries. However, once pregnancy is possible, it may be wise to omit appreciable quantities of bitter melon as a food, because it could promote menstruation and cause miscarriage in pregnant women. Women who eat bitter melon as a regular part of their diet may take some comfort in knowing that the predominant concerns revolve around bitter melon seeds, tablets, capsules, or liquid forms (juice or tea) of bitter melon. More comprehensive study is needed.

- **Bitter orange (synephrine).** Should be safe in quantities commonly found in food (bitter orange oil has GRAS status in food); however, it is best to avoid medicinal amounts promoted for "ephedra-free" weight loss during preconception or pregnancy. Another reason to be careful is that bitter orange poses potential dangers similar to ephedra/ma huang products (banned); may be combined with other stimulants or infused with pharmaceuticals.

- **Camphor.** Likely safe for topical usage (*not* ingestion) for cough suppression when taken according to package instructions, short-term; absolutely avoid use on broken skin or mucous membranes; if there are other ingredients in question, double-check with your physician.

- **Chamomile.** Mild influence on uterus, so limit to one serving per day; avoid completely if allergic to ragweed or aster plants.

- **Chasteberry (*Vitex agnus-castus*).** Under medical supervision, may be effective in decreasing PMS symptoms (especially breast tenderness) and restoring menstrual cycles in women who produce excessive levels of the hormone prolactin, but it is unsafe in pregnancy and should therefore be stopped at least two to four weeks prior to conception. It may prevent successful in vitro fertilization (despite a viable embryo transfer); also interferes with the effectiveness of birth control pills and other hormone-based medications. This herb may dampen libido (hence the name's origin).

- **Chia** (spelling not to be confused with chai, as in chai tea). Edible seeds and sprouts from the *Salvia hispanica* plant are mostly known for the seeds' high fiber, protein, and omega-3 content (alpha-linolenic acid, or ALA); probably safe for people not planning on becoming pregnant. Though there's a lot of hype about chia's potential to reduce the risk of diabetes and cardiovascular disease, there are no reliable studies on its use during pregnancy, so it's best to stay on the safe side and avoid it until more is known. Raw sprouts of any kind should be avoided before and during pregnancy due to their inherent vulnerability to carrying foodborne illness.

- **Chlorella.** Type of seaweed that is highly processed and available mostly in tablets and extracts. Possibly safe for short-term use prior to pregnancy, but not enough safety data available for us to feel comfortable giving the green light for use during pregnancy. Of greatest concern is the fact that chlorella samples vary greatly in their iodine content, and according to a study from the United Kingdom, the amounts can be very high, which could be harmful to future fetal development. Other edible seaweeds such as nori or wakame are healthy alternatives with moderate iodine content.

- **Coffee.** See Chapter 2 on caffeine.

- **Echinacea.** Clinical studies on echinacea and female fertility are limited at this time. One study of men taking echinacea revealed lowered fertility, but the poor methodology of this study casts doubt on the results. A study published in 2000 demonstrated the safety of echinacea during pregnancy. None of the wide variety of echinacea preparations have been definitively proven to protect against catching the common cold or decreasing the severity of symptoms. It is important, however, to avoid echinacea preparations containing goldenseal, as there are no reliable data on goldenseal's safety when ingested.

- **Evening primrose oil.** Appears to be safe and sometimes effective in reducing symptoms of PMS and breast tenderness (but most studies have observed only a strong placebo effect); there is no direct evidence to suggest that short-term use of evening primrose oil could be either harmful or beneficial to fertility or to a fetus; long-term safety data are unavailable; interferes with certain medications such as anticonvulsants and tricyclic antidepressants.

- **Garlic.** Using garlic cloves (fewer than two to three cloves per day) or garlic powder/salt in food preparation is fine, but garlic supplements are discouraged, because it is harder to gauge the amount of active ingredient in them.

- **Ginger.** This common herb with natural antioxidant properties is used in modest quantities for motion sickness and as a digestive aid. It is also used to alleviate morning sickness. Some controversy exists regarding the safety of ginger during preconception and pregnancy in high supplemental doses (i.e., over 10,000 mg [10g] per day). If ginger is part of your diet, do not exceed 1,000–2,000 mg/day. Cut back further if you encounter uncomfortable side effects such as heartburn, stomach discomfort, or diarrhea. The following are some approximate measurements: ginger tea = 250 mg per cup; ginger-spiced Indian entrée = 500 mg; 1-inch-by-¼-inch piece of candied ginger = 500 mg; real ginger ale (not artificially flavored) = 1,000 mg per cup. Those unaccustomed to the taste of real ginger tea may not care for its spiciness at first. However, to get around this you can mellow it by brewing two bags of tea at once—one ginger, the other peach (or similar) according to caffeine guidelines. And if you don't like it hot, an iced version may seem much more refreshing. Another pleasant alternative is to add a dash of rich soy milk or honey to take the edge off.

- **Gingko (*Gingko biloba*).** Strictly limit or avoid because it affects blood-clotting ability.

- **Grape or grape seed extract.** Grapes are an excellent source of polyphenols (proanthocyanidins) that have antioxidant properties (also found in many other fruits, teas, cocoa, and nuts with skins intact, *not* removed). Extracts are probably safe when taken for less than three months, but there are not enough safety data on their use during preconception or pregnancy, so it's best to avoid them. We need to see more data on obesity-related anti-inflammatory properties and possible protective effect against oxidative damage to sperm. Grapes are a healthy food to include in your diet in the form of fresh fruit, raisins, or grape leaves.

- **Guarana.** See Chapter 2 on caffeine.

- **Hawthorn.** Hawthorn has a good record in terms of its extremely low toxicity; as a modest component of popular teas (e.g., Sleepytime), it is likely safe at two or fewer cups per day. Avoid hawthorn extracts packaged as supplements, as dosage can be significantly higher than teas.

- **Isoflavones.** Soybean isoflavones are isolated bioactive compounds available in supplement form, but they are just a single component of a much more complex, healthy food. Isoflavone supplements are not recommended for women or men planning for conception, but traditional soy foods such as soy milk, tofu, edamame, tempeh, and miso may be incorporated into a varied diet.

- **Lavender.** GRAS status for flavoring foods or beverages; lavender oil is likely safe to use during preconception in very modest amounts and only on the skin surface (as part of aromatherapy, lotion, or shampoo, or as a natural bug repellent); toxicity appears low, but that's not a license to use liberally; there are no safety data available for use during pregnancy.

- **Lemongrass.** Likely safe when consumed as an ingredient in a culinary dish and as a supplement prior to pregnancy. Could stimulate the uterus and promote menstrual flow, so avoid medicinal use when pregnancy is possible.

- **Marshmallow (root and leaves).** Long history of use for treating cough and skin sores, though also marketed for diuretic effect. Probably safe in nonpregnant individuals, but little is known about pregnancy safety, so it is best to strictly limit or avoid. This herb interacts with a number of prescription drugs (e.g., diabetes meds).

- **Maté.** See Chapter 2 on caffeine.

- **Melatonin.** Produced in the pineal gland as well as several other tissues in the human body, and is also made by plants or absorbed through the roots from soil. Melatonin has a strong influence on the reproductive function of many animals and plants. For example, melatonin is emerging as a significant player in reducing oxidative stress to the body, improving ovarian function, and possibly reducing free radical damage to the placenta and fetus during pregnancy. In plants, melatonin protects the seeds during germination, and helps protect the plant from oxidative stress and harsh environmental conditions. Scientists are currently beginning to investigate whether supplemental melatonin could improve outcomes for IVF patients by improving egg quality and fertilization rates. However, even though melatonin has very low toxicity, it is not advisable to add this herb as a supplement on your own, and some warn that it could hinder conception. For now, it is prudent to consume plenty of natural plant sources of melatonin (phytomelatonin). Few foods have undergone rigorous testing for their melatonin content, but some of the most commonly eaten ones are nuts and seeds (especially walnuts), tart cherries (especially Montmorency), purslane (an eastern Mediterranean veggie), oats, corn, rice, barley, onion, garlic, ginger, and extra-virgin olive oil (cold-pressed oil only).

- **Nettles.** Stinging nettle leaves can be taken as a tea (less than two cups per day), or the young stinging nettle shoots can be carefully handled, cooked, and eaten as a vegetable serving prior to conception as long as you are not in between pregnancies and still breastfeeding; safety of use longer than six months is unknown. Nettles are lauded as rich sources of vitamin C and beta-carotene (vitamin A precursor). They are said to help prevent anemia, perhaps because vitamin C boosts absorption of one form of iron. If consumed in quantities greater than our limits, a mild increase in urine output could occur. Women with blood coagulation disorders should shun this herb because of nettle's high vitamin K concentration. It is especially important to confirm proper identification of this herb before consuming it, so if you cannot tell, it is better to eat vegetables and fruits that contain similar nutrients. Once pregnancy is possible, avoid nettles, as they may cause uterine contractions; however, under midwife supervision, nettle tea is sometimes used at the end of a full-term pregnancy to "ready the uterus" for delivery.

- **Pycnogenol.** There are still too few data to support claims that it may have antioxidant effects and reduce pelvic pain in women with PMS or endometriosis. It may improve erectile dysfunction and sperm health in men with unexplained fertility problems. A small study demonstrated safety during the third trimester of pregnancy, but no safety data are available for preconception and early-to-mid pregnancy. Pycnogenol is often packaged with other plant extracts that are not recommended in supplement form.

- **Quercetin.** Plant compound (bioflavonoid) that has antioxidant and anti-inflammatory properties when consumed from whole foods. Insufficient evidence is available to support effectiveness or safety of quercetin when extracted and put in supplement form, so it is best to eat only whole food sources such as berries, apples, cruciferous vegetables (broccoli, cauliflower, cabbage, etc.), tea, and onions.

- **Raspberry leaf.** Red raspberry leaf tea has long been a favorite herbal tea among prospective mothers. It is purported to increase fertility, strengthen the uterus to prevent miscarriage, alleviate morning sickness, and aid the uterus in delivery. However, these benefits have not been backed up by scientific proof, and there is nothing known about its long-term safety. Herb experts James Robbers, PhD, and Varro Tyler, PhD, ScD, coauthors of *Tyler's Herbs of Choice,* state that this herb has been shown to have different effects on a woman's uterus depending on whether or not she is pregnant: in pregnant women, raspberry leaf tea may cause uterine contractions late in the first trimester and early second trimester, so we suggest avoiding it once you have begun trying to conceive. Although it is not likely to cause harm before you conceive, its tannin content is reason enough to consume it only in moderation. (Excessive amounts of tannin bind certain minerals, such as iron, rendering them unavailable for the body to use.)

- **SAM-e (S-adenosylmethionine).** Used mostly for the treatment of depression and osteoarthritis on a short-term basis with some success. This herb is possibly safe if used during late pregnancy for pregnancy-related intrahepatic cholestasis, but no studies have been published to our knowledge on pre-pregnancy or early pregnancy. SAM-e can be synthesized internally as long as you have adequate levels of folate and B_{12} (unless you have impaired metabolism of either vitamin), so supplementation shouldn't be necessary. People on certain medications, such as for bipolar disorder, should avoid this herb. Though strictly regulated as a drug in many countries (e.g., Germany, Italy, and Spain), it is considered a supplement in the United States and you therefore cannot be sure of its purity or dosage.

- **Sarsaparilla.** Irresponsibly and falsely marketed as a performance enhancer and tonic, though it is okay in small amounts as a flavoring agent.

- **Stevia.** In countries such as Japan, Brazil, and Australia, stevia has long been approved as a "natural" intense table-top sweetener and food additive. Approval is more limited in the United States, where whole leaf stevia products are more loosely regulated as supplements and bear the inherent risks discussed previously. That said, new purified stevia extracts (rebaudioside A, or Reb A) received no objection from the FDA for safe use in foods and beverages. Though relatively high daily intakes of Reb A appear safe, it's prudent to keep intake modest when reproductive health is at issue. We conservatively define "moderate consumption" for natural *and* synthetic FDA-approved nonnutritive sweeteners as a combined total of no more than three items per day (e.g., one packet of sweetener and a beverage that contains two servings per container).

- **Tea (green, black, white, oolong).** See Chapter 2 on caffeine. See separate listings for herbal teas that contain no caffeine. For example, red bush (rooibos) and peppermint teas are found in Table 8-4, while chamomile, ginger, hawthorn, nettles, and raspberry leaf teas are included in this chart (Table 8-5). Mormon tea and herbal diet teas such as aloe and cascara sagrada are found in Table 8-6.

- **Valerian** (not to be confused with Valium). Minor tranquilizer with no known dangers in pre-pregnancy or pregnancy, but may be best to limit or avoid unnecessary exposure.

- **Wheatgrass.** Attractive nutrient profile, and probably safe for short-term use as a food during preconception. However, safety data is insufficient for use as a supplement, and it is not recommended once pregnancy could be possible.

- **Wild yam.** Different from the yams found in the produce section of a grocery store, which are highly recommended as food. Instead, a wild yam compound called diosgenin can be isolated from wild yam and converted in a laboratory into various steroids, including "natural" estrogen and progesterone. One example of an FDA-approved progesterone product derived from wild yam is Prometrium; another is Crinone gel, prescribed as part of certain infertility treatments. The same compound (diosgenin) is extracted from wild yam, converted in a lab setting, and sold as over-the-counter supplements or cream, falsely claiming that they are a "natural alternative" to estrogens or "natural DHEA." It's unclear whether wild yam estrogen products pose any danger to women as they prepare for conception, although women with endometriosis, uterine fibroids, or PCOS are more strongly cautioned to avoid these supplements. Some "natural DHEA" products are notorious for being tainted as well. Once pregnancy is possible, don't experiment on your own with these supplements; too little is known about their safety and effectiveness.

TABLE 8-6
HERBS AND DIETARY SUPPLEMENTS TO COMPLETELY AVOID DURING PRECONCEPTION AND PREGNANCY

- **Aloe.** An extremely strong laxative when taken orally; often used as an ingredient in herbal diet teas and weight-loss supplements. Aloe vera gel can be used safely as a topical application on the skin or scalp for wound healing or to soothe skin irritation.

- **Angelica.** Promotes menstrual flow.

- **Black cohosh.** Could stimulate uterine contractions. Although we do not advise it, this is sometimes used at the very end of pregnancy under the supervision of a midwife or physician to tone the uterus for contractions. Also, this herb has not been proven effective for PMS.

- **Blue cohosh.** Promotes menstrual flow; stimulates uterine contractions; potentially toxic.

- **Buchu.** Strong diuretic; can cause dehydration.

- **Buckthorn.** Three types of buckthorn—alder, European, and California—are stimulant laxatives and should be avoided; only sea buckthorn berries are likely safe when consumed as food (pies, jam), but no data are available on sea buckthorn teas or extracts, so they are best avoided.

- **Bugleweed.** Insufficient data on short- and long-term safety with reproductive function.

- **Cascara sagrada.** Stimulant laxative; often used as an ingredient in herbal diet teas and weight-loss supplements; safety concerns have arisen over the active constituent of cascara for pregnant women.

- **Coltsfoot.** Toxic to the liver.

- **Comfrey.** Very toxic to the liver.

- **Cottonroot.** May be abortive.

- **Dong quai.** Although not backed by scientific proof, dong quai is often touted for easing menstrual cramps or irregularities; there is also some speculation about its utility in fertility treatment in certain women, but again, there is no proof. It is best to avoid unnecessary exposure unless under close medical supervision, and even then we recommend stopping two weeks prior to trying to conceive. Completely avoid dong quai during pregnancy, as it may interfere with the hormonal milieu.

- **Ephedra sinica or ma huang** (often referred to as "herbal speed"). Strong cardiac stimulant (active ingredient is ephedrine); has antihistamine properties; was a common component of diet pills and dieter's teas as well as fruit smoothies or bottled beverages designated as "energy boosters" before being banned by the FDA in 2004. Note: Mormon tea is made from one ephedra species called *E. nevadensis* that does not appear to contain the dangerous stimulant ephedrine, but it does have a high tannin content. Mormon tea is mildly diuretic and should be limited, but not necessarily avoided altogether.

- **Essential oils (e.g., those extracted from peppermint, rose, and cinnamon).** Intended for external use and potentially dangerous if ingested; this warning applies to the *pure oil* form only. There's no need to ban cinnamon from your baking, for instance, nor do you need to avoid the *occasional* single serving of peppermint or orange spice tea that contains orange oil (a minute amount) in the ingredients list.

- **Fenugreek.** Could stimulate uterine contractions. Fine to consume while breastfeeding to increase milk production (a common practice in some cultures).

- **Feverfew.** Promotes menstrual flow; avoid during pregnancy.

- *Garcinia cambogia* **(hydroxycitric acid).** Found in weight-loss supplements, but more rigorous study is needed to collect safety data and ensure quality control before an informed recommendation for preconception can be made. Regardless of safety and effectiveness, avoid weight-loss herbs during pregnancy.

- **Gentian.** Insufficient data on safety with reproductive function, but may promote menstrual flow and high blood pressure.

- **Ginseng (of the *Panax* genus).** Could accentuate discomforts of pregnancy and interfere with hormones; best to avoid until more is known; caused birth defects to embryos in one animal study; sometimes found in herbal weight-loss supplements.

- **Ginseng, Siberian.** Even less is known about the safety of this form of ginseng than Panax ginseng; best to avoid.

- **Goldenseal.** No reliable data on safety of this herb when ingested; could stimulate uterine contractions; found as a component of certain herbal weight-loss supplements and cold remedies or in injectable form.

- **Gotu kola** (not to be confused with kola/kola nut/cola nut, which contains caffeine). Insufficient data on safety with respect to reproductive function.

- **Hoodia.** Has been identified as potentially having appetite suppressive properties; unfortunately, many crude hoodia weight-loss products in today's market do not contain what they claim or may be adulterated with potentially dangerous substances. More rigorous study to collect safety data and ensure quality control is needed before an informed recommendation for preconception can be made. Regardless of safety and effectiveness, avoid weight-loss herbs during pregnancy.

- **Horsetail.** Weak diuretic.

- **Irvinga gabonesis (seeds; also known as African mango).** A relative newcomer to natural weight-loss supplements, with effectiveness based on poor-quality research; insufficient data on safety with respect to reproductive function.

- **Juniper.** Could stimulate uterine contractions; diuretic; may damage kidneys.

- **Kava (kava-kava).** Toxic to the liver; dulls motor reflexes; insufficient data on safety with respect to reproductive function. Though touted to promote relaxation and sound sleep, there are safer ways to accomplish this, including meditative and relaxation techniques, avoiding alcohol, exercising (but well before bedtime), and drinking warmed milk before bed.

- **Licorice.** Fairly common in herbal cough remedies. Real licorice is seldom found in "licorice" candy sold in the United States; authentic licorice is found in most European markets. May affect hormone and electrolyte balance, especially in large amounts over two to three weeks; contributes to preterm labor. Men may experience sexual dysfunction and lower sex drive.

- **Life root.** Toxic to the liver; may promote menstrual flow.

- **Lobelia.** Potentially dangerous to the central nervous system and lungs.

- **Male fern.** Toxic to intestinal worms, but may pose additional unknown dangers to the person taking the herb.

- **Mandrake, American.** Laxative effect; may be toxic.

- **Mistletoe.** Not safe for consumption, as it may cause uterine contraction; toxicities documented; definitely okay to stand underneath!

- **Mugwort.** May promote menstrual flow.

- **Myrrh.** May promote menstrual flow, but relatively nontoxic.

- **Osha.** May cause uterine contractions.

- **Passionflower.** Insufficient data on safety with human reproduction function.

- **Pennyroyal.** May cause abortion and is potentially lethal.

- **Pokeroot.** Extremely toxic.

- **Red clover.** Insufficient data on safety with reproductive function.

- **Red yeast rice.** Its cholesterol-lowering effects could interfere with normal fetal development, and some companies who manufacture it have been cited by the FDA for adding unauthorized prescription drugs to their formulas.

- **Rhubarb, medicinal** (not to be confused with garden rhubarb). Strong stimulant laxative; related to yellow dock.

- **Rue.** May promote menstrual flow and be abortive; can cause phototoxicity.

- **Saint-John's-wort.** Slight unfavorable effect on uterus during pregnancy; insufficient data on further safety with reproductive function (for both women and men); may interfere with prescription drugs such as the birth control pill (e.g., many women using Saint-John's-wort have reported breakthrough bleeding as well as unexpected pregnancies while faithfully using the birth control pill as their sole method of contraception).

- **Sassafras.** Potentially toxic and cancer-causing; by law, real sassafras is not to be used as a flavoring agent or food additive.

- **Senna.** Strong stimulant laxative; often used as an ingredient in herbal diet teas and weight-loss supplements; safety concerns over the active constituent of senna for pregnant women.

- **Shepherd's purse.** May stimulate uterine contractions.

- **Skullcap.** Often of questionable quality and potentially dangerous; subject to adulteration.

- **Slippery elm.** Though possibly helpful in alleviating sore throats, it has a reputation for being abortive if placed on the cervix; it's best to be cautious and avoid it orally until more is known.

- **Tansy.** Potentially toxic and may be abortive.

- **Uva ursi (bearberry).** Insufficient data on safety with reproductive function; potential for toxicity.

- **Wormwood.** Could stimulate uterine contractions; also produces mind-altering effects similar to those from smoking marijuana.

- **Yarrow.** May be abortive.

- **Yellow dock.** Strong laxative; could worsen anemia due to high tannin content.

- **Yohimbe.** Although marketed as an aphrodisiac (and actually may help with erectile dysfunction), there are insufficient data on safety with reproductive function; new reports of life-threatening side effects outweigh possible benefits.

- **5-HTP (5-hydroxytryptophan, primarily from seeds of the *Griffonia simplicifolia* plant).** Marketed as an aid for fibromyalgia, premenstrual syndrome (PMS), depression and anxiety, and control of binge eating; insufficient safety data regardless of reproductive goals; avoid at least one month prior to trying to conceive.

A WORD ABOUT NONHERB, NONVITAMIN-MINERAL SUPPLEMENTS

What about the safety of popular nonherbal, non-nutrient supplements on the shelves of health food and grocery stores?

A common one is melatonin, a hormone produced naturally in your body or taken in pill form to prevent jet lag and aid in sleeping (synthetic melatonin). In the mid-1990s, scientists discovered that humans and animals are not the only ones who make melatonin. Plants do too, and it's called phytomelatonin, a substance with potent antioxidant properties (discussed in Table 8-4), which also appeals to scientists studying animal and plant reproduction. Synthetic melatonin (pill form) has been shown to slightly lower your body temperature if taken during the day, and may interfere with ease of conception. For this reason, we do not advise self-medicating with melatonin supplements.

Another is bee pollen in supplement form (not the small amount found in honey). Bee pollen has a questionable safety record in some individuals, particularly those with sensitivity to pollen and bee stings (with *and* without a prior history of allergic response) or honey allergies.

Nonfood supplements that claim to enhance sports performance or soothe achy joints (e.g., creatine, pyruvate, DHEA, HMB, glucosamine, chondroitin, glandulars, and MCT oils) are generally not advocated during preconception or pregnancy.

One more popular vitamin-like supplement called coenzyme Q_{10} (CoQ_{10}) will be mentioned in the men's health chapter. Though your body can make CoQ_{10}, it may require supplementation if you are taking a cholesterol-reducing statin drug or if your partner has low sperm motility. Ask your doctor what he or she recommends. Other than those two conditions, natural food sources of CoQ_{10} are your best bets and include meat, poultry, fatty fish (herring and trout), and canola and soybean oil; nuts and vegetables are sources, too, though more modest ones.

FOR FUTURE REFERENCE: During Pregnancy/After Delivery

Not only is it best for your fetus if the womb environment is free from most herbs and non-nutrient supplements, but the same advice is recommended after your baby is born. If use of a product is not advisable during pregnancy, assume that it is best avoided during breastfeeding, unless otherwise specified. Never offer any sort of herbal supplement (either orally or rubbed on the skin) to infants and children unless approved by a pediatrician. Also, be very cautious to store supplements—herbal and otherwise—far out of reach of little hands.

CHAPTER 9

What Men Can Do

*M*ost guys don't really think about preparing for their role in preconception, but in fact, the best gift you—the dad-to-be—can give your future son or daughter is preparing to conceive. Whether you're excited about the prospect of learning more or you're feeling a little cajoled into reading this, two things are certain. First, your odds for an easier conception and a healthier baby will improve if you put our advice into action. Second, by showing a willingness to be involved you will become closer to your partner, not only because of your concern and care but also because you will be working together as a team.

In the course of writing this book, we informally surveyed a group of men and asked them what planning ahead for a future pregnancy meant to them. Their answers may sound familiar:

Andrew, age forty-three: "I guess I'll need to start wearing boxer shorts."

Trent, age thirty-three: "I would offer emotional support to my wife if she has to make some special changes in her lifestyle or with what she eats and drinks."

Dave, age thirty-six: "I don't know. My wife is the one who gets into that sort of thing."

D.J., age twenty-nine: "To me, planning would involve sitting down together and figuring out if we could afford to have a baby. I'd probably want to put in a lot of overtime and save up vacation time, too."

Antonio, age thirty-one: "I've always wondered whether there are things I can do to improve our odds of having a healthier baby. The doctors only talk about what my wife can do, but I haven't heard much on what men can do. I'd like to, though."

If any of these comments reflect your own thoughts or provoke your own questions, we think you'll find the information in this chapter valuable. If you have been frustrated in your search for information, you are not alone. It is only recently that the scientific and medical communities have started examining the role the prospective father plays in fertility and early pregnancy health. Using these latest studies, we will help you to optimize your role in pre-conception. First we cover how sperm are made and exactly what goes on during the ninety days prior to conception. Next we discuss how what you eat and how you exercise affect your ability to conceive. Then we move on to specific medical conditions and how they play a role in your fertility.

WHY MEN NEED TO PLAN AT LEAST NINETY DAYS IN ADVANCE

The factory for sperm production resides in the testicles, opening for operation at puberty and continuing to manufacture sperm for the rest of your life. If all runs smoothly, as it does for 88 percent of men, you can produce up to a hundred million sperm each day.

When a sperm cell begins to develop, it is assigned genes that could someday deliver half of the DNA needed to create a baby. Basic sperm formation takes about seventy-four days. An additional twelve to twenty-one days of maturation are needed for the sperm to acquire the ability to move and be fertile. That is why it is so important to give yourself a minimum of ninety days' preparation time before trying to conceive. What you eat, how you exercise, and what you are exposed to in your environment *today* affects each and every sperm produced during the next ninety days.

Once sperm are fully mature, they congregate in the sperm "waiting room," better known as the epididymis, until duty calls. Newcomers enter the epididymis daily to maximize the number of functional sperm available at any given time. The ejaculate, or semen, is made up of sperm and its nutrient-rich fluid, which is provided by the accessory glands (i.e., prostate, seminal vesicles; see Figure 9-1).

BALANCING YOUR DIET

When you are preparing to conceive a child, what you eat and drink assumes a whole new meaning. After all, you are consuming the nutrients that will be building sperm, and you want to do what you can to encourage the development of the healthiest sperm possible. Modifying your eating habits now is something that you and your partner can do together as part of pre-conception planning to improve fertility, and we all know that it's easier to stick to a healthy diet when you have a buddy to do it with. Of course, the long-term benefits of eating well include better overall health and appearance, increased physical energy, and a greater sense of emotional well-being. Who doesn't want that? Furthermore, if you stick with it, you'll have the

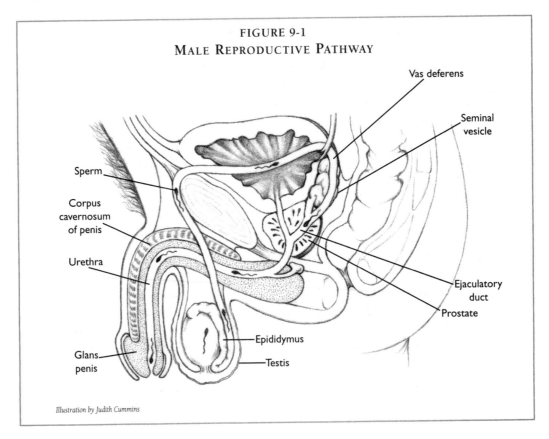

FIGURE 9-1
MALE REPRODUCTIVE PATHWAY

Vas deferens

Seminal vesicle

Sperm

Corpus cavernosum of penis

Urethra

Ejaculatory duct

Prostate

Glans penis

Epididymus

Testis

Illustration by Judith Cummins

added benefit of someday setting a good example for your children to imitate (otherwise they have a way of picking up the habits you least want to pass along). Clearly, your nutrition affects not only you but also those around you and is of the utmost importance in preparing to conceive.

Food and the Health of Your Sperm

Being lean and having the correct balance of nutrients helps optimize sperm development; similarly, inadequate paternal nutrition has a potential negative effect on this process. For instance, did you know that overweight men (body mass index greater than 25) as well as severely undernourished men have lower sperm counts and fewer strong swimmers? Poor nourishment also lowers the amount of nutrient-rich seminal fluid and diminishes sex drive. If your intake of specific nutrients, such as essential fatty acids, selenium, zinc, vitamins E and C, and folate, is very low, sperm health can be compromised. Too much stress may also undermine reproductive function in undernourished men.

Limitations of Nutritional Research on Sperm Health

In developed nations such as ours, extreme single- or multiple-nutrient deficiencies are a rarity. Marginal nutritional deficits are more likely. Unfortunately, large-scale well-controlled studies on marginal deficiencies are seldom done.

We do know, however, that a modest deficiency in one mineral (e.g., zinc) ends up having a greater negative effect on sperm quality if another marginal deficiency coexists (e.g., low selenium status). Subtle deficiencies often go undetected and may have little or no obvious impact on male fertility. Similarly, we do not know whether there is any effect on the offspring—during fetal development or after delivery—of men who remain fertile but have only mediocre nutritional status prior to conception.

It is our hope that future investigations will explore the extent to which something as basic as paternal nutrition during sperm formation influences the lifelong health potential of the baby. Because you do not have the luxury of waiting around until all of this is sorted out, we suggest that you be proactive and assume that good nutrition will prove to be paramount.

Healthy food choices are your surest bet for improving your nutritional status. Modest vitamin or mineral supplementation may also help. Make sure that you don't fall into the foolish practice of snubbing healthy eating and figuring that taking supplements will make up for anything lacking. Careless use of supplements has the potential to do more harm than good. So let's focus on food first and address safe supplementation after that.

Healthful Eating

Healthful eating means consuming a wide variety of foods and beverages in proper proportions to meet your body's needs (see Figure 9-2). There is even room for occasional junk foods as long as the *majority* of your diet is nourishing. The Department of Agriculture's MyPyramid was designed for the general public, and further individualizes it by taking into consideration gender, age, and activity level. Superactive people, particularly men, may have even higher needs than suggested.

A big part of creating a healthy balance in your preconception diet is to have a working knowledge of portion control. On the surface this advice may be obvious, but it often isn't followed. It's too easy to over- or underestimate what you eat if you have little knowledge of serving sizes. For instance, a small banana sliced on your cereal in the morning is great, but you need still more fruit to reach your recommended number of servings for the day. Also, did you know that if you use a whole can of tuna for a sandwich at lunch, that comes close to meeting

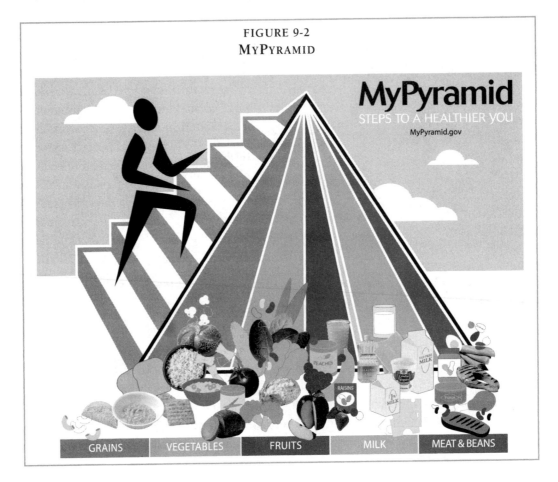

FIGURE 9-2
MYPYRAMID

your body's requirements for protein for the whole day, leaving you little, if any, room for meat or meat alternatives later in the day? Then there are the oil servings of mayonnaise mixed into the tuna. One level tablespoon of regular mayonnaise counts as three oil servings, but many people use a heaping tablespoon, which nearly doubles the servings, leaving little room for other fats that day.

So, how are you supposed to know what food counts where in the MyPyramid? What amount counts as a serving? And how can this be simplified to make the learning curve easier? Because you and your spouse both need to know this information, we suggest that you create your preconception food plans together. To avoid being repetitive, we've saved the in-depth discussion and written exercise on this for Chapters 12 and 13. Remember: the food "plan" part of this is only temporary; once you've been doing it for a while, it becomes automatic.

MyPyramid has been replaced with the new graphic image MyPlate, though the technical information remains essentially unchanged and current. Accessible through the more user-friendly www.ChooseMyPlate.gov.

Two Confident Cooks

If one of you does most or all of the cooking and/or shopping, try to set a date to go to the grocery store together so you can both identify the abundant foods you have to choose from. Talk about what to look for on the labels to find the leanest ground beef or the whole-grain bread instead of its more refined counterpart. Conquer the produce aisle as you discriminate between the cantaloupes that are ripe and the ones that are not. This mutual familiarity will make it less intimidating to share shopping duties or, if need be, take it over completely, if your wife, when pregnant, experiences debilitating fatigue or morning sickness. Also, plan one or two days per week to prepare a well-balanced meal together, and try to include a minimum of four food groups in the meal. If one of you is a rookie in the kitchen, make sure that person gets most of the hands-on experience from start to finish; it's the only way to become comfortable and efficient in the kitchen. Don't forget sanitary preparation and cleanup to protect each other from foodborne illness, as discussed in Chapter 13.

Franz and Joanna were both busy working professionals, and neither knew how to cook or had much interest in learning. They ate almost all their meals out or ordered in. However, having not conceived after six months of trying, they committed to making some changes. Eating habits and unrelenting work schedules were first on their list to tackle.

Amy was the main cook in her family but wanted her husband to take a more active role in cooking and meal planning before they started a family. In a pleasant surprise for both of them, he turned out to be an excellent cook. Though he still doesn't inspect the fresh produce as carefully as Amy might—something she had to get over—to this day his proficiency in the grocery store and kitchen is a boon to their family dynamic. He can pitch in or take over at a moment's notice, and does. And when there's time to really labor over a fancier meal, cooking serves as an enjoyable legitimate escape from everyday chores. He livens it up by listening to a sports broadcast or good podcast.

Vitamins, Minerals, and Male Fertility

Fortunately, a man's body has built-in mechanisms for quality control of sperm development. You assist by offering your body top-grade materials from the foods you eat. Remember, you need *at least* ninety days of good nutrition before you begin trying to conceive (TTC). The following nutrients are worthy of special mention in regard to fertility. (For a general listing of all vitamin and mineral recommendations for men of various ages, see the Dietary Reference Intake tables in Appendix B.)

Zinc

Zinc is a trace mineral present in high concentrations in the male prostate gland and testes. Semen and sperm also have high zinc content. Zinc plays a role in making functional sperm, protecting the genetic material in the sperm head, and allowing the sperm to live as long as possible after ejaculation.

- **Recommended Dietary Allowance (RDA) for men:** 11 mg per day.

- **Food sources of zinc:** Animal products such as meat, seafood, eggs, and dairy products; plant sources such as whole grains, legumes, wheat germ, and many fortified breakfast cereals.

- **Supplement guidelines for men:** Standard supplementation of zinc appears unnecessary for most men. Vegetarians, however, may need up to 50 percent more zinc because a naturally occurring chemical in some plants (phytate) interferes with zinc absorption. If supplementation is recommended, it is best to begin with a multivitamin-mineral supplement, preferably without iron, containing the men's RDA for zinc (11 mg) along with 2 mg of copper. Infertile men, especially those with inflammation of the prostate gland and low zinc levels in their semen, may benefit from higher supplemental dosages of 30 mg of zinc per day. This amount of supplemental zinc combined with zinc-containing foods will likely tip your total zinc intake over the safe upper limit (40 mg), which could interfere with copper absorption. Do not exceed this zinc dosage without physician approval. Zinc-containing cold lozenges should be limited for the same reason.

Selenium

Selenium is a trace mineral that is also important for proper sperm production. As a component of the sperm midpiece, selenium is essential for sperm motility and prevention of tail breakage. It also works with vitamin E to protect cells from being damaged.

- **RDA for males over nineteen years old:** 55 mcg per day.

- **Food sources of selenium:** Seafood, meat, chicken, eggs, all grains, and plants grown in selenium-rich soils. Brazil nuts are so high in selenium that more than one per day (on average) is too many.

- **Supplement guidelines for men:** Standard supplementation is unnecessary for most men with normal fertility. However, supplementation up to 100 mcg may be helpful for men with a history of infertility. We recommend focusing on foods for these higher needs; see page 347 for ideas. More than 400 mcg per day from foods and supplements combined is not advisable due to its potential toxicity.

Vitamin E

Vitamin E is thought to play a protective role in male fertility by guarding the outer covering (cell membrane) of the sperm from damage. This is important because even if the DNA or genetic material inside the sperm is healthy, fertilization cannot occur if the sperm cell membrane gets damaged. Plus, if the sperm cell membrane is damaged, the DNA inside the sperm can also be damaged.

- **RDA for men:** 15 mg per day of alpha-tocopherol from food (equals 22 IU of natural vitamin E or 33 IU of the synthetic form, dl-alpha-tocopherol).

- **Food sources of vitamin E:** Vegetable oils, nuts and nut butters, seeds, margarine (with no trans fats), wheat germ, whole grains, tomato sauce, spinach.

- **Supplement guidelines for men:** Standard supplementation is unnecessary for most men with normal fertility. While there is burgeoning research on vitamin E's potential for improving fertility, with the most promise in improving sperm motility, it is unclear if pregnancy outcome is ultimately improved. A little caution is warranted, though. It appears that increasing food sources of vitamin E for at least ninety days may be a much better starting point than supplements (food sources of vitamin E likely contain synergistic nutrients to promote fertility). A Johns Hopkins University study (published in the *Annals of Internal Medicine* in 2005) found an increase in all-cause mortality in adults with suboptimal health who had been taking more than 400 IU/day supplemental vitamin E for longer than one year; whether this has any bearing on healthy men is unknown. Because it is very difficult to get higher amounts of vitamin E from diet alone and most fertility specialists see merit in antioxidant supplementation, including vitamin E, it may be worthwhile to consider separate supplementation equivalent to 150 to 400 IU of natural vitamin E per day (along with approximately 500 mg of vitamin C per day). Supplementing above this level confers no additional benefits and is strongly discouraged. There is a maximum safe upper limit of 1,000 mg per day regardless of the supplement form.

Vitamin C

Vitamin C, or ascorbic acid, plays a protective role inside the sperm cell and in the surrounding seminal fluid. Inside, vitamin C guards the sperm's genetic material during cell divisions early in the ninety-day period of sperm formation. The high concentration of vitamin C in the seminal fluid that eventually mixes with sperm suggests that it helps protect sperm once they have been released on their journey toward fertilization. Smokers use up vitamin C at a higher rate than nonsmokers, which is one of many reasons they often have lowered fertility.

- **RDA for men:** 90 mg per day. Smokers are advised to stop smoking and, in the process of quitting, add an additional 35 mg per day.

- **Food sources of vitamin C:** Citrus fruits, tomatoes, melon, berries, bell peppers, papaya, orange juice, potatoes, broccoli, cauliflower, Brussels sprouts.

- **Supplement guidelines for men:** Standard supplementation is unnecessary for men with normal fertility. However, because male smokers often have lower sperm counts and more abnormal sperm, some studies advise smokers to consume 200 to 1,000 mg vitamin C from a supplement in the months prior to conception. Nonsmokers with infertility issues, including sperm agglutination (abnormal clumping together), may experience improvements in sperm parameters from vitamin C supplementation of 250 to 500 mg per day as well. Another reason to take vitamin C is if vitamin E is also supplemented. The two work together as antioxidants (fending off damage by volatile oxygen molecules) and are experimentally being used to protect sperm during in vitro fertilization.

Folate or Folic Acid

Folate is a B vitamin found in many foods. When it is synthetically manufactured for supplements, it's called folic acid; we'll use the terms synonymously. Most research on folate and reproduction is conducted on women, and woefully little is known about folate's role in male reproductive health. However, folate is necessary to make new cells, and it works at the genetic level. So as your body makes new DNA-bearing sperm around the clock, folate is being utilized in every step along the way. A recent study on nonsmoking men done at the University of California, Berkeley, looked at folate's role in DNA synthesis in sperm. They found that men with the highest intakes of folate had the fewest chromosome-number defects. It makes sense to eat folate-rich foods such as leafy greens, fruits, legumes, and fortified grains, since many are also rich in the antioxidant vitamins and minerals that we just finished talking about.

- **RDA for men:** 400 mcg folate per day, but it appears that almost double this amount could be more beneficial for sperm health.

- **Food sources of folate:** See Table 11-1 for a detailed list.

> ## Practical Application
>
> If you choose to supplement with vitamins and minerals, it may be simplest to look for a multivitamin-mineral supplement low in iron (men's formula or senior formula) that has approximately 100 percent of the Daily Value for most nutrients. (Men easily meet iron needs through foods, and extra iron can promote oxidative damage, be counterproductive to sperm health, and be constipating.) Never take more than one of these to achieve higher doses of vitamins E or C. Instead, add separate supplements of these, and shop for the lowest doses available so you do not exceed the limits that we advise.

- **Supplement guidelines for men:** Supplement with 400 mcg folic acid if your dietary intake does not approach 700–800 mcg folate in the ninety days before conception.

Other Compounds and Nutrients

The following compounds and nutrients have had relatively less attention devoted to them in the current literature on male fertility, but they may eventually prove to be of some benefit. It is important to ask a medical doctor about the safety and effectiveness of these and other supplements. (We'll touch on herbs at the end of this chapter.)

Coenzyme Q_{10} (CoQ$_{10}$), also known as ubiquinone, cannot be called a nutrient because it is not a true vitamin, but it acts similarly to the antioxidant vitamin E. CoQ$_{10}$ may be beneficial for infertile men, particularly those with impaired sperm motility and a varicocele (a dilated blood vessel around the testicle that increases the temperature near ducts where sperm are made, which then decreases healthy sperm production). Men (and women) taking statin drugs to lower cholesterol may also have depleted stores of CoQ$_{10}$ and may be candidates for supplementation under physician supervision. Food sources of CoQ$_{10}$ include meat, poultry, fatty fish (herring and trout), canola and soybean oil, nuts, and vegetables.

Certain individual *amino acids* (e.g., arginine) have been investigated for their role in fertility. Although preliminary results are intriguing, we do not advise taking them. More research is needed, especially as very little is known about the adverse affects of supplementing with single amino acids. These same amino acids can easily be obtained through a well-balanced regular or vegetarian diet. One's body can build carnitine and glutathione too.

EXERCISE AND THE PROSPECTIVE FATHER: THE IMPORTANCE OF BEING FIT

Being physically active and in good health is something you, your wife, and your future child(ren) will certainly value, especially over time. But there are also a few aspects of fitness that are especially pertinent for men preparing for conception. First, there is evidence that very high levels of physical activity (e.g., ultradistance running of more than 100 kilometers, or 62 miles, per week) may actually alter sperm quality and decrease sperm counts, not necessarily to below normal standards but below the individual's norms. Second, a handful of sports are associated with practices that can be detrimental to fertility: those that encourage steroid abuse or dramatic drops in precompetition or "in-season" body weight.

Third, and probably more important than these extremes, is how important it is to make fitness a part of your lifestyle right now. After the baby is born, your life will become even more beautifully complex—if you already have a child, you know this. The best way to deal with these changes is to establish an exercise habit now, while you have the time to focus on self-discipline and adapt your priorities. Once regular activity becomes an integral part of your present life, you are less likely to let it go in the future. It is *really* tough to make this type of lifestyle change after the baby is born.

It Doesn't Take Much: Your Minimum Exercise Requirements

As you read the next paragraph you may catch yourself thinking, "Will this small amount of exercise really do any good?" Yes. Research consistently shows that this *is* all you have to do, unless you take it to an extreme and do nothing but sit for the rest of the day (in which case your body continues to act more like a couch potato metabolically). The following guideline is reasonable enough that it can be incorporated into almost anyone's lifestyle. Of course, if you want to do more, great! But this should serve as your goal in case grander intentions are not consistently realized.

Moderate amounts of physical activity over the course of a lifetime yield major health benefits. According to the U.S. Department of Health and Human Services (2008), just 150 minutes of moderate-intensity aerobic exercise per week improves psychological well-being and offers protection against premature death, heart disease, diabetes, high blood pressure, obesity, and colon cancer. This works out to be an average of 20 to 30 minutes a day! The basis for this recommendation is that this amount of exercise expends roughly 150 calories of energy per day or 1,000 calories per week and leads to measurable health improvements. Examples that meet the moderate-intensity criteria include shooting baskets for 30 minutes or bicycling 5 miles in 30 minutes. If you are already fit and lean, you can do the same volume of aerobic exercise at a higher intensity in less time overall, just 75 minutes over the course of a week. Examples that fit this higher-intensity criteria are running at a 10-minute-mile pace or jumping rope.

If possible, spreading exercise out over several days with a mix of moderate- and vigorous-intensity activity is better than the weekend warrior mentality of exercising *only* one day per week (that is, a long hike or bike ride). Conversely, if you are new to exercising or just don't feel exercise is worthwhile unless you put in a good 30 to 60 minutes at a time, here's a helpful tip. Anything over 10 minutes of moderate-intensity activity counts toward your 150-minute weekly total. The benefits remain the same. The key is to treat your body to some type of physical activity nearly every day. See Chapter 16 for more details.

For those of you who need help keeping your weight under control or simply enjoy greater amounts of physical activity, exercising moderately for 300 minutes per week (or vigorously for 150 minutes), expending 2,000 calories per week will make you even more fit and healthy. But moderate amounts of physical activity are all it takes to reap most health benefits.

Muscle-strengthening activities are an important complement to aerobic exercise, especially as we age, because muscle mass and metabolism begin to naturally decline. Current *Physical Activity Guidelines* suggest incorporating strength-training activities into two or more days per week to complement your aerobic fitness. With proper form to protect your ligaments and joints, fifteen minutes of strength training with free weights or yoga after your run can give your body a well-rounded workout and help shed stubborn pounds.

Hydration for Men

When large muscle groups are recruited for exercise, such as in running and swimming, they generate heat that is circulated throughout the body to the skin's surface. People who exercise regularly are better able to dissipate this extra internal body heat. For instance, if you do yard work or home improvements involving physical labor during the heat of summer, a physically fit body is better able to handle the heat stress than an unfit body. Because it is important to keep sperm from overheating inside the testicles, this athletic training becomes even more beneficial during the preconception months.

This "training effect" will only work, though, if you maintain good hydration. Studies on athletes have shown that men, more than women, tend to drink less during exercise, resulting in dehydration. So it is imperative that you drink plenty of cool water before, during, and after exercise or any other physical work, regardless of the ambient conditions (see Table 9-1). Some athletes (e.g., distance runners, cyclists, basketball players) don't drink enough during exercise because they dislike the feeling of fullness or "sloshing" that sometimes accompanies drinking enough fluids. However, these sensations will diminish over time, and the body will function and train at its best when it is well hydrated.

Keeping cool from the inside out by maintaining good hydration is half of the strategy for keeping scrotal temperature optimal for sperm to thrive (see "Whew . . . It's Hot Down Here" later in this chapter). The other half is to minimize influences that cause overheating from the outside in, such as lounging in a Jacuzzi or extended wearing of protective gear such as athletic cups and jockstraps.

FOR FUTURE REFERENCE: Family Life

Pushing a Stroller Boosts Fitness and Hydration!

Pushing a jogging stroller boosts the core muscle workout you get from running and is a great way to carry water and a snack, for yourself and the kids! You've seen the CamelBak packs that contain water reservoirs and tubes for use while hiking or biking? Just drop a couple of water tanks into the stroller's mesh cargo net and you've got water on the go for you and baby. (Plus you won't have to chase sippy cups thrown from the stroller!) While most parents find themselves sharing utensils and drinking gear with the little ones, experts caution against this practice because you pass oral bacteria to your child. Pack snacks, a small toy, and a book and you should be good to go for a run. If you time it during naptime, you may not even need to stop!

You might be impressed to learn that a recent study led by researchers at the University of Wisconsin found that pushing a stroller while walking 3½ miles per hour boosts the cardiovascular benefit (and calorie burn) 20 percent compared to walking without a copilot. Joggers should anticipate an even greater relative benefit. So, grab the stroller any chance you get and call it modern-day chivalry. You might also encourage your wife to try StrollerStrides (www.strollerstrides.com). It's a great way to connect with other new mothers and get a fitness boost at the same time. If there isn't one in your area, she could start a franchise and earn some money, too!

What to Drink While Exercising

Sports beverages—4 to 8 percent carbohydrate solutions, often with electrolytes, such as Gatorade—are a safe and legitimate way for serious athletes to achieve a competitive edge as well as preserve good hydration. They should be the workout beverage of choice for athletes who strive for optimal performance gains during exercise lasting over one hour, and perhaps as little as thirty minutes, provided the exercise intensity is very high or performed in very hot conditions. For ordinary workouts, water is perfectly fine.

Caffeinated beverages such as tea, coffee, and ordinary soft drinks can be included and will not induce dehydration, provided you adhere to the male preconception recommendation of less than 300 mg of caffeine per day. (But the ratio of water to caffeine in something like a straight shot of espresso *will* have a net dehydrating effect.)

TABLE 9-1
HOW TO MAINTAIN GOOD HYDRATION WHEN YOU EXERCISE

The following strategies are the same for men and women, but men sweat more profusely than women even when the ambient temperature and fitness level are similar. Therefore, in Step 2, you may need to consume the higher amount of fluid more frequently to keep up with your sweat losses.

1. Drink about 16 ounces of water 2 hours before exercise. This allows time for the excess water to be excreted before you begin exercising.
2. Drink 4 to 8 ounces of cool fluid every fifteen to twenty minutes during exercise. (See "What to Drink While Exercising" on page 258.) If you need to remind yourself to begin drinking before you get thirsty (thirst indicates partial dehydration), set your wristwatch alarm to beep at you at fifteen- to twenty-minute intervals. Both chilled and room-temperature beverages will have a cooling effect on your core body temperature, but athletes tend to drink more of a liquid if it is chilled.
3. After exercising, drink 16 ounces of water for every pound of water weight lost during exercise. To determine sweat losses, weigh yourself before and after exercise to gauge how well you're compensating for losses.
4. Monitoring your urine color and volume is good feedback on your level of hydration at all times. Urine should be pale yellow, not dark yellow or brown. (Note: Your urine may be brighter yellow if you are taking B-complex vitamins.) Those who participate in ultra-endurance sports probably already know this, but too much water can cause serious problems, including stroke, coma, or seizures. Use common sense and follow your body's cues to ensure balanced hydration.

The Male Endurance Athlete

Is there such a thing as too much exercise when preparing for conception? Maybe. Most research on this topic has focused on male long-distance runners. Researchers found a trend of declining reproductive indicators in endurance runners who run more than 62 miles (100 km) a week. Once this exercise threshold is crossed, testosterone levels decrease and other changes in reproductive function occur (and bear with us while we make a few obvious man-jokes to lighten things up!):

- Fewer sperm are produced. Remember, the sperm must swim en masse in the race to the finish line (the egg); there's power in numbers.
- A greater percentage of the sperm are immature, ill equipped for fertilization.
- The number of good swimmers declines and those that do swim well often lack the innate drive to swim in the direction of the egg. (A high percentage of sperm would rather die than ask for directions; sounds familiar, doesn't it?)
- A greater percentage of those who make it to the finish line find themselves incapable of penetrating the egg to activate fertilization.

Overtraining in any sport may have a similar effect on reproductive capacity. Why? One explanation is that it is challenging for the body to replenish the energy stores necessary for sperm production when energy expenditure in other areas is so high. When calories are chronically or acutely deprived, the body may interpret this as starvation. Animal studies have shown that fasting and undernutrition may prompt an early warning system in the body to switch into conservation mode. This effectively slows down reproductive function, because reproduction is energy-demanding and nonessential for immediate survival. This slowdown, or even shutdown, occurs independently of body weight changes. So even if you don't look like you're starving, your body will "think" it is. Female athletes have tangible evidence, such as loss of or change in normal menstrual periods, to signal when their reproductive functioning is being affected. For male athletes, evidence of changes in reproductive functioning is not so obvious. So it is vitally important that highly trained men eat enough to maintain an energy balance that will prevent their body from thinking they are being calorie-deprived. A good sports nutritionist (especially one who is a registered dietitian) can be extremely helpful in these situations.

Gaining the Edge Without Harming Fertility

You have likely seen it happen, maybe even to yourself. The guy who was a high school or college athlete suddenly finds himself fifteen, even thirty pounds heavier after having gotten married and settled into domestic bliss. Busy with a demanding job as well, he has little or no time left for exercise. Then he decides he wants to get in shape to play in an adult sports league or train for a half marathon or triathlon.

If you are a fan of professional sports, you are familiar with this scenario at an elite level. A professional player reports to preseason training camp twenty pounds heavier than his usual weight. There is often pressure from the coaches, trainers, and the athlete himself to quickly get into shape by shedding the extra weight. Despite the availability and advice of team dietitians, some athletes fall prey to crash dieting and fasting. That certainly gives them rapid drops in weight from loss of body fat, muscle, and water—but it *prolongs* the time it takes to get fit. Returning to our average guy, this can negatively impact fertility because the body interprets sudden weight loss as an internal energy crisis; it must channel dwindling resources toward immediate survival needs and away from energy-draining reproductive functions. A healthy weight-loss regimen is one that promotes a loss of no more than two pounds per week. This pace allows you to draw on fat reserves while at the same time ensuring sufficient calories to replenish basic energy needs and maintain muscle integrity.

In the quest to get into good physical condition, it can sometimes be tempting to try things that promise better physical performance, stronger muscles, or a speedier metabolism. There is always something new and better that you can pop in pill form or mix with your favorite

BICYCLISTS: FEELING NUMB?

If you are an avid cyclist, perhaps you occasionally experience numbness, tingling, and/or weakness in the hands or fingers, particularly during longer training rides or tours. Although it is less common, these same sensations can occur in the genital area, that is, numbness or tightness in the head of the penis or in the scrotum. Sometimes this numbness can persist for hours, days, or even weeks after being off the bike. And occasionally regular cyclists experience difficulty in achieving or maintaining an erection. Impairments in sexual potency can persist for weeks, several months, or more rarely indefinitely. Pain does not usually accompany these symptoms, and some men experience erectile dysfunction without preceding groin numbness. The majority of the men who report these problems are ultraendurance cyclists, but there have been isolated cases in men who simply enjoy riding a stationary bike for twelve to twenty minutes per day.

Sexual dysfunction in cyclists is often ascribed to exercise fatigue. However, two other factors also come into play. The bike seat appears to compress both the nerves important for erection as well as the main blood supply to the penis. The symptoms sometimes go away when your bicycle seat height is lowered, but this adjustment can place too much strain on the knees. One alternative is to tilt the front of the seat downward, take frequent pauses, and make shifts from sitting to standing position while riding. Researcher Dr. Irwin Goldstein at Boston University pioneered the development of an ergonomic bicycle seat designed to fit your anatomy and alleviate the pressure in the groin area. These seats are now readily available at most bicycle shops.

Usually a rest from biking for three to ten days should eliminate the numbness that may exist around the perineum (the area between the penis and the anus that rests on the bike seat) and the penis. If you've made the alterations described above but sexual dysfunction persists and impedes baby making, you may have to discontinue cycling. Physician consultation is strongly advised to assess persistent problems and to make sure you avoid permanent damage.

juice. Some are harmful, some are not, but very few are completely without risk. Also, most can be a waste of money. For example, adding a little protein powder into a fruit smoothie can be a way to get extra protein into your diet. However, men can easily cover their protein needs with a well-rounded diet. Protein powders are usually just powdered egg whites or powdered milk (and maybe a few popular vitamins) with a hefty price tag. The protein frenzy can also quickly lead to taking high doses of single amino acids, which at this time have no proven safety record. If you are still tempted to take a dietary supplement with the intention of improving sports performance, beware that what appears legitimate may not be. Too many manufacturers (roughly one in four, by one estimate) take advantage of lax regulations and add prohibited substances (steroids or stimulants) to dazzle you with dramatic results, but these could cause serious side effects (including, but not limited to, lowered fertility and damage to your future child's DNA encased in your sperm) and cause positive urine drug tests.

The preconception months are not the right time to be a human guinea pig for any substances (legal or illegal) that promise better and quicker physical results. We urge you to take a conservative approach to getting in shape. In other words, rely on a well-balanced diet and an exercise routine tailored to reasonable athletic ambitions.

WHAT HAPPENS NOW?

Now that we've discussed the effects of nutrition and fitness on sperm production, let's move on to what happens once your sperm are ready to go. The best or healthiest sperm will get to be part of the process known as fertilization. Of the twenty million or more sperm released in an ejaculation, only approximately two hundred make it to the proximity of the finish line (i.e., the egg) and *only one* hardy sperm can usually cross it! Sperm live for forty-eight to ninety-six hours in the female reproductive system. They can usually fertilize an egg (provided that one is there to rendezvous with) up to seventy-two hours after ejaculation. This means conception can occur even if you have sex a couple of days before or the day ovulation occurs.

Cindy and Matt, both thirty-four, went to see Cindy's gynecologist after trying to get pregnant for seven months without success. They worried that they might have fertility trouble. During the consultation, they revealed that they had been having sex daily around the time of ovulation, usually twice a day. "It's a supply-and-demand thing, right?" Matt wanted to know.

The answer to this question is a resounding no. If you make love multiple times within a twenty-four-hour period, the first ejaculation releases 60 to 75 percent of the fully mature sperm present in the epididymis. Each subsequent ejaculation releases fluid with fewer sperm, making it less effective for fertilization. Millions of newly mature sperm enter the epididymis daily, but it can take one or two days to replenish the stores of sperm; allow for the latter, especially if sperm count is low or unknown (while your wife monitors herself for peak fertile days). Mature sperm that are never called into action are retired only two weeks after their arrival in the waiting area, replaced by new sperm.

Regardless of your sperm count, the odds of conception are highest if you shoot for a frequency of three to four times a week, spread out over several days; deterring from this approach might make it take longer for some.

Do You Need a Semen Analysis?

Let's face it: few men relish the thought of going into a small room at a clinic and mastur-bating into a cup to produce a semen sample. The whole process can seem undignified. Add to that the social stigma that's placed on male infertility. However, there can be many reasons for male infertility and it is by far one of the easiest things to fix so a couple can conceive. In addition to having too few sperm, you can have too many, causing a "traffic jam."

One patient, Melissa, wanted to know if there was any way to obtain a sample from her husband without his knowledge, as he was too self-conscious to agree to visit the clinic. At the other end of the spectrum, Andrea and Michael, a couple in their late thirties who had not conceived after thirteen months, discovered low sperm counts on two semen analyses conducted a few weeks apart. Michael, keeping his focus on the goal of conceiving a baby, viewed the process of semen collection as a step toward that goal. He was relieved that the cause of their infertility had been identified, and he was excited about moving ahead with assisted conception. They were able to get pregnant the following month using intrauterine insemination.

If you and your partner have not conceived after twelve months of trying (six months if your partner is over thirty-five years of age) or if you are concerned about your fertility po-tential, you should have a semen analysis, which evaluates sperm on four criteria: motility, or the ability to move well (which requires a normal sperm tail); quantity of fluid to swim in; morphology, or the shape of the sperm's head, which is necessary to guide it into the egg; and the total number of sperm in the ejaculate. Normal sperm parameters (that will result in a pregnancy) are:

- A sperm count of at least twenty million is required for normal fertility.
- More than 63 percent of the sperm have to be able to move normally.
- More than 35 percent of the sperm should be normally shaped.
- Subfertile ranges in semen analysis are noted if fewer than thirteen thousand sperm are present in each ejaculate, fewer than 32 percent of sperm move well, and fewer than 9 percent of the sperm shapes are normal.

A semen sample is best collected after two to three days of abstinence and analyzed within one hour of ejaculation. If a question arises about sperm normalcy, testing should be per-formed at least twice, with samples produced two to three weeks apart (see Figure 9-3).

THE MODERN SPERM

Men today seem to produce many fewer sperm than they used to. If it's true, why isn't there an obvious change in the incidence of male infertility? Why are there fewer sperm now? Clinical research proposes that increased exposure to tobacco, alcohol, recreational drugs, heat, and environmental toxins may all contribute. We discussed the effects of these substances on male fertility in Chapters 2 and 3. Suffice it to say that when sperm are excessively exposed to these substances, they are rendered incapable of carrying out their purpose of fertilization. Sperm can't swim well without a tail or easily enter the egg without a normally functioning head. Unfortunately, in some cases, a damaged sperm does fertilize an egg, which can lead to a higher incidence of miscarriage, infertility, birth defects, and various childhood cancers. It used to be thought that any problems with the fetus could be traced back to a faulty egg. It is now apparent that both the sperm and the egg are equally important in providing a foundation for a healthy baby.

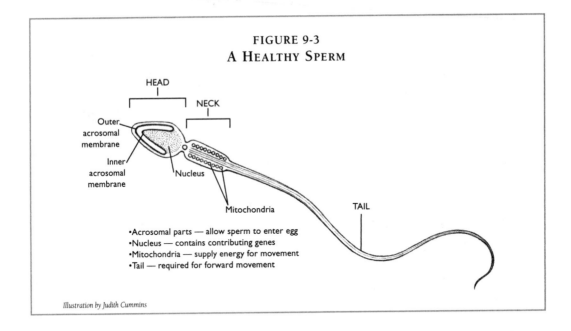

FIGURE 9-3
A HEALTHY SPERM

HEAD

NECK

Outer acrosomal membrane

Inner acrosomal membrane

Nucleus

Mitochondria

TAIL

• Acrosomal parts — allow sperm to enter egg
• Nucleus — contains contributing genes
• Mitochondria — supply energy for movement
• Tail — required for forward movement

Illustration by Judith Cummins

WHEW . . . IT'S HOT DOWN HERE!

Have you ever wondered why your testicles are located outside of your body? Actually, your testicles start out residing inside the body early in fetal development and eventually migrate to the scrotum. If this descent doesn't occur, the testicles produce less effective sperm. In other words, the migration of the testicles to a cooler spot in the scrotum is a practical design feature intended to keep sperm at an optimal temperature for healthy development, generally one to two degrees cooler than the rest of the body.

Can a healthy male be too hot to produce the healthiest sperm for conception? The answer is yes. In one study, professional athletes were evaluated to determine if their protective genital gear affected testicular temperature and sperm function. These athletes were asked to wear cups and jockstraps for twelve to twenty-four hours a day, for six to fourteen weeks. Among the athletes in the study, the longer the protective gear was worn, the higher the testicular temperature. This was associated with a 20 percent decrease in sperm count. Other studies that examined heat and its effect on sperm health revealed reduced conception rates in men who had occupations in a hot environment, such as firefighters, bakers, and truck drivers. So temperature does make a difference in sperm count, although it may not affect fertility unless repeated, excessive exposure is the norm.

Are Boxers Really Better?

Everyone (except, probably, your doctor) tells you that you should wear boxer shorts to reduce everyday heat in the testes while trying to conceive. In one recent study, ninety men were asked to wear boxers or briefs for at least twelve hours a day. Their testicular temperature was taken every two hours and no significant differences were found; wearing the briefs didn't raise the temperature of the testicles, as many suspected it would. Other studies have reported no significant difference in potency and sperm counts between the wearers of boxers and briefs. We think you can wear whatever type of underwear you like.

What Can You Do to Limit Your Exposure to Extended or Extreme Heat?

- Minimize your exposure to Jacuzzis, steam rooms, and saunas; don't exceed fifteen minutes twice a week, and while you're there take two-to-three-minute intermissions to cool down. (Some urologists recommend completely avoiding Jacuzzis when you are trying to conceive.)
- If you sit for the majority of your workday, try to walk around the office every two hours for ten to fifteen minutes.
- If you drive most of the day, stop and walk around every two hours and make sure the vehicle you are in is temperature-regulated to keep your overall body temperature comfortable. Cranking up the seat warmer on a long winter drive might not be a wise idea, either.
- Work out in a protective cup or jockstrap, but limit the time you wear it to less than six hours a day and remove it immediately after you complete your exercise. Also, keep well hydrated during the workout to maintain overall body temperature control.

- Men with a lot of excess adipose tissue (fat) in the groin area experience warmer testicular temperatures. Gradual weight loss and regular moderate exercise help minimize this.

Certain anatomical situations increase testicular temperature, resulting in a significant reduction in sperm count. Cryptorchidism, or undescended testes, is one situation, usually diagnosed at birth or prior to puberty. If one or both testicles do not descend during fetal development, they will remain exposed to higher temperatures, which significantly reduce sperm production. Cryptorchidism can be surgically corrected and normal sperm function fully restored. Another is a *varicocele,* a dilated vein within the spermatic cord, which also raises the temperature in the testicles. In fact, a varicocele is one of the most common correctable causes of male infertility, accounting for about 15 percent of cases. Your doctor can diagnose this condition via physical exam or testicular ultrasound. Surgical repair often results in an improvement in normal sperm production within three to six months. If your testicles are overheated due to anatomical or environmental reasons, improvement is often seen as early as ninety days after correction of the problem as new sperm are produced in the new "climate."

Practical Application

When was the last time you enjoyed a soak in the sauna, steam room, or Jacuzzi? Are you planning a vacation soon that will include using these spa services? In a usual workday, how many hours do you spend in a sitting position? Think of how you can modify these circumstances to get ready for conception. Remember, begin these changes at least three months before trying to conceive.

YOU'RE A FINE SPECIMEN OF A MAN!

Because fertility problems sometimes do originate with men, we strongly recommend a checkup, especially if you haven't had one in two or three years. Remember, the healthier the man, the healthier the sperm. A routine preconception evaluation for men will begin with your comprehensive medical history. The Men's Preconception Medical Checklist (see Figure 9-4) can assist you and your doctor in evaluating your health risk and the impact your family history can have on your fertility and general health. Your doctor will also ask you about:

- Current physical complaints
- Pertinent sexual history, including previous sexually transmitted diseases, difficulty with

FIGURE 9-4
WHAT TO TALK ABOUT AT THE DOCTOR'S OFFICE:
THE MEN'S PRECONCEPTION MEDICAL CHECKLIST

Fill this out now and bring it with you to your scheduled appointment.

Name: _____

Age: _____ Height: _____ Weight: _____

1. Here is my past medical history. (Put an X by anything you have **now** or had **in the past**)
___ Asthma
___ Cancer (type of: _____)
___ Chicken pox (at what age? ___)
___ Diabetes
___ Depression
___ Epilepsy
___ High blood pressure or heart disease
___ HIV/AIDS
___ Iron overload or "high iron" (hemochromatosis)
___ Kidney disease
___ Lupus
___ Mumps
___ Sexually transmitted disease
___ Testicular infection or surgery
___ Thyroid problems

2. Yes / No   I currently experience some sexual dysfunction (i.e, trouble with getting an erection). If yes, explain: _____
_____
(note whether you are an avid cyclist)

3. Some inherited diseases are more common among certain ethnicities. My ethnic origin is: _____
My partner's ethnic origin is: _____ -

4. I <u>do / do not</u> know my blood type. _____

5. I have a blood relative who has or had (put X):
___ Bleeding disorder (e.g., hemophilia)
___ Birth defects
___ Mental retardation
___ Sickle-cell disease
___ Tay-Sachs
___ Muscular dystrophy
___ Cystic fibrosis
___ Huntington's chorea

6. Yes/No   I use medication for hair loss (or have used them in the past, and still have some left at home)

7. I take the following oral or topical prescription medications, over-the-counter medications, herbs, natural cold/flu remedies: (include anything within the past 6 months)
_____
_____
(Ask) Should I be avoiding any of these while we're trying to conceive? _____

8. I <u>do/do not</u> know whether my mother took DES (diethylstilbesterol) while she was pregnant with me.

9. We now practice _____ method of birth control (if any). Between now and the time to "start trying," we plan to use _____ method of contraception.*(If your partner is going off birth control medication for a few months prior to conception, you will need to choose a barrier method such as condoms.)*

10.   (Circle one)
Yes / No   I work around chemicals, solvents, lead, or other potential hazards.
Yes / No   We own a cat who uses a litter box. Who cleans the kitty litter box now? _____
Yes / No   I like to lounge in a Jacuzzi or sauna periodically.
Yes / No   I use one or more recreational drugs such as marijuana, cocaine, "meth," IV drugs, etc.
Yes / No   I may find it difficult to cut down on alcoholic beverages (including beer, wine, hard alcohol)
Yes / No   I smoke cigarettes. How many? _____ and how often? _____
Yes / No   I smoke cigars (and/or a pipe)? How many? _____ and how often? _____

11. (Circle one: everyday - often - sometimes - never) I drink more than 1 to 2 alcoholic beverages within a 24-hour period.

12. Have you ever fathered a child in the past? _____

13. What best describes your current lifestyle: mostly sedentary; sporadically active; regularly active (exercise workouts or daily manual labor)?

14. *(Ask)* Are there any tests that I should have before I begin to increase my exercise regimen or prepare for conception?

erection or ejaculation, pain with sexual activity, pain with urination, or lack of sexual desire
- Previous infections, such as postadolescent mumps, that can impact fertility
- Review of past medical problems as an adult, as well as any childhood history of hernias and/or urinary problems
- Past experience with inflammation of the urethra, which, in addition to passing urine, is the conduit through which your sperm travel on their vital mission
- Any history of infection of the prostate
- Family history of fertility problems
- Family history of diabetes, high cholesterol, or heart disease; if so, you should be screened with simple blood tests for blood sugar and cholesterol and have your blood pressure checked to assess you for long-term disease risk

Many medical problems can influence your fertility, so be candid with your doctor about details of your overall health, even if they don't seem relevant to you at the moment. In addition to your medical history, a thorough physical exam and complete reproductive organ evaluation is recommended to determine:

- The presence of abnormal lesions on your penis
- Possible hernia, which is a weakening in the fascia of the abdominal wall where the bowel can poke through
- Testicular swelling or suspicious masses in the scrotum or in the lymph nodes of the groin that can help in early diagnosis of cancers, benign masses, or infections of the reproductive system

Careful examination of the prostate is also recommended, especially if you are over forty. The prostate exam is done via a digital rectal exam. One man I know says he spent twenty years in fear of this exam and ultimately found it anticlimactic: *"I was so edgy about the exam, and then it was over in an instant. The great news that I had no prostate problem was almost lost in my amazement that the examination was really no big deal."*

Your doctor may also want to screen you for a sexually transmitted disease (chlamydia, gonorrhea, syphilis, herpes, and warts caused by the human papillomavirus), because they can affect the male reproductive system.

Symptoms of STDs include:

- Burning with urination
- Copious discharge from the penis not during urination or arousal
- Difficulty ejaculating or painful erection and ejaculation
- Changes in the penis or scrotal skin, such as blisters or sores

Immunization History of the Prospective Father

To minimize the risk of passing on a preventable infection to your partner or simply to improve your own health, your doctor will need information on your vaccination history. Give careful consideration to the following:

- If you were vaccinated before the 1970s, it's very unlikely you've had measles, mumps, or rubella (MMR). You might want to be sure you've had two doses of MMR. Mumps used to be a significant source of sterility for men. More than 25 percent of men who contracted mumps during or after puberty risked sterility. But since the advent of immunization for mumps in 1957, there are not many men at risk for this disease. Rubella (German measles) can be contagious; if you contract it and give it to your partner during pregnancy, serious fetal damage can occur. Simple vaccination against rubella can prevent this.

- Have you had chicken pox? If not, you should consider being vaccinated, especially if your partner is not immune or has chosen not to be vaccinated herself.

- When was your last tetanus shot? And have you seen the news about pertussis (whooping cough)? If you are uncertain about your last tetanus shot, or if it has been at least two years since your last booster, ask for the Tdap—it adds protection against pertussis to the usual tetanus and diphtheria (Td) shot (see Table 1-2). Pertussis is one disease you really don't want—a hacking cough for a month with lingering effects for up to six months. This vaccination has the added benefit of ensuring that you won't pass these diseases on to your future offspring in the first six months of life.

- Do you have any of the following risk factors for exposure to hepatitis B or A? If yes, and if it has been more than five years since your last vaccination, your doctor may wish to give you a booster shot or check your immunity by drawing a blood sample to check antibody levels.

Hepatitis B Risk Factors
- Intravenous street drug use or sex with an IV drug user
- History of multiple sex partners
- Being a health care worker
- Having received clotting factors or blood transfusions

Hepatitis A Risk Factors
- Exposure to contaminated water supply, unsanitary food preparation, or general poor hygiene
- Travel to foreign countries where hepatitis A outbreaks occur

There is little known about the optimal timing of vaccination for men before conception, but we recommend pursuing vaccination at least three to six months before trying to conceive, just as we recommend for women.

If chronic infections are allowed to continue, tubules in the testicles or epididymis can eventually be scarred, reducing the number of sperm available for ejaculation. In some men, this obstruction can be so severe that it affects both testicles, resulting in a total absence of live sperm in their ejaculate. Prompt treatment of these infections, however, will eliminate these concerns. Screening for HIV infection is also recommended prior to conception to reduce the health risks to you, your spouse, and your baby.

WHEN THE PROBLEM IS ERECTILE DYSFUNCTION

Julia is a thirty-three-year-old sales executive who at her annual gynecological exam confided that she would like to get pregnant but was concerned because she and her husband, Rick, had sex only once or twice a month, and he just didn't seem interested in her "that way." As they continued to try to conceive, their relationship grew more strained and lovemaking became even more infrequent. In couples counseling, Julia learned that while she felt ready to start a family, Rick was growing increasingly anxious about financial pressures. Julia eventually agreed to postpone her baby plans for a year so that she and Rick could address their overspending and reduce their debt. Once Rick felt that their finances were under control, he became much more sexually interested and Julia became pregnant a few months ahead of schedule.

Marianne, a thirty-seven-year-old pastry chef, came to the office complaining of reduced libido. After careful questioning, she revealed that her lack of sexual desire began after her husband, Elliot, no longer seemed to desire her. She was convinced that he was seeing another woman. Only after she threatened him with divorce did he admit that he was having difficulty sustaining an erection. His embarrassment had kept him from sharing this secret with her. They sought both medical and psychological help, and Elliot was prescribed some medication, which restored his sexual functioning. Now they're both more relaxed and look forward to making a baby.

Erectile dysfunction (ED) means an inability to achieve or maintain an erection satisfactory for sexual intercourse. It affects more than thirty million American men of all ages. The causes of erectile dysfunction include:

- Substance abuse, including tobacco, alcohol, and illegal drugs
- Psychological reasons
- Medical conditions (such as diabetes, hypertension, or obesity with BMI $\geq$ 30)
- Previous trauma or surgery

- Certain medications
- Frequent long-distance biking
- Sedentary lifestyle, especially when obesity is a factor

The good news is that the majority of causes of erectile dysfunction can be treated. The first step is to have an open and honest discussion with your partner. Society places incredible sexual pressure on men from the time they are prepubescent boys. They are judged (and judge each other) on the size of their genitals and on their sexual prowess. Erectile dysfunction can be devastating to a man's self-image, leading to shame and secrecy; facing ED as partners starts you on the way to solving your problem.

Erectile dysfunction usually comes on gradually; at first, men are unable to achieve an erection for lovemaking only some of the time, but then the episodes become more frequent. It is usually not the result of an anatomical defect, nor is it usually a permanent problem. If you experience spontaneous erections without arousal, especially in the morning, be assured that the nerves and blood vessels that connect the penis to the brain and the rest of the body are still intact.

Substances such as tobacco, alcohol, and marijuana can reduce the blood flow to the penis, causing a temporary lack of erection and, over time, permanent impairment of erectile function. (More about this later in the chapter.) Nerve injury in men who undergo surgery to the prostate, bladder, or rectum can cause ED, resulting in temporary or permanent problems. Men who have suffered trauma to the spine or pelvis as a result of a motor vehicle or horseback-riding accident, for example, sometimes experience ED. Most ED problems require a urology evaluation, which often includes a thorough exam of the external genitalia, urinalysis, semen analysis, and hormonal blood testing.

Purely psychological reasons account for 10 to 15 percent of all ED cases. Reversing psychological ED almost always requires a team effort, including the man, his partner, and a medical expert with training in psychology and sexual dysfunction. If the prospective father suffers from depression, this in itself may affect his libido. The ambivalence about fatherhood that many men experience can also have an effect on their sexual functioning. Extreme emotional stress relating to work, relationships, or finances is also a possible cause of psychological ED. Counseling alone can often restore normal sexual functioning.

Some medications prescribed for the treatment of depression and anxiety have the unwanted side effects of dampening libido and inhibiting normal ejaculatory functioning (e.g., there is a longer time from arousal to ejaculation if SSRIs are used such as Prozac or Zoloft), which can end up compounding already existing sexual issues. Good communication with your counselor and/or prescribing physician is vital to maintain a careful balance between the psychological benefits and physical side effects of your medication therapy.

Erectile Dysfunction Due to a Medical Condition

Men with diabetes, obesity, significant vascular disease, hypertension, arteriosclerosis (clogged blood vessels), arrhythmia (abnormal heartbeat), or chronic liver disease may experience difficulty maintaining and obtaining an erection. Control of these medical problems with good medical care, a healthy diet, and compliance with medical regimens will reduce the risk of impotence and infertility. Let's consider some medical conditions.

Diabetes

Diabetes can affect male potency by causing neurological and vascular changes in the male genitals. Good blood sugar control is essential in limiting the detrimental effects on sexual function and can also lower the risk of long-term heart disease and kidney dysfunction. Treatment with diet, insulin, or blood-sugar-lowering medication will not reduce your potency or fertility.

Hypertension

High blood pressure causes problems throughout your organ systems, including vascular changes that reduce penile blood flow, resulting in impotence; the medication used to treat high blood pressure can also dampen sexual functioning. Hypertension is easily diagnosed with a routine blood pressure reading during a medical checkup. Prompt treatment can reduce the risk of heart attack, stroke, kidney damage, and penile dysfunction. If you experience sexual difficulties due to your medical regimen, your doctor can adjust your medication accordingly. (See Table 9-2 for more about safe medication options.) Dietary changes, including fat and salt reduction, and exercise are the first line of therapy for heart diseases of all types. Some of the medical therapies for erectile dysfunction can actually lower blood pressure.

Hypercholesterolemia

High cholesterol levels can result in obstruction of the arteries, which in turn leads to reduced circulation. If blood flow to the penis is affected, the result may be an inability to achieve and maintain an erection. At best, diet and exercise can lower cholesterol levels by only 25 percent. The remainder tends to depend on genetic predisposition. Blood testing not only can measure your overall cholesterol level but also can give you your cardiac risk profile. This is the ratio of HDL ("good") cholesterol to LDL ("bad") cholesterol, which can help determine the risk to your heart health. Your doctor will then suggest specific modifications to your diet for at least three to six months; then, if needed, medication may be prescribed to further improve your cholesterol levels. Also, C-reactive protein blood levels can predict your risk of future heart disease, which in turn can allow you to optimize healthy eating habits, regular exercise, and appropriate medical surveillance.

TABLE 9-2
MEDICATIONS THAT AFFECT MALE PERFORMANCE

Medication	*Effect on Male Fertility*
Antihypertensives *Clonidine*	Impaired ejaculation, temporary erectile dysfunction (ED)
Diuretics *Spironolactone*	Affects steroid metabolism; ED, reduced testosterone levels
Antidepressants *Paxil, Zoloft, Xanax*	ED, reduced libido, increased time to climax
Antiseizure medications *Dilantin (phenytoin)*[a]	Reduced sperm counts
Antihistamines *Tagamet (cimetidine)*	H2 blocker, stomach acid reduction, binds to the testosterone receptor; temporary ED, reduced sperm counts, increased prolactin levels

Antibiotics
   Macrodantin (nitrofurantoin)
   Ketoconazole (treats yeast infection)
	Reduced sperm counts
	Reduced testosterone

Chemotherapeutic drugs[b]
   Cytoxan (cyclophosphamide)
 	
   Methotrexate (used to treat cancer and psoriasis)
	Interferes with sperm development; reduced sperm counts, sperm motility, and normalcy
	Reduced sperm counts, damages DNA in sperm

Immunosuppressive drugs *Azulfidine (sulfasalazine, used to treat ulcerative colitis)*	Reduced sperm counts, damage to sperm DNA

Gout therapy
   Colchicine
   Zyloprim (allopurinol)
	Reduced sperm production
	Reduced sperm production

a. A small study reports increased incidence of Peyronie's disease with the use of Dilantin.
b. Normal testicular function may take one to three years to return after discontinuation of chemotherapeutic medications. If you know you will need chemotherapy, you will often be advised to save sperm beforehand, which can then be used later when you prefer to conceive via intrauterine insemination (IUI).

Treating Erectile Dysfunction

The first step in treating ED is to remove any possible physical cause: tobacco, alcohol, recreational drugs, and long-distance biking. If a particular prescription drug is the culprit, ask your doctor to change the medication if possible. If ED persists, counseling can be helpful to resolve any underlying psychological issues. Last, there are surgical and medical options. None of the following is guaranteed to restore ejaculation and fertility, but they do provide a starting point. It is also important to note that all of these medical options require arousal to get an erection in the first place—foreplay and lovemaking count for *both* partners.

- **Viagra** (sildenafil) is one of the most commonly used medical therapies available for erectile dysfunction. In studies of men suffering from impotence due to diabetes, vascular problems, and psychological sources, 50 to 75 percent found they were able to maintain an erection using Viagra. There was no change in number or motility of sperm with the use of Viagra. There are no risks to the fetus and no birth defects associated with the use of Viagra by men. It is usually taken thirty minutes to four hours before intercourse would be desired. Side effects can include headache and flushing.

If you have any heart disease or high blood pressure, check with your physician before considering the use of this medicine. In fact, any man considering the use of Viagra should first consult with his physician. Men with a history of heart disease or who take medications with nitrates (e.g., nitroglycerine) should avoid Viagra due to a possibly severe blood pressure drop. Also, if you take Nexium or Protonix for indigestion, you will need to lower the dose of Viagra to maximize its safety. Do not, under any circumstances, try one from a friend or secure your own medication from an online source unless you've previously discussed this with your physician.

- **Cialis** (tadalafil) is another oral medication that can be used to assist in temporarily restoring potency. The advantage of this medication is that it can be taken up to twenty-four hours in advance of planned intercourse (and with twenty-four hours to spare, it can also allow intercourse to be more spontaneous). The same precautions discussed above for Viagra, including heart disease precautions and medical advice before use of this product, apply with Cialis. The most common side effects are muscle aches and indigestion or gastric upset.

- **Levitra** (vardenafil) is the latest in the armamentarium of oral drugs for the treatment of erectile dysfunction. This medication has shown a 65 percent increase in the ability to achieve a sustainable erection compared to baseline.

If you have difficulty with one of these medications for erectile dysfunction, a different one may agree with you. It may also depend on which of these your insurance company will cover.

- **Testosterone topical gel** can be used to restore male hormone levels for those with an impairment of testicular function. This doesn't change sperm quality but does improve erection ability and male libido.

- **Papaverine** is an injectable agent that was used with success before the current medications were available and now is offered to those who can't tolerate the medical options. It increases blood vessel dilation around the penile muscles and aids in achieving an erection. The effect lasts forty-five to sixty minutes and the treatment is not costly.

- **Penile implants** are available at a cost of $10,000 to $20,000. While there is a small risk of infection, these are an excellent option for many men who have erectile dysfunction that is totally unresponsive to other forms of therapy.

- **Vascular surgery** to improve blood flow has been attempted with limited success. It is recommended only if there is a specific arterial narrowing, usually associated with a previous history of pelvic trauma. Surgery is accompanied by considerable discomfort and is quite costly.

EJACULATION DISTURBANCES: TIMING IS EVERYTHING

When we assess men's fertility, the first question is: "Is an erection possible?" The next is: "Does the ability to ejaculate exist?" To ejaculate after arousal and erection, the nerves, blood vessels, and glands in the male reproductive system have to work together to release the semen that carries the sperm. There is a broad range of what is considered normal for ejaculation. But if it occurs too rapidly, takes too long, flows backward (what we call retrograde), or is painful, fertility can be compromised.

Premature Ejaculation

Premature ejaculation is ejaculation that occurs very soon after arousal, often before vaginal penetration is possible. Without penetration, of course, the sperm is unable to get to the egg for fertilization. One evolutionary explanation for premature ejaculation is that prehistoric men had to be quick to impregnate their chosen women before their rivals did. In more recent times, young men may have grown to be quick because of a fear of discovery when they are adolescents: Mom might enter the room without knocking, for example, or that nosy little brother may barge into the bathroom. There is a slightly higher risk of premature ejaculation if you have been circumcised, because of increased sensitivity at the head of the penis. If you are concerned that you may suffer from premature ejaculation, you may have noticed the following:

- Early ejaculation has been an issue since your initial sexual experience
- Erection issues have remained similar since your first experience
- Ejaculation occurs within thirty to sixty seconds of vaginal penetration
- Early ejaculation is present with different partners

Treatment options include behavioral therapy to retrain men to maintain an erection longer and topical anesthetics to reduce the intensity of stimulation so that ejaculation can be delayed. Steroids may be recommended to treat underlying medical problems. Also, antidepressants have been found to be helpful, as they can lengthen the time it takes to reach climax during sexual stimulation. Ultimately, as long as ejaculation does occur, semen can be collected, making intrauterine insemination and in vitro fertilization excellent alternatives for those seeking conception.

Retrograde Ejaculation

For some men, ejaculation occurs in a timely fashion, but instead of being released outside of the body, sperm is released backward into the bladder, interfering with fertility. This is usually seen in men who are diabetic, men who have suffered physical trauma, or men who have undergone a surgical procedure called TURP (transurethral resection of the prostate). Treatment with alpha agonists such as pseudoephedrine (e.g., Sudafed) is very successful. A procedure called retrograde sperm retrieval from the bladder is a common way to allow for fertility.

Painful Ejaculation

Painful ejaculation is usually the result of infection or inflammation. Treatment of the underlying condition often alleviates the symptoms. A man's partner should also be treated if an STD is discovered.

A non-STD-related condition that causes pain during intercourse in 1 percent of men is *Peyronie's disease,* an abnormality of the fibrous tissue that causes nodules to develop within the penis. This results in an erection that is curved rather than straight, in some cases making vaginal penetration difficult and uncomfortable. Diagnosis is made by physical exam, patient history, and ultrasound. Treatment options include medication, electrical therapy, and surgical correction. If intercourse remains unattainable, masturbation can provide sperm for artificial insemination.

Can a Vasectomy Be Reversed?

Men who have previously undergone a vasectomy and wish to consider a reversal have excellent prospects. Although the reversal of a vasectomy is more successful if performed within ten years of the original procedure, successful reversals have been performed up to twenty-five years afterward. The greatest problem is if the testicular tubules are blocked to any degree. If so, impaired sperm counts and mobility can be expected. The cost of a vasectomy reversal is between $8,500 and $15,000, and success rates (assuming unobstructed tubules in the testicles) range from 69 to 95 percent. Pregnancy rates hinge on female factors as well.

SPECIAL MEDICAL CIRCUMSTANCES AND FERTILITY

Testicular Cancer

If you have suffered in the past from testicular cancer, you may have had a testicle removed (usually just one), chemotherapy, or radiation therapy. Testicular cancer has a very high survival rate, and because it often occurs in men under thirty, it leaves a large number of survivors who are eager to become fathers. During and after treatment, your sperm may suffer in terms of form, quantity, and motility, but over time many men recover their pretreatment sperm values. Others, however, may experience a persistent reduction of their sperm count. Before either chemotherapy or radiation, we recommend you have a supply of sperm cryopreserved (frozen). Radiation therapy is particularly toxic to the testicles; the higher the radiation dose used to treat the cancer, the longer the expected recovery of testicular function. A cancer-free interval of at least six to twelve months is recommended prior to trying to conceive.

Spinal Injury or Pelvic Trauma

Spinal injury or significant pelvic trauma can also prevent erection or ejaculation. Men who suffer from paraplegia may be able to get an involuntary erection but have little or no control over its timing. Sperm can be retrieved by electroejaculation: the pelvic nerves controlling ejaculation are stimulated and the harvested sperm are used for intrauterine insemination (IUI) and in vitro fertilization (IVF). This method can be effective more than 50 percent of the time if your partner is under thirty and 40 percent of the time if she is over thirty. In IVF, your partner undergoes egg retrieval to allow sperm to be introduced into the egg in the laboratory. Costs can range from $20,000 to $40,000 for both the male and female components of the fertilization procedure, which may have to be repeated more than once to achieve pregnancy. Your health insurance may cover part, all, or none of this treatment.

Cystic fibrosis

Cystic fibrosis is the result of a genetic mutation that causes an increase in mucus production in all the glands of the body, reducing sperm motility and hence reducing fertility. If you don't have this condition but know a close family member who does, you may carry the genetic material for this disease and can pass it to your offspring. Sometimes carriers of cystic fibrosis have been born with a condition known as bilateral absence of the vas deferens. These men have normal sperm production, but the sperm are not part of the ejaculate because without the vas deferens, they have no way to get to the outside world.

Conditions that Affect Testosterone Levels

There are a number of genetic and medical problems that can alter testosterone production, which in turn has a negative impact on fertility. The majority of medical conditions presented here may complicate your fertility, but they will not stand as an insurmountable obstacle between you and fatherhood. When it comes to becoming a parent, where there's a will, there is almost always a way.

- **Klinefelter's syndrome** is a genetic disease denoted by the presence of an extra X chromosome (every man usually has one X chromosome and one Y chromosome; these men have two X chromosomes and one Y). This results in a constellation of physical features and hormonal changes that lead to significantly reduced testosterone levels and infertility.

- **Congenital adrenal hyperplasia** is a genetic defect that affects male hormone and steroid metabolism. This causes an increase in testosterone but not in any of the other steroid hormones that work in concert with the testicles. If this disorder diagnosed early, medical treatment can help maintain good health and fertility.

- **DES (diethylstilbestrol)** was a medication used by expectant mothers in the 1930s through 1970 to reduce the rate of miscarriages. Some male offspring of these mothers have a reduced testosterone level, leading to a reduction in libido and sperm production. DES has been off the market since 1971.

- **Obesity (BMI of 30 or more)**, extra estrogen in your fat cells will be produced, which changes the male hormonal milieu, risking sperm counts and function.

- **Severe kidney disease** impacts testosterone, causing reduced libido, impotence, and infertility. Sperm counts are lowered for six to twelve months after a kidney transplant, often as a side effect of antirejection medications. (This can be viewed as a built-in safety factor, to stabilize health before a new baby joins you.)

Severe liver disease can result in a natural increase in estrogen production, which reduces testosterone in men. This can be accompanied by breast formation and testicular atrophy and unfortunately may not be reversible.

- **Cushing's syndrome** is a defect in steroid metabolism resulting in decreased testosterone levels. Cushing's also reduces sperm production and virilization (e.g., body hair growth and deepness of voice) in men.

- **Hemochromatosis** is an overaccumulation of iron from red blood cells. This condition directly affects the pituitary gland, causing testosterone levels to drop and reducing the amount of sperm produced by the testicles. Iron deposits in the testicle itself can also be damaging. Dietary modifications such as carefully limiting iron intake and taking advantage of foods and beverages that naturally inhibit iron absorption are imperative (see Chapter 7). Occasional donation of blood may also help treat this disease in adults. Consulting a registered dietitian is essential in the management of this problem.

- **Celiac disease** may result in "unexplained" infertility related to either malabsorption of nutrients involved in sperm development or low androgen hormone levels.

How Do Medications Affect Male Performance?

If you are taking any medications during preconception, discuss them with your doctor to identify which ones may have a detrimental effect on your sexual performance, your fertility, or even the health of your offspring. Your doctor will probably be able to offer you safe alternatives while you and your spouse are trying to conceive. Because this is an area of research where many unknowns still exist, being medication-free three months prior to conception is optimal, although we know it is not always possible.

Medications for Male Pattern Baldness

The FDA-approved medications for male pattern baldness include *minoxidil* (Rogaine) and Propecia. Minoxidil has been on the market for twenty years and comes in a liquid form that is rubbed on the scalp twice a day. The annual cost is $200 to $350 and its success rate in creating new hair growth is about 25 percent. When the medication is discontinued, the hair growth stops, and slow loss of the new hair will take place. There is little known about the fetal effects of this medication, but you should discuss it with your doctor. Propecia has been on the market for ten years in pill form. If you are using this medication for hair loss, or another formulation of the same drug known as Proscar for treatment of prostate problems, *your partner must not handle it at all.* It can be absorbed through the skin and has been known to cause birth defects if fetal exposure occurs during early pregnancy. We recommend discontinuing this medication at least three months prior to pregnancy, because its effect on sperm is unknown. Non-FDA-approved hair-growth products should be avoided for three months before conception, as there is no regulation of these products or information available on their potential effects on fertility.

HERBS AND THE PROSPECTIVE FATHER

A discussion of medications must also include herbal remedies, which have become a popular alternative to conventional medications. However, it's important to understand that the production and sale of herbal products in the United States are not subject to extensive scrutiny by the FDA.

How does it affect conception when a prospective father takes herbal supplements? Of all the herbal remedies available, only a handful have been studied with this question in mind, and even these small studies have been unable to reveal the true impact of herbal exposure. However, it is generally accepted that if potential risks exist, they increase with the dosage.

One highly publicized study of three very popular herbal remedies—Saint-John's-wort, ginkgo biloba, and echinacea—demonstrated that each may actually lower male fertility. However, there were many objections from the scientific community about how this study was conducted, making the results questionable. More research is needed on these and other herbs before we can draw definite conclusions.

In the previous chapter, we advised women to avoid most herbs if they are trying to conceive or are pregnant. Perhaps a similar recommendation should be instituted for prospective fathers for at least three months prior to conception, at least until more light is shed on the risks and benefits of herbal supplements on male reproductive capacity. Even then, it is probably best to err on the side of caution until uniform standards of quality are implemented in the United States.

ALL SYSTEMS GO

If you are like most men, there are only a few simple guidelines to follow to ensure a safe and healthy conception. A balanced diet and staying fit are essential. Even if your fertility has been compromised by a medical condition, illness, or injury, you still have a very good chance of fathering a child. With the amazing breakthroughs in reproductive technology, there are many other ways to aid conception—after all, it takes only one sperm. So, eat right, be fit, and have fun. And get ready to be a dad!

CHAPTER 10

Pre-pregnancy Nutrition

YOU ARE WHAT YOU EAT: GETTING THE NUTRITIONAL EDGE

Jean-Anthèlme Brillat-Savarin (1755–1826) once said, "Tell me what you eat and I will tell you what you are." Nowhere is this more true than for babies, who must rely on their mothers to provide their nourishment in the womb. A prospective mother who gets nutritionally fit one to three months *before* pregnancy ensures that the right mix of nutrients is ready and waiting for the fetus, thus giving him or her a head start in life.

Being nutritionally healthy before you conceive encompasses eating a balance of baby-friendly foods, knowing what supplements can and cannot do for you, achieving a healthy pre-pregnancy body weight, and being committed to gaining the recommended pregnancy weight. Knowing that food is your ally will give you freedom to enjoy what you eat, too. The next five chapters take you through the steps to do this. *Bon appétit!*

The Interplay Between Genetics and Nutrition

Genetically, your future child will inherit tendencies and traits from you and your husband as well as your parents, grandparents, and generations of ancestors who preceded them. However, the baby's future wellness is not determined solely by biological ancestors. Your baby will be a product of both nature (genetics) and nurture (environment, lifestyle). Nutrition is a vital element in the nurture part of the equation. The rapidly growing field of nutritional genomics explores how one's diet can favorably (or unfavorably) change the expression of nurture-sensitive genes. By changing the milieu in the baby's first environment, your womb, with optimal nutrition choices, the result is a healthier baby-to-be. In other words, with the same DNA, improved eating habits can mean a better outcome for you and your baby.

This concept of nutrition affecting developing genetic material in your future fetus is known as "developmental plasticity" or "metabolic programming" or "fetal origins of health and disease." This does *not* mean that if you change your dietary habits you can then influence the shape of your child's nose or the color of her eyes. This *does* mean, though, that if you have a tendency to gain weight easily, you might make it easier on the next generation (and even your children's children) by having your body at its personal best upon conception so their weight-gain habits may be less challenging. The bottom line is that a healthy diet and body weight can help maximize your future baby's health from the moment of conception to when she's a robust eighty-year-old. (If the topic of weight predisposition particularly interests you, take your time reading Chapter 14, "Body Weight, Body Image.")

Certain nutrients are involved in organizing the genetic material inside your egg before it is released. One key player is the B vitamin folate, which helps those preparatory steps go smoothly. Later, upon conception, genetics provide the blueprint for the general course of fetal development and adulthood potential, much like an orderly set of building instructions with a very strict time-line. During critical windows of fetal development, certain nutrients must be present in order for the step to be properly completed. It is a common misperception that a developing baby can get anything it needs from its mother at any given moment. Aside from a few exceptions (e.g., the fetus can leach as much calcium as it needs at the expense of the mother's bones), the mother's basic needs must be met before the baby's because the mother must end up healthy enough after pregnancy to be able to care for her infant. This fact of nature is more pronounced when the pregnant mother herself is still maturing, as when teenagers become pregnant.

When you are at your healthiest, you make it easier on your body to live up to its reproductive potential. In effect, you can reduce factors that are out of your control (e.g., maternal age or preexisting medical condition) to a position of lesser significance. All of this may have a positive impact on your stress level, too, which is a sign to your body that you're up to the challenge of childbearing.

FOR FUTURE REFERENCE: During Pregnancy

A small percentage of women suffer extreme nausea and vomiting during some or all of pregnancy. Even with the best medical care, there may be days or weeks when excellent nutrition is impossible to sustain. There are encouraging indications that offspring of women who are well nourished prior to conception will be protected against or only minimally affected by severe morning sickness as long as they receive medical assistance to stay as well nourished as possible, prevent severe dehydration, and avoid significant weight loss. If you find yourself at the point where you can hardly keep down food or beverages, do take it seriously enough to seek medical attention. Also, focus on eating foods that sound somewhat appealing instead of worrying about how perfect your diet is. If that means having tacos for breakfast or choosing sugary lemonade over a whole-some glass of milk, so be it. By veering from your typical food choices and eating according to what will stay down, you may interrupt the cycle of nausea and vomiting long enough to restore hydration and energy balance.

THE FOUNDATION NUTRIENTS: IT ALL STARTS HERE

Our bodies depend on food and beverages for survival. A sumptuous meal is made accessible internally by the process of digestion, which breaks down foods into water, carbohydrates, proteins, fats, vitamins, and minerals so they can be absorbed into the bloodstream and delivered to sites in the body where they are needed. Although some nutrients can be partially made inside the body, we mostly rely on outside food sources to get the proper balance. Of these nutrients, carbohydrates, proteins, and fats have calories; water, vitamins, and minerals do not.

Before discussing how to design a preconception-friendly meal plan, it helps to have an understanding of the nuts and bolts—the foundation nutrients—of foods and beverages. By learning about the functions and sources of individual nutrients in this and the next chapter, you can begin identifying deficiencies or excesses of individual nutrients in your daily diet.

Water

As much as 55 to 80 percent of your body is composed of water, making it the most abundant nutrient in the human body (the leaner you are, the higher the percentage). It fills many nooks and crannies in the body and makes up the majority of muscle and blood. Even fat and bone cells are about 25 percent water by weight. So essential is water to our health that we typically cannot survive without it for more than a week.

Water is also the medium in which many nutrients travel and interact with one another. Natural chemical reactions in the body are dependent on it. Water helps transport excess heat, waste products, and toxins safely out of the body. It aids in digestion, lubricates joints, and moistens the eyes, nose, and mouth. Once you are pregnant, amniotic fluid, which is 99 percent water, plays a vital role in fetal growth and development.

To meet pre-pregnancy needs, most women need to drink approximately eight 8-ounce glasses of fluid over the course of a day. You may be able to stay hydrated on a little less (say, seven glasses) if you are petite or not very active. (Men, by the way, need about eight to ten glasses per day.) Drink more if you are in a climate that is very hot, dry, or at high altitude; if you eat a very high-fiber diet; or if you are very athletic. It is often easier to drink more water when you carry a refillable water bottle to work, the fitness club, or other activities. Please refer to Chapter 3, which complements pages 285–286.

Your fluid needs can be met in more ways than by just drinking water. Beverages such as milk and an occasional glass of fruit juice may take the place of a few water servings as long as you adhere to recommended portion sizes. You may even notice that your need for beverages isn't quite as high if you consume lots of foods with high water content such as whole fruits and veggies. Caffeinated beverages (unsweetened iced or hot tea, coffee) have a mild diuretic effect on your body—they increase urine output. However, if you stay within the pre-pregnancy limitations for these two beverages (limit of 100-200 mg of caffeine per day), the diuretic effect is negligible, and they can be counted toward your daily fluid requirements.

Enhanced water products (vitamin- or electrolyte-enhanced waters) are popular but aren't in the same league as plain water. Sleek packaging and star-studded marketing aside, recognize enhanced waters for what they often are—discretionary calories from sugar made to look "healthier" by tossing in a few vitamins or electrolytes. Watch for caffeine and/or natural herbal compounds, especially if marketed as "energy drinks" or "naturally sweetened." As long as the ingredient list jibes with our preconception safety guidelines, then your choice of discretionary calories is up to you; just watch that serving size and multiply the calories per serving by the appropriate number if you intend to drink the whole container (more on discretionary calories in Chapters 12 and 13). Above all, make sure that your taste buds remain most familiar with the taste of good old-fashioned water. If you are a huge fan of soft drinks, the occasional indulgence is okay, but again, you may need to cut back to limit overall sugar intake, and cross-check with Chapter 8 if any contain herbs or natural supplements.

Practical Application

Hydration and the Unglamorous Art of Color Analysis

How can you tell whether you are drinking enough fluids? The simplest gauge is the color of your urine, which should be pale yellow. (If you take a vitamin supplement, it may be a little brighter in color.) Odorous, darker yellow urine (the color of apple juice) in relatively small volume indicates partial dehydration. Do not rely on thirst to tell you whether you are well hydrated, because once thirst kicks in, you are already 1 to 2 percent dehydrated (equivalent to a loss of one to four pounds of water weight for most women). On the flip side, if you are urinating excessively day and night, the urine is clear, and you have no discomfort indicating an infection, you are likely overhydrating yourself and should cut back a bit. Sometimes frequent urination and undiminished thirst can be a sign that you are having a fluctuation in your sugar metabolism and may be at risk for diabetes. If you think your drinking habits do not explain the amount and frequency that you are having to urinate, discuss it with your health care provider.

Over the next few days, take note of whether you are well hydrated at all times. It is normal to have slightly deeper-colored urine first thing in the morning after a good night's sleep. However, try to get to the point where light yellow urine is the norm.

Water Supply

Water is a precious resource, and the U.S. Environmental Protection Agency (EPA) does its best to make sure that your tap water is safe at all times. Unless there have been concerns raised in your community about the quality of your water supply, tap water should be safe for drinking and cooking.

If you have concerns about your tap water, call your local health department for further information. Another resource is your water utility company, which must upon request provide you with a copy of the *Annual Drinking Water Quality Report,* also known as the *Consumer Confidence Report* (CCR). The phone numbers should be at the front of your phone book in the government section, and all reports are accessible online.

You may feel even more confident about your water supply if you put a NSF-certified activated-carbon filter on your tap. Follow filter maintenance instructions to maintain optimal safety. Another option is to use commercially bottled water, particularly if the provider is certified by the International Bottled Water Association (IBWA). Bottled or filtered water may have the added benefit of tasting, looking, or smelling better than some municipal waters, even though their safety may be comparable.[1] Many bottled-water companies offer fluoridated water. Mineral waters and sparkling bottled waters are safe options. But overall, keep in mind that tap water is least expensive, highly regulated for safety, and least demanding of precious fossil fuels to produce.

The debate over the safety of bisphenol A (BPA) was discussed in Chapter 3. BPA is an industrial chemical that is a component of most rigid clear plastic containers and is a common ingredient in the resin lining food and beverage cans (where it protects against corrosion and leaching of dangerous metals or bacteria into the food). However, most disposable plastic water bottles, as well as juice and soft drink bottles, do not contain BPA. Whether you choose to buy bottled water in disposable plastic containers or switch to a metal reusable water bot-

---

1. Drinking water needs to be purified as one method of protecting the public from infectious disease. The safety of drinking water disinfection by-products (DBPs) in municipal water sources has received careful scientific scrutiny. To date, the most thorough research conducted, by Savitz et al. of the University of North Carolina, found very low threat, if any, to prospective mothers and future risk of miscarriage. However, the authors note that not all women are reassured by this data and may choose to use water filters. Carbon filters significantly lower DBPs, while bottled water is typically free of DBPs due to alternative sanitizing methods that are not feasible for municipal water departments to use. As a point of comparison with municipal water sources, you may request a report on contaminant levels, if any, from bottlers. Alternatively, your local health department can offer referrals to independent labs that test water quality.

tle, keep in mind that uncontrolled growth of bacteria is what experts are most concerned with. Disposable containers aren't designed for safe use over an extended period of time, and stainless steel or aluminum containers should be routinely washed with warm water and mild detergent to avoid introducing unwanted bacteria into your system.

FOR FUTURE REFERENCE: During Pregnancy

Drinking enough water can become more of a challenge than you might anticipate. Even women who are accustomed to drinking plenty of water find that they have to continuously remind themselves to drink more than usual while pregnant (and later, when breastfeeding). Keeping well hydrated during pregnancy is very important to allow optimal blood flow for amniotic fluid production and nutrient delivery, to reduce muscle cramping, and to maintain a safe body temperature while exercising. Dehydration can also stimulate early uterine contractions. Interestingly, drinking excessive water during labor can present its own challenges to uterine contractility, so it's important to seek a balance.

Carbohydrates

Carbohydrates ("carbs") are your mind and body's main source of energy. They will also be the primary source of energy for your baby in the womb. Carbs come in two forms: simple and complex. The simplest carbohydrates come from naturally occurring sugars such as in fruits and milk, as well as added sugars such as table sugar and honey. The most complex forms of carbohydrate are starch and dietary fiber. The process of digestion breaks complex forms of carbohydrates down into the simplest forms. Three simple forms of carbohydrate—glucose (the body's favorite fuel source), fructose, and galactose—are absorbed from the intestine into the bloodstream. The latter two are eventually converted to glucose at cell sites, where energy is produced or stored for later use.

Carbohydrates should comprise roughly half (45 to 65 percent) of the total calories you ingest. If you are athletic, the higher percentage may be advantageous. If you have diabetes or polycystic ovary syndrome (PCOS), the lower percentage may be better. Your remaining calories should come from protein (10 to 35 percent) and fat (20 to 35 percent). There is no need to rush to get your calculator to determine whether your intake fits this profile. By eating according to the Food Guide Pyramid, which we discuss in Chapters 12 and 13, you will automatically eat the right proportions of carbohydrate, protein, and fat. This is not the time to experiment with low-carbohydrate, high-protein diets. You will need the energy provided by carbs as your body conceives and nurtures a baby.

Calories in Carbohydrates

There are 4 calories per gram of carbohydrate. The Nutrition Facts label on a bread package might state "Total Carbohydrate 15g" for one piece of bread, so multiply the 15 grams of carbohydrates by 4 calories/gram = 60 calories from carbohydrate in that slice.

You should not need to meticulously count grams of carbohydrate to eat well. However, if you are diabetic and manage your blood sugars by counting carbs, you may subtract half of any sugar alcohol grams (explained on the next page), if any, from total carbohydrate grams. If the serving of food contains more than 5 grams of fiber, subtract those grams, too. This is slightly different from how manufacturers calculate "net carbs," a term that has no standardized FDA definition at this time. The American Diabetes Association publishes excellent guides on how to accurately count carbs for insulin dosage management.

Familiar Food Sources of Carbohydrates

Carbohydrates are the major components in breads, cereals, and other grains, vegetables, fruits, nuts, legumes, and milk. These are naturally occurring carbs. Carbohydrates may also take the form of added sugars such as table sugar, honey, syrup, molasses, and fruit juice concentrate. Be on the lookout for these in candy and other desserts (even low-fat ones) and sugary beverages such as lemonade, regular sodas, sweetened teas, and fruit-flavored drinks. One way to begin improving the quality of your carb intake is to replace foods that have added sugars or "enriched wheat flour" (a.k.a. white flour), substituting a variety of naturally occurring carbohydrates—the less processed, the better. Research is murky on whether people benefit further by preferentially choosing carbs with a low glycemic index, but research is ongoing to see if low-glycemic-index foods assist in management of weight and PCOS—more on this next.

Glycemic Index

A full explanation of the glycemic index (GI) and glycemic load (GL) of foods is beyond the scope of this book. So, consider this a brief introduction to a topic of debate among scientists and nutrition professionals. When you eat, not all carbohydrate-containing foods act the same during the process of digestion. Some, the high-GI foods, spike blood glucose levels before they go back down, promoting greater release of insulin into the bloodstream; others, the low-GI foods, promote a more modest rise and fall in blood sugar and require less insulin release for the same amount of carbohydrate. Foods considered for inclusion in the GI charts must contain at least 10 grams of carbohydrate per serving. Foods with fewer than 10 grams don't get tested; this is why you won't see healthy foods such as leafy green vegetables, nuts, seeds, avocados, and so on listed in the GI tables. Low-GI foods are typically, but not always,

What About No-Sugar-Added and Sugar-Free Products?

Some food items contain polyls (labeled as sugar alcohols) in place of sucrose so the label can still state that the product has "no sugar added" or is "sugar-free." Polyls are not the same as sugar or alcohol, nor are they artificial sweeteners. These sugar alcohols include mannitol, sorbitol, xylitol, isomalt, erythritol, hydrogenated starch hydrolysates or polyglycitol, lactitol, and maltitol—look for these on the label the next time you pick up a pack of sugar-free gum, jam, hard candy, breath mints, or dessert. Polyls are deemed safe for consumption at all times. The only drawback to sugar alcohols is that they are very slowly and incompletely digested. This can result in uncomfortable side effects such as gas, bloating, and diarrhea in certain people. To some, these symptoms are not worth the few calories saved—approximately 2 calories per gram instead of 4. This may be especially true during pregnancy, a time when gastrointestinal discomforts can be exaggerated.

If you see the term "net carb" on a food label that contains sugar alcohols, the manufacturer has most likely subtracted all grams of sugar alcohol (as well as fiber), but serious carb counters should subtract only half that amount to account for partial digestion.

One last sweetener that deserves mention is the natural, no-calorie sweetener called stevia. This plant-derived sweetener has been used in countries such as Brazil, Japan, and China for many years, but due to lack of safety data it formerly was available in the United States only as a dietary supplement (and therefore only loosely regulated for purity). Recently, a highly purified food-grade stevia extract has been approved by the FDA as generally recognized as safe (GRAS) as a sweetener for food and beverages.

higher in fiber and not as processed (two things we already recommend). For the most part, the low-GI foods (e.g., lentils, most vegetables, low-fat milk/yogurt, pasta) are what you'd typically call healthy. However, the reason why some countries (the United States in particular) and organizations (such as the American Diabetes Association) are hesitant to recommend a low-GI diet for health promotion is that some of the low-GI foods are very high in saturated fats, which are unhealthy if eaten in excess. The real downside, however, may be when saturated fats get replaced by refined grains and sugars instead of mono- or polyunsaturated fats.

Meanwhile, the Food and Agriculture Organization (FAO) of the United Nations and the World Health Organization (WHO), as well as countries such as Canada and Australia, are moving forward to educate the public on how to integrate low-GI diet selections into already established dietary recommendations. Though we would still like to see more research in this area, it is very worthy of consideration, particularly for people who already have some degree of insulin resistance, cardiovascular risks, and excess body weight. If you wish to pursue this further on your own, a good free reference is the International Table of Glycemic Index and

What About Foods and Beverages Containing Nonnutritive or Artificial Sweeteners?

Nonnutritive (artificial, very-low-calorie, or intense) sweeteners are noncaloric sweeteners that are so intense in flavor that you need use only a small amount. Like many women, you may consume artificially sweetened diet soft drinks, flavored yogurts, or sweeteners in your coffee or tea. Now that you're considering conceiving, it has probably crossed your mind to ask whether these foods and drinks are still safe.

There has been an extensive amount of research on their safety, particularly in the area of reproduction. The FDA has approved the use of six nonnutritive sweeteners as safe for most women during preconception, pregnancy, and breastfeeding.[a] We find these particularly nice for women with diabetes or women keeping tabs on their weight.

The six nonnutritive sweeteners are:

- Aspartame (formerly known only as NutraSweet or Equal)
- Acesulfame K (Sunette, Sweet One)
- Sucralose (Splenda)
- Saccharin (Sweet'n Low, SweeTen, Sugar Twin)
- Neotame
- Stevia-based rebaudioside A, reb A, or rebiana (Truvia, Sun Crystals, PureVia)[b]

Of these, saccharin has been the most controversial, so some women choose to avoid it. It is reassuring, however, that the federal government removed saccharin from its list of cancer-causing substances in humans many years ago.

The amounts of nonnutritive sweeteners that have generally been deemed safe are typically much higher than most people consume. If you prefer some sort of guideline as to how much is well within safety limits for preconception, we loosely define moderate consumption as no more than three servings in a day from different food sources. Examples of one serving include a cup of light yogurt, a mug of sugar-free hot cocoa, or a diet soft drink. Our reasoning for such a conservative limit goes beyond the proven safety record. This modest amount encourages people to experience most of their food flavors as they naturally exist instead of disguising them with an extra sweet taste.

a. Women diagnosed with the very rare genetic disorder phenylketonuria (PKU) must avoid aspartame.
b. The first food-grade stevia extract received GRAS approval in 2008, which meant it was generally recognized as safe. Other food-grade stevia derivatives are pending GRAS approval. See Chapter 8, herbal section, for more detail.

Glycemic Load Values (available in the *American Journal of Clinical Nutrition* 76, no. 1 [2002], pp. 5–56) and do a Google search for Jennie Brand-Miller and colleagues from the University of Sydney in Australia and Harvard University in Massachusetts.

Dietary Fiber

Noel: "I have figured that I eat about 16 to 19 grams of fiber from my current diet. Why is it important to increase my fiber intake to at least 25 grams per day? After all, my bowel habits are perfectly normal now."

Dana: "Within a year of delivering my son by C-section, I was diagnosed with irritable bowel syndrome after experiencing symptoms of mild constipation interspersed with periods of painful cramping, gas, diarrhea, and debilitating dizziness at the peak of feeling rotten. However, when I changed my diet after reading the book IBS Relief, by Dawn Burstall, RD, et al., my symptoms vanished. For me, that meant religiously drinking enough water and steering clear of obvious offenders (beans, nuts, and popcorn, to name the main ones, though I am finally able to have these in small doses) while gradually increasing other high-fiber foods, including a daily serving of old-fashioned oats or oatmeal, cooked oat bran cereal, or All-Bran cereal. Symptoms do still creep back when I slack off on my diet for a few days. What amazed my doctor and me was that I was able to control my IBS naturally, without medications."

Unlike some animals, humans cannot digest fiber from whole grains, vegetables, fruits, and legumes, so this form of carbohydrate does not provide energy. However, fiber does plenty of good while in transit through the digestive tract. Dietary fiber is most commonly known for its role in gut health, aiding friendly gut bacteria and easing problems with constipation and hemorrhoids. During pregnancy this will take on more meaning, because most pregnant women experience some degree of constipation; the resultant straining during bowel movements may lead to painful hemorrhoids or exacerbate existing ones (hemorroids are dilated veins in the rectal/anal region). Fiber-rich foods also appear to normalize insulin and blood glucose levels, lower cholesterol levels, aid in the removal of potential toxins, make weight loss or maintenance easier, and reduce the risk of colon cancer and possibly breast cancer. Other health-promoting substances in fiber-rich foods enhance the risk reduction.

How to Comfortably Add Fiber to Your Diet

Most Americans average only 14 to 15 grams of dietary fiber daily, whereas optimal fiber intake is 25 to 35 grams per day. Fruits, vegetables, legumes, nuts, and whole grains are some common sources of dietary fiber, as outlined in Table 10-1. These whole foods are natural sources of additional nutrients as well. Supplemental sources of fiber—see "Fiber in Disguise"—such as chicory root or guar gum are added to certain processed foods, such as low-calorie desserts. Isolated fiber (e.g., psyllium) can be found in products such as Metamucil, but these should not be used in place of a high-fiber diet. Fiber pills are discouraged but may be used at your doctor's discretion during preconception and pregnancy.

It takes time to get used to eating a variety of high-fiber foods. The following tactics will help alleviate the unpleasant gassy, bloated symptoms that accompany a too-rapid addition of fiber to the diet. First, identify the low-fiber carbohydrates that are part of your diet, including sweets. Don't be fooled by wheat crackers and breads that derive their rich brown hue from added molasses or food coloring! If the ingredient list says only "enriched wheat flour" instead of whole-wheat flour (or whole oat, rye, etc.), you have been duped. Out of curiosity, get up for a minute and go check your favorite cereal, bread, or cracker label. For a product to qualify as "whole-grain," the word *whole* should be first in line in the ingredient list (or at least in the second and third ingredients, effectively adding up to a respectable fiber content). With help from the Practical Application below, try to replace some of your low-fiber foods with the higher-fiber foods that you like in Table 10-1 (also see page 362). Incorporate these into your diet gradually: for the first week add approximately 4–5 grams of fiber per day, then an additional 4–5 grams per day the next week, until you reach 25–35 grams/day total. Drink sufficient liquids, too, or else the extra fiber will have the opposite effect of being constipating.

Many women find it easy to gradually add one-third to one-half cup of bran cereal (about 8 to 12 grams of fiber per serving) into their daily food plan. You can munch on it plain, eat it with yogurt or milk, mix it with cottage cheese (sounds weird but tastes great), or add it to trail mix with walnuts and dried fruit.

Practical Application

1. With a pen or pencil, highlight all of the foods that appeal to you in Table 10-1. Tally an estimate of what you normally consume in a given day, paying particular attention to how your serving size compares with the amount we're using as a reference. Halve or double values as needed.

2. Do you see opportunities to replace low-fiber foods with higher-fiber choices that you like just as well? Add some of these to the blank shopping list in Appendix E. If you want to double-check the actual grams of fiber in your favorite packaged foods, look at the Nutrition Facts panel. Compare how much you eat to what they use as the reference serving size (at the top of the panel). Now scan down to "Total Carbohydrates" and circle the number listed to the right of "Dietary Fiber." That's how much total fiber is in a serving of their food.

Even if Table 10-1 doesn't appear particularly useful at this moment, flag it for later when those pregnancy hormones begin slowing down your gastrointestinal tract, creating a traffic jam in your normal bowel habits.

TABLE 10-1
DIETARY FIBER CONTENT OF FOODS
(LISTED CATEGORICALLY FROM HIGHEST FIBER CONTENT TO LOWEST)

Food	Amount	Dietary Fiber (grams)	Calories
FRUITS			
Figs	5 medium	8.0	185
Blackberries	1 cup	7.6	74
Raspberries	1 cup	6.8	60
Boysenberries	1 cup	5.1	66
Pear	1 medium	4.0	45
Blueberries	1 cup	3.9	81
Apple, with skin	1 medium	3.7	81
Strawberries	1 cup	3.4	45
Orange, with membrane	1 medium	3.1	60
Prunes, dried	6	3.0	110
Banana	1 medium	2.7	105
Avocado	¼ medium	2.1	77
Raisins	¼ cup	2.0	130
Peach	1 medium	1.7	37
Melon	1 cup	1.2	57
VEGETABLES			
Potato, baked, with skin	1 medium	4.8	220
Collard greens, cooked	½ cup	3.6	18
Broccoli, cooked	½ cup	2.3	22
Corn, whole kernel, cooked	½ cup	2.3	89
Carrot, raw	1 medium	2.2	31
Spinach, cooked	½ cup	2.2	21
Brussels sprouts, cooked	½ cup	2.0	30
Cabbage, raw, shredded	1 cup	1.6	18
Tomato, raw	1 medium	1.4	26

Food	Amount	Dietary Fiber (grams)	Calories
Asparagus, cooked	½ cup	1.4	22
Kale, cooked	½ cup	1.3	21
Lettuce, romaine, shredded	1 cup	1.0	8

COOKED LEGUMES AND SHELLED NUTS

Lentils	½ cup	7.8	115
Kidney beans, black beans, pinto beans	½ cup	7.5	115
White beans	½ cup	5.7	125
Lima beans	½ cup	4.9	85
Edamame or soybeans, green, boiled	½ cup	3.8	127
Green peas, petite	½ cup	2.7	47
Almonds, with skin, 12	½ ounce	2.0	83
Peanuts, 20	½ ounce	1.2	83
Peanut butter	1 tbsp	1.1	94

BREAKFAST CEREALS[a] (Note: Some low-fiber foods are listed purely for comparison)

Fiber One, General Mills	½ cup	13.0	60
Bran Buds, Kellogg's	⅓ cup	12.0	83
All-Bran, Kellogg's	⅓ cup	10.0	81
100% Bran, Post	⅓ cup	8.3	75
Kashi, Good Friends	¾ cup	8.0	90
Bran flakes	⅔ cup	6.0	90
Raisin bran	½ cup	4.0	95
Wheat germ, toasted	¼ cup	3.7	111
Cheerios, General Mills	1 cup	3.0	110
Grape-Nuts, Post	¼ cup	2.5	100
Corn flakes	1 cup	1.1	102

Food	Amount	Dietary Fiber (grams)	Calories
OTHER GRAINS AND GRAIN PRODUCTS (Note: Some low-fiber foods are listed purely for comparison)			
Rye (whole grain), crispbread	3 crackers	5.1	111
Bulgur (cracked wheat), cooked	½ cup	4.1	76
Popcorn, air-popped	3 cups	3.6	92
Barley, cooked	½ cup	3.1	99
Whole wheat crackers[b]	1 oz	2.8	126
Oatmeal, cooked	½ cup	2.0	73
Whole wheat bread	1 slice	1.9	69
Rice, brown, cooked	½ cup	1.8	108
Wild rice, cooked	½ cup	1.5	83
Corn tortilla (6–7-inch diameter)	1 medium	1.3	56
Couscous, cooked	½ cup	1.2	100
Spaghetti noodles, cooked	½ cup	1.2	99
Grits, cooked	½ cup	0.3	73
Rice, white, cooked[c]	½ cup	0.3	103

a. Portion sizes of cereals represent approximately 1 ounce, and may differ from portion sizes mentioned on food labels.

b. Many mainstream brand names are making lower-fat, trans-fat-free versions of their full-fat counterparts. Read the Nutrition Facts panel to determine whether your favorite brands make the cut (and watch that a bunch of sugar isn't added to compensate for taste).

c. Read labels to identify new converted white rice products that are processed to have much higher fiber content.

Sources: Industry data, accessed 2009; J.A.T. Pennington, *Bowes & Church's Food Values of Portions Commonly Used,* 16th ed. (Philadelphia: Lippincott, 1994)

Protein

Often, we think of protein only in terms of building muscle. In fact, protein is an essential part of all human and animal cells. Proteins provide structure for each cell and serve as enzymes that are fundamental to proper cell function. During times of growth, development, or repair—such as pregnancy—there is more demand for protein. When you conceive, your body begins to build the cell mass that becomes the fetus; it is also building the uterus (a

Fiber in Disguise

It's easy to know you are getting dietary fiber from a cup of fresh blackberries. But how can you identify hidden fiber, the ones extracted from a natural source or synthetically manufactured, then added to thicken, bulk, or stabilize a cereal or cereal bar, low-calorie cake, or ice cream? These types of fiber are healthy, but too much of a good thing can add up and contribute to gas and bloating, especially if paired with any of the sugar alcohols discussed earlier. Look for disguised fiber in the ingredient list as any of the following terms:

- Cellulose or methylcellulose
- Chitin or chitosan
- Beta-glucans (barley; oats)
- Guar gums
- Hemicellulose
- Polydextrose
- Inulin, oligofructose, and fructo-oligosaccharides (chicory root; fructan; Jerusalem artichoke)
- Lignan
- Pectin
- Psyllium (plantago seed or ispaghula husk)
- Resistant dextrins or maltodextrins
- Resistant starch

Source: H. Grabitske and J. L. Slavin, "Low-Digestible Carbohydrates in Practice," *Journal of the American Dietetic Association* 108 (2008): 1677–81.

muscle), the placenta, more blood, and other necessary tissue for pregnancy. Proteins are also part of most hormones, and they make up antibodies, some of which are passed to the fetus to strengthen its immune system. Eat too much protein and the excess is stored as fat. Eat too little and you could affect your fetus's development.

Animal studies have specifically examined the impact of very-low-protein diets prior to conception and throughout pregnancy. Even though caloric intake was sufficient, the protein-deficient diet diminished optimal formation of the fetal kidneys and pancreas. This led to greater difficulty in maintaining normal blood pressure and blood sugar levels later in life. However, we rarely, if ever, see women who eat too little protein unless they are recovering from bariatric surgery, are severely restricting calories, have an eating disorder, or go on all-fruit crash diets. Nauseated pregnant women are at risk, too, if they exclusively rely on ginger ale and saltines (or the like) for weeks on end.

Individual protein molecules are made up of tinier building blocks called amino acids. There are twenty different amino acids. Just as the twenty-six letters in the alphabet can be put together to spell out countless words and phrases to form poems, short stories, and novels, the twenty amino acids can be linked together in a number of ways to form various proteins. The arrangement of the amino acids acts like a code that dictates its unique function. Nine of the twenty amino acids are essential, meaning we must get them from our foods; our body cannot make them. The remaining eleven are available from foods, too, but can also be assembled inside the body as long as you eat a balanced diet.

Women who are nineteen years or older have a recommended dietary allowance (RDA) of 46 grams of protein per day. Athletic women may need between 20 and 30 grams of additional protein per day, depending on their body weight and degree of training; elite and/or strength-trained athletes may require even higher amounts. Most women—even athletes—still easily meet their basic protein requirements by eating a balanced diet. Remember: neither very-low-protein (fewer than 40 grams per day) nor very-high-protein diets (more than 110 grams per day) are advised for preconception.

Familiar Food Sources of Proteins

Ample protein is found in meats, poultry, seafood, eggs (both yolk and white), and dairy products, legumes (beans, lentils, peas), nuts, and seeds. Small servings of these over the course of the day help us feel satisfied, potentially decreasing hunger between meals. Vegetables and grains also contain smaller amounts of protein (see Table 10-2).

TABLE 10-2
HOW MUCH PROTEIN IS IN EACH?

Dairy	8 grams per serving, such as 1 cup milk or 1 slice cheese
Meat, poultry, fish, egg, nuts, legumes	7 grams per 1-ounce equivalent,[a] such as one jumbo shrimp, one whole egg (don't throw away the yolk), or 1/2 cup baked beans
Grains	2–3 grams per serving, such as 1 slice bread or ½ cup of cooked rice or noodles
Vegetables	2 grams per serving, such as 1 cup raw spinach or ½ cup cooked carrots

a. A chicken drumstick or small fish fillet is 2 to 3 ounces in size, so a typical serving provides 14 to 21 grams of protein.

Calories in Protein

One gram of protein contains 4 calories. For example, a golf-ball-size meatball (1 ounce) contains about 7 grams of protein, so 7 grams × 4 calories/gram equals 28 calories from protein. Guidance on how many grams of protein during preconception and pregnancy begins on this page.

Both plant and animal sources of proteins contain varying amounts of all twenty of the amino acids. Animal and soybean proteins have very high amounts of all the amino acids. However, most plant sources are low in one or two essential amino acids. This is not a problem for vegetarians as long as a wide variety of vegetarian foods is eaten over the course of a day. (Chapter 12 discusses vegetarianism and preconception in more depth.)

FOR FUTURE REFERENCE: During Pregnancy/After Delivery

The RDA for protein goes up to approximately 71 grams during pregnancy and through the postpartum months if breastfeeding, though your clinician may opt to calculate your daily needs based specifically on 0.5 grams protein per pound of your pre-pregnancy weight. This does not include the additional protein needs of very active women. If you start adding up how much protein you currently get from your diet, you'll see that you probably already exceed the pregnancy RDA for protein. It is just fine to consume 100 to 125 grams per day of protein (preferably from foods, not from protein supplements) during pregnancy and/or breastfeeding. In fact, this higher amount of protein may even be beneficial if the pregnancy becomes higher-risk. If you're expecting twins or triplets, protein intakes of 150 and 200 grams per day, respectively, are commonly advised, especially in the second and third trimesters. Refer to Table 10-2 to get ideas for the extra grams of protein; Chapters 12 and 13 further explain serving sizes.

You may discover that pregnancy alters your taste for some of your favorite sources of protein. For example, many pregnant women suddenly can't stand the thought of chicken or fish, but luckily salty nuts or scrambled eggs sound great. Then there's the vegetarian who suddenly craves a hamburger instead of a veggie burger. Know the alternative sources of protein so you can incorporate them into your diet if this happens. If you still have difficulty meeting your protein needs, supplemental sources of protein such as a whey protein isolate or hydrolyzed whey protein concentrate (look for WPC80 or higher) may boost your protein intake.

Fats

Fats are finally shedding their bad image as food enemy number one as we've come to recognize their positive qualities. When eaten in moderation, fats play an important role in your health and fertility. They are primarily used for energy. They also transport the fat-soluble vitamins A, D, E, and K and provide essential fatty acids that cannot be synthesized in the liver from other fats. Fats provide cushioning to protect internal organs, insulation to regulate body temperature, and structure for every cell.

You should get approximately 20 to 35 percent of your daily calories from fat. Fat calories come from a combination of added fats—salad dressings, oil, margarine or butter, and mayonnaise—and hidden sources of fat, including regular and low-fat dairy or soy products, fattier cuts of meat and poultry, snack chips, bakery goods, avocados, and nuts.

How will you know whether you are getting the recommended amount of fat without going overboard? Should you count fat grams? Although counting fat grams may be a valuable educational tool initially, it has been our observation that it tends to make people paranoid, and often takes the enjoyment out of eating. Granted, it is good to have a general awareness about the fat content of foods, but you are better off learning about which *types* of fat to choose while following the USDA's MyPyramid in Chapter 12. By consciously choosing a wide variety of foods in the appropriate portions, your fat intake will automatically fall in line.

Familiar Food Sources of Fat

Fats usually come in two forms: either solid or liquid at room temperature. Those that are solid at room temperature typically contain high amounts of saturated fats (which give them the structure to stay firm at room temperature). The "sat fats" are not very good for your overall health, particularly your cardiovascular health. Most are of animal origin, such as butter, lard, meat and poultry fat, and high-fat dairy products, though tropical oils (coconut, palm, and palm kernel oils) are plant-derived sources. You don't have to completely shun them, but limit your intake, and use the type of fat discussed next as a substitute.

The other type of fat is typically liquid at room temperature and is called unsaturated fat (the "un-" part being key here), specifically monounsaturated and polyunsaturated fats (fatty acids, really, but we will use the terms interchangeably). These are better for your health and generally come from plant sources or fish and other marine foods. The polyunsaturated fatty acids (PUFAs) are essential for mammals to consume because our livers cannot synthesize them.

Unfortunately, in processed foods, unsaturated oils are frequently either partially or fully hydrogenated (hydrogen is added) to make them more solid at room temperature, like margarine, or to extend their shelf life, as in snack chips, microwave popcorn, high-fat crackers, store-bought cookies, and baked goods. The process of partial hydrogenation creates the notorious trans fats, which, through legislation and public pressure have largely been cut back or eliminated from processsed foods and restaurant fare. Trans fats appear to reduce the healthy unsaturated fats in the womb; they may also affect ovulation, harm the placenta (potentially causing miscarriage), and reduce birth weights. Oust as many man-made trans fats from your diet as you can before conception. But when avoiding trans fats, don't make the mistake of replacing them with saturated or fully hydrogenated fats; instead, opt for healthy poly- and monounsaturated fats, and try lower-fat substitutes (not ones with refined carbs, though).

Note: In the section that follows we'll delve into how to balance your fat intake and avoid the chronic, low-grade inflammation brought on by the typical North American diet. The detail that follows is for all of you science nuts and clinicians who cannot get enough of this stuff. And if that's not for you, first scan the highlighted box, "Fatsville's Main Cast of Characters" and then use the Practical Application (page 302) and points numbered 1–7 (pages 303–307) to better stock your fridge and pantry to keep the fats in the right proportions.

It's not easy keeping the names of the fats and oils straight, so we created a "cast of characters" to help. This lighthearted way to distinguish the good guys from the villains is interspersed with footnotes to clarify some of the subtle scientific references. If this is too silly for you right now, please forgive us, but do dog-ear the page so you can come back to it when your head is spinning with terms and acronyms you'd really like to remember!

FATSVILLE'S MAIN CAST OF CHARACTERS

The Sat Fats

A simple, solid lot, aside from a few slick characters; prone to taking up residence in places where they aren't wanted; irresistibly charming, but good company only in small doses. Favorite hangout: deli counter, ice cream parlor, or snack food aisle.

The Un Families (Monos and Polys)

The Mono Uns. Calm, understated guys of medium height and Mediterranean good looks, whose steady presence makes everyone's lives run smoothly. The Mono Uns are ardent protectors when cold pressed to take action. Favorite foods: olive oil and avocados.

The Poly Uns. A diverse lot, not indigenous[a] to the community, but introduced from the outside world to live in Fatsville. Unique aptitudes as mind-body wellness gurus make them essential to the community's health. As novices, the two most well-known Poly Uns are nicknamed Lin and Alpha. They adopt new names if and when they blossom into fully productive adults.
- *Lin (or LA) Poly Un:* Fond of long, delicate chain necklaces and decked out in their omega-6 brand of jeans. Fatsville is most harmonious[b] when the Lins outnumber their counterparts, the

Alphas, by about 5:1. However, when too many Lins move in at once, overcrowding causes in-flamed tempers[c] (a growing concern in Fatsville). If Lins reach full maturity, most adopt the name AA or A-Rac; amicable intentions go awry when too many Lins vie for mature status at once. Favorite food during youth: liquid vegetable oils.

- *Alpha (or ALA) Poly Un:* Similarly fond of long, delicate chain necklaces,[d] but prefer the omega-3 brand of jeans. These energetic gals work hard to champion their small, but rightful spot at the communal table. A precious few Alphas make it to elder status, distinguishing themselves in the community as the peacekeeper[b]/neuroscientist duo, EPA and DHA. To signify their right of passage, EPAs and DHAs wear even longer chain necklaces. Favorite food during youth: wal-nuts. Favorite food in adulthood: fish ("brain food").

The Trans Clan

The Trans clan are distant relatives of the Poly Uns, but you would hardly know it. The Trans clan have undergone too many transformations since being plucked out of Fatsville and given free makeovers to make them stay young forever. Except for a few who refused the treatments and stuck to raising livestock and dairy cows back home,[e] the majority of the Trans clan were banned from participating in community events. They were bad news. Favorite foods: just about anything that would survive a nuclear disaster, especially processed baked goods.

a. Poly Uns "not indigenous": Our body can piece together all the other fatty acids except for the two essential fatty acids ALA and LA, so these must be provided externally from food.
b. Words such as *peacekeeping* or *harmonious:* When omega-3s and omega-6s are in balance, they promote blood vessel health and an anti-inflammatory tone (this is what we want).
c. "Inflamed tempers": There's a tipping point beyond which pro-inflammatory reponses occur and the vascular system rebels (chronic internal inflammation is the concern here).
d. Long chain necklaces: Poly Uns are all long-chain fatty acids, some of which can add more carbon atoms to the existing chain and achieve new "fully productive" functions.
e. Reference to trans fats who stick to raising dairy cows, etc.: fat found in dairy and meat has a tiny amount of naturally occurring trans fat that is of negligible health concern compared to artificially manufactured trans fats.

Balancing Your Omega Fatty Acids

From a few short weeks after conception through the first two years after birth, two long-chain polyunsaturated fats, called arachidonic acid (AA, an omega-6 fatty acid) and docosa-hexaenoic acid (DHA, a omega-3 fatty acid), are especially important for a baby's development. For example, AA plays a dominant role as the most prominent essential fat in the placenta from the earliest weeks of pregnancy through delivery. The omega-3s, on the other hand, take the spotlight when it comes to the baby's brain, nervous system, and eye development. Babies develop optimally when there is a fine balance of AA and DHA. AA has to be made from a fellow omega-6 called linoleic acid (LA), one of two essential fats. DHA, on the other hand, can be derived with "no assembly required" directly from eating fish, fish oil, or supplements containing omega-3s made by marine algae (which is mostly in the form of DHA); in humans only, a scant amount of DHA can be assembled from the other essential fat, a fellow omega-3 called alpha-linolenic acid (ALA).

But there's one more long-chain omega-3 that we should emphasize here: eicosapentaenoic acid (EPA). Ample EPA in your body may suppress abnormal inflammatory processes and eventually help prevent the uterine contractions of premature labor, though the science on the latter is especially young. Interestingly, EPA and DHA can interconvert when one is needed more than the other, but retroconversion from DHA back to EPA is extremely slow. Things work best when both of these long-chain omega-3s are plentiful. You don't want internal competition for omega-3s before your pregnancy, nor do you want maternal-fetal competition after you conceive. Let's make sure you have plenty to share, both for the known benefits and in case preliminary evidence is confirmed that the fetus uses omega-3s to strengthen its developing immune system, thereby reducing chances of childhood asthma, allergies, and infections.

The problem with achieving a balance of readily available AA and DHA (and EPA) for pregnancy is that the North American diet typically provides way too many omega-6s and too few omega-3s. In fact, it is not uncommon for the omega-6 fatty acids to outnumber the omega-3s by at least a ratio of 25:1. It is far better to keep this ratio closer to 5:1 (or 10:1 if you follow the more lenient recommended intakes set in the United States). Why does a smaller ratio matter?

Eating excessive omega-6s may have a pro-inflammatory downside when you do not eat enough omega-3s to counterbalance them. It is speculated that overabundant omega-6s crowd out synthesis of the scarcer omega-3 fatty acid DHA. But what does this mean for your body? If dietary omega-6s are overly abundant in your diet and stored in your tissues, they compete with the enzymes needed to make DHA. When this happens during pregnancy the maternal body does all it can to maintain stable DHA levels for your baby's brain development, but if there isn't enough readily available DHA, it will make it from EPA that should be focusing on anti-inflammatory protection. A domino effect ensues.

The omega-3s DHA and EPA are found together in a small handful of foods, so take it in stride when our charts of (preformed) omega-3-rich foods include both; many omega-3 supplements will contain them together, too. Aim for a daily average intake of 500 to 650 mg DHA plus EPA from foods, supplements, or a mixture of both, preferably beginning at least ninety days before trying to conceive. At least 300 mg of this should come from DHA; the other 200–350 mg should come from EPA.[2] There are no Dietary Reference Intakes (DRIs) for

2. International recommendations vary, but the figures given here were established by the International Society for the Study of Fatty Acids and Lipids and the National Institutes of Health and are among the most heavily supported by current research. Another omega-3 called docosapentaenoic acid (DPA; an intermediary long-chain molecule, also called clupanodonic acid to distinguish it from a different DPA in the omega-6 family) should also be included in the mix but is usually not mentioned.

these two long-chain omega-3s yet, but the U.S. Food and Drug Administration suggests not exceeding 3,000 mg per day, with fewer than 2,000 mg from supplements, due to risk of excessive bleeding, so supplement users should be cautious. Fortunately, several well-designed studies on pregnant women have tested this upper limit and haven't identified significant risks, so it appears there's a cushion if you approach that level. Prescription dosages of omega-3s at this magnitude may be warranted if there are special circumstances (e.g., recurrent miscarriages due to antiphospholipid syndrome or exceptionally high triglyceride levels); however, this should be considered only under strict medical supervision. Table 10-3 outlines seven steps toward improving your fatty acid balance, so have your shopping list handy or go to Appendix E, "Shopping List."

Tweaking your balance of omega-6s and omega-3s will optimize your future baby's visual and neural development in the womb and eventually make your breastmilk optimal, too. The evidence is compelling that you'll also be lowering your risk for preeclampsia and preterm delivery as well as inflammation, depression (including postpartum depression), cardiovascular disease, Alzheimer's, certain cancers, and possibly joint pain.

Bottom line: your two goals to restore tissue fat balance during these preconceptional months are to (1) increase direct dietary sources of the omega-3s EPA and DHA to a combined total of 500 to 650 mg/day, while making sure the other essential fatty acids are in balance, and (2) decrease saturated and trans fat intake.

Practical Application

Do you answer yes to any of the following? If so, pay even more attention to how you can boost your levels of DHA and EPA before conception. See Table 10-3 for helpful hints.

Yes / No   I currently eat fewer than two servings of fish per week.

Yes / No   If I eat fish at all, it's usually fried fish or fish sticks.

Yes / No   I eat a lot of processed, prepackaged, or fast foods.

Yes / No   I am a vegan or strict vegetarian.

Yes / No   I strictly avoid fat or have a medical condition that impacts fat absorption.

Yes / No   I already have an infant or twins/triplets under the age of eighteen months and want to become pregnant again soon.

Yes / No   I've recently been pregnant but lost the baby after the first trimester or soon after giving birth.

Yes / No   I had preeclampsia or premature labor/delivery in a prior pregnancy.

Yes / No   I have a history of depression or postpartum depression.

Yes / No   I have a history of high blood pressure or high cholesterol (or a family history).

TABLE 10-3
GET YOUR SHOPPING LIST AND MAKE WAY FOR OMEGA-3s: DHA AND EPA

1. **Get some or most of your DHA and EPA from whole foods, meaning fish and seafood.**
   Don't let anyone convince you otherwise. Research overwhelmingly supports this
   recommendation, with safety and benefits to you and the future baby as guiding forces.
   Unless you're allergic, increase your consumption of oily fish and seafood such as salmon
   (preferably wild), herring, sardines, light tuna (or albacore in smaller amounts), mackerel
   (too "fishy" tasting for some), lake trout, and halibut. These food sources contain already
   formed DHA and EPA and are by far the most efficient way of getting these omega-3s. Plus
   scientists are identifying numerous nutrient synergies and built-in protection mechanisms
   that come from eating whole foods. Aim for three to four servings of different fish or
   shellfish per week for a **goal of 12 ounces per week, no less.** Use the chart below to help
   vary your selection of safe fish and seafoods. Always cook your fish to avoid foodborne
   illnesses. (See Chapter 13, pages 414–420, for safe fish and sustainability.)

DHA AND EPA OMEGA-3 FATTY ACID PROFILES OF PRECONCEPTION- AND PREGNANCY-
FRIENDLY SEAFOODS

Amount	Food, Cooked	DHA mg	EPA mg
3 oz	Mackerel (only small; avoid king)	774	400
3 oz	Salmon	750	400
3 oz	Trout	500	320
3 oz	Tuna, canned, albacore (<6 oz/week)	535	198
3 oz	Sea bass	473	175
3 oz	Mussels	430	235
3 oz	Freshwater bass	389	259
1 oz	Anchovy, canned, drained	360	216
1 oz	Herring	279	302
3 oz	Halibut	318	77
3 oz	Squid (calamari)	323	138
1.5 oz	Oysters, eastern (6 medium)	245	225
3 oz	Sole, flounder	219	207
3 oz	Oysters, canned	194	179
3 oz	Perch	210	87
3 oz	Surimi made from *fish* (not crab)	205	133
3 oz	Tuna, canned light (chunk light)	190	40

Amount	Food, Cooked	DHA mg	EPA mg
3 oz	Lobster, shell off	118	290
3 oz	Crab	98	240
1 oz	Sardines, canned	144	134
3 oz	Shrimp	122	145
3 oz	Clams	124	117
3 oz	Cod, haddock	139	65
3oz	Catfish	112	54
3 oz	Eel	69	92
3 oz	Scallops	66	55
3 oz	Tilapia	43	2

Source: USDA Searchable Database on Food Content. Accessed February 2010. Data was averaged for some fish with a common name representing more than one species (e.g., numbers for salmon are averaged from several species of salmon).

Reference for measurement: A 3 oz portion of fish is approximately as compact as a deck of cards. A 1 oz portion is approximately the size of four dice side by side.

2. **Omega-3 supplements.** You can meet the daily goal of 650 mg of the preformed/mature omega-3 fats from foods alone, but if you're not a fish lover, it can be really tough. High-quality fish oil supplements may be a low-mercury yet rich source of omega-3 fatty acids, though their safety and effectiveness during preconception and pregnancy are only recently attracting vigorous scientific scrutiny. (Note: Fish *liver* oils may contain unsafe levels of the fat-soluble vitamins A and D. Do not take them during this phase of your life.) If you decide to choose a fish oil supplement with physician approval to partially or fully meet your omega-3 goals, store them according to package instructions.

There are a dizzying number of fish oil supplements on the market, and they vary in quality, stability, taste, and palatability. Two over-the-counter brands in particular, Nordic Naturals and Coromega (a gel packet, for those who don't like to swallow pills), pass our scrutiny and could be good ones to try. Pharmaceutical companies are also developing prescription-only prenatal vitamin supplements with separate fish oil capsules (e.g., DuetDHA by StuartNatal); since these fall under the prescription drug laws, they are regulated for safety and purity. Vegetarian alternatives to fish oil supplements are appearing on the market at an increasing pace. The source of DHA in the vegetarian supplements is marine algae, but algae is not a good source of EPA, and your body is inefficient at converting DHA back into EPA (though it will try as best it can). Examples of algae DHA supplements include Martek DHA Neuromins and Mead Johnson Expecta Lipil.

3. **Vegan food sources of omega-3s.** Some plant foods contain the essential polyunsaturated fatty acid alpha-linolenic acid (ALA), which must mature into the longer-chain omega-3s (EPA

and DHA) before they can do their critically important jobs during pregnancy. However, this conversion process is inefficient or even absent in a small percentage of the population. Evelyn Tribole, MS, RD, author of *The Omega-3 Diet,* points to recent research showing that only about 2.7 percent of the ALA you eat is turned into EPA, and virtually none of it makes it to the next step, DHA. According to Tribole, "Pregnant women need at least 650 milligrams a day of EPA plus DHA and unless you eat fish regularly or take fish oil, you will not likely meet this amount." So eat your plant food sources of ALA because they help the whole-body balance of essential fats (remember that 5:1 ratio). Food sources that contain small but significant amounts of ALA include walnuts and walnut oil, butternuts (the nuts, not the squash), canola oil, non-genetically modified soybean oil, soybeans and soy products, pumpkin seeds, and pumpkin seed oil. They have the added benefit of being more resistant to rancidity than fish oils (though walnut and pumpkin oils need refrigeration), and are usually void of the mercury or polychlorinated biphenyl (PCB) contamination that taints some fish. Aim for at least one serving of ALA-rich food per day, and vary the choices as much as possible. One note: You may know that ground flaxseeds and flaxseed oil are the best sources of ALA. However, the well-known flaxseed researcher Lilian Thompson, PhD, from the University of Toronto remains cautious and advises pregnant women to avoid or strictly limit eating flaxseed products (especially the flax flour or meal; eggs from flax-fed hens should be okay). Too little is known about flaxseed and safety to the fetus, so until we see fewer conflicting study results, begin choosing other ALA sources now and through your pregnancy.

4. **Omega-3s in disguise.** Eat up to one "designer egg" per day from hens fed diets enriched with flaxseed, canola oil, or, best of all, marine algae. The carton will say "omega-3" on it. Whether or not the eggs are organic, free-range, or brown or white is a personal choice that does not alter the omega-3 potential of the egg. A few examples of reputable brands are Gold Circle Farms (boasting 150 mg DHA per egg, compared to 20 mg in a regular egg), Eggland's Best, Chino Valley Ranchers, and Organic Valley. In the United States, cattle are mainly grain-fed and have no DHA, but if the cattle are grass-fed, a 3-ounce serving of lean beef has approximately 30 mg DHA. DHA-fortified milk or yogurt has 32 mg DHA per serving. Check the labels of other products that claim to be DHA-fortified.

5. **Best plant-derived oils.** Plant oils contain mixtures of fatty acids, including varying amounts of omega-3s, omega-6s, monounsaturated fats (which are also called omega-9s), and saturated fats. Some plant oils are outstanding sources of one predominant fatty acid (e.g., olive oil, for its monounsaturated fat). But when you see the same plant oil discussed more than once in the next three paragraphs, it's because there is more than one thing that makes the oil a good choice (e.g., canola oil is desirable for both its omega-3s and its monounsaturated fats). Since different plant-derived oils are needed to fulfill different needs, we ask you to choose a few for your stock of healthy oils.

    Omega-3s (choose one or two for your pantry). Not many preconception-friendly oils contain the omega-3 ALA as part of their fatty acid profile, but that's okay. A few do. And you don't need much. The pregnancy DRI is only 1.4 grams per day, though a little more is welcome. Our favorite recommendations are canola, walnut, and pumpkin seed oils. (Recall from item 3 that flaxseeds and flaxseed oil have the highest amount of ALA but are probably best left alone until after your pregnancy.) Your body will convert some of the oil's ALA directly into the anti-inflammatory EPA, and the rest is used for other functions or is burned for energy. Some non-genetically modified soybean oils and soybean oil blends meet the criteria as viable substitutes, but our favorites still stand. Canola oil (and the soybean oil) are great for cooking, while walnut and pumpkin oils are best reserved for cold preparations such as salad dressings.

Omega-6s are an optional pantry item because many are already part of your diet. For example, soybean oil is the predominant oil used by food manufacturers and restaurants. Read labels and inquire at restaurants to confirm what you're getting. Oils that are rich in the essential omega-6 fat linoleic acid (LA) include sunflower, grapeseed, soybean (non-GMO and, even more so, GMO), peanut, sesame, corn, cottonseed, and most vegetable oils. They can be chosen in more modest quantities than most people do these days, but you still need approximately five to ten times more LA than ALA. For example, the DRI charts recommend 11 grams per day for a nonpregnant woman and 13 grams per day during pregnancy, which you can get from just over a tablespoon of store-bought salad dressing that contains soybean or sunflower oil (go open your refrigerator and check!). There should be room in your diet for these liquid oils because you have minimized your intake of spreads, shortenings, and fried foods containing these oils, particularly in their synthetically altered form (the trans fats). A variety of nuts and seeds are other excellent sources of these polyunsaturated oils and may be eaten regularly in serving sizes consistent with the USDA MyPyramid (food guidance system). Remember, LA is the starting material for arachidonic acid (AA), defined earlier as the omega-6 that is essential for robust placental and fetal development.

Monounsaturated fat (choose one or two for your pantry). Olive oil should be one of your primary go-to oils to add variety to your oil portfolio. It's mostly monounsaturated fat (omega-9), which serves as an energy source, is kind to your cardiovascular system, and does not antagonize the balance between the essential omega-3 and omega-6 fats. Unrefined or extra-virgin olive oil retains natural phytochemicals and other healthy substances that most refined oils lose during processing. Quite similar to olive oil but harder to find are tea seed, avocado, and almond oils. Safflower (labeled high monounsaturated or high oleic), canola, sesame, and peanut oils also have a nice amount of monounsaturated fat. Olive oil is versatile and stable for most cooking. For high-heat cooking, tea seed oil is remarkably stable (though canola is almost as stable and way more cost-effective).

All oils, nuts, and seeds should be eaten in serving sizes consistent with MyPyramid (in Chapter 12). You have lots of choices, so keep a few kinds in your cupboard or refrigerator, and alternate eating them. If you follow these recommendations, you need not be any more precise to meet your needs.

6. **Track down trans fats.** Cut way back on industrially produced trans fats from baked goods, shortening, margarine, and packaged foods that contain hydrogenated or partially hydrogenated oils in the ingredient list. If a serving of the food contains 1 gram or more of trans fat, according to the Nutrition Facts label, it's a food to drop from your repertoire. Nutrition Facts panels may state 0 grams of fat if a serving provides less than 0.5 grams per serving, but if you notice it's still in the ingredient list, it should not be eaten in multiple servings lest that negligible amount adds up to too much. If a product contains fully hydrogenated vegetable oil, the American Heart Association (AHA) currently says to count

Fat Calories and Fat Grams

Fat is a very concentrated source of calories. Each gram of fat, regardless of whether it's unsaturated or saturated, contains 9 calories. For example, a McDonald's Quarter Pounder with cheese offers a whopping 510 calories and 26 grams of fat. That is 26 grams × 9 calories/gram = 234 calories from fat—much of it saturated. One tablespoon of canola oil or olive oil tossed in a salad or with cooked pasta has 14 grams of fat, so 14 grams × 9 calories/gram = 126 calories per tablespoon, mostly monounsaturated—a better choice, as it's associated with lower risk for coronary artery disease. A modest 3-ounce serving of baked salmon has about 155 calories and 7 grams of fat, 63 calories from primarily the omega-3 fatty acids EPA and DHA.

these as a source of saturated fat, not trans. However, the AHA concedes that these fully hydrogenated oils, also called interesterified fats, may have a different physiological effect from traditional saturated fats, and more research is needed.

7. **Limit saturated fat sources.** Reduce your intake of saturated fats by eating only small amounts of fatty meats and high-fat dairy products such as full-fat cheeses, butter, ice cream, and whole milk. Coconut oil and other tropical oils should be limited to small amounts because they are higher in saturated fat than most other plant oils discussed in item 5.

FOR FUTURE REFERENCE: After Delivery

Breastmilk is typically a good source of all essential fatty acids for infants (the maternal diet considerably influences the balance). Unfortunately, breastmilk tested from women in the United States has among the lowest essential fatty-acid levels in the world due to our comparatively lower intake of DHA and EPA omega-3 fats. What a wake-up call to implement the recommendations in Table 10-3! Prior to 2002 the FDA allowed infant formulas to include only the precursors to DHA and AA, which at best are inefficiently used by infants, particularly preemies. In many other countries, formula manufacturers have long been required to add fully formed DHA and AA. In a smart move, the U.S. FDA is now permitting the same here.

Cholesterol

Cholesterol and fat are closely related, but they are really two different substances that happen to be found in many of the same foods. Cholesterol has no calories, whereas fat is a dense source of calories. Cholesterol functions as a structural part of every cell membrane in our bodies, so during times of rapid cell division and growth (such as pregnancy) cholesterol is especially important. It is also essential for making certain hormones and vitamin D as well as a digestive compound called bile acid. But as essential as cholesterol is, diets that are too high in saturated fat and cholesterol have been implicated in heart disease.

You get cholesterol from dietary sources, but your body can make sufficient amounts, too. So no extra effort is needed to get enough cholesterol. Fat comes from plant and animal sources; cholesterol is found *only* in animal foods such as organ meats, meat, poultry, seafood, egg yolks, cheese, and other dairy products. Thus, foods such as peanut butter and olive oil contain no cholesterol, but do have a significant amount of fat and calories.

The only high-cholesterol foods that should be limited from the month before conception through pregnancy are liver and giblets. This has more to do with their excessively high levels of vitamin A than their cholesterol content. An occasional small amount of liver and giblets in homemade stuffing or gravy is fine. However, an average portion of liver, chicken livers, liverwurst, foie gras, or liver cheese is better left alone when considering conceiving.

HOW TO READ A LABEL

To simplify label reading for the general public, the FDA came up with reference values for certain nutrients. These daily dietary intake standards are called Daily Values (DV). Many labels list the DV toward the base of the label panel for both a 2,000- and 2,500-calorie daily "reference diet." In addition to what you see on an ordinary food label, a number of food manufacturers and supermarkets are participating in nutrient profiling by using on-pack rating symbols or shelf tags; many are based on high nutrition standards (e.g., the Guiding Stars system), but you'll now be able to identify which ones are more heavily influenced by commercialism than good nutrition. Restaurants, too, are beginning to provide nutrient analyses on menus or have it available upon request or online.

Amounts of individual nutrients in a single serving of food are expressed as a percentage of the total DV. The percentage of Daily Values (%DVs) for total fat, saturated fat, total carbohydrate, dietary fiber, and protein are based on a 2,000-calorie reference diet. Therefore, your needs may vary somewhat, depending on your personal calorie requirements and pre-pregnancy weight. There may be no %DV stated for protein because its listing is optional; however, the DV for protein is 50 grams if you want to calculate it yourself. There is no DV for unhealthy trans fats, so it's best to compare rival products and choose the version with the lowest amount or forgo it if none fit your needs. There is also no DV for sugars, because it would be difficult to pin down an appropriate amount to have in the diet. Keep in mind that sugars include natural sugar found in fruits and lactose (the simple carbohydrate in milk) as well as table sugar, corn syrup, and honey.

Knowing the %DV helps consumers compare how certain nutrients in a serving of a food match up to the model 2,000-calorie reference diet. People who meet 100 percent of the DVs for each nutrient from a variety of healthy foods over the course of a day can feel reasonably comfortable that their diet favorably resembles the reference diet on which the government bases its guidelines.

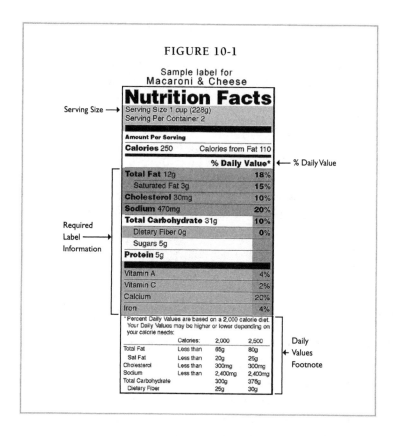

FIGURE 10-1

In this example, one serving of the food has 12 grams of fat and the %DV is 18 percent. In other words, if a consumer has one serving—though who eats only *half* of this type of meal?—the 12 grams of fat count as almost one-fifth of her total daily fat. The amounts of unhealthy fats are the real deal breakers here, with 3 grams of trans fat and 3 more grams of saturated fat, both doubled when the whole entrée is consumed.

Similarly, this product contains 0 grams of dietary fiber, which fulfills none of her DV for fiber based on a requirement of 25 grams, as noted at the base of the label.

Also listed on the Nutrition Facts label are %DVs for cholesterol, sodium, and often potassium; the DVs for these are the same no matter what your calorie intake. The FDA determined DVs for an additional nineteen vitamins and minerals based on previous government recommendations that meet most people's needs. They're still good broad recommendations, despite the fact that they aren't as individualized as the age- and gender-geared Dietary Reference Intakes (DRIs), discussed later. Of the nineteen DVs, only two minerals (calcium and iron) and two vitamins (A and C) are required to be listed as a %DV on food labels. Others may be voluntarily listed by the food manufacturers.

Supplements, on the other hand, must represent each amount of ingredient as a %DV on the Supplement Facts label. As a rule of thumb, a woman planning for pregnancy should try not to exceed 100 percent of the DV for vitamins or minerals in supplement form (including frequently eaten fortified foods) unless her physician has approved it.

Practical Application

Look at some of the food labels of packaged foods in your refrigerator, pantry, or cupboard. Notice the %DVs. Compare foods based on their similarities and differences in nutrient composition. Use this valuable label information along with what you are learning in these chapters to adjust your shopping list in Appendix E to include items that will create better balance and variety.

ENOUGH BUT NOT TOO MUCH: RATIONALE FOR DIETARY REFERENCE INTAKES

The National Research Council of the National Academy of Sciences advises the federal government on matters pertaining to adequate nutrient intakes. Historically, they have been responsible for establishing the Recommended Dietary Allowances (RDAs). The RDAs are only one component of the updated and expanded Dietary Reference Intakes (DRIs). In Chapter 11 we use the information from the DRI charts to set nutrient goals for vitamins and minerals for optimal preconception health; we also include information on absolute upper levels of safety that you shouldn't exceed if you choose to consume more than the recommended amount. The complete DRI tables for different ages and genders are found in Appendix B.

If you note discrepancies between DRIs and the DVs, don't worry. Remember that the DVs are for label reading on food packages and do not apply to a specific age or gender. Don't let the minor differences concern you. We will let you know if one recommendation is more applicable to preconception than the other.

CHAPTER 11

Vitamins, Minerals, and Supplements

*N*ever before has there been such enthusiasm about the impressive properties of vitamins and minerals. Historically, scientists knew only that a lack of these essential nutrients created serious health conditions. Today, marginal nutritional deficiencies remain a public health concern for certain at-risk individuals, but life-threatening deficiencies are almost unheard of. Instead, now that vitamins and minerals are widely available in supplement form, it is more common to see toxic overdoses.

Occasionally, a patient dumps an arsenal of supplements from her purse onto the desk and asks, "What do you think of these?" A typical collection includes several individual packets of high-potency prenatal supplements ordered through the Internet, a few vitamin supplements prescribed by her chiropractor, and numerous herbal products. It quickly becomes apparent that, taken daily, they either add up to megadoses or create unhealthy imbalances. Increasingly, dietitians and doctors are having to temper the public's attitude that supplements can do no wrong. More is not necessarily better, especially when planning for conception.

In the following pages we address your most frequently asked questions about individual vitamins and minerals:

> What do vitamins and minerals do, and how are conception and early fetal development affected by them?
> How much of each does the body need in preparation for making a baby?
> Will extra amounts be helpful or harmful?
> What foods are highest in selected nutrients?
> Should certain foods or supplements be avoided due to their vitamin or mineral content?

What can be done to maximize the effectiveness of particular micronutrients from foods or supplements?

Once you've familiarized yourself with the answers to these questions, you'll be able to make a more informed decision about whether you need a supplement and, if so, what the guidelines are for choosing and safely taking one. This discussion begins on page 353.

As you read the following pages, understand that your body never absorbs 100 percent of the vitamins or minerals you consume, regardless of the source. This is partially a natural outcome of eating a healthy mix of foods, but it's also a built-in protective mechanism. If you absorbed every bit of the vitamins and minerals from what you eat, you could get too much of certain ones, so your body guards against nutrient toxicities as best it can (megadosing overwhelms this capability). Therefore, contrary to the implication that a fortified cereal or pill can give you everything you need for the day, we offer guidance on how to optimize your intake of micronutrients—with the understanding that this cannot be accomplished in one fell swoop. You need a whole day's worth of meals and snacks. Also, avoid the temptation to zero in on one "magic" food, vitamin, or mineral. Your job is to eat a variety and balance of foods—and perhaps an approved supplement. Your body naturally works out the details of making the best use of what you've offered it, within reason.

VITAMINS

Water-Soluble Vitamins

There are two categories of vitamins, water-soluble and fat-soluble, depending on their structure. This determines how they are transported, stored, and excreted within the human body. There are nine essential water-soluble vitamins. Key vitamins for pregnancy are folate and vitamins C, B_6, and B_{12}. The body does not maintain large reserves of water-soluble vitamins, so they must be consumed regularly to prevent deficiencies. These vitamins are also more vulnerable to destruction by light and heat. If they are added to a food by being sprayed on the food surface (e.g., on a cereal flake), they can dissolve in liquid (so drink the milk in your cereal bowl instead of discarding it).

Folate or Folic Acid

Description and Function. Folate is a B vitamin that occurs naturally in foods. The synthetic form of folate is called folic acid. Folic acid is what is added to supplements or fortified foods and is considered to be 1.7 to 2 times as potent as natural folate.

Folate is required to decode and synthesize the genetic material (DNA) and to make new cells. During pregnancy the rapid growth of the fetus and placenta as well as the de-

Facts About Neural Tube Defects

The incidence of neural tube defects (NTDs) in the United States is 7.2–15.6 per 10,000 live-born and stillborn infants (this estimate doesn't include early miscarriages).

The two most common NTDs are:

- **Spina bifida.** Birth defect where the neural tube of the spine doesn't get completely enclosed; spinal cord membranes are pushed through the incomplete closures and form protrusions that look like tumors but are not true tumors. Paralysis as well as bowel and bladder incontinence may occur; mental capacity may diminish with secondary complications.
- **Anencephaly.** Also a birth defect, an essential part of the brain never develops; babies rarely survive longer than a few hours after birth.

velopment of maternal tissues mean greater demands for folate. Many important metabolic reactions, including some that regulate blood clotting and placenta development, also require folate as a participant. Formation of hemoglobin, which carries oxygen in red blood cells, depends on cooperation between folate and vitamin B_{12}. There is new interest in how folate may play a role in preventing preterm births (especially births that occur eight or more weeks early), which most often have their origin in unrecognized maternal infections that occurred at or near the time of conception.

Of all the vitamins and minerals, folate is the only one that currently has unanimous public health support to take now, before you get pregnant. Why? Because poor folate intake increases the risk of neural tube defects (NTDs)—birth defects of the brain and spinal cord—and it is hard to get enough from food alone. It is estimated that up to 70 percent of NTDs can be prevented by folic acid supplementation combined with a folate-rich diet.[1] Neural tube development must be completed by the twenty-eighth day after conception. So the timing of folic acid supplementation is critical. It can reduce the risk of NTDs only if taken beginning at least one month before conception through the first two missed periods, to ensure that the first four weeks after conception are covered in women with irregular menstrual cycles. If you begin supplementation after that time, it doesn't mean an NTD is destined, but the fetus misses out on this extra protection. Looking beyond the time of neural tube closure, optimal folate intake continues to support healthy growth of the fetus, placenta, and maternal tissues (uterine muscle, blood volume, breast tissue, and more).

1. The only women who do not appear to gain protection against NTDs from folic acid supplementation are women who enter pregnancy obese. This may be because obesity is an independent risk factor for NTDs—too complex for folic acid supplementation to override. The only known antidote is to healthfully lose weight to a BMI below 30 before conceiving.

There is also speculation that adequate folate and B_{12} before conception could reduce the risk of random genetic events, such as Down syndrome. Every month right before ovulation, the egg intended for release resumes preparation of the chromosomes, which carry genetic material. If a complication occurs in this process, an extra chromosome may find its way into the fertilized embryo, causing Down syndrome (this was discussed in more detail in Chapter 6). It is possible that women could be at higher risk for this chromosomal abnormality if they can't metabolize folate very well. So getting enough folate before ovulation and conception occur may be even more important than we ever knew. This possible dietary link, however, is only one piece of the puzzle. Other influences on the fetus's first environment include high alcohol consumption, crash dieting near the time of conception, advanced maternal age, and heredity. For example, Hispanic women are more likely to have folate metabolism defects, and African Americans are least likely to have this problem; perhaps not coincidentally, the prevalence of Down syndrome and NTDs are highest in Hispanic babies and lowest in African American babies.

Women's Preconception Recommendation. The RDA is 400 mcg per day of synthetic folic acid from fortified foods, supplements, or a combination of both for at least one month prior to conception.[2] Some public health advocates recommend taking folic acid in the range of 400 to 800 mcg per day, to better cover women in countries where routine fortification is absent. The higher end of the range may also better protect women at higher risk for NTDs (Hispanic and non-Hispanic white women, obese women, and women who have diabetes or a family member affected by an NTD), though this still needs more study. If you're like some of our patients who prefer to get vitamins and minerals "naturally," with no supplements whatsoever, you can most likely get the same protection solely from naturally occurring folate, but that would be equivalent to eating a minimum of 680 to 800 mcg of folate-rich foods every day—very challenging for most people.[3] More recent research published in the *American Journal of Clinical Nutrition* (2007) suggests that the bioavailability of folate is only about 20 percent less than synthetic folic acid instead of 40 or 50 percent lower. This is encouraging, but further substantiation is needed before any changes are made to current recommendations.

Pregnancy Recommendation. Keep taking the 400 mcg per day of folic acid through your first two missed periods. It might help to simply keep this up through the remainder of your pregnancy, though the RDA states that the equivalent of 600 mcg per day of naturally occurring folate[4] is fine after the first trimester. You can meet your pregnancy needs from foods, supplements, or a combination of both.

2. The current recommended intakes for folate may also safeguard against coronary heart disease, stroke, cervical cancer, colon cancer, and Alzheimer's, so it's not just for women of childbearing potential.

3. We cannot be certain that food folate confers the exact protection that synthetic folic acid does, since the RDA was established from research using synthetic folic acid to guarantee that study participants got the standard dosage. This doesn't diminish the importance of eating healthy food sources of folate.

4. The equivalent of 300 to 350 mcg of synthetic folic acid (per DRI charts in Appendix B).

EXCEPTIONS TO THE RULE:
WHO MAY NEED MORE THAN THE ORDINARY FOLIC ACID DOSAGE?

• Women who have previously had a pregnancy involving an NTD are currently advised to take 4,000 mcg of folic acid per day, or ten times the usual amount, under doctor supervision; most other exceptions do not require this high a dose.
• Women with seizure disorders or those on certain psychiatric medications may have higher needs that should be individually assessed.
• Women with recurrent pregnancy loss related to the MTHFR genetic variant, which affects folate metabolism, also should be individually assessed. Ask whether a supplement containing L-methylfolate could be a better form of folic acid if this describes you.

All of these patients should get their extra folic acid from a separate single vitamin pill, not from multivitamin-mineral supplements. Physician consultation is imperative, and one's vitamin B12 status and homocysteine status should be concurrently monitored.

Daily Value (DV) for Food Labeling. The DV has always been 400 mcg of synthetic folic acid. The %DV on a Nutrition Facts food label does not distinguish whether the food contains preexisting natural folate or added folic acid; however, the separate Ingredient List should specify folic acid if it has been added.

Best Food Sources of Folate. Because there is a difference in potency between natural and synthetic versions of folate, it is expressed in units called dietary folate equivalents (DFEs). We have to make this distinction because there is an upper limit of safety of 1,000 mcg for synthetic folic acid from supplements and fortified foods (excluding women with a prior history of an NTD-affected pregnancy or seizure disorders and excluding women on certain psychiatric medications). There is no upper limit on consumption of naturally occurring folate. Synthetic folic acid added to food (such as a fortified grain product) is 1.7 times more potent than natural folate; synthetic folic acid in pill form taken on an empty stomach is 2 times more potent than natural folate. For example, your body gets the same amount of usable folate from 25 mcg of folic acid in a pill, 30 mcg folic acid in a bagel made from fortified flour, or 50 mcg folate from an orange. In Table 11-1 we've listed foods in terms of DFEs so you can compare them on a level playing field.

Practical Application

Using a pen or marker, highlight all the foods in Table 11-1 you currently consume. Then look at the foods that you rarely, if ever, eat and try to think of ways to incorporate these into your pre-conception diet. For instance, try lentil or black bean soup, fix yourself a bean burrito, and steam or grill asparagus more often. Try a spinach salad instead of the Caesar salad next time you go out, drink orange juice instead of apple juice, and put raspberries on your breakfast cereal instead of a banana.

TABLE 11-1
FOOD SOURCES OF NATURAL FOLATE AND SYNTHETIC FOLIC ACID, IN DIETARY
FOLATE EQUIVALENTS (DFEs)

Since 1998 the Food and Drug Administration has required that all enriched breads, flour, cornmeal, pasta, rice, and some other grain products be fortified with modest amounts of folic acid. These are indicated by an asterisk (*). Some products, particularly certain breakfast cereals, are fortified with up to four times the FDA-mandated amount, which can be helpful for women who don't take folic acid in pill form. However, if you are taking 400 mcg of supplemental folic acid to satisfy your preconception requirement, try not to regularly exceed 600 mcg (equal to 1,020 mcg DFE) from the asterisk-marked foods. Why? Because the combined total would surpass the daily upper limit of 1,000 mcg of synthetic folic acid. Remember: there is no daily limit on natural folate (the ones without an asterisk).

Food Source	Folate Content (mcg DFE)
HIGHEST (MORE THAN 150 MCG DFE PER SERVING)[a]	
*1 serving (size varies; see Nutrition Facts label) ready-to-eat cold cereals or packaged hot cereals fortified with:	
• 25% of the Daily Value	170
• 50% of the Daily Value	340
• 100% of the Daily Value	680
*1 cup rice, enriched, cooked	170
*1 cup macaroni product, enriched, cooked	160
*1 serving liquid meal replacements	170
½ cup, cooked:	
lentils	179
mung beans, not sprouted	160

Food Source	Folate Content (mcg DFE)
HIGH (101–150 MCG DFE PER SERVING)	
*1 10-inch-diameter flour tortilla, enriched	140
6 spears asparagus	132
½ cup, cooked from fresh or frozen (canned foods lose about half of their folate):	
baby lima beans, pinto beans	136–147
spinach, turnip greens	131–134
kidney beans, white beans, navy beans, and black beans	114–128
MEDIUM (51–100 MCG DFE PER SERVING)	
*½ cup grits, enriched, cooked	70
¼ cup soybean nuts	90
¼ cup wheat germ	75
1 cup blackberries, raspberries, boysenberries	51–84
½ cup, cooked from fresh or frozen (unless otherwise noted):	
broad beans, great northern beans	88–90
turnip greens	85
chickpeas (garbanzo beans), navy beans, canned	80–81
kidney beans, canned	64
split peas	63
homemade baked beans	61
green peas	51
½ cup, raw:	
collards, chopped, frozen	65
spinach, turnip greens, raw, chopped	54
1 medium artichoke, boiled	61
4 oz orange juice from frozen concentrate	54
1 oz seaweed (nori or wakami; see section on iodine, pages 348–349), raw	51

Food Sources	Folate Content (mcg DFE)
STILL GOOD, BUT LOWER (26–50 MCG DFE PER SERVING)	
*1 3-inch-diameter bagel, enriched	50
1 navel orange	47
½ cup tempeh, miso	43–46
1 cup plantain slices, cooked	40
½ cup, cooked from fresh or frozen:	
Brussels sprouts	47
beets	45
parsnips	45
cauliflower, broccoli, okra	32–39
½ cup romaine lettuce, shredded	38
½ cup tofu, raw, firm	37
½ cup endive, raw and chopped	36
¼ cup hummus	36
*1 waffle, frozen	35
*1 slice bread, enriched	35
*1 small roll, biscuit, pita, cornbread, muffin, English muffin (half), enriched	25–45
¼ medium avocado	34
1 oz most nuts and seeds	30
1 cup strawberries, cantaloupe	26–27

a. Although an excellent source of folate, liver should be strictly limited or avoided due to its extremely high vitamin A content. For this reason, it is omitted from this category of the table.

Sources: J. A. T. Pennington, *Bowes & Church's Food Values of Portions Commonly Used,* 16th ed. (Philadelphia: Lippincott, 1994); U.S. Department of Agriculture data interpreted by C. W. Suitor and L.B. Bailey, "Dietary Folate Equivalents: Interpretation and Application," *Journal of the American Dietetic Association* 100 (2000): 88–94.

Folate and Prenatal Vitamins

Women often ask, "Why did my doctor prescribe a prenatal supplement containing 1,000 mcg of folic acid if I only need 400 to 800 mcg?" It's true, many prenatal vitamins contain 1,000 mcg (1 mg), and fortified foods typically provide an additional 100 to 200 mcg of folic acid per day to the average woman's diet. We still recommend finding one with only 400 to 800 mcg, but this is one instance when health care practitioners tend to be lenient about that upper limit.

Choline

Description and Function. Choline, an essential nutrient, but not a true vitamin, is included here because it plays a role similar to folate. It bolsters the health of cell membranes and is needed to make the neurotransmitter acetylcholine, a chemical messenger in the brain. It is critical for developing fetal brain structures and healthy memory for mom and baby. Studies show that, as with folate, women who have low intakes of choline are at a higher risk for having a baby with a neural tube defect, and higher circulating levels of choline are protective against NTDs. Interestingly, the metabolic pathways of choline and folate are intermingled—a deficiency of one places extra demand on the other. Some women (and men) are born with a poorer ability to process choline, folate, or both, and with the extra demands of pregnancy and breastfeeding looming near, the ninety days prior to conception should be used to boost intake to current recommendations. Unlike folic acid, which is found in most vitamin supplements and fortified grains, very few vitamin supplements contain choline, and only one in ten women reach choline goals, so pay close attention to how you can beat this statistic.

Choline is relatively new to the Dietary Reference Intake (DRI) charts, because prior to the late 1990s scientists thought your body could make all it needed. However, choline is now recognized as an essential nutrient that must be partially obtained from the diet, even though the body makes some of its own choline.

Women's Preconception Recommendation. Though 425 mg of choline per day is considered adequate for nonpregnant women, in our opinion it's best to be somewhere between the pregnancy and breastfeeding goals during the preconception months to provide better coverage during the earliest weeks of spinal cord and brain development.

Pregnancy Recommendation. An adequate intake for pregnant women is considered to be 450 milligrams per day. Once you deliver the baby and begin breastfeeding, 550 mg per day is considered to be an adequate intake. (See the box "A Little Help from Choline's Friends.")

Daily Value (DV) for Food Labeling. The DV is 550 mg.

A Little Help from Choline's Friends

An eye-opening study supported by the March of Dimes Birth Defects Foundation in Berkeley, California, found that women with choline intakes near or above 500 mg/day had the lowest risk of a baby with an NTD. But that wasn't the only take-home message. You and your future baby might get a little more "health insurance" when your diet incorporates direct food sources of betaine. In animal studies the body uses betaine to protect cells against environmental stresses as well as incorporating betaine into biochemical pathways. Though our body turns choline into betaine, we can free up some of that choline to do its other jobs by consuming dietary betaine as part of a well-balanced diet. (A good balance of dietary protein derived from a variety of legumes, nuts, soy, and/or animal products helped, too.) Best food sources of betaine include beets, spinach, wheat germ, and wheat-based products (both whole and refined) such as cereals, bread, pancakes, pasta, crackers, and very specific types of fish and shellfish (e.g., shrimp, tilapia).

Best Food Sources of Choline. Liver is an excellent source but should be very limited or avoided preconceptionally. The best concentrated source of choline is found in eggs, with 125 mg in the yolk of one large egg. Good sources of choline include beef, poultry, lamb, pork, fish and shellfish, and soybeans (roughly 60 to 120 mg per serving); modest sources include broccoli, cauliflower, Brussels sprouts, soy milk, milk, yogurt, cottage cheese, and ricotta cheese.

Vitamin C (Ascorbic Acid)

Description and Function. Vitamin C is involved in the collagen formation essential for healthy bones, teeth, skin, ligaments, and cartilage. It helps keep the immune system strong and aids in wound healing. Vitamin C plays a role in protein metabolism, and a particular form of iron is absorbed better in vitamin C's presence. Healthy blood levels of vitamin C are suspected to protect against lead toxicity, too. Vitamin C also has antioxidant properties that appear to block unstable molecules from causing damage and disease in the body. For women, significant deficiencies of vitamin C may play a role in prompting premature delivery. Vitamin C is also important for male fertility because it protects the interior and exterior of male sperm cells. Birth control pills, cigarette smoking, and alcohol tend to deplete stores of vitamin C more rapidly than normal.

Women's Preconception Recommendation. The RDA is 75 mg of vitamin C per day, preferably from foods. A balanced diet that includes a variety of fruits and vegetables will make it easy to meet or exceed this goal. If you are trying to quit smoking prior to conception, add an extra 35 mg per day.

Pregnancy Recommendation. The pregnancy RDA is 85 mg per day.

Daily Value (DV) for Food Labeling. The DV is 60 mg.

Best Food Sources of Vitamin C. Some foods are fortified with ascorbic acid, but fruits and vegetables are the major source for natural vitamin C. Good fruit sources of vitamin C, providing between 25 and 75 mg per serving, include kiwi fruit, citrus fruits (oranges, grapefruit, lime, lemon) and their juices, melon, berries, mango, lychee, cherimoya, and breadfruit. Papaya and guava are standouts, with 188 mg and 165 mg per serving, respectively. Good vegetable sources of vitamin C include broccoli, cauliflower, peppers, tomatoes, cassava, kale, cabbage, kohlrabi, spinach, potatoes, and collard greens. Make it a goal to choose at least one of your fruit or vegetable servings from this list every day.

Note: The maximum upper limit of safety for vitamin C from foods and other sources during preconception and pregnancy is 2,000 mg per day. Women (and men) with a medical condition called hemochromatosis (see page 193) should avoid supplemental vitamin C and seldom exceed the RDA of vitamin C food sources.

FOR FUTURE REFERENCE: During Pregnancy

Researchers who study antioxidant vitamins are interested in the pregnancy complication called preeclampsia (sometimes referred to as toxemia) that can flare in the latter half of pregnancy. Forty percent of women who develop preeclampsia are forced to deliver their babies prematurely. Many studies have searched for a potential preventive role for supplemental vitamins C (1,000 mg) and E (400 IU) beginning in midpregnancy in women at risk for preeclampsia and found no favorable improvements. It appears we are not intervening early enough. Few, if any, nutrition-oriented studies look at what could be done prophylactically—meaning three months before and after conception (long before preeclamptic symptoms begin). This is perplexing given the growing knowledge that preeclampsia stems primarily from early complications with implantation in the womb and is followed by a compromised placental connection with the baby. To date, the best preventative nutrition interventions associated with decreasing the risk of preeclampsia are to take a daily multivitamin or prenatal vitamin supplement beginning in the months before conception and continued after conception.[a] Vegetable and fruit consumption on the high end of the recommended ranges helps, too. Importantly, women who are overweight (body mass index over 25) don't reap this protection, providing greater motivation to get as close to being within their BMI goal as possible.

a. This study by Bodnar and colleagues, published in the *American Journal of Epidemiology* in 2006, didn't specifically note the content of the vitamin supplements. In addition, most multivitamin supplements contain folic acid, which may have a role in ameliorating infection. Minerals such as calcium, too, cannot be ruled out as a possible factor in controlling the high blood pressure that accompanies preeclampsia.

Vitamin B₆ (Pyridoxine)

Description and Function. Vitamin B₆ is important for amino acid and protein metabolism as well as conversion of the amino acid tryptophan into niacin. Adequate vitamin B₆ promotes a healthier nervous system, immune system, red blood cells, and cardiovascular system.

It remains controversial whether supplemental doses of B₆ can diminish symptoms of PMS, but it does help lessen the severity of morning sickness. If you're interested in supplementation, discuss it with a qualified health care professional and never exceed 100 mg per day prior to or during pregnancy, due to toxicity concerns; this upper limit includes food sources as well as supplements.

Vitamin B₆ requirements are higher for pregnant women than for nonpregnant women; B₆ is also one of the vitamins which pregnant women tend to have inadequate intakes, so make sure to optimize pre-pregnancy B₆ intake by consuming a variety of the best food sources. Recent studies demonstrate that the mother's B₆ status prior to conception is just as critical to healthy development of the baby as her B₆ status during pregnancy.

Alcohol and caffeine as well as certain medications (e.g., birth control pills and theophylline for asthma patients) may compete with vitamin B₆ and therefore slightly increase a woman's needs. To make up for the loss of B₆ due to past or present use of these substances, a supplement with approximately 100 percent of the DV for B₆ may be appropriate. Some medications may necessitate as much as 10 mg supplemental B₆ per day.

Women's Preconception Recommendation. Aim for the pregnancy RDA of 1.9 mg per day, as B₆ deficiencies are fairly common in pregnant women. The RDA for women not planning pregnancy is 1.3 mg per day.

Pregnancy Recommendation. The pregnancy RDA is 1.9 mg per day.

Daily Value (DV) for Food Labeling: The DV is 2 mg.

Best Food Sources of Vitamin B₆. Foods that contain 0.4 to 0.7 mg per serving include fortified hot and cold cereals, potatoes with skin, bananas, poultry, and meat (limit organ meats). More modest amounts of B₆ (0.2 to 0.4 mg) are found in legumes, fish (especially fatty fish such as salmon, tuna, or trout), avocado, mango, watermelon, and sunflower seeds. Numerous vegetables provide lower amounts of B₆.

Vitamin B₁₂ (Cyanocobalamin)

Description and Function. Like folate, vitamin B₁₂ is needed for DNA synthesis and is necessary for normal red blood cell formation. Vitamin B₁₂ also helps maintain cardiovascular and nervous system health. Some researchers advocate adding a conservative dose of B₁₂ to folic acid supplements, believing that a balanced combination of the two may synergistically reduce the risk of NTDs.

Vitamin B₁₂ deficiencies are seen almost exclusively in people over age fifty, but strict vegetarians (especially vegans) are also at risk because they don't always get enough B₁₂ in their diet. Anyone with a history of gastric bypass or women who have just stopped taking certain birth control pills may be a little low on B_{12}, too. And lastly, if you have been taking metformin for diabetes or PCOS in daily doses over 1,000 mg or for more than two years, there's a greater risk of becoming B_{12} deficient. A mother's deficiency increases the potential damage to a baby in the womb and when exclusively breastfeeding. If you fall into one of these at-risk groups, make sure that your doctor monitors your vitamin B_{12} status and see "Best Food Sources of Vitamin B_{12}" below. Also avoid excess supplementation of folic acid, which can mask a B_{12} deficiency (hence the recommended upper limit of 1,000 mcg of folic acid mentioned earlier).

Women's Preconception Recommendation. The RDA is 2.4 mcg per day.

Pregnancy Recommendation. The RDA is 2.6 mcg per day.

Daily Value (DV) for Food Labeling: The DV is 6 mcg.

Best Food Sources of Vitamin B_{12}. The natural form of Vitamin B_{12} that humans can use is found exclusively in animal foods. Meats, poultry, fish, seafood, eggs, and dairy products are all good sources. For vegans, nutritional yeast and foods fortified with synthetic vitamin B_{12} (some soy milks, meat analogues, and cereals) are reliable sources. Spirulina, tempeh, miso, and sea vegetables may contain B_{12}, but it is not in a form that humans can use. A vitamin supplement containing 100 percent or less of the DV is another option for vegans.

Other Water-Soluble Vitamins

The remaining five water-soluble vitamins are important for your reproductive health but require no extra attention provided you follow a reasonably healthy diet.

Vitamin B₁ (Thiamin)

Description and Function. Helps convert carbohydrates into energy; essential for proper function of nervous system; despite manufacturers' claims, does not "reduce fatigue" or provide an "extra energy boost" in supplemental doses.

Women's Preconception Recommendation. The RDA is 1.1 mg per day.

Pregnancy Recommendation. The pregnancy RDA is 1.4 mg per day.

Daily Value (DV) for Food Labeling: The DV is 1.5 mg.

Best Food Sources of Thiamin. Whole-wheat products (such as 100 percent whole-wheat cereals and breads) and other grains and grain products (oat cereals, rye bread, pastas, and rice) all provide between 0.1 and 0.3 mg per serving. Often thiamin is added back in similar amounts to grains after the refining process. Other good sources include lean pork, peas, dried beans, nuts, milk, and soy milk. Liver and other organ meats are thiamin sources but are not advised in appreciable quantities for preconception or early pregnancy. Thiamin deficiencies are rare in the United States, except among alcoholics.

Vitamin B₂ (Riboflavin)

Description and Function. Helps the body use energy from all types of foods; essential for growth (so pregnant women, infants, and children all have increased requirements). Riboflavin is destroyed by light, so foods containing this B vitamin need to be packaged and stored properly (this is the rationale for milk in cardboard or opaque containers and not glass).

Women's Preconception Recommendation. The RDA is 1.1 mg per day.

Pregnancy Recommendation. The pregnancy RDA is 1.4 mg per day.

Daily Value (DV) for Food Labeling: The DV is 1.7 mg.

Best Food Sources of Riboflavin. The best natural sources of riboflavin are milk, yogurt, mushrooms, cheese, meat, poultry, fish, eggs, and dry-roasted soybean nuts, each containing approximately 0.2 to 0.4 mg per serving. Grains and grain products (cereal, bread, pasta, and rice) are also good sources. Again, liver should be strictly limited. Riboflavin deficiencies are extremely rare except in severely malnourished individuals.

Niacin

Description and Function. This B vitamin helps body cells produce and use energy from food. It is necessary to maintain the health of the nervous system, skin, and digestive tract.

Women's Preconception Recommendation: The RDA is 14 mg per day.

Pregnancy Recommendation. The pregnancy RDA is 18 mg per day.

Daily Value (DV) for Food Labeling: The DV is 20 mg.

Best Food Sources of Niacin. Niacin is found in ample amounts in meats, poultry, and fish; legumes (including peanuts), grains, and grain products (cereal, bread, pasta, and rice) are also good sources. Niacin can also be manufactured in the body from the amino acid tryptophan, so protein-rich foods (meats, meat substitutes, dairy foods) are reliable indirect sources of niacin. A specific form of niacin is sometimes prescribed under medical supervision for its cholesterol-lowering effect, but women planning for pregnancy are advised against this.

Biotin

Description and Function. This B vitamin is required for metabolism of fats, protein, and carbohydrates. Biotin is getting more attention because new information suggests it has important functions in DNA replication and gene expression. Biotin is not typically found in multivitamin supplements, but may be in the future. For now, emphasis should be on food sources.

Women's Preconception Recommendation. Until an RDA can be established, 30 mcg of biotin per day is considered to be an adequate intake.

Pregnancy Recommendation: An adequate intake is considered to be 30 mcg (.03 mg) per day.

Daily Value (DV) for Food Labeling: The DV is 30 mcg per day.

Best Food Sources of Biotin. This B vitamin is widely distributed in food sources, especially cooked egg, yeast, meat (avoid organ meats), legumes, nuts, and cereal. A relatively balanced diet ensures adequate intake. Excesses of biotin are exceedingly rare.

Fat-Soluble Vitamins

There are four fat-soluble vitamins: A, D, E, and K. As their classification suggests, these vitamins dissolve in fats instead of water. This means that in order to travel in the body, they have to hook on to a fat-like substance. Any excess fat-soluble vitamins are stored inside your body fat for later use instead of being excreted in the urine. The ability to store fat-soluble vitamins is helpful in preventing shortages, but it also carries the potential for vitamin toxicity if too much is consumed over time.

Of the four fat-soluble vitamins, the first three—A, D, and E—are the ones you'll need to be most aware of regarding preconception readiness. Vitamin K deficiencies and excesses are rare, so we'll only touch on it at the end.

Vitamin A

Description and Function. Vitamin A is best known for its essential role in vision. It also helps build and maintain the health of bones, skin, and the gastrointestinal and urinary tracts. In addition, it indirectly helps to ward off infection by maintaining the health of internal barriers to disease-carrying organisms.

Vitamin A can be consumed in a fully formed, or preformed, state, or in precursor forms that require transformation within the body into vitamin A. The precursor forms of vitamin A—those found in plant foods such as carrots—are discussed separately below, as they have unique functions and food sources of their own. Fully formed vitamin A is called retinol. It is found naturally in some animal foods and is also used to fortify a small number of foods (e.g., ready-to-eat cereals, milk). When retinol is added to fortified foods or supplements, it is in a more stable form called vitamin A acetate or vitamin A palmitate. Therefore, when you're label reading, fully formed vitamin A may be expressed as vitamin A, retinol, vitamin A acetate, vitamin A palmitate, or retinyl palmitate. All five are essentially the same thing (and worthy of a bright yellow highlighter pen mark right now, to catch your eye later for a quick reference).

Proper intake of vitamin A is extremely important, especially during the initial weeks of pregnancy. Although vitamin A deficiency is a serious issue for women in developing countries, we tend to have the opposite problem: vitamin A toxicity. Overdoses of vitamin A, most commonly from supplements, potentially disrupt fetal development. Birth defects related to vitamin A overdoses include damage to the skull, eyes, brain, heart, and spinal cord. These babies are often spontaneously lost early in the pregnancy, but many are carried to term. The defects may be devastatingly apparent at birth or not identified until later in life. The good news is that vitamin A toxicity is easily preventable.

How much is too much? Daily intake of fully formed vitamin A in excess of 10,000 IU per day may pose a danger, although most studies indicate that the potentially harmful level is closer to a regular intake of 25,000 to 30,000 IU per day. Vitamin A–related birth defects most commonly appear when the mother ingests excess vitamin A during the two weeks prior to conception and/or during the first six weeks of pregnancy. For this reason, we query all childbearing-age patients—even those not intending to conceive for a while—about their intake of vitamin A–containing medications, vitamins, and foods listed in the lower half of Table 11-2. The risk of birth defects increases at a steeper rate when the excess comes from supplements as opposed to foods. To their credit, most reputable supplement companies have voluntarily lowered their preformed vitamin A content or have partially or completely substituted the nontoxic beta-carotene form of vitamin A. We still see some that offer 10,000 IU per dose, though. The few fortified cereals that used to contain 100 percent of the RDA for vitamin A no longer do so either, to our knowledge. Regardless, it's prudent to check the label.

Women's Preconception Recommendation. The RDA is 2,300 IU, also expressed as 700 mcg RAE (retinol activity equivalents). Make sure to meet the RDA, but stay below the safe upper limit of 10,000 IU (3,000 mcg RAE) per day at least one month prior to conception.

Pregnancy Recommendation. The pregnancy RDA is 2,550 IU. Meet this RDA, but stay below 10,000 IU per day.

Daily Value (DV) for Food Labeling: The DV is 5,000 IU per day, about twice the RDA for women (see the note following Table 11-2).

Best Food Sources of Vitamin A. Healthy levels of preformed Vitamin A are found in fortified foods such as some breakfast cereals; dairy products such as milk, most cheeses, butter, and margarine; fortified soy milk; eggs; chicken; fish; and shellfish. Foods such as mashed potatoes are sources of vitamin A, too, because they are generally made with milk and butter. In addition, products in your kitchen that claim to be liquid or bar meal/snack replacements contain some form of vitamin A, so look at the Ingredients List, keeping in mind those five highlighted terms from the previous page.

Liver, which can be extraordinarily high in fully formed vitamin A, is one of the best sources of iron and is frequently recommended for women with iron-deficiency anemia. It's also a nutritious, inexpensive source of folate and other nutrients. However, due to its excessive vitamin A content, we recommend that liver not be consumed in any appreciable quantity beginning in the month before pregnancy through the end of the first trimester, unless you're working with a dietitian to regulate portions and stay within safe limits. Don't worry: a single slice of Braunschweiger, a tiny serving of pâté or foie gras, or a serving of homemade stuffing and gravy containing small bits of chicken or turkey liver periodically will not elevate your risks. To include the very highest iron sources but get around the liver/vitamin A issue entirely, Jean Cox, MS, RD, LN, from the Department of Obstetrics and Gynecology at the University of New Mexico, suggests eating clams, mussels, oysters, and nutritious organ meat substitutes, such as spleen, kidney, heart, and gizzards that are low in vitamin A but excellent sources of highly absorbable iron, in addition to animal proteins listed later in this chapter in Table 11-3.

Below, Table 11-2 lists the preformed vitamin A content of foods that are safe to consume in ordinary quantities and those that should be limited. Rest assured that you could have three servings of milk, a serving or two of breakfast cereal, a breast of chicken or two-egg omelet, and a pat of butter all in one day and still be way under the upper limit, leaving ample cushion for vitamin A found in certain multivitamin supplements.

TABLE 11-2
FULLY FORMED VITAMIN A SOURCES

Amount	Item Name	Vitamin A Content (IU)
SAFE AND RECOMMENDED FOODS		
1 cup	Fortified milk (dairy, soy, rice)	500
1 serving[a]	Fortified ready-to-eat cereals	500–1,250
1 oz	Cheese (most types)	100–500
1	Egg yolk	500
3 oz	Chicken, fish, or shellfish	~50–250
1 tsp	Butter or margarine	165
SAFE NONFOODS (SUPPLEMENTS)		
1 dose[a]	Certain vitamin supplements: those with less than 5,000 IU	
FOODS WARRANTING CAUTION/LIMITATION		
3.5 oz	Liver (chicken, turkey)	12,000–17,000
3.5 oz	Liver (veal, pork, lamb, and beef)	20,000–36,000
3.5 oz	Foie gras (duck or goose liver)	30,000–40,000
1 slice	Braunschweiger and liverwurst, pork liver sausage	4,000–7,500
1-oz slice	Liver cheese (pork liver)	5,000–6,000

Amount	Item Name	Vitamin A Content (IU)
3.5 oz	Giblets (chicken or turkey)	6,000–12,000
1 serving[a]	Meal replacement bars or energy bars: those exceeding 1,250	

SUPPLEMENTS TO AVOID

1 tbsp	Cod liver oil	400–14,000 (these vary too greatly from batch to batch and from brand to brand)
1 dose	Certain vitamin supplements: those exceeding 5,000 IU	

MEDICATIONS TO AVOID

Medications containing vitamin A–derived compounds (the generic isotretinoin, as well as brand names Claravis, Accutane, Roaccutane, and Retin-A topical cream) should be discontinued under the guidance of your physician before you conceive. Usually we recommend quitting oral medications at least three months in advance, skin creams one month in advance.

a. Serving sizes vary. See Nutrition Facts label on foods and Supplement Facts label on supplements.

Note: The DV on food and supplement labels is 5,000 IU per day for vitamin A—roughly twice the RDA for women. The DV does not differentiate between fully formed vitamin A and the provitamin A carotenoids, but during preconception the difference does matter. As a rule of thumb, unless a Nutrition Facts label, Supplements Facts label, or Ingredients List states specifically that a carotenoid such as beta-carotene is the source of vitamin A, assume that all other types of vitamin A are the fully formed or retinol type. For example, the Nutrition Facts label of Brand X breakfast cereal states that a single serving contains 10 percent of the DV for vitamin A; therefore, it contains 500 IU fully formed vitamin A. Or a popular multivitamin supplement contains 100 percent of the DV for vitamin A, but it states "40 percent from beta-carotene." There is really only 60 percent of the DV (3,000 IU) of vitamin A in the retinol form, which is what you count to stay below 10,000 IU day to day.

If a multivitamin supplement has been recommended for you, make sure it contains less than 5,000 IU of vitamin A, preferably with some or all from beta-carotene instead of retinol. This amount of supplemental vitamin A should not take you over the 10,000 IU daily limit as long as you follow a healthy diet.

Practical Application

Periodically we see patients who have already started trying to conceive and realize that on isolated occasions they consumed more than 10,000 IU of vitamin A, primarily from foods (e.g., "a couple of Braunschweiger sandwiches last week" or "a foie gras appetizer at our favorite restaurant"). If this pertains to you, do three things: do not panic, discontinue the foods and supplements in the second half of Table 11-2, and try to stay closer to the RDA of 2,300 IU per day for the following two weeks by eating foods in the top half of that table, then liberalize as desired to no more than 10,000 IU thereafter. If you find that you need to stop taking a multivitamin supplement to adhere to these guidelines, it's important to continue taking a separate supplement containing only folic acid. The only time we recommend that couples stop trying to conceive for an extra one to three months is when the woman has been consistently exceeding 10,000 IU of fully formed vitamin A (primarily from oversupplementation) for several weeks or months.

Provitamin A Carotenoids (Precursors to Vitamin A)

Description and Function. The six hundred or more known plant-synthesized pigments are collectively called carotenoids. Three well-known ones—beta-carotene, alpha-carotene, and beta-cryptoxanthin—as well as fifty other carotenoids can turn into the active form of vitamin A when eaten. To avoid creation of too much vitamin A, the body converts it on an as-needed basis. To date, provitamin A carotenoids are not known to be toxic to humans. Excesses simply turn the skin a harmless shade of orange (reminiscent of the early days of the tan-in-a-bottle for those of us old enough to remember).

Some carotenoids (including the increasingly popular lycopene and lutein) have antioxidant properties that appear to protect against processes inside the body involved in disease and aging.

Women's Preconception Recommendation. No optimal level of intake has been set. However, we suggest that you eat at least two carotenoid-rich vegetables or fruits daily; this is considered to be the best way to get a healthy mix of carotenoids. It is acceptable to take up to 5,000 IU of vitamin A wholly or partially in the form of a precursor, usually beta-carotene, if a vitamin supplement contains it.

Pregnancy Recommendation. Same as preconception recommendation.

Daily Value (DV) for Food Labeling: On food or supplement labels provitamin A carotenoids are counted together with fully formed vitamin A as part of the DV for vitamin A, despite the differences between the two. Usually, manufacturers like to note in parentheses if all or a portion of the vitamin A DV comes from a vitamin A precursor; for example, on a label you might see "Vitamin A (as beta-carotene)," meaning none of the vitamin A is fully formed.

Best Food Sources of Provitamin A Carotenoids. Vegetables and fruits that are colored deep orange, yellow, or green are generally carotene-rich. These include carrots, pumpkin, sweet potatoes, greens (collards, mustard, kale, spinach), broccoli, and peppers. Fruits high in carotenoids are mango, papaya, cantaloupe, guava, apricots, mandarin oranges, nectarines, peaches, persimmons, loquats, and pitanga (Surinam cherry). Carotenoids are not lost through the processing or canning of any of these foods. The full health benefits of eating mixed carotenoids from vegetables and fruits have yet to be replicated in pill form.

Vitamin D

Description and Function. Strangely enough, vitamin D functions as both a vitamin and a hormone. It helps make bones and teeth strong in both you and your baby-to-be. Perhaps more interesting is the way vitamin D assists the immune system and genes that orchestrate repair of damaged cells. Also of interest to women who want to conceive soon is vitamin D's important role in healthy oocyte (egg) formation and insulin sensitivity (insulin-resistant women often have problems with irregular ovulation). Judy Simon, MS, RD, CD, a dietitian and fertility specialist in Seattle, Washington, notes how strikingly many of her female clients are vitamin D deficient: "Here in the Pacific Northwest, vitamin D deficiencies are common, especially in women with polycystic ovary syndrome or those who are overweight and have ovulatory difficulties." She points out that excess fat sequesters or locks up vitamin D, making it less available to do its job. Women who have undergone gastric bypass surgery for weight reduction are also at high risk for vitamin D deficiency. "Once we resolve the vitamin D deficiency through aggressive, supervised supplementation, many of these women begin ovulating spontaneously. It appears critical to improving fertility," she says. Fast-forwarding a bit, during pregnancy your body will freely give calcium to the baby, but it won't be as generous with vitamin D, which needs to be plentiful in your system to support a healthy pregnancy and supply vitamin D in breastmilk for your newborn.

Fortunately, the world has an abundant source of vitamin D: the sun! Your skin can make its own vitamin D when it is directly exposed to UV rays from sunshine. Anything that gets between your skin and the sun (clothing, veil, sunscreen, or glass windows) will significantly impair the ability of the skin to make vitamin D. But exposure to your face, hands, and arms for ten to fifteen minutes at midday for three days per week may be all it takes during the summer months, and this is widely received through incidental exposure. The exposed skin maxes out its daily vitamin D production within twenty minutes' time; slightly before that, it is better to cover up or apply sunscreen.

You cannot depend on the sun year-round for vitamin D since winter sun may seldom or never get intense enough. Nor should you believe claims that a tanning booth is a safer route (it's not), partially because of the known risks for skin cancer. In addition, melanin in darker-skinned women acts as a natural sunscreen, so too much sun exposure is needed to stimulate skin production of vitamin D, leaving most deeply pigmented women in the United States vitamin D deficient and at an inherent risk for maternal and fetal complications.[5] This trend is getting worse, not better, as we spend fewer hours outside and drink less milk (sometimes due to lactose intolerance, or simply in favor of soft drinks). A preconception remedy to this has experts wondering if this could be an important factor in the racial/ethnic disparity in pregnancy outcomes, including vulnerability to infection and rates of preeclampsia, premature birth, and low birth weight. In the northern states and Canada during the winter, the UV rays are often too weak to stimulate the manufacture of vitamin D in the skin. Until recently, it was thought that stored vitamin D along with a healthy diet would suffice to give you what you need during the winter months. However, this is being seriously debated and disproven, and recommended intakes will be raised accordingly. Most women end up needing some degree of vitamin D supplementation, despite good dietary intake.

It has been suggested that sunshine-derived vitamin D plays a role with certain reproductive hormones, making for seasonal variations in fertility. Although little human research has been done to test the theory, it could help explain why decreased conception rates have been observed in women from northern countries during the winter months.

Women's Preconception Recommendation. Although at this writing 200 IU per day from foods is the official recommendation, this amount is described by prominent vitamin D researcher Bruce Hollis, PhD, of Medical University of South Carolina, as "useless for maintaining nutritional vitamin D status, let alone improving it." Newer scientific consensus suggests increasing the recommendation to 400–1,000 IU per day, probably higher for women of childbearing age who are dark-skinned, overweight or obese, recently pregnant, or otherwise at risk for vitamin D deficiency.

Pregnancy Recommendation. Same as preconception. The previous pregnancy recommendation was 400 IU per day and should be reinstated or, preferably, raised.

Daily Value (DV) for Food Labeling: The DV is 400 IU.

Food Sources of Vitamin D. Vitamin D is found in very few foods. Fortified milk (including liquid, powdered, and evaporated) and fortified soy milk provide 100 IU per serving. With the exception of a few yogurt brands (e.g., Yoplait), other dairy products do not. Fortified orange juice may contain 100 IU per serving, but check labels to be sure. Some fortified cereals contain 40 to 80 IU of vitamin D per serving. Fatty fish, egg yolks, butter, and margarine provide slightly lower amounts. Fresh or dried mushrooms contain 30 IU per

---

5. Exposure time for sufficient skin production of vitamin D can vary greatly depending on pigmentation and can amount to up to five or six hours of summer sun in deeply pigmented individuals, versus five to fifteen minutes in lighter-skinned individuals.

ounce of vitamin D, a good vegan choice. Fish liver oils (e.g., cod liver oil) and liver are not recommended as safe sources of vitamin D for pre-pregnancy or pregnancy but are fine postpartum.

Note: If you recognize yourself as possibly being low on vitamin D, go ahead and request a blood test from your doctor. Currently, the best measure is serum 25-hydroxyvitamin D, and ideally, anything below 30 ng/mL should be a red flag for supplementation. If you are hovering right at 30 ng/mL, the typical vitamin D supplement (usually as part of a multivitamin) contains 400 IU and could be sufficient, but higher amounts from a single-ingredient supplement might be necessary—perhaps 1,000–2,000 IU daily. Individual calcium supplements such as Citrical Plus often contain vitamin D too and may be used to provide part of the supplemental vitamin D. If you find that you are vitamin D deficient (below 20 ng/mL, and particularly if below 12 ng/mL), you will need to supplement with even higher amounts, under careful medical supervision. Toxicities of vitamin D are possible, but most research supports increasing the tolerable upper limit to 10,000 IU (it's now set at 2,000 IU per day). Going above the current 2,000 IU limit is okay when you are being treated for deficiency, but otherwise do not.

Sometimes vitamin D is measured in micrograms of cholecalciferol per day; 1 mcg equals 40 IU.

VITAMIN D SUPPLEMENTATION: WHAT FORM OF VITAMIN D IS BEST?

Much of the limelight has been cast on D_3, which is the form most commonly found in foods, but D_2 is another possibility. Hollis has pointed out that daily D_3 supplementation may be the better choice of supplement during breastfeeding, because that's the dominant vitamin form that is transferred to human breastmilk; to our knowledge, no data are available on whether the placenta prefers to transfer one form over the other to the fetus. D_3 also has a reputation for being more easily absorbed, but it may be more important to pay attention to this little-known fact: either form of vitamin D is best absorbed when consumed *with* a little bit of fat. Could this partially explain why researchers at the Harvard School of Public Health found that women with high-fat dairy intake (which always contains vitamin D and fat consumed together) had fewer problems with infertility due to lack of ovulation than those who reported lower-fat dairy substitutes? We're not against enjoying dairy fat, but we do advocate substituting healthier fats when possible. So, would a bowl of fortified cereal with 1 percent milk (both excellent vitamin D sources), topped with crushed walnuts, a great source of healthier omega-3 fat, be just as effective as whole milk or ice cream? Both scenarios provide the combination of vitamin D and fat, but you just have to work harder to remember to eat the fat source *together with* the vitamin D food. The answer remains unclear, but the book *The Fertility Diet* by researchers Chavarro and Willett is a targeted, thoughtful read for women with infertility related specifically to difficulty with ovulation.

Is there a "best" time to take a vitamin D supplement? As long as you have your D_3 or D_2 along with something fatty, the timing shouldn't matter. The best timing is what's easiest for you to remember and be compliant with. So some doctors prefer to give their patients a daily supplement (usually D_3), while others are more comfortable with a single but much higher weekly or monthly dose of D_2; some combination of the two is not uncommon.

Vitamin E

Description and Function. Vitamin E refers to eight compounds called tocopherols and tocotrienols. The name comes from the Greek words *tokos* (childbirth) and *phero* (to bear), because the initial discovery of vitamin E revolved around its ability to prevent sterility in vitamin E–deficient male and female animal subjects. Today vitamin E is best known for its powerful antioxidant properties. It works together with vitamin C and other antioxidants to protect cell membranes from damage inside the body. High-dose vitamin E supplementation (more than 400 IU) can be detrimental to health and is no longer recommended, though lower doses and different forms of vitamin E are still under investigation for potential roles in strengthening the immune system and placental connection between mom and baby, cutting the risk of cardiovascular disease and cancer, and slowing the progression of Alzheimer's disease and age-related macular degeneration.

True vitamin E deficiencies and excesses are uncommon; however, mild deficiencies are possible. It's better to get your vitamin E through natural food sources, especially if you have chronically followed a very low-fat diet, but if you need to take more than the RDA you'll probably want to take a supplement. Because vitamin E is stored in the fatty portion of foods, ingesting a lot of vitamin E–rich foods would provide an overabundance of dietary fat and calories.

The form of vitamin E that the body most readily uses, referred to as d-alpha-tocopherol, is found in foods. When it's incorporated into a supplement, it is called "natural-source" vitamin E. A number of other natural forms are being studied to determine whether they are more healthful mixed with d-alpha-tocopherol or alone. The label should state what you are getting. Synthetic forms of vitamin E are less expensive but more difficult for the body to use; therefore, you must take higher amounts to make up for the inefficiency. Most multivitamin supplements contain the synthetic form.

Women's Preconception Recommendation. The RDA is 15 mg per day as alpha-tocopherol, preferably from foods (approximately 22 IU natural-source d-alpha-tocopherol, or 33 IU synthetic d-alpha-tocopherol). Separate supplementation above the RDA in doses of 100 to 400 IU natural-source vitamin E along with 200 to 1,000 mg of vitamin C has no proven benefits for female fertility and is not generally advised for pre-pregnancy.

Pregnancy Recommendation. The RDA is the same as the preconception recommendation. Current research suggests no additional protection from supplemental vitamin E and C (they were hopeful) begun midpregnancy for women with a pregnancy history of preeclampsia (refer back to "For Future Reference" on page 321). A plant-based diet and broad-spectrum multivitamin begun *before* pregnancy and continued through pregnancy appears to be a more sound choice for risk reduction.

Daily Value (DV) for Food Labeling. The DV is 30 IU.

Food Sources of Vitamin E. Wheat germ oil is the highest source, providing 27 mg per tablespoon. Other vegetable oils contain 2.5 to 6 mg per tablespoon. Nuts—whole nuts, nut butters, and oils derived from them—are also excellent sources, especially sunflower seed kernels (14 mg per ounce) and almonds, hazelnuts, or filberts (7 mg per ounce). Mixed nuts, tomato sauce, spinach, and whole grains have a modest vitamin E content, with the exception of high amounts in toasted wheat germ (5 mg per ¼ cup).

Note: Consuming more than the maximum upper safety limit of 1,000 mg from either food or a supplement (equal to 1,500 IU natural-source vitamin E or 1,000 IU synthetic vitamin E) can cause severe bleeding risks.

One Last Fat-Soluble Vitamin: Vitamin K

Description and Function. Vitamin K plays an essential role in normal blood clotting and aids proteins that put calcium into bone. Half of the vitamin K you need is made inside your digestive tract by friendly bacteria that normally live there.

Women's Preconception Recommendation. Until an RDA can be established, 90 mcg per day is considered to be the adequate intake.

Pregnancy Recommendation. Same as preconception.

Daily Value (DV) for Food Labeling: The DV is 80 mcg.

Food Sources of Vitamin K. Vitamin K is widely found in foods; green leafy vegetables and legumes are particularly rich sources.

Note: Deficiencies and excesses of vitamin K are rare. Women who are on anticoagulant medications must be more vigilant about having a steady intake of vitamin K, not too high and not too low (see Chapter 7, pages 183–184). Women who have been given broad-spectrum antibiotics for more than a month are also at risk for deficiencies.

MINERALS

Minerals make up approximately 4 percent of adult body weight, most of them performing structural roles in the bones and teeth. Many are involved in metabolic processes that regulate our energy. Others help to regulate muscle contractions, nerve impulses, and fluid balance.

There is no way to prevent some degree of competition among the nutrients we ingest for absorption by our body. But there is also synergy among others. So, as with any nutrient, when you provide your body with a reasonably healthy and balanced preconception diet, over time it will make the best use of the minerals discussed here. Simply do what you can to prevent "dietary monotony" so different minerals can shine at different times.

We primarily focus our discussion on the five minerals most pertinent for reproductive health: iron, zinc, calcium, selenium, and iodine. The others are no less essential, but with the exception of chromium, they require very little effort to prevent deficiencies and excesses.

Iron

Description and Function. Iron's primary function is to assist the oxygen-carrying compounds hemoglobin (in red blood cells) and myoglobin (in muscles). It also plays a role in our immune system. Both iron and calcium partially protect the body from lead poisoning. Adequate stores of iron are necessary prior to conception to cope with the 45 percent increase in maternal blood volume during pregnancy.

As discussed in Chapter 7, both too low and too high maternal reserves of iron carry serious implications for women who want to bear children. Anemic women should seek medical attention and completely resolve their iron deficiencies *prior* to trying to get pregnant. If the cause of the anemia is not a true iron deficiency but instead an anemia of inflammation, recall that the two require totally different interventions; only the former requires iron replenishment.[6] Measuring the serum ferritin level should distinguish between those two types of anemia, but it gets tricky when the two overlap (newer tests should help with diagnosis). Women with the less common problem of iron overload (a genetic disorder) should also be under the care of a medical doctor and dietitian prior to conception.

Women's Preconception Recommendation. The RDA is 18 mg per day. When the National Academy of Sciences set the RDA for iron, they set it high enough to account for the fact that only about 10 to 18 percent of this daily iron intake would be absorbed. Women taking oral contraceptives need slightly less than the RDA because their menstrual iron loss is lighter; vegetarians with limited vitamin C intake and women with very heavy periods or

---

6. In medical parlance, anemia of inflammation is called anemia of chronic disease, or ACD. It is usually due to the body's response to a recent or current infection or an underlying source of inflammation (e.g., obesity, autoimmune disease).

closely spaced pregnancies all may need up to twice the iron RDA. The maximum upper limit of safety from foods and supplements is 45 mg iron per day unless a doctor prescribes more for a specific reason.

Pregnancy Recommendation. The pregnancy RDA is 27 mg per day. A supplement with approximately 100 percent of the pregnancy RDA is usually recommended in nonanemic pregnant women beginning in the second trimester, when maternal blood volume expands the most. However, if anemia is detected, you should eat high-iron foods for the fastest rebound, and the doctor may prescribe 60 to 120 mg iron along with an extra 2 mg copper and 15 mg zinc until the anemia is resolved.[7] If your doctor is willing, a single weekly dose of iron or a lower daily dose of iron will be as (or almost as) effective, is easier to comply with, and will not set up a situation where free iron radicals are hanging around, up to no good. Once the anemia is improved or resolved, the daily dose can then be lowered to 27 mg. After the twelfth week of pregnancy, hemoglobin levels normally decrease to some degree. A hemoglobin level that remains unchanged (above 13 g/dl) alerts your physician to consider stopping routine iron supplementation.

Daily Value (DV) for Food Labeling: The DV is 18 mg.

Best Food Sources of Iron. See Table 11-3.

TABLE 11-3
IRON CONTENT OF FOODS

Food Source	Iron Content (mg)
ANIMAL PROTEINS, COOKED[a]	
Spleen from beef, lamb, pork, 3.5 oz	22–40
Clams, 3 oz	23
Kidney or heart from beef, lamb, or pork, 3.5 oz	5–12
Mussels, oysters, 3 oz	5–8
Turkey or chicken gizzard, 3.5 oz	5
Beef, 3.5 oz	1.9–3.8
Lamb, 3.5 oz	1.6–2.8
Pork, 3.5 oz	1.8–2.2

7. The percentage of iron absorbed from high supplemental doses can be significantly lower than 10 percent, which is why supplemental doses close to the pregnancy RDA of 27 mg per day are often as effective as higher supplemental doses in treating anemia (and compliance is better). Iron supplements can be taken with water or a vitamin C food source such as orange or tomato juice. If you notice that your bowel habits change (development of constipation or diarrhea) soon after starting a supplement that contains iron, see pages 355–357 for more information on beating side effects.

Food Source	Iron Content (mg)
Chicken, 3.5 oz	0.9–1.4
Fish, shellfish, most varieties, 3 oz	0.5–2
Eggs, 1 whole	0.7
LEGUMES, ½ CUP, COOKED	
Tofu, soybean product	6.5–13
Soybeans	4.4
Lentils, white beans	3.3
Pinto, navy, and baked beans	2.2–2.5
Textured vegetable protein (TVP)	2
Lima, garbanzo, and refried beans	2
Tempeh, soybean product	1.9
Black-eyed peas, black and kidney beans	1.5–1.8
GRAINS	
Ready-to-eat cold cereal, 1 serving (see label)	Varies (avg 4.5)
Individually packed instant hot cereals, 1 pkt.	3–8
Cream of Wheat, cooked, ½ cup	5.5
Waffle, 1 frozen	1.5
Corn grits, enriched	1.3
Bagel, ½ (3-inch diameter)	1.3
Wheat germ, 2 tbsp	1.1
Bread, most kinds, 1 slice	0.7–1.3
Rice, most kinds, ½ cup	0.8–1.3
Pasta noodles, ½ cup	0.8
Oatmeal, old fashioned, ½ cup	0.8
VEGETABLES, ½ CUP COOKED, UNLESS STATED OTHERWISE	
Sea vegetables, raw	2–22
Potato, baked with skin, 1 medium	2.7

Food Source	Iron Content (mg)
Swiss chard, chopped	2
Pumpkin	1.7
Spinach	1.4
Green peas	1.3
Hearts of palm, 1 heart	1
Collards and Brussels sprouts	0.9
Tomato paste, sundried tomato, approx. 2 tbsp	0.7
Broccoli	0.5
FRUITS, RAW	
Figs, 2–3, dried	1.3
Avocado, ½	1.1
Raisins, ⅓ cup	1.1
Prunes, 5	1.1
Apricots, dried, 5 halves	0.8
NUTS AND SEEDS, ¼ CUP	
Mixed nuts	2
Seeds (pumpkin, sunflower)	2–4
MISCELLANEOUS	
Blackstrap molasses, 1 tbsp	3.5
Soy milk beverage, 8 oz	1.4

a. Although an excellent source of iron, liver should be strictly limited or avoided due to its extremely high vitamin A content. Other organ meats such as spleen, kidney, heart, and gizzard contain low levels of vitamin A and are featured in the chart.

Source: J. A. T. Pennington, *Bowes & Church's Food Values of Portions Commonly Used,* 17th ed. (Philadelphia: Lippincott-Raven, 1998).

A nutritious diet will contain foods that naturally enhance and inhibit iron absorption. These factors are listed here for your interest, but there is considerable protection against iron deficiency in just eating a wide assortment of foods. If your diet is limited in food choices, for example, because of food allergies or self-imposed food restrictions, the iron inhibitors make a greater impact. Women and men who overstore iron should consult a registered dietitian to create an acceptable meal plan that limits iron enhancers while still maintaining good nutrition. (Also see Chapter 7, page 193.)

There are two forms of iron. Non-heme iron is the predominant dietary form, but heme iron is the real powerhouse. The heme form of iron, found only in some animal proteins (e.g., red meats, clams, poultry, and fish), is dramatically easier for the body to use than non-heme iron, found in plant sources (e.g., fortified cereals, spinach, nuts and seeds, prune juice, and dried beans).

Adding even a small amount of a heme source of iron to a vegetarian meal helps the non-heme source of iron be more absorbable, such as in the following meal: Heme iron from meat sauce or red clam sauce would trump plain marinara or cream sauce; serve it over pasta enriched with non-heme iron.

Another way to enhance non-heme iron's absorption is to eat vitamin C–rich foods along with the iron source. For example, vitamin C–rich tomato sauce consumed in a vegetarian chili can increase the absorption of iron by four times! Fruits and vegetables have small amounts of other natural acids such as citric acid that add to this vitamin C effect.

Just as some foods enhance iron absorption, others partially inhibit it. Calcium-rich foods or supplements (including antacids) partially inhibit iron absorption, so try to limit calcium in the couple of hours surrounding your iron-richest meal of the day.[8] Calcium-fortified orange juice, however, does not inhibit iron absorption very much, probably because of the high vitamin C content.

Polyphenols, including tannins (all very healthy compounds), in black and herbal teas and coffee also inhibit iron absorption; caffeine is not the culprit here. Get around the iron-binding dilemma by drinking these beverages between meals rather than at meals; if not, include meat, fish, poultry, or vitamin C–rich foods at the same time.

Dietary fiber (as discussed in Chapter 10) also reduces the body's absorption of iron, but don't cut down, as it's necessary to counteract the constipating effects of supplemental iron.

Other inhibitors include naturally occurring phytates, found in whole grains and legumes; soy protein; and a compound in eggs. Again, keep in mind that ample heme iron and vitamin C intake from foods can largely counteract many of these inhibitors of iron, so don't let them stop you from eating these healthy foods.

Zinc

Description and Function. More than a hundred zinc-dependent enzymes participate in essential metabolic processes that occur inside the body. Gene expression, growth, immune system function, tissue health, our sense of taste, and our appetite also rely on zinc's presence. Although zinc is found in all tissues of the body, it is especially concentrated in tis-

---

8. Multivitamin-mineral supplements contain iron and should count as a good iron source as long as they contain less than 250 mg of calcium in the same pill.

sues that are constantly re-creating healthy new cells, such as the male reproductive organs with their high rate of sperm turnover.

It is of utmost importance, then, that zinc be adequately available from the moment conception occurs. The fetus needs it for the fast rate of cell growth and organ development.

It's estimated that women of childbearing age average 9 mg of zinc per day from foods—barely meeting nonpregnant needs, and sometimes not even that. Pregnant and breastfeeding women have higher zinc requirements, and several studies have found that they often do not meet these.

Women with optimal zinc intakes before getting pregnant may be at lower risk for NTDs (as with folate and choline). Interestingly, improving zinc intake does not reduce this risk nearly as well in women who enter pregnancy overweight as in women who are in the normal weight range. Also, in a comparison between pregnant women who had either sufficient or inadequate dietary zinc intake, women with sufficient intake showed better birth weights in their offspring and fewer preterm deliveries. Because most animal foods have ample zinc readily available for the body to put to use, it could be that more than just the zinc is acting as the protective factor.[9] Maybe the animal product's concentrated source of protein is the key; maybe the relatively higher levels of the amino acid methionine, with its tie to folate metabolism, is beneficial in preventing NTDs. Also, it's been found that when zinc-deficient people are given adequate zinc, it enlivens their appetite. This may cause them to eat better, which also improves birth outcomes, including birth weight. Happily, supplemental forms of zinc are readily absorbed by our bodies.

Women who have a very low consumption of animal products combined with a very high consumption of legumes and unrefined grains are most at risk for zinc deficiency. Naturally occurring phytates in legumes and whole grains make the zinc in these foods much less bioavailable. Therefore, those of you who are vegetarians should try to consume more than the recommended daily amount.

Women's Preconception Recommendation. The RDA is 8 mg per day. The maximum upper limit of safety from foods and supplements is 40 mg per day.

Pregnancy Recommendation. The pregnancy RDA is 12 mg per day. The maximum limit is still 40 mg. Consistent intake of zinc keeps it circulating in the maternal system for easy access by the fetus. Stored zinc does not mobilize well during times of deficiency.

Daily Value (DV) for Food Labeling: The DV is 15 mg.

Best Food Sources of Zinc. All meats, poultry, crab, and lobster contain 2 to 4 mg per 3-ounce serving. Cooked oysters are even higher (1 medium = 8 mg), but you should limit your intake to no more than one or two in a day, with a maximum of six in a week, to

---

9. The high calcium content of milk may render some of its abundant zinc unavailable, so vegetarians who exclude all animal products except dairy may still be at risk for marginal zinc deficiency. This can be overcome with good planning.

stay under the safe limit. Milk and milk products have around 1 mg per serving. Whole grains, legumes, and nuts contain approximately 1 to 2 mg per serving, but absorption is lower.

Note: Nausea and vomiting are usually the first signs of too much zinc. An excess of zinc can also lead to copper deficiency. Taking cold lozenges supplemented with zinc as directed far exceeds the safe upper limit and should be strictly limited beginning at least one month prior to conception.

Calcium

Description and Function. Calcium is well-known for keeping bones and teeth strong. It also assists in muscle contraction, blood pressure regulation, and immunity. Any potential danger posed by environmental lead exposure is significantly lessened in people who have healthy levels of calcium in their bodies. Leg muscle cramps are sometimes related to low calcium intake as well as other factors. Relatively new research is investigating the potential for modest calcium supplementation (between 1,000 and 1,200 mg per day) in reducing PMS symptoms; some studies have shown promising results.

The demand for calcium goes up during pregnancy and breastfeeding, yet the recommended intake is the same for childbearing-age women whether pregnant or not. This is because the female body amazingly adapts to make better use of the calcium gained from dietary and supplemental sources during this time. Nevertheless, that level should be met while concurrently meeting vitamin D requirements. If a pregnant woman does not consume adequate calcium during pregnancy, the baby is actually able to drain most of the calcium it needs from the maternal stores, to the detriment of the mom's bones.

Women who enter pregnancy with calcium intake close to the recommended level appear not to need supplemental calcium. However, supplementation may be helpful for pregnant women with chronically low calcium intake. When given supplemental calcium of between 1,500 and 2,000 mg per day, calcium-deficient women show improved control of blood pressure and lower incidence of preeclampsia compared to similar pregnant women who have gone untreated; the baby's future blood pressure may benefit similarly.

Women's Preconception Recommendation. The safe and adequate intake is 1,000 mg per day for calcium until an RDA can be established. The maximum upper limit of calcium from foods and supplements is 2,500 mg per day. Also see recommendations for vitamin D.

Pregnancy Recommendation. Same as for preconception.

Daily Value (DV) for Food Labeling: The DV is 1,000 mg. Do not be fooled by foods or supplements that claim to offer 100 percent of the DV for calcium in one serving—your body can absorb only up to 500 mg at a time, and the extra is wasted.

Best Food Sources of Calcium. Table 11-4 lists foods and beverages that are good calcium sources. Dairy sources generally have the highest amounts of calcium and are usually easiest for the body to absorb.

Be aware that excessive amounts of sodium and protein promote loss of calcium through urinary excretion. High caffeine intake interferes with calcium retention in bones. Partial inhibitors of calcium absorption include oxalates (natural substances found in spinach, tea, beets, rhubarb, peanuts—and chocolate to a small degree), phytates (natural compounds found in whole grains and legumes), and dietary fiber. However, if you plan a reasonably balanced diet in which the recommended calcium intake is met, none of these substances will pose a threat to your calcium status.

TABLE 11-4
CALCIUM CONTENT OF FOODS

Food Source	Calcium Content (mg)
HIGHEST (GREATER THAN 200 MG PER SERVING)	
Yogurt, plain or sweetened, 1 cup	300–400
Milk (nonfat, 1%, 2%, or whole), 1 cup	288–302
Lactose-free milk, 1 cup	300
Evaporated milk, canned, ½ cup	320
Citrus (orange, grapefruit) juice, calcium-fortified, 1 cup	350
Milkshake, average fast-food	330
Soy milk, fortified with calcium, 1 cup	200–300
Fortified Rice Dream beverage, 1 cup	300
Chocolate milk, 2%, 1 cup	284
Buttermilk, 1 cup	285
Cheese (Swiss), 1-oz slice	272
Firm tofu, fortified with calcium, ½ cup	258
Salmon canned with edible bones, 3 oz	212
Cheese (cheddar, mozzarella, provolone), 1 oz	204–212
HIGH (100–199 MG CALCIUM PER SERVING)	
Sardines, 2 oz (4 Atlantic or 2 Pacific)	183
Collard greens, cooked, ½ cup	179
Rhubarb, cooked, ½ cup	174
Blackstrap molasses, 1 tbsp	172

Food Source	Calcium Content (mg)
Ricotta cheese, part skim, ¼ cup (~2 oz)	169
Cornbread, homemade with milk, 2½ inches × 1½ inches	162
Parmesan cheese, grated, 2 tbsp	140
Ice milk, soft-serve vanilla, ½ cup	138
Regular tofu (not set with calcium), ½ cup	130
Edamame (green soybeans), boiled, ½ cup	130
Turnip greens, cooked, ½ cup	125
Cheese (American), 1 oz	124
Spinach, cooked, ½ cup	122
Soy nuts, dry-roasted, ¼ cup	116
Frozen yogurt, soft-serve, ½ cup	105

MEDIUM (40–99 MG PER SERVING)

Kale, cooked, ½ cup	90
Sesame seeds, 1 tbsp	88
Bok choy, cooked, ½ cup	79
Cottage cheese, ½ cup	73
Hot cocoa mixes (vary greatly), 1 serving	45–120
Figs, 2 dried	54
Seaweed, wakame, 1 oz raw	43
Corn tortilla, 1	42
Almonds, ½ oz or ~11 nuts	42
Broccoli, cooked, ½ cup	40
Garbanzo beans, ½ cup	40

Sources: J. A. T. Pennington, *Bowes & Church's Food Values of Portions Commonly Used,* 16th and 17th eds. (Philadelphia: Lippincott, 1994, 1998)

Practical Application

Using Table 11-4, consider your typical daily diet and tally your daily calcium intake for seven days. Enter the range you typically consume from lowest to highest: _____ milligrams to _____ milligrams per day. If you go to www.MyPyramid.gov, it'll do this for you.

Do you regularly get 1,000 mg calcium? If your answer is yes, congratulations and keep up the good work! If your answer is no or only occasionally, you are not alone. Unfortunately, the majority of women in the United States do not meet their optimum calcium needs. They simply do not consume enough sources of calcium. Here are some sneaky ways of adding more calcium into your diet:

• Eat meals and snacks that have milk hidden inside them, such as French toast, waffles, and pudding made with low-fat or nonfat milk or buttermilk.
• Try calcium-fortified orange and grapefruit juice.
• Add extra nonfat powdered milk to hot cereals or mashed potatoes. Because it is powdered, it does not add to the volume of the food as liquid milk does.
• Blend up a refreshing fruit smoothie using yogurt or calcium-fortified vanilla soy milk along with fresh and frozen fruits. A little calcium-fortified OJ adds a nice touch, too.
• Use evaporated nonfat or low-fat milk in place of cream or half-and-half in "cream" soups, sauces, and casseroles; as these don't thicken much, use flour or cornstarch to thicken as desired. Evaporated milk has double the calcium of regular milk.
• Add moderate amounts of cheese to sandwiches, tacos, casseroles, and lean burgers.
• Sneak high-calcium veggies and legumes into soups. Try hummus dip too!
• As a higher-calcium alternative to peanut butter, try almond butter or soy nut butter.
• Try a cappuccino or soy latte in the morning instead of a coffee (ask for "half-caff" so the regular espresso doesn't bump you over your daily caffeine limit).
• If you really dislike drinking plain milk, go ahead and have chocolate- or strawberry-flavored milk in moderation (consider diluting it with extra nonfat milk). Hot cocoa with extra powdered milk also makes a tasty cold-weather snack.
• If you avoid plain milk because of the discomforts of lactose intolerance, try a lactose-free milk. (More on lactose intolerance in Chapter 12.)

Note: To prevent calcium from significantly inhibiting your iron absorption, each day plan one meal (or snack) that is high in calcium (between 300 and 500 mg) and another that is relatively low in calcium but high in iron. Don't worry: it isn't necessary to be this calculated with the remainder of your calcium and iron intake, unless you have iron-deficiency anemia.

Practical Application

Do you answer yes to any of the following? If so, pay even more attention to how you can meet or modestly exceed the daily goal of 1,000 mg calcium per day. You may very well need the help of a calcium supplement.

Yes / No   I am an athlete with very inconsistent or absent periods (now or in the recent past).

Yes / No   I don't drink milk and/or eat many dairy products, nor do I sufficiently substitute calcium-fortified beverages such as soy milk in place of milk.

Yes / No   I am lactose intolerant.

Yes / No   I have a medical condition such as milk allergy, Crohn's disease, or ulcerative colitis that necessitates avoidance of milk or dairy products on a permanent or temporary basis.

Yes / No   I take certain medications that increase calcium loss, according to my doctor.

Yes / No   I'm a smoker.

Yes / No   I have had weight-loss surgery (bariatric surgery).

Yes / No   I am at risk for osteoporosis (family history; persons with limited mobility).

If you are still concerned that your dietary intake of calcium is under 1,000 mg per day, take supplemental calcium to cover the deficit.[10] Choose a supplement with calcium carbonate or calcium citrate (not oyster shell calcium, due to the risk of contamination with heavy metals). Unless stated otherwise, true elemental calcium content per tablet is 40 percent for calcium carbonate and 21 percent for calcium citrate. Calcium carbonate *must* be taken with food for best absorption, but calcium citrate is highly absorbed between or with meals as long as it dissolves properly in the stomach.

It is important that the calcium supplement dissolve properly in your stomach or it will be of little use to you. The U.S. Pharmacopeia (USP) symbol on the container ensures that the supplement will dissolve in a timely manner. If you have already spent money on a calcium supplement that doesn't boast the USP symbol, try dissolving one tablet in a few ounces of vinegar; if it remains intact after thirty minutes, you need to find a better calcium supplement. Chewable calcium carbonate supplements such as Viactiv chews obviously pass the dissolution test. But be aware that Viactiv products contain vitamin K and are not recommended for women with blood coagulation disorders.

10. It's okay if your calcium supplement contains supplemental vitamin D or magnesium, but neither is requisite as long as you follow the separate recommendations for the individual nutrients.

Some women experience uncomfortable side effects such as constipation, bloating, or gas when taking calcium supplements. The best way to combat these symptoms is to drink adequate amounts of fluids, eat enough dietary fiber, and not oversupplement.

Selenium

Description and Function. Selenium is an essential element that is required by a series of enzymes (selenoenzymes) that have important antioxidant functions. These enzymes recycle vitamin C and work together with vitamin E to prevent and reverse oxidative damage in cells. There is evidence, first identified in the 1960s and 1970s and currently receiving renewed interest, that an optimal intake of selenium either minimizes or prevents the adverse effects of high mercury exposures. It was initially thought that mercury and selenium bind together to form a nontoxic new compound, making mercury unable to cause harm to tissues. This would appear to be very good news, except for one catch: the body is glad to be rid of the mercury, but it still needs the selenium. It turns out that instead of selenium binding to mercury to keep mercury from causing harm, it is *because* mercury binds to selenium that mercury is so harmful. When there is too much mercury in the body, it binds to the selenium in the selenoenzymes, making them unable to defend highly active tissues of the body.

The best news is that it's easy to get ample selenium from your diet and keep selenoenzymes functioning at optimal levels. This way selenium is free to carry out its protective role as an antioxidant in the brain and neuroendocrine tissues (including ovaries and testes); this is crucially important in the fetal brain, which, because of its high rate of oxygen use, produces potentially damaging by-products. Selenium-dependent enzymes help stop and even reverse oxidative damage from those by-products.

Nick Ralston, PhD, a researcher at the Energy and Environmental Research Center, University of North Dakota, states, "Scientific evidence is mounting that only when mercury outnumbers selenium do we see the physical impairments and cognitive delays attributed to methylmercury toxicity in developing humans (and animals). When this is the case, selenium is outnumbered and can no longer make the enzymes that are needed to detoxify the reactive oxygen species (ROS) being produced in tissues with high metabolic rates. If the ROSs aren't detoxified, they will ultimately cause severe damage." The implications of this knowledge may extend beyond protecting our health to improving that of our planet. The EPA is currently pursuing methods to clean up troubling levels of mercury in our environment. As you might deduce, mercury is a more extensive problem in low-selenium soils. Ralston notes that "volcanic soils are naturally low in selenium, and fish that live in lakes and streams of these areas can often be higher in mercury. Pollution from coal-powered electrical plants and industrial wastes have made mercury more ubiquitous in the environment, but mercury accumulations in fish are lower where selenium is richest. Fish from lakes that are selenium-deficient accumulate far more mercury than fish from lakes with normal selenium levels. Studies in Sweden and Canada show that selenium enrichment reduces the amount of mercury that accumulates in fish from these lakes. Studies are investigating how selenium helps plants clean up mercury-contaminated soil and water through natural processes."

See more on this fascinating subject in Chapter 13, when we discuss safe fish and seafood choices for preconception and pregnancy.

Having adequate dietary intake of selenium during pregnancy and between pregnancies is also good for thyroid health. Although selenium assists some infertile men in improving their fertility (see Chapter 9), results from small studies investigating selenium status and/or supplementation in women with recurrent miscarriages have been mixed. For women of childbearing age there is no clear evidence to support supplementation of selenium above 100 percent of the Daily Value. Although it may sound tempting to supplement with selenium for its antioxidant properties, research discourages it except under very controlled circumstances due to the relatively narrow margin of safety. Get the majority of your selenium from a wide variety of food sources.

Deficiencies and excesses of selenium are uncommon in the United States.

Women's Preconception Recommendation. The RDA is 55 mcg of selenium per day, primarily from foods. The upper limit is 400 mcg per day.

Pregnancy Recommendation. The pregnancy RDA is 60 mcg per day, primarily from foods. The upper limit is no different than the preconception recommendation.

Daily Value (DV) for Food Labeling. The DV is 70 mcg.

Food Sources of Selenium. Seafood (ocean water has abundant selenium) and many freshwater fish are the best sources, averaging 45 to 130 mcg per average modest serving size (approximately 3 ounces); meat and poultry average 25 to 45 mcg for a 3-ounce portion. Nuts, eggs, cereals, and other grain products (both unrefined and refined) provide good amounts of selenium, averaging 15 to 20 mcg per serving.[11] The selenium content of soil varies from place to place, affecting the selenium content of foods grown in those soils. By buying grains grown in a variety of geographical areas, you will likely consume adequate selenium; locavores (people who only eat locally grown food) take notice.[12] Cheeses and a variety of other foods contain lower amounts.

11. Most nuts are good sources of selenium. Brazil nuts are the only nuts that are off-the-charts high (543 mcg for 6–8 nuts), so eat these only occasionally and in small amounts.
12. Soils are low in selenium in many parts of the United States (much of the western Pacific Northwest and Florida, for starters), as well as in Finland, New Zealand, and certain parts of China. However, certain locations of the United States (parts of Arkansas and Louisiana) and abroad in Caracas (Venezuela) have soil selenium levels that are too high and wildlife and livestock, and (rarely) humans, are at risk as a result.

Iodine

Description and Function. Thyroid hormones, which regulate the rate at which the body expends energy, require iodine. Very low intake of iodine causes lowered activity of the thyroid gland, sometimes resulting in a goiter in the neck. Severe iodine deficiency during pregnancy causes an easily preventable form of mental retardation, dwarfism, and thyroid problems in offspring. A more realistic concern for women in developed nations is mild to moderate iodine deficiency, which could be related to slightly lowered intelligence in offspring and is very worthy of your attention.

Women's Preconception Recommendation. The RDA is 150 mcg of iodine per day. Because iodine in very high amounts can be harmful, an upper limit of 1,100 mcg per day is advised.

Pregnancy Recommendation. The pregnancy RDA is 220 mcg per day. The same upper limit applies.

Daily Value (DV) for Food Labeling. The DV is 150 mcg.

Best Food Sources of Iodine. Dairy products, seafood, eggs, commercially made breads, and cured products are the primary sources of iodine. (See the sidebar "Sea Vegetables" for safety information.) The USDA has yet to compile a comprehensive nutrient database of iodine in foods, but this is no easy task, considering the variability within foods. As a point of reference, researchers from the Boston Medical Center state that cows' milk is a leading source of dietary iodine in the United States, averaging 110 mcg iodine per cup (data based on a variety of milks sold in the Boston area).

Iodized table salt is a reliable source of iodine, too. Groups such as the World Health Organization and the Micronutrient Initiative are working hard to ensure that all women of childbearing age receive sufficient iodine, and universal salt iodization is the ultimate goal. It's that important. Salt harvested from soil needs to be iodized, usually in the form of potassium iodide. As long as you are not on a strict low-sodium diet, iodized table salt (make sure the label says "iodized") should be your salt of choice during this time of your life. It contains approximately 69 to 114 mcg iodine per quarter teaspoon of salt, according to Dr. Elizabeth Pearce, associate professor of medicine at Boston University School of Medicine. Kosher salt does not contain iodine. Salt water is naturally rich in iodine, yet all the tantalizing varieties of sea salt contain no iodine, either (unless otherwise stated). You don't have to give up your favorite fleur de sel, but use it more sparingly, and have iodized salt on hand.

So what is the take-home message about salt and iodine? Remember to preferentially use iodized salt when you are following a recipe or adding a dash of salt to a scrambled egg or tomato sandwich. And if you tend to eat a lot of processed foods, as many busy women do, recognize that you may be at risk for iodine deficiency. While many processed foods contain salt, manufacturers typically do not use iodized salt. Be extra vigilant to eat the

Sea Vegetables and Iodine

Experts caution that even though the sea vegetable kelp is a natural source of iodine, it is too high a source of iodine and should not be routinely consumed, especially before and after conception. Other sea vegetables that are either too high in iodine or vary too greatly include kombu, arame, and hiziki (it's unclear if dulse is too high). Alternative dietary sea vegetables such as nori and wakame are good sources of iodine, and not nearly as variable in their composition; the overall iodine content is low enough to be safe to consume in a varied diet.

aforementioned best sources of iodine (knowing that milk is a reliable source for daily consumption).

The American Thyroid Association now recommends that all pregnant and breast-feeding women take a multivitamin containing at least 150 mcg iodine per day, but consensus is building to extend this recommendation to all women of childbearing potential. Intervention—beginning before conception—has the greatest protective effects.

In recent years, scientists at the Boston University Iodine Research Laboratory have investigated a variety of prescription and nonprescription prenatal multivitamins and found that roughly half contained iodine. However, the amounts on the labels often were not what was found in the pills. The supplements that contained potassium iodide were most likely to contain the stated amount, whereas when kelp was the listed source of iodine, amounts varied too much. USP-certified brands of multivitamins verify that their products contain what the labels claim, so these are good bets, too.

Other Minerals

Magnesium

Description and Function. Activates hundreds of enzymes; required for making energy and proteins; helps muscles and nerves function and is a component of bones. Preliminary data also suggest that magnesium may lessen mild PMS symptoms related to headache, mood, and fluid retention.

Women's Preconception Recommendation. The RDA is 310 to 320 mg of magnesium per day, primarily from foods. There are no upper limits on magnesium from food sources. However, if you take a magnesium-containing supplement or pharmacological agent (e.g., milk of magnesia), do not exceed 350 mg per day from these sources.

Pregnancy Recommendation. The pregnancy RDA is 350 to 360 mg per day. The same limit on supplements and pharmacological agents applies. Severe morning sickness during pregnancy may cause significant loss of magnesium (via the stomach's gastric juices). This is one of many reasons to seek adequate medical attention under these circumstances.

Daily Value (DV) for Food Labeling: The DV is 400 mg.

Best Food Sources of Magnesium. Magnesium is found in a variety of foods, particularly legumes, nuts, and whole grains (often more than 100 mg per serving). Vegetables, especially green leafy ones such as spinach, are also good sources. Milk, fish, meat, and poultry contain modest amounts. A well-rounded diet easily prevents marginal intake of magnesium.

Copper

Description and Function. Required component of many enzymes, connective tissue, and the protective sheath surrounding nerves; needed for proper utilization of iron. Excessive intakes of zinc or vitamin C have been shown to interfere with copper utilization.

Women's Preconception Recommendation: The RDA is 900 mcg of copper per day. The tolerable upper limit is 10,000 mcg per day.

Pregnancy Recommendation: The pregnancy RDA is 1,000 mcg. The upper limit is the same.

Daily Value (DV) for Food Labeling: The DV is 2 mg.

Best Food Sources of Copper. Good sources include seafood, nuts and seeds, and legumes. Grains and some vegetables provide noteworthy amounts. Organ meats are extremely rich in copper but should be strictly limited during preconception and pregnancy. Significant deficiencies and toxicities are rare.

Fluoride

Description and Function. Necessary for maintaining healthy teeth and bones.

Women's Preconception Recommendation. Until an RDA can be established, 3 mg of fluoride per day is recommended. The safe upper limit is 10 mg per day.

Pregnancy Recommendation. Same as preconception recommendation.

Daily Value (DV) for Food Labeling: No DV for fluoride has been established.

Food Sources of Fluoride. Fluoride is not readily found in foods unless they have been cooked in or mixed with fluoridated water. Natural sources include tea (from fluoride in the leaves), marine fish with edible bones, shellfish, and gelatin. Tap water is fluoridated in some parts of the country and not in others. Bottled water is available with or without added fluoride, so if your tap water is not fluoridated, you may want to consider buying fluoridated drinking water if you seldom eat the natural sources. Fluoridated toothpastes and other dental care products are nonfood items that contain fluoride in concentrated amounts. Avoid swallowing appreciable amounts of these to prevent fluoride excess that can cause problems with your future baby's tooth development. Please refer to "Dental Health and Hygiene" in Chapter 4 for more information.

Chromium

Description and Function. Influences overall metabolism by increasing the effectiveness of insulin. Most research does not support the recent marketing claim that chromium increases muscle mass or decreases body fat.

Women's Preconception Recommendation. Until an RDA can be established, 25 mcg of chromium per day is recommended. More research is needed to determine the upper level of safety.

Pregnancy Recommendation: Until an RDA can be established, 30 mcg per day is recommended.

Daily Value (DV) for Food Labeling: The DV is 120 mcg, reflective of previous recommended intakes.

Best Food Sources of Chromium. Good sources include whole grains (refining removes chromium), brewer's yeast, egg yolks, meat, oysters, cheese, nuts, and some veggies (broccoli, asparagus, mushrooms, spinach). Limit liver despite its rich chromium content. Your chromium intake will be less than optimal if you neglect to eat whole grains regularly. Diabetics and athletes should be especially sure to consume adequate amounts of chromium, but there is insufficient evidence to recommend supplemental doses for these people.

Sodium

Description and Function. A type of mineral known as an electrolyte, sodium helps regulate the fine balance of fluids and acid/base equilibrium in the body. It is critical to helping the plasma volume expand properly once pregnancy occurs. Sodium plays a role in muscle contraction, including that of the heart, and nerve impulse transmission. Significant losses of sodium through excessive sweating or vomiting can have adverse effects on the body if the accompanying water and electrolyte losses are not replenished.

Women's Preconception Recommendation. No RDA has been established. However, an adequate intake of 1,500 mg of sodium per day is recommended for all healthy adults. This is considerably less than most people consume through nutritious eating.

Pregnancy Recommendation. Pregnant women are discouraged from significantly restricting their sodium intake unless their physician instructs them differently. Moderation is the preferred course of action. Sodium is found in salt, and severe salt restriction can worsen water retention and further complicate preeclampsia.

Daily Value (DV) for Food Labeling: The DV is 2,400 mg.

Food Sources of Sodium. The majority of dietary sodium comes from hidden salt in processed foods such as soups, salty snack items, fast foods, frozen entrées, and dairy products. It is also found in cured foods such as lunch meat, ham, bacon, and pickles. Most condiments, such as soy sauce, ketchup, and garlic salt, also count in this category. Table salt contains approximately 2,300 mg of pure sodium per level teaspoon; iodized salts should be the preferred type for preconception and pregnancy. Kosher salt (and some sea salt) usually has larger grains than table salt, and therefore less sodium per teaspoon, but as you may recall, they seldom are iodized. Processed meats that are preserved with sodium nitrite or sodium nitrate should be limited due to the nitrite/nitrates, not the sodium content. See "Food Safety" in Chapter 13.

FOR FUTURE REFERENCE: During Pregnancy

The natural changes in physiology that occur during pregnancy cause the fluid volume in the body to increase (because you expand your blood volume and create amniotic fluid) and cause sodium to be less easily conserved. Under normal circumstances, healthy dietary intake covers any dilutional effect, and the body adjusts to the changes.

Interestingly, the symptoms of morning sickness—nausea, vomiting, and fatigue that can occur at all hours of the day—match some of the symptoms of low blood sodium, although there are not yet studies confirming any connection. Morning sickness expert Miriam Erick, MS, RD, author of *Managing Morning Sickness: A Survival Guide for Pregnant Women,* has made an intriguing discovery that salty potato chips and lemonade often sit well with her patients when almost nothing else does. Perhaps there is a partially biological explanation behind this. By the way, Erick's book is an excellent resource for pregnant women who struggle with severe nausea and vomiting during pregnancy.

Potassium

Description and Function. Potassium is an electrolyte that helps regulate the fine balance of fluids and the acid/base equilibrium in the body. It plays a role in muscle contraction, including that of the heart, and nerve impulse transmission and blood pressure. Also, a number of enzymes need potassium to work to their best effect. Significant losses of potassium through excessive vomiting or diuretic use or abuse can have adverse effects on the body if the water and electrolyte losses are not replenished.

Women's Preconception Recommendation. No RDA has been established. However, an adequate intake of 4,700 mg potassium per day is recommended for all adults, with particular emphasis on potassium-rich foods for African Americans, who as a group reportedly have diets lower in potassium. No upper limit has been set, but supplemental potassium should be taken only under doctor supervision.

Pregnancy Recommendation. Same as preconception. Women who experience severe morning sickness must replenish electrolytes, including potassium, from dietary sources; in extreme cases, intravenous electrolyte replacement may need to be administered.

Daily Value (DV) for Food Labeling: The DV is 3,500 mg.

Best Food Sources of Potassium: Many foods are excellent sources of potassium, especially in their natural, unprocessed state. It is easy to get plenty of potassium from potatoes (approximately 800 mg in one baked potato) and other vegetables including mushrooms, bananas (450 mg in one medium banana) and other fruits, fruit juices, legumes, dairy foods, meat, poultry, and fish.

DO YOU NEED A SUPPLEMENT?

A significant number of women of childbearing age could likely benefit from taking a daily multivitamin-mineral supplement, including:

- Vegans
- Women who are on calorie-restricted diets or who have recently lost a significant amount of weight
- Women who have pregnancies fewer than eighteen months apart
- Those at high risk for a poor dietary intake, particularly women of lower socioeconomic status and sexually active teenagers[13]
- Women with certain preexisting health conditions that increase nutrient needs above ordinary levels and also require medically supervised vitamin/mineral supplementation (see Chapter 7 for more information on medical issues, Chapter 14 for post-bariatric-surgery tips)
- Women who smoke or abuse drugs or alcohol. These women should also take an appropriate supplement while they focus on stopping their destructive habits before considering pregnancy.

All generally healthy women planning on becoming pregnant should consume 400 mcg of supplemental folic acid daily, and although the jury is still out on whether they should also take a multivitamin-mineral supplement, it may be prudent to do so. There is intriguing evidence that a daily multivitamin supplement (that includes folic acid) taken one to three months during preconception through early pregnancy (mainly the first month) might help

13. The nutrition information in this book does not take into account the specific nutritional needs of teenagers (eighteen and under) who are capable of becoming pregnant. DRI tables in Appendix B are included to serve as a source of comparison.

reduce the incidence of preeclampsia and risk for other types of birth defects: those of the lip and palate, limbs, heart, urinary tract, and brain, in addition to NTDs. In one study, even using multivitamin supplementation three or four times per week significantly reduced the risk of a severe type of heart birth defect. Unfortunately, being overweight or obese largely cancels out this extra protection, and the only way to get it back is to de-stress your body by getting as close to a healthy pre-pregnancy body weight as possible (BMI between 18.5 and 24.9). Most of the studies focused solely on their participants' use of multivitamins, but many common multivitamin supplements contain minerals, too. It does not appear that the potential benefits apply exclusively to women with poor diets, although it is commonly understood that people with primary nutrient deficiencies benefit most from replenishment.

So, although we prefer food as the safest and most natural source of vitamins and minerals for you as you prepare your body for pregnancy, we see no reason to discourage the addition of a modest safety net. This may come from either a general multivitamin with minerals or a prenatal supplement taken daily (or at least most days per week), begun during the pre-pregnancy months. The main difference between the two is that prenatal supplements are generally more expensive (although sometimes they are covered by insurance) and may provide higher than necessary amounts of iron, folic acid, and certain other micronutrients for preconception and early pregnancy; virtually none contain enough choline or iodine, though this is improving in the prenatal supplement market (and some children's chewables contain them, too).

Should you decide to take a supplement in addition to eating healthfully, refer to Table 11-5 to make sure that the supplement does not contain excessive levels of selected nutrients. This risk is not trivial, as some manufacturers' formulations operate on the misguided principle that more must be better. The potential for overuse of supplements is also a significant reason why health officials are reluctant to recommend supplements more widely.

TABLE 11-5
GUIDELINES FOR PRECONCEPTION AND PRENATAL SUPPLEMENT FORMULAS

The following is a summary of what we look for in a multivitamin-mineral supplement formula. For an explanation of when exceptions are safe and when they are not, see the detailed information on individual vitamins and minerals in this chapter, and refer to Chapter 10 for advice on omega-3 fats. Confer with your health care provider to verify whether a supplement is appropriate for you, and take only as prescribed.

Folic acid: 400–800 mcg
Iron: 18–27 mg; the higher amount of iron is not absolutely recommended until the twelfth week of pregnancy, so nonpregnant women with normal iron stores don't need to rush into getting a supplement with more than 18 mg of iron.

Calcium and magnesium: no more than 250 mg of calcium and 25 mg of magnesium

Vitamin A: less than 5,000 IU. The beta-carotene form as part or all of the vitamin A is preferred over the retinol form to lessen the chance of toxicity (more than 10,000 IU/day)

Zinc: 8–15 mg

Vitamin D: 200–400 IU

Vitamin C: 60–85 mg

Vitamin B$_6$: 1.3–2 mg

Vitamin B$_{12}$: 2.4–6 mcg

Copper: 0.9–2 mg

Iodine: 150 mcg. This is a new recommendation. Not all multivitamins or prenatals contain iodine, but they should.

Choline and biotin: a typical multivitamin will not routinely provide much, if any, of these, and only a handful of prenatals do, but if available, less than or equal to 100% RDA or 100% of the DV would be a welcome addition. If neither are included, purchase a separate choline supplement, and just be sure you're eating a balanced diet to get sufficient biotin.

Any other vitamins and minerals, such as selenium, vitamin E, and vitamin K: less than or equal to 100% of the RDA or 100% of the DV.

Sources: National Academy of Sciences, Year 2001 & 2004 Dietary Reference Intakes (these DRIs are the most current, though new vitamin D recommendations are anticipated to be released in the latter half of 2010); Institute of Medicine, Subcommittee for a Clinical Application Guide, Committee on Nutritional Status During Pregnancy and Lactation, Food and Nutrition Board, *Nutrition During Pregnancy and Lactation* (Washington, D.C.: National Academy Press, 1992, and updated with newer recommendations); American Thyroid Association.

Best Time and Way to Take a Multivitamin-Mineral Supplement

The best time to take this type of supplement is with a low-calcium meal any time of day to minimize interference with iron absorption.[14] That includes any meal with which you might take a calcium supplement, too. For practical purposes, we typically advise taking the multivitamin-mineral supplement with a low-calcium dinner or evening snack, because if you subsequently experience nausea as a side effect, you may be able to sleep through it. This side effect is accentuated during early pregnancy, when queasiness is common. Constipation is another common side effect, so take the supplement with a big glass of water in addition to a high-fiber diet. Diarrhea is a less common side effect.

---

14. A few prescription prenatal supplements are specially formulated to release their iron and calcium at separate times to avoid interference, but most just don't have enough calcium to cause much trouble.

WARNING

Vitamin or mineral toxicities stem almost exclusively from excess intake of synthetic versions; rarely do they come from naturally occurring vitamins and minerals in foods. So, never take double or triple doses of multivitamin-mineral supplements. Even if a health care professional suggests it or you see it recommended in a fertility/pregnancy book, get a second opinion. This is an area where ignorance is all too common. Exceeding proper doses of broad-spectrum vitamin-mineral supplements has the potential to raise your intake close to or above recommended levels. For example:

- If you've been told to take a prenatal supplement and you forget to take it one day, do not take two the next day. Just get back to your regular daily schedule.
- If you have trouble swallowing pills and have been told to take children's chewable vitamins (with iron, especially after the twelfth week of pregnancy), it is still most prudent to take only *one* of these daily in addition to a well-rounded diet, including folate-rich foods listed in Table 11-1. Instead of children's chewables, there are now adult versions of over-the-counter chewable multivitamin-mineral supplements, as well as chewable prenatal supplements available by prescription. Ask your doctor for a prescription, as this may even make it more likely that insurance will pay for this. Liquid supplements are another option to discuss with your physician, but these are typically reserved for special circumstances such as women who have had gastric surgery.
- If you've been told that you do need to take more of a single vitamin or mineral than is available in your multivitamin-mineral supplement, take a separate pill containing only that micronutrient. For example, anemic women may need a separate iron pill; vitamin D–deficient women need very large amounts of separate supplemental vitamin D; women who have previously had a pregnancy involving an NTD need considerably more folic acid in separate pill form; women who cannot get enough calcium from foods may need supplemental calcium because multivitamin-mineral supplements often have very little.
- If you are really drawn to the convenience and taste of snack bars or meal replacement bars, just keep in mind that most are fortified with synthetic vitamins and minerals, some with as much as a multivitamin-mineral supplement. There are even designer nutrition bars for pre-pregnant, pregnant, or breastfeeding women (Bellybar is a reputable one). If you want to include an occasional one of these in your diet, take a close look at the wrapper to critique the label information. Make sure it won't bump you over the tolerable limits for any micronutrients, two examples being vitamin A and iron. Armed with this information, your health care professional can help decide if you need to adjust how frequently you take your vitamin-mineral (pill) supplement.

Persistent Side Effects from Multivitamin-Mineral Supplements

Most women tolerate multivitamin supplements quite well. However, some pre-pregnant women will find themselves thinking, "I've never been so constipated in my life!" while her friend, taking the same supplement, develops diarrhea. And later on, an exasperated pregnant patient asks, "Why even take this supplement when I seem to throw it up only minutes later?"

What should you do if side effects from multivitamin-mineral supplements remain bothersome or even debilitating? First, recognize that the often higher-than-recommended dose of iron in many prescription prenatal formulas is most responsible for the aforementioned side effects. For relief, switch to a general multivitamin supplement with or without minerals that contains no more than 100 percent of the Daily Value for each vitamin or mineral. If you prefer to stick with a prenatal formula, ask for one with less iron; an over-the-counter prenatal formula may fit the bill, too. Instead of 60 to 90 mg of iron per dose, look for one with 18 to 27 mg of iron; this is plenty for women who are not anemic or only mildly iron depleted. If this still doesn't agree with your stomach, consult your doctor to see if you can stop taking the supplement and switch over to one with no iron (a men's multivitamin or one children's chewable without iron). If this, too, fails, at least make sure to get 400 mcg folic acid in a separate pill through your first two missed periods.

CHAPTER 12

Using MyPyramid as a Guide: Ready to Provide Womb Service?

*W*e just spent the last two chapters exploring the qualities of individual nutrients such as carbohydrates, proteins, fats and oils, vitamins, and minerals. You can always refer back to those if you have a targeted question, say, on how to get a good balance of omega-3s or the latest research on the glycemic index of foods. Now let's take a look at the more practical concepts for diet and preconception. What happens when individual nutrients come together as components of whole foods?

It is actually a favorable trait that we humans are dependent on a balance of foods for good health. Our senses are delighted daily. Our taste buds relish the abundant flavors that foods have to offer. We have the opportunity to smell the aromas of freshly baked goods and savory entrées. We enjoy the sight of beautifully prepared food in all colors, sizes, and shapes. We salivate at the sound of a crisp apple being bitten into or the sizzle of a perfect steak on the grill. Our hands are rewarded by the feel of a fuzzy peach or the snap of a pea pod. And then there is the satisfaction of enjoying a meal with good company or alone in a peaceful setting.

Many of us have spent at least some of our adult life stressed out about what we eat—watching our weight, feeling guilty about eating fast food or junk food, vowing every day to adopt a more healthful diet. Preparing for pregnancy is an ideal time to adjust your attitude toward food and remind yourself that eating is one of life's greatest pleasures, not its greatest chore. To help people along, most countries use some form of pictorial food guide—in the shape of a pyramid, circle (or plate), pagoda, or rainbow—to illustrate food categories and recommend wholesome diet patterns. The USDA's MyPyramid (Figure 12-1) is a great tool to use in guiding your food choices not only now—prior to conception—but also during pregnancy, postpartum, and eventually when you must make decisions about how to feed your own children. The online component at www.MyPyramid.gov allows people to use an inter-

MyPyramid has been replaced with the new graphic image MyPlate, though the technical information remains essentially unchanged and current. Accessible through the more user-friendly www.ChooseMyPlate.gov.

active, tailored approach based on age, gender, height, current weight, and activity level. Or if you just want a quick snapshot of how to count one food or compare two foods side-by-side, the relatively new MyFoodapedia feature on this same website will accommodate your need for a quick reference, bypassing the slightly more time-consuming features.

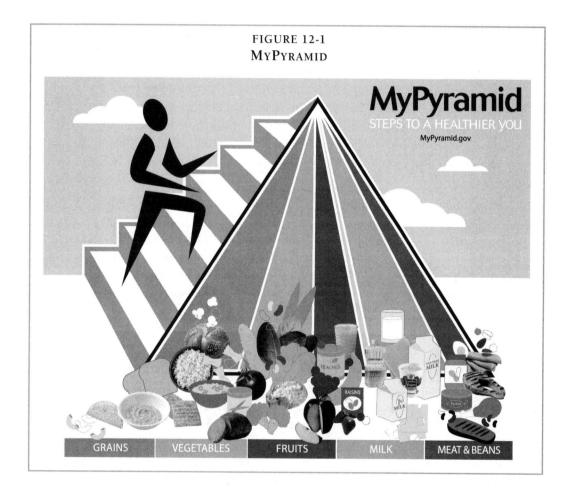

FIGURE 12-1
MyPyramid

MyPyramid replaced the Food Guide Pyramid in 2005, which replaced the "Basic Four" food groups (remember those?) in 1992. It categorizes foods and beverages according to their key nutrient similarities, yet advocates varying food choices within each group from meal to meal. The body of the Pyramid is made up of six color bands of varying widths to illustrate proportionality. The bands represent the five major food groups (from widest to narrowest: grains, vegetables, fruits, dairy, and concentrated proteins), and the sixth sliver represents a healthy balance of oils, which we'll categorize as the honorary sixth food group that we make a point of using in meal makeovers beginning in the middle of Chapter 13.

Each food group has its own redeeming qualities, and too much or too little of any group places a strain on the nutrient equilibrium needed for pre-pregnancy. MyPyramid visually represents how foods proportionately fit into a healthy diet. More emphasis is placed on grains, vegetables, fruits, and low-fat dairy in terms of volume of food. Then smaller portions of concentrated proteins and healthy oils (alone or as a component of another food such as nuts or fatty fish) complete the balance. Solid fats and sugars (and alcohol)[1] aren't even represented by a category. Instead, they are relegated to the status of discretionary calories (extras) that may be included when you've met your body's needs through nutrient-dense foods and still have room for a few more calories. When trying to eat exceptionally well, people don't typically have that many calories left to their discretion and often use them up as a component of the other groups (e.g., ice cream or sugar-sweetened low-fat yogurt instead of nonfat plain yogurt; a fattier cut of meat instead of a lean one; baked goods that include hidden fat and sugar). If you are a saint, discretionary calories can always be used to eat more of the healthier choices as well, but most people want to know how the occasional not-so-healthy indulgence fits in.

Although Helena considered herself relatively healthy and informed about nutrition, eating well had never been a strong point for her, and she seemed daunted by the prospect of using this book in conjunction with the MyPyramid Menu Planner as the basis for her nutrition makeover. However, after a short demo on the computer, she warmed to the fact that there was more to MyPyramid than meets the eye. It could serve as the basis of what she really wanted—knowledge that she was getting the most nutritious diet to promote fertility and get geared up for pregnancy. So we began talking about what she had eaten so far that day, and how her intake stacked up to her body's requirements. Helena learned to work with MyPyramid. She even tinkered with the vitamin-mineral analysis that it would do for her! For many combination items such as lasagna, Helena liked that the program knew how to allocate the ingredients to their respective food groups, and she even found a listing for her half-caff "latté," which served as a milk serving or two, depending on the size she ordered. She also learned to work with the program's quirks—for example, she enjoyed candied walnuts on salads, and she learned that she needed to break them down as "walnuts" and "honey" (and count the honey partially toward her discretionary calories). Later she could go to her cupboards, refrigerator, and nearby grocery store and compare what she considered to be a serving with what MyPyramid said. She realized that she hadn't fully appreciated the information contained in the triangular graphic she'd so often dismissed. Soon she was using the MyPyramid Menu Planner as the template for all her meal and snack decisions. "Why didn't I do this a long time ago? It's so much easier now!" she said.

---

1. For women, limit consumption to one alcoholic beverage per day as long as you are more than two weeks from conceiving. For men, limit consumption to two servings per day. See Chapter 2 for more specifics.

To follow MyPyramid successfully, understand that it is designed to estimate the needs of fairly average, healthy people. If that doesn't describe you, don't worry. You'll just need a little additional guidance from a health care professional with nutrition expertise to determine your needs. Another plus is that you don't need to know which foods fall into each group. You'll learn as the graphics on the screen spell it out for you. However, not everyone has access to the Internet, and some people get frustrated with learning a new computer program and quit before getting hooked. The key here is to click on the "SuperTracker" button and try it out. Navigate the site with your partner as you both will benefit from using the MyPyramid before and after conception to optimize healthy eating and to offer moral support to each other as you pursue this goal.

To give you insight into what MyPyramid is based on, we'll help you get to know the food groups and what constitutes a single serving of each. The "Inside the Food Pyramid" option on www.MyPyramid.gov is excellent for learning this (you can even view photos of portion sizes in the "food gallery" for each group). It is quite common for people to unknowingly eat several portions when they think they are eating only one. A perfect example of this is a bagel, which is the equivalent of three or four bread servings. (This is not to say that you'll be limited to one serving at a time. But be aware that MyPyramid's individual portion sizes are not necessarily the same serving sizes that appear on nutrition labels; the USDA and FDA haven't coordinated that yet.) MyPyramid estimates the total number of daily servings to aim for, and this is individualized based on your gender, age, weight, height, and activity level. For now, pay attention to what constitutes a single portion so you can get used to judging how many portions you consume—or should consume—every time you eat.

The simplest way to construct a balanced preconception diet is to include all six food groups in the recommended amounts each day. No food group is easily expendable. This is why vegetarians who avoid dairy products must be vigilant in choosing various nondairy products that, when accounted for as a whole, cover the nutrients missed from dairy foods.

FROM MARKET TO HOME: MAKING YOUR SHOPPING LIST AND STOCKING YOUR KITCHEN

Let's start from the left side of MyPyramid and work our way through all the food groups.

Grain Group (Bread, Cereal, Rice, and Pasta)

Grains are carbohydrate-rich foods that make up the biggest part of a healthy preconception diet. At least half of your choices should be whole grains—those that retain the bran and germ as well as the endosperm after milling—as the best source of fiber, vitamins, minerals, and health-promoting essential fatty acids and phytonutrients (refining takes most of these out). There is room for some refined grains but, in general, the less refined, the better they are for you.

QUICK TIP

Some manufacturers display a Whole Grain Stamp to help consumers identify products that contain healthy amounts of whole grains, the highest being products with 100 percent whole grains. However, many excellent whole-grain products (including those made by many small producers who opt out of membership in this nonprofit organization) are not using the symbol, so you'll need to use your knowledge from this chapter and Chapter 10 to read ingredient lists. And always probe further into the Nutrition Facts panel for "Total Fiber" grams.

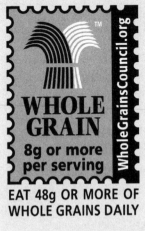 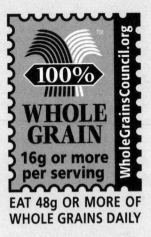

Courtesy of Whole Grains Council, www.wholegrainscouncil.org

Grain-based foods that are prepared with fat (e.g., muffins, pancakes, stuffing, taco shells) should count in the grain group; count the fat as part of your discretionary calories. Cakes, cookies, and ice cream cones count similarly—as grain plus added fat and sugar. Even though popcorn and fried corn chips are technically made from the vegetable corn, these snack foods are counted in the grain group (plus fat again).

The following items each count as one serving of grain:

1 slice of bread or small (6-inch) corn or flour tortilla
½ cup cooked cereal, pasta, rice, or barley
1 ounce ready-to-eat cereal (1 oz = 28 grams)
4–6 small crackers or pretzels
½ mini bagel, English muffin, pita, or bun (a regular-sized bagel is almost 4 servings)
3 tbsp wheat germ

Vegetable Group

Notice that the vegetable group on MyPyramid is wider than the fruit group to its right. This is to encourage a slightly higher consumption of veggies, equivalent to at least 2½ cups per day. Try to choose from each of the five subcategories of vegetables: dark green, bright orange, legumes, starchy, and "others" (deep red tomatoes and peppers, onions, and possible infection- and cancer-fighting cruciferous powerhouses such as Brussels sprouts, cauliflower, cabbage, radicchio, and turnip). The deeply colorful veggies are generally higher in healthy carotenoids and/or vitamin C plus other vitamins and minerals (refer to Chapter 11 for specific examples). Vegetables also contain a variety of other natural phytochemicals (also called phytonutrients) that may improve long-term health. Researchers are only beginning to understand the healthful potential of phytochemicals, so consume a wide variety of veggies (and culinary herbs and spices) to reap known and undiscovered benefits.

Often, one meal will contain two or three vegetable servings. Starchy vegetables such as potatoes, peas, corn, and winter squash are very nutritious but have more calories than other vegetables. When you choose to have something like a small baked potato as a side dish, try to make a point of including a less starchy vegetable (sliced tomato, salad, or steamed broccoli) instead of another starchy veggie, such as corn or peas. To turn your taste buds on to the most flavorful vegetables at the least expensive price, eat mostly ones that are in season; for terrific seasonal recipes, start with Jill Nussinow's cookbook *The Veggie Queen*—a real gem.

The following items each count as 1 cup equivalent of vegetables in MyPyramid:

1 cup raw chopped or cooked vegetables

1 large sweet potato or medium baked potato

1 cup whole or mashed dry beans or peas, cooked

1 cup vegetable juice

¾ cup vegetarian spaghetti sauce (less than 1 cup because it's more concentrated)

2 cups raw leafy vegetables, such as spinach or lettuce leaves (not as compact, so it takes more to be equivalent to the others)

Fruit Group

Try to get your fruit servings primarily from a variety of whole fruits. We prefer to limit fruit juices to no more than one-half serving per day because they are typically lower in fiber, higher in calories, and easy to overconsume because they go down so easily!

Regularly include fruits that are noted for their vitamin C, potassium, and/or carotenoid content as well as those high in other vitamins and minerals. Fruits, like vegetables, contain a variety of naturally occurring phytochemicals that have antioxidant and potential anti-inflammatory activity. By routinely varying your choices of fruits (and vegetables), you get the benefits of thousands of these molecules. Variety balances the calorie variation, too.

The following items each count as 1 cup equivalent in MyPyramid:

> 1 medium fresh fruit (pear, apple, or avocado) or 3 smallish fruits (plum, kiwi)
> 1 large fruit (grapefruit, papaya, orange); 1 large banana
> 1 cup cooked or canned fruit (preferably with very little or no sugar added)
> 1 cup berries, grapes, or melon
> 1 cup 100 percent fruit juice (e.g., orange, pomegranate, blueberry, grape)[2]
> ½ cup dried fruit such as açai, blueberry, cranberry (remember, these fruits were much bigger before they lost most of their moisture content)

Milk Group

Dairy foods are a rich source of minerals, especially calcium, as well as vitamin A, vitamin D, and riboflavin. Dairy foods unfortunately have the reputation of being high in fat. Indeed, some are, but there are also numerous low-fat and even fat-free choices. Choose with the knowledge that some dairy fat is acceptable—even potentially helpful in cases of ovulatory infertility—in the preconception food plan but that most of your choices should be low-fat. One notable exception here is for soy milk drinkers. Always buy regular (full-fat) soy milk as a great source of healthy oil that is underrepresented in most people's diets.

The following items each count as 1 cup equivalent in MyPyramid—and notice that when butterfat is integral to a product (e.g., 1%, 2%, and whole milk; cheeses), it counts as both milk *and* solid fat in the "discretionary calories" section:

> 1 cup of milk (fat-free/nonfat/skim, 1% low-fat/light, 2% reduced-fat, or whole); includes lactose-reduced milk; regular enriched soy milk (unsweetened) may be substituted, but technically these count in the meat and beans group of MyPyramid
> 1 cup of fermented probiotic milk beverage such as kefir, acidophilus milk, buttermilk
> 1 cup of fat-free or low-fat yogurt
> ½ cup evaporated milk (try fat-free or low-fat)
> ⅓ cup powdered dry milk
> 1½ ounces natural cheese or 2 ounces processed cheese (American)[3]
> 2 cups cottage cheese

---

2. Don't count drinks such as lemonade, cranberry juice cocktail, Hi-C, Tang, or Kool-Aid in the fruit group. These are counted primarily as added sugar, in the extras category.
3. Remember, some of this will count towards solid fat ("extras"). An exception is cream cheese, which is *all* solid fat, no milk.

Foods such as ice cream, instant breakfasts, pudding, custard, and frozen yogurt count here, in the dairy group. But ½ cup of one of these items counts as half of a milk serving with 70–110 more calories tagging along; these remaining calories count as discretionary, meaning calories from solid fat and sugar.

If you follow a vegan lifestyle, you can still eat healthfully without dairy foods, but nondairy sources for calcium, vitamins A and D, riboflavin, iodine, and phosphorus deserve special attention. For starters, 1 cup of fortified soy milk can be counted as a milk substitute, although MyPyramid formally classifies this in the meat and beans group, as it is derived from soybeans.

LACTOSE INTOLERANCE

If you cannot drink milk or eat other dairy products without getting bloated and gassy afterward, you may be lactose intolerant. This is different from having a milk allergy. An intolerance to the milk sugar called lactose—a carbohydrate—normally manifests anywhere from age two to twenty. It is quite common all over the world, particularly among blacks, Asians, Hispanics, Pacific Islanders, and Native Americans.

What causes these uncomfortable symptoms? Lactose-intolerant individuals have little or none of the intestinal enzyme that normally digests the lactose. Instead, the lactose molecules travel through the gut and attract more water (leading to diarrhea), while bacteria in the colon ferment the lactose (creating gas and bloating). Such discomfort is enough to steer anyone away from these calcium-rich foods!

Fortunately, very few people are completely lactose intolerant, meaning that smaller portions of dairy products may be well tolerated if distributed throughout the day's meals. This way your smaller amount of functioning enzyme can keep up with the amount of lactose you eat. Also, tolerance of lactose naturally improves during pregnancy. See how much you can build your tolerance to lactose by gradually including a few small portions of dairy foods throughout the day. If you still come up short, see Chapter 11 specifically for nondairy food sources and supplement ideas for calcium, vitamin D, and iodine.

Hard cheeses, cottage cheese, yogurt, and ice cream are often better tolerated than cow's milk. Lactose-free cow's milk is readily available at the grocery store, as are soy milk and rice milk. These do not contain lactose (nor does coconut milk, but be aware of its high level of saturated fat). Pay attention to the calcium and vitamin D content in the nondairy alternatives to cow's milk, because many are naturally poor sources of both unless they are fortified; rice milk is also lower in protein than soy milk.

Meat and Beans Group

MyPyramid uses 1-ounce *equivalents* for portion sizes, although each of the items listed below doesn't weigh exactly 1 ounce. Don't worry; it's simpler than it looks. For example, visualize 1 ounce as the same as an egg or one golf-ball-sized meatball. If you eat two eggs or two meatballs, you've eaten two 1-ounce equivalents. It's common to eat three to six 1-ounce equivalents at a sitting if you have a fillet of fish, a chicken breast, or a small steak; it can quickly add up! The following are 1-ounce equivalents:

> 1 oz cooked beef, lamb, pork, poultry, fish, and shellfish[4]
> 1 egg (eat up to 7 yolks per week for an excellent source of choline; no limit on whites)
> ¼ cup egg substitute (though whole eggs are preferred for nutritional balance)
> ¼ cup cooked dried beans, lentils, or other legume
> ¼ cup tofu, tempeh, seitan, textured vegetable protein (TVP)
> 1 cup unsweetened soy milk; soy yogurt
> 1 tbsp peanut butter or other nut butter (also see "For Future Reference" on page 380)
> ½ ounce nuts or seeds (7 walnuts, 12 almonds; ¼ cup pumpkin or sunflower seeds)

Good sources of protein are found in other foods outside of the meat and beans group, but this group contributes the greatest proportion of protein in a well-rounded diet. *Each 1-ounce equivalent in this group contains approximately 7 grams of protein.* Most people meet well over half of their protein needs from this one group of foods.

If you consume six or fewer ounce equivalents of these concentrated proteins before conception, you may need to add more ounce equivalents per day during pregnancy (as discussed in Chapter 13). Very high-protein fad diets are not advisable because they are low in folate and usually don't permit adequate intake of energy from carbohydrates; if the body has to resort to getting energy from sources other than carbohydrates, it forms ketones that can be harmful in high amounts to the mom and even more to a fetus. Very high protein intakes (especially of animal protein) might cause your body to excrete calcium in your urine.

By eating a variety of foods from the meat and beans group you get nutrients such as iron, zinc, choline, and some of the B vitamins (thiamin, niacin, B12). Some selections yield a little more hidden, solid fat than you bargained for, but moderate portion sizes, leaner selections, and leaner cooking methods can keep that in check. Do try to reserve one or more protein selections for nuts and seeds, which double as a good way to fill your need for oils (see next section).

---

4. If the concept of ounces of meat is Greek to you, use the traditional "deck of cards" as a point of reference for what a 3-ounce portion looks like in size and thickness after cooking.

Oils

The narrowest band in the MyPyramid visually sends the message that oils—the lipids that are liquid at room temperature—should play a modest but integral role in our everyday diet. For example, a healthy balance of oils and fats plays an indispensable role in hormone production and fertility in these preconception months. To emphasize this importance for you, we take it one semantic step further and count oils as the honorary sixth food group when doing meal makeovers in Chapter 13.

If the majority of your food choices tend to be lean or low-fat, then there should easily be room for around six servings of added oil per day, adjusted downward if you have meals with significant hidden oil or fat. To guide the majority of your choices toward the healthier varieties of oils, we mention just a sampling of the monounsaturated and polyunsaturated fat sources that are available to you (our favorites are denoted with a ♥). Check Chapter 10 for a more complete listing of healthy liquid oils and foods that are naturally rich in them.

The following items each count as a 1-teaspoon equivalent of oil:

1 tsp oil (such as canola♥ or olive♥ oil)
1 tsp margarine (always trans fat free)
1 tsp mayonnaise, aioli♥ (made with extra virgin olive oil)
1 tbsp lite margarine, mayonnaise
1 tbsp oil-based salad dressing♥ such as Italian
1 tbsp mayonnaise-based salad dressing (ranch, blue cheese)
1½ tbsp thousand island dressing
2 tbsp reduced-fat salad dressing
¼ to ½ ounce nuts♥ and seeds♥; ½ to 1 tsp nut butters♥ and seeds♥ (see explanation below)

Nuts and seeds are concentrated sources of healthy oils, and they count mostly as oil, but also as members the meat and beans group. It's an inexact science, but good enough over time. For example, if you choose an amount of ¼ ounce (~5–6 nuts) almonds, it is equivalent to ½ ounce "meats" plus 1 tsp oil, whereas ½ ounce (11 nuts) still counts as 1 tsp oil but bumps up the protein enough for a 1-ounce "meat" credit. Give MyPyramid a try to see how these are automatically divvied up—the program keeps track of these confusing details so you don't have to. You are smart to look here for avocados because they are rich in healthy oils, but MyPyramid counts them in the fruit group only.

Practical Application

MyPyramid's free computer program (www.mypyramid.gov) does not chastise you if discretionary calories are a problem area for you, but once your allotment of daily discretionary calories is used up, you spill over from your green ("go for it") zone to a red ("whoa, Nelly!") zone. While you read this, head over to your computer if you haven't already. Even if you don't want to enter what you eat into the "Menu Planner" function, just navigate to the "Inside the Pyramid" choice (on the left-side menu bar)." Then look at the right-side menu bar and choose "Discretionary Calories." Go directly to "How Do I Count Discretionary Calories?" for an eye-opener. If you decide you want to see this in action, you can always go back to the beginning and use the Menu Planner function. It's really interesting to tinker with and see how these extras can add up unexpectedly quickly (e.g., that one glazed doughnut that you mindlessly ate at the office the other day added a whopping 165 calories to your "extras" tally in addition to the one serving of grains). The "Report" function will show you exactly where the indiscretions came from, and offers nonjudgmental tips for better balance.

DISCRETIONARY OR "EXTRA" CALORIES: SOLID FATS, SWEETS, AND ALCOHOL

Solid Fats

Butter, stick margarine, and shortening are all conspicuously absent from the "oils" category of MyPyramid, because they contain solid fats (either naturally or through the process of hydrogenation, making it a trans fat). So, too, are things such as cream, sour cream, cream cheese, gravy, and bacon. This is a departure from the older Pyramid version, where all concentrated fats and oils were sequestered in the attic of the Food Guide Pyramid. Now the USDA's new MyPyramid has visually retained oils alongside the five primary food groups but relegated solid fats (and sweets and alcohol) to the sidelines. The sidelined foods are not banned, though. They count in a separate "calorie bank account," the "extras." When you eat something like ten steak-cut dinner fries, you will notice that they do count toward ½ cup of a vegetable, but the "extra" calories add up to 147 calories; those represent the fat calories from the frying vat. The whole milk you added to your cereal counted as one milk serving, but also 65 calories more in the "extras" category. Keep tuned in to when your "extras" category is being maxed out before your real food group requirements are being met.

You may begin to see a pattern forming here. Much of the solid fat that we consume is hidden in whole foods, so we often overdo it or forget to count it separately. The more hidden fats you consume, the fewer obvious added fats you should eat (such as that pat of butter or dash of cream), and vice versa. Keep in mind that most people get thrown for a loop when they eat out a lot: there is a great deal of disguised fat (as well as larger portions) in restaurant servings. Ditto for many premade, prepackaged foods, unless you have studied the label with a keen eye on what constitutes a portion, total fat, saturated fat, and trans fats. As a rule of thumb, you can outsmart all of this by eating foods that have been minimally processed; then you are in control of whether you add "extras" to them.

Sweets

As you know from the introduction to carbohydrates in Chapter 10, sugar takes different forms and may be present to some degree in the five major food groups—as naturally occurring sugar (in milk and fruits) and as added sugar. The discretionary calories in MyPyramid cover added sugars and syrups. With the knowledge that added sugars are nutrient poor, use them only sparingly. But what does this really mean?

Most women can still meet their nutrient needs and maintain their weight while including sparing amounts of disguised and added sugars in their diet. For instance, if your weekly diet includes foods such as sugar-sweetened cereals, muffins, sugar-sweetened yogurt, or occasional pie or ice cream, then your intake of concentrated added sweets such as jam or jelly, honey, sugar, and syrups will need to be very limited. Items such as sweetened soft drinks, fruit-flavored drinks, sweetened teas, regular Jell-O, Cool Whip, and candy should be a rare treat. As an example, a canned soft drink contains close to 8 teaspoons of sugar! Instead of debating the purported evils of real sugar versus high-fructose corn syrup (both are void of the redeeming qualities of true food groups), it is better to choose nutrient-dense, whole foods. You also have the option of eating "no sugar added" or "sugar-free" products in an attempt to satisfy your sweet tooth (Chapter 10 covers the difference between these products and their safety records).

Alcohol

All calories consumed from wine, beer, and distilled spirits count in the discretionary calorie category. See Chapter 2 for a full overview of how alcohol fits into your preconception plan, if you choose to drink at all.

Mixed Dishes

Meals and snacks are often a combination of many food groups. In these cases, you have the extra challenge of considering what all of the main ingredients are, and then estimating how much of each is in the item. This task is relatively easy once you break the meal into the basics, and you don't have to be exact—www.MyPyramid.gov does it all for you. If you are not near your computer or Internet-enabled phone, here's how to guesstimate in your head. For example, a large piece of thin crust cheese pizza with vegetable topping would count as 1 to 1½ grains (crust), ¼ to ½ cup equivalent of vegetable (tomato sauce and veggies on top), and ¼ to ½ cup milk servings plus "extra" calories (cheese), depending on how generous they are. A 1-cup serving of seafood pasta salad might be counted as 1 ounce grain (noodles), 1 ounce meat substitute (seafood), ¼ cup vegetable (chopped veggies), and 2 added oils (mayonnaise or salad dressing).

CUSTOMIZING YOUR PYRAMID

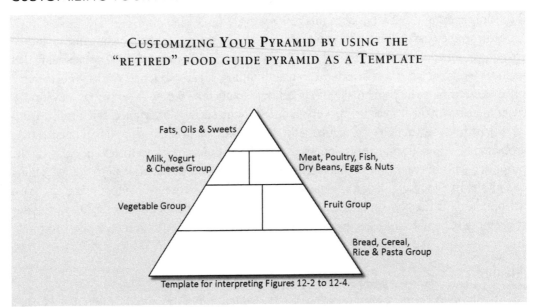

CUSTOMIZING YOUR PYRAMID BY USING THE "RETIRED" FOOD GUIDE PYRAMID AS A TEMPLATE

Fats, Oils & Sweets

Milk, Yogurt & Cheese Group

Meat, Poultry, Fish, Dry Beans, Eggs & Nuts

Vegetable Group

Fruit Group

Bread, Cereal, Rice & Pasta Group

Template for interpreting Figures 12-2 to 12-4.

Every culture has food traditions that are very healthy and based on the region's native foods, culinary herbs, and spices. From a nutritional perspective, the least processed, freshest local ingredients were what nourished people through the childbearing years and into old age because the local foods retained more nutrients. The personal touch to your preconception diet comes from finding out how recipes or restaurants that honor local food traditions fit within the existing model. So what's different about what you see on the next few pages? The template you see was adapted from the original Food Guide Pyramid layout that was retired in 2005. Both that version and the current one are generic templates from which to work, the only major difference now is how oils, solid fats, and sweets are categorized, but you have enough information on how to count those differences (using your discretionary calorie category) to still appreciate these timeless resources. We've simply found no other resource that contains such an extensive categorization of cultural food preferences by name (no ambiguous food drawings here; it's all spelled out clearly).

Virtually every type of food imaginable can be easily incorporated into one of the five food groups, oils, or discretionary "extras." To demonstrate how MyPyramid can be customized to meet different food preferences, Figures 12-2, 12-3, and 12-4 feature "world foods" placed in the traditional food Pyramid to create multicultural food Pyramids. This same exercise can be done for foods that are characteristic of other regions. There is no limit to the diversity of foods that you can place in your own personal MyPyramid. As long as you know what food group the basic item counts as, you can probably almost guess if discretionary calories need to be accounted for, too (for example, a biscuit counts as grain as well as discretionary calories from solid fat). Chances are you'll be pleasantly surprised to find many of these items in the current MyPyramid database, so you can check how close you are to eyeballing where foods fit into your meal plan.

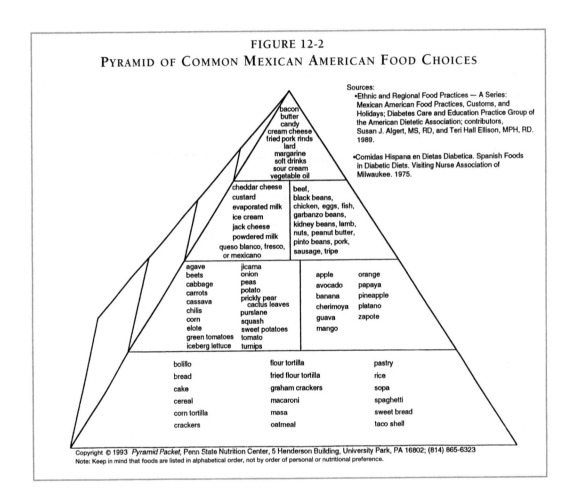

FIGURE 12-2
PYRAMID OF COMMON MEXICAN AMERICAN FOOD CHOICES

Sources:
• Ethnic and Regional Food Practices — A Series: Mexican American Food Practices, Customs, and Holidays; Diabetes Care and Education Practice Group of the American Dietetic Association; contributors, Susan J. Algert, MS, RD, and Teri Hall Ellison, MPH, RD. 1989.

• Comidas Hispana en Dietas Diabetica. Spanish Foods in Diabetic Diets. Visiting Nurse Association of Milwaukee. 1975.

bacon
butter
candy
cream cheese
fried pork rinds
lard
margarine
soft drinks
sour cream
vegetable oil

cheddar cheese
custard
evaporated milk
ice cream
jack cheese
powdered milk
queso blanco, fresco, or mexicano

beef,
black beans,
chicken, eggs, fish,
garbanzo beans,
kidney beans, lamb,
nuts, peanut butter,
pinto beans, pork,
sausage, tripe

agave
beets
cabbage
carrots
cassava
chilis
corn
elote
green tomatoes
iceberg lettuce

jicama
onion
peas
potato
prickly pear cactus leaves
purslane
squash
sweet potatoes
tomato
turnips

apple
avocado
banana
cherimoya
guava
mango

orange
papaya
pineapple
platano
zapote

bolillo
bread
cake
cereal
corn tortilla
crackers

flour tortilla
fried flour tortilla
graham crackers
macaroni
masa
oatmeal

pastry
rice
sopa
spaghetti
sweet bread
taco shell

Copyright © 1993 *Pyramid Packet*, Penn State Nutrition Center, 5 Henderson Building, University Park, PA 16802; (814) 865-6323
Note: Keep in mind that foods are listed in alphabetical order, not by order of personal or nutritional preference.

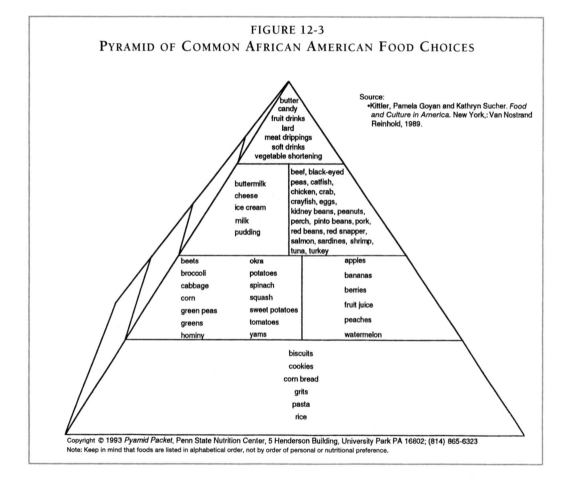

FIGURE 12-3
PYRAMID OF COMMON AFRICAN AMERICAN FOOD CHOICES

butter
candy
fruit drinks
lard
meat drippings
soft drinks
vegetable shortening

Source:
•Kittler, Pamela Goyan and Kathryn Sucher. *Food and Culture in America*. New York,: Van Nostrand Reinhold, 1989.

buttermilk
cheese
ice cream
milk
pudding

beef, black-eyed peas, catfish, chicken, crab, crayfish, eggs, kidney beans, peanuts, perch, pinto beans, pork, red beans, red snapper, salmon, sardines, shrimp, tuna, turkey

beets
broccoli
cabbage
corn
green peas
greens
hominy

okra
potatoes
spinach
squash
sweet potatoes
tomatoes
yams

apples
bananas
berries
fruit juice
peaches
watermelon

biscuits
cookies
corn bread
grits
pasta
rice

Copyright © 1993 *Pyamid Packet*, Penn State Nutrition Center, 5 Henderson Building, University Park PA 16802; (814) 865-6323
Note: Keep in mind that foods are listed in alphabetical order, not by order of personal or nutritional preference.

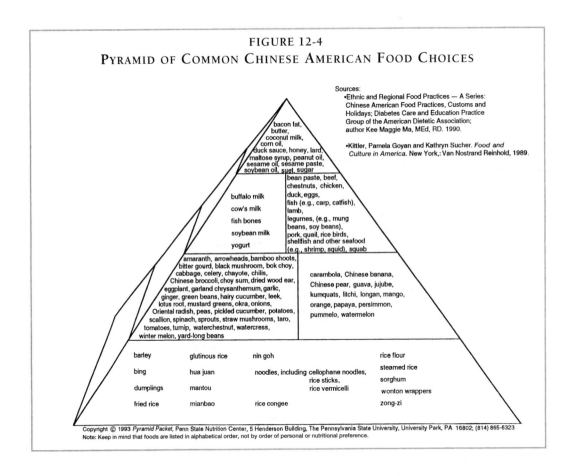

FIGURE 12-4
PYRAMID OF COMMON CHINESE AMERICAN FOOD CHOICES

Sources:
•Ethnic and Regional Food Practices — A Series: Chinese American Food Practices, Customs and Holidays; Diabetes Care and Education Practice Group of the American Dietetic Association; author Kee Maggie Ma, MEd, RD. 1990.

•Kittler, Pamela Goyan and Kathryn Sucher. *Food and Culture in America.* New York,: Van Nostrand Reinhold, 1989.

bacon fat, butter, coconut milk, corn oil, duck sauce, honey, lard, maltose syrup, peanut oil, sesame oil, sesame paste, soybean oil, suet, sugar

buffalo milk
cow's milk
fish bones
soybean milk
yogurt

bean paste, beef, chestnuts, chicken, duck, eggs, fish (e.g., carp, catfish), lamb, legumes, (e.g., mung beans, soy beans), pork, quail, rice birds, shellfish and other seafood (e.g., shrimp, squid), squab

amaranth, arrowheads, bamboo shoots, bitter gourd, black mushroom, bok choy, cabbage, celery, chayote, chilis, Chinese broccoli, choy sum, dried wood ear, eggplant, garland chrysanthemum, garlic, ginger, green beans, hairy cucumber, leek, lotus root, mustard greens, okra, onions, Oriental radish, peas, pickled cucumber, potatoes, scallion, spinach, sprouts, straw mushrooms, taro, tomatoes, turnip, waterchestnut, watercress, winter melon, yard-long beans

carambola, Chinese banana, Chinese pear, guava, jujube, kumquats, litchi, longan, mango, orange, papaya, persimmon, pummelo, watermelon

barley	glutinous rice	nin goh	rice flour
bing	hua juan	noodles, including cellophane noodles, rice sticks, rice vermicelli	steamed rice, sorghum
dumplings	mantou		wonton wrappers
fried rice	mianbao	rice congee	zong-zi

Copyright © 1993 *Pyramid Packet*, Penn State Nutrition Center, 5 Henderson Building, The Pennsylvania State University, University Park, PA 16802; (814) 865-6323
Note: Keep in mind that foods are listed in alphabetical order, not by order of personal or nutritional preference.

Our thanks to Penn State Nutrition Center for permitting us to reprint three of the eight culturally diverse food pyramids it developed. Though they are laid out differently than the new MyPyramid design, which uses narrow bands without room for detailed wording or pictures (disallowed in their copyrighted graphics), these Penn State ones work splendidly for that very purpose. The other Pyramids are Asian Indian, Jewish, Navajo Indian, Puerto Rican, and Vietnamese American.

FOR VEGETARIANS

Women who choose a well-balanced vegetarian lifestyle are no different from nonvegetarians in their ability to support a healthy conception and pregnancy. On the other hand, a poorly balanced vegetarian diet, one that lacks variety, adequate fat, and sufficient calories, is not enough to support normal ovulation and menstrual cycles and a healthy womb environment. It is crucial that dietary variety be high and that the USDA's MyPyramid be used as the guideline (Figure 12-1). If you are completely avoiding the dairy group, those nutrients can be compensated for. It just takes extra work and creativity to cover your nutrient requirements. However, vegans may need to be particularly resourceful to make this work.

Vitamin D, calcium, zinc, and iron are often potentially low in the vegetarian diet; vitamin B_{12} and iodine may be particularly low in the vegan diet. These nutrients can be deliberately sought out in a variety of vegetarian food choices. Please read Chapter 11 carefully if you are following a vegetarian diet.

Vitamin B_{12} is found naturally only in animal products, so vegans will need to consciously include vitamin B_{12}–fortified foods such as certain ready-to-eat cereals, soy milk, and some veggie burgers and meat substitutes (check the label). A supplement that contains B_{12}, or cyanocobalamin, is also an option. Another reliable B_{12} source is nutritional yeast (Red Star Vegetarian Support Formula, formerly T6635). Many vegans have been misled into thinking that algae, seaweed, spirulina, and specially fermented soy products, such as miso and tempeh, are good sources of vitamin B_{12} because the bacteria used in the fermentation process produce B_{12}. However, humans cannot utilize the type of vitamin B_{12} in these products.

What about protein? Both plant and animal sources of protein (except gelatin) contain all of the amino acids, the individual building blocks of proteins. Animal proteins have high amounts of all the amino acids; plant sources are usually low in one or two essential amino acids. This needn't be a problem. As long as strict vegetarians consume a variety of legumes, nuts, seeds, grains, and vegetables over the course of a day according to MyPyramid, they will meet their protein needs. It's no longer believed necessary to combine plant foods in the same meal to get high amounts of essential and nonessential amino acids at once, as the body can also draw from its "reserve" pool of free amino acids to complement shifts in plant protein composition.

Beginning in the months prior to conception, the essential fatty acid alpha-linolenic acid (ALA), which must be converted into the active omega-3s EPA and DHA, should also receive greater attention in the vegetarian's diet to prepare for fetal brain and eye development. Because strict vegetarians avoid fish (fatty fish are the best source of EPA and DHA), it is extra important to eat ALA food sources such as walnuts and walnut oil, butternuts, canola oil, soybean oil, soybeans, and soy products, as discussed in Chapter 10. However, it's important to note that most ALA conversion to the long-chain omega-3 fatty acids stops at EPA, and very

Types of Vegetarians

- **Semivegetarian or flexitarian:** Loose term encompassing people who are simply limiting meat in their diet as well as those who exclude meat and/or poultry, but include fish
- **Lacto-ovo vegetarian:** Includes dairy products and eggs, but no meat, poultry, or fish; this is the most common category of vegetarian
- **Lacto-vegetarian:** Includes dairy products, but no meat, poultry, fish, or eggs
- **Ovo-vegetarian:** Includes eggs, but no meat, poultry, fish, or dairy products
- **Vegan or strict vegetarian:** Avoidance of all animal products (and possibly honey, sugar, vinegar, wine, and beer)
- **Other vegetarian:** Macrobiotic, fruitarian, raw foods, or natural hygiene diets. (not recommended for women or their partners while trying to conceive)

little ends up as DHA. Some brands of soy milk and snack bars are fortified with DHA, and if you are willing to eat eggs, try ones from hens supplemented with feed containing marine algae. Eggs from hens who are fed canola oil or flaxseed (both are ALA-rich) could be alternated, though they don't offer a comparable DHA boost. Marine algae, the only source of the "brain food" omega-3 DHA, is also being used in omega-3 supplements as a vegan alternative to fish oil; however, not much DHA is converted backward (retroconversion) into EPA, making the aforementioned ALA food sources all the more valuable to achieve omega-3 balance.

Vegetarians or vegans who have specific questions about resources or recipes would do well to start by looking at the Vegetarian Resource Group website, www.vrg.org.

You now have the basics to identify what food groups your food choices fall into. In the next chapter you'll get to evaluate your current intake through a written exercise and give your and your partner's meal plan a preconception tune-up.

CHAPTER 13

Tailoring Your Preconception Diet to Meet Your Needs

To eat is a necessity, but to eat intelligently is an art.
　　—*François de La Rochefoucauld*

Formulating a practical, nutritious, and enticing pre-pregnancy diet is the ultimate in self-care. After all, you are preparing your body to be at its very best. With just a few adjustments, your healthy diet can carry you not only through pre-pregnancy and pregnancy but to postpartum and beyond. The same goes for your partner, but he won't need to anticipate adding extra calories during the pregnancy part, unless he gains "sympathy pounds" with you!

To easily maneuver through your preconception diet makeover, you need to build on the information you learned in Chapter 12. We'll gradually move from the general to the specific— to what you currently eat and how that compares to your body's physical needs and food preferences. Then we'll look at convenient, affordable meal makeover ideas taken from our clients, and add a touch of food safety savvy.

If you are adept at cooking and have always had a handle on eating wholesomely, this part of your preconception plan will be a breeze. You'll need no convincing that it can be fun to figure out how to make "breakfast for dinner" with, say, four to five food groups in it (think whole-wheat toast, scrambled egg, cheese, thick wedges of tomato, and a small side salad topped with orange slices and walnuts—voilà!). But not everyone has a flair for cooking. So our aim is for all prospective parents to know food prep basics and food safety precautions, so they eventually feel comfortable enough to wing it healthfully. But believe it or not, it's empowering to have a few culinary tricks up your sleeve if you want to nourish yourself and your future family well. You *can* do this!

Let's begin by looking at Table 13-1. This table corresponds to how many food group servings prospective parents need every day, according to the MyPyramid guidelines and Estimated Energy Requirements (EER) formulas for women and men at various ages.[1] A

---

1. EER formulas come from the current Institute of Medicine Dietary Reference Intakes macronutrients report and are built into the simple fill-in-the-blank introductory page on www.MyPyramid.com to estimate your calorie needs more exactly.

moderately active woman in her twenties, thirties, and early forties would look to the middle range of the chart as a guide for what she should be eating. Not every individual fits that profile, so estimates are given for minimum and maximum calorie patterns to suit varying needs. For instance, starting at the top of the table, you see that you could need anywhere from five to ten servings from the grain group each day. Before you get too excited about all those carbs, remember that this amount is spread throughout the day and should include whole grains from cereal and pasta as well as many other options we introduced to you to in the last few chapters (in particular, Chapter 10's section "Carbohydrates," as well as "Dietary Fiber"; Chapter 12's section on the grain category of MyPyramid). More suggestions await you in the meal makeovers of this chapter. And keep in mind that for many ordinary meals, it's not uncommon that the amount you put on your plate may technically be equivalent to two or three servings at once.

TABLE 13-1
RECOMMENDED FOOD SERVINGS FOR PRE-PREGNANCY

Food Group	Minimum	Midrange	High
	1,600 calories	2,200 calories	2,800 calories
Grain servings (ounces)	5	7	10
Vegetable servings (cups)	2	3	3½
Fruit servings (cups)	1½	2	2½
Milk servings (cups)	3	3	3
Meat and beans (ounces or equivalents)	5	6	7
Oil servings (tsp)	5	6	7
Discretionary calories ("extras")	132	290	426

Source: U.S. Department of Agriculture, Center for Nutrition Policy and Promotion

Consider Maggie, a client who, when we reviewed her previous day's diet, was amazed to find that she had easily eaten about eight servings from the grain group: her giant muffin from the coffee cart at work counted as three (plus "extra" sugar and fats), her small whole-wheat roll with her lunch salad counted as approximately one or one and a half, the popcorn shared with a coworker counted as two (plus fats), and her cup of rice with dinner counted as two. As we reviewed her diet further, we identified other food groups where she either fell short or exceeded the recommended amounts. She also realized that her food choices were sometimes narrow, that she hadn't had this or that fruit or vegetable in a while. She tended to get into baked chicken ruts, when she could have been substituting seafood, lean meats, and vegetarian sources of protein more often. As you take a look at your and your partner's diet and do the upcoming Practical Applications, you, too, will make similar discoveries—small or large—about where and how to focus your preconception efforts.

YOUR CALORIE REQUIREMENTS

There is obviously a broad difference in calories taken in by someone who eats the most versus the least number of recommended daily servings in Table 13-1. Consumption of the minimum number of daily servings from each food group provides approximately 1,600 calories. This low calorie level along with an increase in activity level is appropriate only for women who are trying to lose weight well before trying to conceive (see Chapter 14 for details). Even a very petite woman will need more than this, as long as she is moderately active. The middle of the range provides closer to 2,200 calories. Most reproductive-age women of average height, weight, and moderate activity level can maintain their weight at this level; being tall or muscular will tip your needs higher. Underweight women who want to gain and very active women may easily require more calories and should choose additional foods to reach the higher end—from 2,400 to 2,800 calories. Most men need between the middle and high end of the range of food servings, sometimes more. To gauge whether your average calorie intake is right for you, pay attention to your weight, how your clothes fit, and how you feel.

FOR FUTURE REFERENCE: During Pregnancy/After Delivery

Most pregnant women need more than 300 to 400 extra calories per day, primarily in the second and third trimesters, to gain an average of twenty-eight pounds. In comparison to your preconception requirements in Table 13-1, your intake of dairy foods should increase from three to four servings per day, and meat/meat alternatives should be six to seven ounce equivalents per day. Modest additions from the remaining food groups should satisfy any additional energy needs of pregnancy. Keep in mind that carbohydrates should provide more than half of the extra calories; protein and fat provide the rest.

Exclusive breastfeeding requires 330 to 400 calories above maintenance requirements; however, most postpartum moms can shed their pregnancy weight by drawing these calorie needs from their maternal fat stores (part of the weight put on during pregnancy). This allows a comfortable weight loss—around one half to one pound a week, which will not affect breastmilk supply or quality. In other words, go back to your pre-pregnancy approach in Table 13-1 and 13-2 to guide your selection of foods.

When you eat a wide variety of foods within MyPyramid, you may notice different calorie compositions of foods within each group. A few examples will make this clearer. For instance, one portion (1 cup) of nonfat milk contains 90 calories, whereas one portion of cheddar cheese (1½-ounce slice) contains 160 calories and one portion (1 cup) of nonfat yogurt has 100 to 200 calories (depending on whether it is sugar-sweetened), yet each counts as a milk serving. When there is that much discrepancy, and you know that the difference comes from added sugar (the flavored yogurt) or high amounts of solid fat (the cheese), count it as one milk plus any excess as discretionary calories. A 1-ounce equivalent of Atlantic halibut contains about 40 calories, whereas a 1-ounce equivalent of black beans (¼ cup) has 55 calories, and a 1-ounce equivalent of peanut butter (1 tbsp) contains about 95 calories (this time the extra calories count as oil, not discretionary). Again, mix up your choices to find the middle ground. All qualify as healthy choices, and if you use MyPyramid's computer program, it will know where to count the discrepancies and instantly shows you what your body will receive.

At first glance, these differences can be disconcerting to anyone who really wants to keep track of her calorie intake. But by taking full advantage of the variety that a balanced diet has to offer, you can get away from calorie counting. Just count whether you have had the proper number of servings from each food group. Once you get the hang of this approach, you will realize that a wide range of food choices really is the solution. You will find that high-, low-, and medium-calorie choices naturally blend into moderation. This moderate approach becomes even more evident when you step back and mentally note the variety of nutrients you consume over the course of a week or a month. Short periods of poor food variety or the occasional junk food selection or overeating won't pack much punch when the overall variety and portion control in a diet are good.

FOR FUTURE REFERENCE: During Pregnancy/After Delivery

Women who eat a wide variety of foods during pregnancy get top ratings for unforgettable womb service! They do their babies the favor of introducing a variety of food and spice flavors while in the womb. The fetus can actually taste new flavors in the amniotic fluid late in pregnancy. Similarly, breastfed babies are exposed to certain flavors through breastmilk. When solid foods are slowly introduced at six months of age, these infants end up being more accepting of a similar variety of food tastes.

You may also wonder if your pregnancy and/or breastfeeding diet could have an impact on your future baby's risk of developing food allergies, asthma, or atopic dermatitis. The American Academy of Pediatrics reported in 2008 that "current evidence does not support a major role for maternal dietary restrictions, including peanuts, during pregnancy or lactation," but you may want to speak with your obstetrician or a pediatrician about this if you, your husband, or other children have significant allergic disease.

Practical Application

We recommend sitting down side by side and going over these pages together, while logged into www.MyPyramid.gov. Have a little fun, and don't get too bogged down in details like whether a tomato is a fruit or a veggie. MyPyramid operates more by what people commonly count as foods rather than pure science, so tomatoes are typically counted as veggies. The take-home message is that the goal isn't perfection. The overarching purpose is variety, moderation, balance, and learning what works for you as a couple. If you are both used to eating and preparing most of your meals separately, this is the time to talk about how you can develop some traditions that revolve around eating together more often, as you will likely aim to do as a family—one common meal for everyone, with two parents who have a working knowledge of how to plan healthy meals and snacks.

If you're doing this exercise by hand, not computer, first, recall what you both ate yesterday from the moment you got up to the time you crawled back into bed. If you snacked during the night, remember that, too. Write down everything you ate and drank (including alcohol) and the amounts. Include incognito ingredients in mixed dishes, too. For instance, in one medium slice of thick crust pepperoni pizza, count the crust as two grain portions, the tomato sauce as ¼ cup vegetable portion, the cheese as ¼ cup milk portion, and the pepperoni as a half ounce equivalent of meat (cheese and pepperoni are fatty choices, so you've used around 80 discretionary calories too). If you had two slices, double the portions, and so on. (Flip back to Chapter 12 to help determine portions.) Then mark in Figure 13-1 how many portions you had from a particular food group(s). A single portion counts as an ⊠, two as ⊠⊠. Half portions count as a ◻. The solid line boxes in Figure 13-1 represent the minimum number of servings for each group, so you can see at a glance whether you're at least meeting the minimum requirements from each group. If you have a copy machine handy, you can make extra copies of the template before filling it in. Repeat the exercise for the next two days, trying to include one weekend day to give a fuller picture. By looking closely at three days' worth of what you eat and drink, you get a sense of trends.

Compare your dietary strengths and weaknesses with those of your partner, and see if together you can come up with some creative solutions to improve your diets in and out of the home environment.

Prior to conception, most women need the number of food servings near the *middle* of the recommended range (Table 13-2) to maintain their weight. Most men need the number of foods between the *middle* and *high* end of the recommended range (Table 13-3) to maintain their weight. From what you record next on your "One-Day Food Intake," circle or write on the chart below the number of servings closest to what you consumed. See if what you normally consume jibes with what MyPyramid would calculate for you.

Women's Exercise

FIGURE 13-1
ONE-DAY FOOD INTAKE

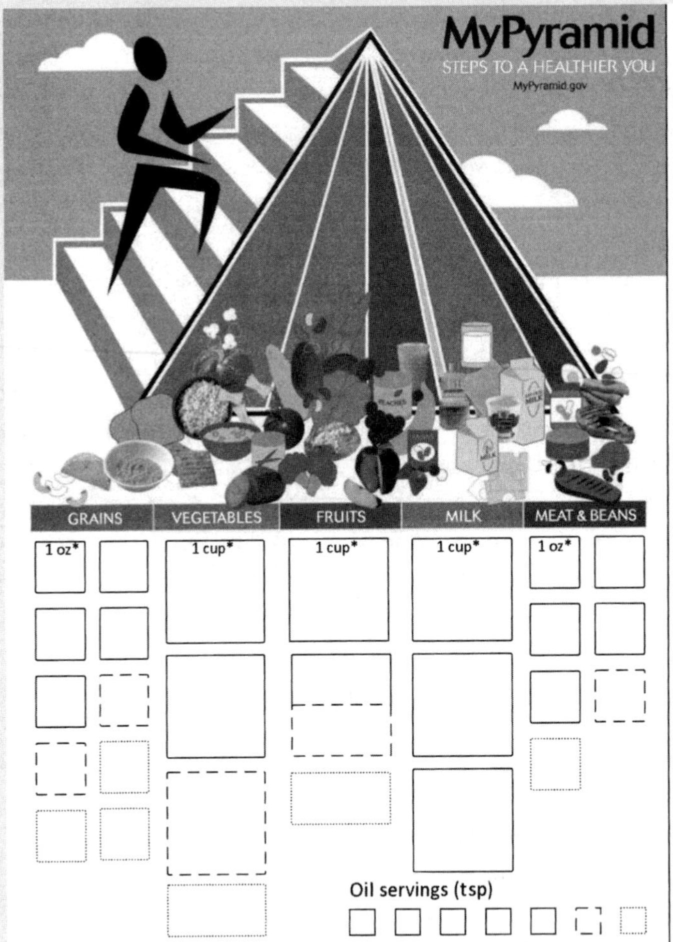

MyPyramid
STEPS TO A HEALTHIER YOU
MyPyramid.gov

Yesterday . . .
List food or beverage amount.

Breakfast

Snack (optional)

Lunch

Snack (optional)

Dinner

Snack (optional)

GRAINS	VEGETABLES	FRUITS	MILK	MEAT & BEANS
1 oz*	1 cup*	1 cup*	1 cup*	1 oz*

Oil servings (tsp)

Key:

Calorie ranges provided in Table 13-1.

☐ Minimum calorie consumption (everyone eats at least this much).

☐ Add these servings for midrange.

☐ Add above plus these for high range.

Discretionary Calories ("extras"):

Allowances for solid fats, sweets, alcohol, etc.:

minimum range	132 calories
midrange	290 calories
high range	426 calories

Note:
This tool will be easiest to use if you have read all the material, beginning with Table 13-1.

*Flip back to Chapter 12 for a review of serving sizes — with a little practice it will be second nature.

TABLE 13-2
DAILY RECOMMENDATIONS FOR FOOD SERVINGS
FOR MOST PRE-PREGNANT WOMEN

Food Group	Minimum	Midrange	High
Grain servings (ounces)	5	7	10
Vegetable servings (cups)	2	3	3½
Fruit servings (cups)	1½	2	2½
Milk servings (cups)	3	3	3
Meat and beans (ounce equivalents)	5	6	7
Oil servings (teaspoons)	5	6	7
Discretionary calories ("extras")	132	290	426

Note: Alcoholic beverages are counted only in the discretionary part of the Pyramid, but wines and distilled liquors are metabolized similarly to 2 or 3 fat servings, respectively; beer as 1½ fat plus ½ grain; cocktails as 4 or 5 fats and, potentially, ½ grain. Discontinue all alcoholic beverages two weeks prior to trying to get pregnant.

Source: U.S. Department of Agriculture, Center for Nutrition Policy and Promotion

Now see how your diet measures up by filling in the following blanks:

My dietary strong points are _____

_____

My weaker dietary points are _____

_____

Two food groups that could particularly use an infusion of variety include the _____

group and the _____ group.

If I need to trim some beverages or foods to make way for healthier ones, I could cut down on

the following: _____

_____

and then add more of these choices: _____

_____

Notes: _____

_____

_____

Men's Exercise

FIGURE 13-2
ONE-DAY FOOD INTAKE

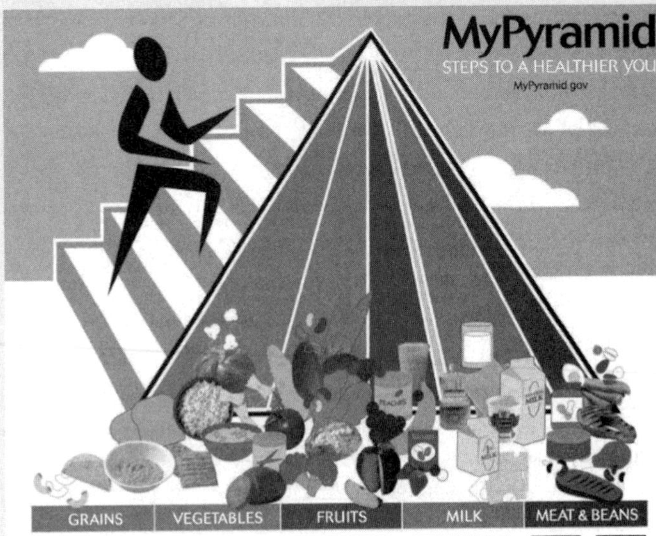

MyPyramid
STEPS TO A HEALTHIER YOU
MyPyramid.gov

Yesterday . . .
List food or beverage amount.

Breakfast

Snack (optional)

Lunch

Snack (optional)

Dinner

Snack (optional)

GRAINS	VEGETABLES	FRUITS	MILK	MEAT & BEANS
1 oz*	1 cup*	1 cup*	1 cup*	1 oz*

Oil servings (tsp)

Key:

Calorie ranges provided in Table 13-1.

☐ Minimum calorie consumption (everyone eats at least this much).

☐ Add these servings for midrange.

☐ Add above plus these for high range.

Discretionary Calories ("extras"):

Allowances for solid fats, sweets, alcohol, etc.:

minimum range	132 calories
midrange	290 calories
high range	426 calories

Note:
This tool will be easiest to use if you have read all the material, beginning with Table 13-1.

*Flip back to Chapter 12 for a review of serving sizes — with a little practice it will be second nature.

TABLE 13-3

DAILY RECOMMENDATIONS FOR FOOD SERVINGS
FOR MOST PROSPECTIVE DADS

Food Group	Minimum	Midrange	High
Grain servings (ounces)	5	7	10
Vegetable servings (cups)	2	3	3½
Fruit servings (cups)	1½	2	2½
Milk servings (cups)	3	3	3
Meat and beans (ounce equivalent)	5	6	7
Oil servings (teaspoons)	5	6	7
Discretionary calories ("extras")	132	290	426

Note: Alcoholic beverages are counted only in the discretionary part of the Pyramid, but wines and distilled liquors are metabolized similarly to 2 or 3 fat servings, respectively; beer as 1½ fat + ½ grain; cocktails as 4 or 5 fats and, potentially, ½ grain.

Source: U.S. Department of Agriculture, Center for Nutrition Policy and Promotion

Now see how your diet measures up by filling in the following blanks:

My dietary strong points are _____

_____

My weaker dietary points are _____

_____

Two food groups that could particularly use an infusion of variety include the _____

group and the _____ group.

If I need to trim some beverages or foods to make way for healthier ones, I could cut down on

the following: _____

_____

and then add more of these choices: _____

_____

Notes: _____

_____

_____

Foolproof Tips for a Preconception-Friendly Diet

1. Intentionally create meals and snacks that include several food groups at one time.
   - Try to include *four or more* food groups *at every meal.*
   - Try to include small amounts of *at least two* food groups *at every snack* (if you snack).

2. Vary your choices regularly, while keeping portions moderate.

3. Take pride in how you shop and dine to make eating pleasurable and wholesome. Consider what's in season to maximize flavor, and buy locally grown foods when you can; buying organic is an added bonus. Fresher foods look and taste so good that it's almost sinful not to give them a little of your time and attention. They also beg for simple preparation methods that accentuate Mother Nature's influence and make rookie cooks look like seasoned veterans. If you haven't already done so, Google Carlo Petrini's Slow Food movement to bring out the foodie in you.

4. Get unstuck in your ways. Be open to trying new foods, or learn to cook if you don't know how. Often a cookbook for beginners or viewing a cooking demo (e.g., Food Network) can inspire you to try something in a way you hadn't thought of or were unsure how to prepare.

5. Get the recommended number of servings from each food category according to the MyPyramid system. Increase the availability of foods you don't get enough of and limit access to foods that you overindulge in.

6. Never skip meals! Instead, care for your body by eating at regular intervals, and avoid grazing in between. Accomplish this by eating from three to as many as six times per day based on your personal preference. Once you're pregnant, it is best to eat five to six times per day.

PRECONCEPTION MEAL MAKEOVERS

Chances are you will occasionally fall short in certain food groups—usually it's the veggies, low-fat dairy, and fruits. There will be other times when you go over the top too often—usually fats and sweets and sometimes starches and meats. The following meal makeovers are all real examples taken from patients who came in for nutrition consultations. In the right-hand column, you'll either see what's discussed with a patient, what we jot down for a patient to read, or interesting background that might help you empathize with the person's situation. We always focus on dietary patterns using MyPyramid as a prompt, often with no initial emphasis on single nutrients such as folate, calcium, or iron. However, as food choices are broadened, foods containing these nutrients inevitably assume more prominent roles in the new preconception diet. Also, note how portion sizes can be manipulated to stabilize the caloric intake even as the number of food groups is increased.

BREAKFAST

BEFORE:

- A bagel from a bagel shop
- 2 tbsp cream cheese
- 16 oz bottled flavored and sweetened tea

Food groups represented: only 1
Total calories = 531, of which 232 are discretionary ("extra")

This bagel is typical of most bagel-shop bagels, though some are even bigger than four grain servings. Whole bagels are still nice as a treat, but really should not be routinely eaten, particularly for anyone watching the glycemic load of their meals. Recall that cream cheese counts as solid fat (an extra), not as milk (dairy) or oil. The tea beverage contains "2 servings per container," so the 70 calories per serving from sugar must be doubled because she drinks the whole beverage, providing a total of 140 calories of added sugars. The drink and large amount of cream cheese max out most of her discretionary calories, and her day has hardly begun.

Key: The one food group represented here is 4 grains (refined, not whole). The 232 discretionary calories are from solid fat and added sugars.

AFTER:

- 2 pieces whole wheat toast (not oversized)
- 1–2 tbsp all-natural peanut butter
- 1 cup strawberries
- 1 cup plain unsweetened yogurt sweetened with 1 tsp jam or honey
- Water (usually) or hot tea

Food groups: 5
Calories = approximately 407–524, of which 58–79 are discretionary

When proposed as a substitute for the original bagel meal, this breakfast sounds like an awful lot of food. However, it is similar or lower in calories, and the nutrient value is dramatically better. This client did need to buy more normal-sized bread, or if she bought oversized slices, she ate only 1–1½ pieces to equal two regular-sized pieces. She could also save money and sugar calories by buying large containers of plain yogurt and lightly sweetening it herself. Recall from Chapter 12 that nut butters count as meat alternatives plus healthy oil servings, so leaner protein sources are recommended for the rest of the day.

Key: The five food groups represented here are 2 whole grains, 1–2 meat and beans, 1 cup fruit, 1 milk, and 1–2 oils. The reasonable number of discretionary calories come from the whole grain bread's small amount of hidden fat and sugar; jam or honey adds another 18–21 calories, which is minor compared to the amount of sugar hidden in presweetened yogurt.

BREAKFAST

BEFORE:

- 1½ cups cottage cheese
- large coffee with ½ cup reduced-fat 2% milk and artificial sweetener

Food groups: 1
Calories: 303, of which 50 are discretionary

This client had put herself on a strict high-protein diet, had lost a lot of weight, was regaining some of it despite being more active in a boot camp workout, and was feeling absolutely exhausted and hungry most of the time. She was terrified to eat anything other than this mound of cottage cheese for breakfast. Her remaining meals were limited to 2 or 3 food groups (also with disproportionate portion sizes). She desperately needed a change.

Key: The one food group represented here is 1¼ milk equivalents (not much credit; seems like it should count for more). The 50 discretionary calories are from solid fat hidden in the two milk items.

AFTER:

- ½ sprouted wheat bagel (open-face) with 1 tbsp cream cheese
- Tomato slices or sun-dried tomato
- ¾ cup orange juice or 1 whole orange in segments
- 1 cup nonfat or 1% low-fat milk (some saved for a smaller serving of coffee, with 1 packet of sweetener to accommodate personal preferences)

Food groups: 4
Calories = 348–391, of which 46 are discretionary

Her goal was to further lose weight until she reached the lowest-risk BMI range (before conception), so a modest breakfast was fine. However, she needed a more even distribution of calories and all food groups, including carbohydrate sources that she had formerly banned. By doing so, she would have the energy to work out, remain moderately active for the entire day, and not overeat later in the day. Whereas a whole bagel is too much (as in the first example), the bagel half is a good alternative, and we found a hearty whole-grain one at her local farmer's market. This might be a nice meal for a small midday appetite, too.

Key: The four food groups represented here are 2 whole grains, ¼–½ cup vegetable, ¾ cup fruit, and 1 milk. The discretionary calories are from the modest amount of cream cheese and the 1% milk fat.

BREAKFAST

BEFORE:

- 1–2 packets instant oatmeal (presweetened)
- Coffee (half decaf) with dash (2 tbsp) of creamer and 1 packet sugar

Food groups: 1
Calories = 186–316, of which 86 to 116 are discretionary

Oatmeal is an excellent focal point of any breakfast (or lunch or dinner!), and this type counts as a fortified cereal. However, with all the added sugar and no other food groups added to round out the meal, this choice is too nutritionally limited. You could well be hungry by midmorning, too. Instead of creamer in coffee, try switching to 2% milk or soy milk.

Key: The one food group represented here is 1–2 whole grains. The discretionary calories come from hidden sugar in the presweetened instant oatmeal as well as added sugar and saturated (or often hydrogenated) fat from the creamer.

AFTER:

- ½–1 cup old-fashioned oatmeal (cooked)
- 1 cup nonfat or 1% milk substituted for some of the oatmeal's cooking water
- 2 rounded tbsp chopped walnuts
- ½ cup fresh berries or ¼ cup dried fruit
- 1 tsp brown sugar (optional)
- Water or tea (usually) or coffee (occasionally)

Food groups: 5
Calories = 290–444, of which 0–36 could be discretionary

Highlights here include less sugar, and since it is not fortified, it's low in iron, too (recall that a low-iron meal is a good place for higher calcium intake and absorption); higher calcium and vitamin D (milk), essential omega-3 oil and protein source (walnuts), folate and vitamin C (berries), protein, fiber, and zinc, and can still be cooked in the microwave (if stirred periodically to prevent it from overflowing); could use instant plain oatmeal if the fortified vitamins and minerals are desired. Instead of adding the milk serving to the oatmeal, you could have tea au lait or "half-caff" café latte.

Key: The five food groups represented here are 1–2 whole grains, ½ cup fruit, 1 milk, ½ meat and beans, and 1 hidden oil. The discretionary calories come from 1% milk and brown sugar.

OR

- 1–2 ounce equivalents (a 1-ounce equivalent is usually a ½–1 cup portion or roughly 30 grams) of ready-to-eat breakfast cereal (look on the label for less than 5 grams "sugar," like Cheerios)
- 11 almonds (½ ounce)

- 1 cup nonfat or low-fat (1%) milk
- 1 medium sliced peach or nectarine
- Water

Food groups: 5
Calories = 273–403, of which 4–20 are discretionary

This cold alternative includes less sugar and is higher in protein and calcium, too. Almonds contain healthy fat, and the cereal is fortified. If you're unable to sit down to eat, this meal can easily be packaged into portable containers and insulated beverage cups.

Key: The five food groups represented here are 1–2 whole grains, ½ cup fruit, 1 milk, ½ meat and beans, and ½ hidden oil. The discretionary calories are mostly from the 1% milk.

LUNCH

BEFORE:

- Turkey (4 oz) sandwich (ready-to-eat from a café at work)
- 2 slices sourdough bread (plus 1 mustard packet, no mayo)
- Iceberg lettuce slices
- Small snack-size tortilla chips or pretzels
- Diet soft drink

Food groups: 3–4 (barely)
Calories = 369–412, of which only about 20 are discretionary

This patient had gotten into a rut of having the same meal every day at work because it "seemed like a healthy choice, except for the potato chips." She was open to adding more variety and higher-fiber carbohydrates. She also needed an alternative to the ready-to-eat sandwich, because made-to-order sandwiches weren't available (to control for risk of listeria food poisoning during preconception and pregnancy, women need to follow specific guidelines for luncheon meats and ready-made sandwiches; see pages 406–414. The tortilla chips are equivalent to 1½ servings of refined grain and 2 oil choices, whereas pretzels are 1½ refined grain. She found herself craving candy by midafternoon, which blew her "healthy" lunch.

Key: The four food groups represented here are 3½ grains (not whole), ¼ vegetables, 4 meat and beans, and 0–2 oils. The discretionary calories are from the lunch meat.

AFTER:

- From home, 2–3 oz deli sliced turkey breast, chicken, lean roast beef, all heated to steaming and cooled before sandwich assembly; canned tuna is another option
- Fresh lettuce or spinach leaves, plus tomato or red bell pepper slices
- 0–1 slices of cheese on sandwich from home (sometimes)
- 2 slices of whole grain bread
- Mustard and ½–1 tbsp lite mayonnaise
- 1 cup of vegetable or tomato soup (not creamy or bisque)
- 2 peeled and sliced kiwi fruits or whole junior-size banana
- Water (usually), or unsweetened iced tea; diet soft drink (less often)

Food groups: 5–6
Calories = 450–646, of which 0–84 are discretionary

No longer in a rut, this patient made her lunch the night before and refrigerated it until the next morning (then transferred it to her insulated lunch bag with ice pack). On days when this patient knew she was going to go out to dinner with her husband after work, she'd choose the leaner meats and leave the cheese off her sandwich. Her fruit choice was from home or the café and saved for her midafternoon pick-me-up snack, which tided her over until dinnertime.

Key: The five to six food groups represented here are 2–2½ grains (mostly whole, except tomato soup thickener), 1–1¼ cups vegetable, ¾ cup fruit, ½–1 milk, 2–3 meat and beans, and ½–1 oil. The 84 discretionary calories are present only when she includes cheese on her sandwich.

LUNCH

BEFORE:

- 1½ cups steamed white rice
- 4 oz stir-fried chicken teriyaki (dark and breast meat), including sauce

Food groups: 3
Calories = approximately 800, with 50 or more as discretionary calories from dark poultry meat. This chef used 2–3 tbsp cottonseed oil (6–9 tsp), though this is an estimate because the amount was arbitrarily measured; sodium content of this meal is quite high.

Key: The three food groups represented here are 3 grains (not whole), 4 meat and bean, and 6–9 oil. The discretionary calories are from the dark meat, and any oil choices that exceed one's allotment for the day should count as discretionary calories, too.

AFTER:

- 1 cup steamed brown rice
- 2 oz stir-fried chicken breast, shrimp, or extra-firm tofu with soy and fresh ginger sauce
- 1 cup steamed Oriental vegetables
- ½ mango
- Water

Food groups: 5
Calories = 453–505, 0 discretionary

For a more balanced meal, find another restaurant that offers whole-grain brown rice and more options including veggies, tofu, seafood, poultry breast meat, and less oil for stir-frying (or at least less sauce). For even more control, try stir-frying at home using approximately 2 tsp canola oil per person; this healthier version can be made for dinner the night before and makes a good microwavable lunch the next day; veggies were added for their nutrients as well as to add bulk to the meal for satiety; choose a deep orange/yellow fruit for the healthy carotenoid-rich food choice.

Key: The five food groups represented here are 2 grains (whole), 1 cup vegetable, ¾ cup fruit, 2 meat and beans, and 2 oils.

DINNER

BEFORE:

- 1½ cups three-bean chili (meatless)
- Iceberg lettuce salad with tomato, cucumber, and 3 tbsp regular ranch salad dressing
- 12 oz cranberry juice cocktail

Food groups: 4
Calories = 815, of which 277 or more are discretionary

This dinner was off to a very good start, but the large juice portion is mostly added sugar and there is an excess of ranch dressing (mayo-based, so it counts as oil), both of which take the place of what could have been a high-fiber, phytonutrient-rich fruit choice, plus another food group or two. If juice is a frequent fruit choice, it should be halved and substituted with a variety of 100% juices for fewer calories and a better variety of plant nutrients. Another caveat here is that this woman was told that she needed to increase her iron intake, and the legumes with vitamin C–rich tomato sauce weren't enough to quickly help her iron status.

Key: The four food groups represented here are 2½ cups vegetable (note that you could count the beans as more meat/bean, but most people will need credit toward veggies), 1¼ cups fruit, 2½ meat and beans, and 6 oils. Most of the discretionary calories come from the cranberry juice cocktail; any excess oil will count as discretionary, too.

AFTER:

- ¾–1¼ cup vegetarian bean chili, plus 2 oz lean ground beef for heme iron is recommended for women with iron-deficiency anemia (in addition to supplemental iron)
- Topped with ½ oz cheddar cheese
- 1½ cup spinach salad
- Topped with ½ sliced hard-boiled egg, and 2 tbsp pistachio nuts, plus 1–2 tbsp homemade balsamic vinaigrette (or light dressing if you need to watch oil portions)
- 1 small whole wheat dinner roll with 1 tsp no-trans-fat margarine or butter
- ½ papaya with lime
- Water

Food groups: 6
Calories = 660–854, of which up to 67 are discretionary

Look at how much more variety and balance are here, and for almost the same (or fewer) calories. This meal is packed with basically every essential nutrient there is, including a lot of naturally occurring folate and choline, and is fairly high in protein. With the addition of a couple of frozen meatballs, the amount of available iron goes up, too; this should offset some of the healthy components that inevitably inhibit some of the meal's iron.

Key: The six food groups represented here are 1 whole grain, 2–2¼ vegetable, 1 cup fruit, ⅓ dairy, 4–5 meat and beans, and ½–3 oils. The discretionary calories are mostly hidden sources of solid fat.

DINNER

BEFORE:

- 6 oz grilled steak
- Medium baked potato with butter (2 tbsp) and light sour cream (1 tbsp)
- 1 ear corn or ¾ cup cut corn with 1 tsp butter
- Lemonade (8 oz)

Food groups: 2
Calories = 976, of which 432 are discretionary

It's terrific that this meal contains so many vegetables; however, the choices are both from the starchy vegetable group and lend themselves to too much added butter, especially considering the steak's hidden contribution of saturated fat. See how we keep part of this theme but vary it with green and orange vegetables below. The lemonade contains 100 calories of added sugar (which is okay if the rest of the day is very low in sugar).

Key: The two food groups represented here are 2¼ cup vegetables and 6 meat and beans. The discretionary calories come from the high amount of butter, the solid fat hidden in steak and sour cream, and the sugar in the lemonade.

AFTER:

- 3–4 oz grilled steak or salmon
- "Open face" whole 5-inch sweet potato brushed with 1 tsp olive or canola oil and lightly salted before baking
- 1 cup chopped asparagus spears, red bell pepper or tomato, and onion, and ¼ diced avocado mixed with 1 tbsp extra virgin olive or canola oil vinaigrette
- 1 piece (2½ by 1½ inches) of whole-grain cornbread and 1 tsp honey (using a whole-grain cornmeal)
- Water

Food groups: 4
Calories = 581–669, of which 93–123 are discretionary

Notice how healthy oils have replaced most of the fats, though some remain disguised in the meat and cornbread servings. The avocado counts as a vegetable that has healthy monounsaturated fat. The salmon option is rich in DHA and EPA omega-3s instead of saturated fat. This meal substituted a lower glycemic index vegetable, the sweet potato, instead of a regular potato. Folate-rich asparagus and phytonutrient-rich tomatoes and onions also add taste and visual appeal.

Key: The four food groups represented here are 1 grain (part whole grain), 2 cups vegetable, 3–4 meat and beans, and 2 oils. Most of the discretionary calories come from the meat, cornbread, and honey—much better than the "before" example.

SNACK

BEFORE:

• Whole bag of light microwave popcorn

Food groups: 1
Calories = 327, of which 39 are discretionary

As a snack food popcorn is classified in the grain group (much like fried corn chips and taco shells), not the veggie group, plus added fat. Fact: A small movie theater popcorn contains 450–650 calories, including at least half as solid fat, often trans fat, so it isn't a better option. Home-popped popcorn using oil, salt, and seasoning such as paprika, is a healthier whole-grain option, and the portion size could be cut in half.

Key: The one food group represented here is 4 whole grains. The 39 discretionary calories are from the bright yellow–dyed solid fat.

AFTER:

• 6–12 small no-trans-fat whole-wheat crackers (e.g., Kashi TLC Original 7 Grain crackers) or 100% whole-wheat pita wedges
• 3 tbsp hummus (Hummus is a Middle Eastern dip made from chickpeas, lemon juice, tahini, olive oil, and garlic. It counts as 1 oil and ½ meat and beans or as oil and ¼ cup veggies.) Low-fat bean dip can be a substitute.
• 1 cup baby carrots, raw broccoli or cauliflower, or zucchini wedges
• Water

Food groups: 4
Calories = Approximately 130–230, of which less than 5 calories are discretionary

Hummus or low-fat bean dip can be a substitute for less healthy dips (such as ranch dressing or onion soup dip) if you dislike plain raw veggies. Look for crackers with no saturated or trans fats and 3 or fewer grams of total fat (which will count as healthy oil). To make this snack into a quick, easy meal, add more food groups—a little fruit and/or yogurt.

Key: The four food groups represented here are ¾–2 whole grains, 1 cup vegetables, ½ meat and beans, and approximately 1–2 oils.

SNACK/DESSERT

BEFORE:

• ½ package red "licorice" twists (approximately 11 pieces)

Food groups: 0
Calories = 210, all discretionary

Remember, many packaged candies contain several servings per package—the information on the Nutrition Facts label is for one serving only. Red licorice is marketed as a fat-free candy, which is true, but most preconception meal plans don't have much room for nutrient-poor sources of calories. If you are a licorice fan, be sure to see Chapter 8 for safety concerns over black licorice during pregnancy.

Key: All the discretionary calories come from sugar.

AFTER:

Blended fruit smoothie made with
• ½ cup plain or sweetened nonfat yogurt (try a mix of both to reduce the added sugar)
• ¼ cup 100% orange juice or grape juice (fortified with vitamin C)
• ¼ cup fresh or frozen banana, peach, or mango chunks
• ½ cup frozen or fresh raspberries or blackberries
• ¼ cup calcium-enriched soy milk (vanilla flavor) or tofu
• 1 tbsp wheat germ
• Tiny splash of vanilla extract to add the final taste touch
• Blend in ice if you prefer a thicker consistency

Food groups: 4
Calories = 170–220, of which 0–60 calories are discretionary

This snack or dessert was designed to emphasize calcium, folate, and vitamin C; it can be made into a bigger snack by increasing portion sizes. If you're in need of a modest calcium supplement (e.g., 200–250 mg calcium carbonate), this would be a good snack to take it with.

Key: The four food groups represented here are less than ½ grain, approximately 1–1¼ cup fruit, ½ milk, and 1 meat and beans (from soy products). Discretionary calories are from pre-sweetened yogurt and flavored soy milk.

OR
• 1 whole rectangular graham cracker (2 smaller square sections equal one whole)
• 1 tbsp natural peanut butter, walnut butter, or almond butter
• 1 cup nonfat or low-fat milk or calcium-fortified citrus juice (or ½ sliced banana to top nut butter), preferably covering two food groups

Food groups: 4 or 5
Calories = Approximately 260, of which 30 are discretionary

A nutritious but higher-calorie snack or dessert, but do make an effort to include higher-fiber grains and fruits elsewhere.

Key: The four or five food groups represented here are ½ grain (refined, not whole), preferably ½ cup fruit and ½ milk, 1 meat and beans, and 1 oil. Discretionary calories come from the graham cracker's sugar content.

We hope the Foolproof Tips #1–6 from page 386 and these before-and-after exercises will help you plan ahead and keep your diet healthier than ever. Every day will be a little different, but that keeps it interesting as well as nutritionally balanced over the course of time. Isn't it wonderful to have so many choices?

Our book is not intended to be the only book you need once you become pregnant, nor is it a cookbook, so if you want nutrition-focused resources that have more recipes to pick up where we leave off, watch for books by Elizabeth Ward, MS, RD, or Bridget Swinney, MS, RD, and for pregnancy with multiples Barbara Luke, ScD, MPH, RD. Once you start your family, there's nobody better than Ellyn Satter, MS, RD, LCSW, BCD, to get you off to a great start and see you through the toddler, childhood, and teen years.

CONVENIENCE AND AFFORDABILITY: MAKE YOUR PRECONCEPTION DIET FIT YOUR LIFESTYLE

After good taste, convenience and affordability are the qualities that most people look for when deciding whether healthy eating habits are worth keeping. And more often than not, you'll have to pay more for the convenience factor. But a healthy, delicious diet need not tap your wallet dry, nor should being frugal and simplifying your diet mean forfeiting nutritional value. The following suggestions are intended to add convenience and affordability to your preconception meal plans.

Convenience

- Make sure that you always have healthy food choices readily available: fresh and frozen veggies and fruits, seafood, peanut butter, hummus, whole-grain cereals and breads, pasta, canned tomatoes and beans, eggs, nonfat yogurt, and lowfat cottage cheese. One way to make this happen is to have a shopping list posted in a prominent place in your kitchen and add to it as you go (recall the shopping list in Appendix E). Before going to the store, sit down with your partner and outline what you both might like to have for dinners that week, allowing for when you might eat out or order in. After planning dinners, work backward to gauge what foods you'll need for lunches, breakfasts, and snacks. Don't forget to keep in mind your MyPyramid template for each day.

- You can have food delivered right to your home. Many grocery stores have home delivery options, and the delivery fee is often waived if you spend over a certain dollar amount. This is an option if you foresee a baby hindering your ability to regularly grocery shop. It also helps prevent impulse buying. Another option is to look into getting a CSA (community-supported agriculture) farm share, akin to being one step closer to your local farmer than visiting the farmer's market (also a potentially convenient option for you). CSAs foster a link between local and regional farmers and local consumers. Your membership entitles you to baskets of fresh foods—from produce to farm-fresh eggs—picked up at a convenient spot near you during the growing season. You have direct access to the farms if you choose to visit, and can decide for yourself how you feel about the care of their animals and farming practices (many follow organic farming practices but do not pursue USDA certification). Many CSAs are working to "extend the harvest" and are equipped to vacuum-pack, freeze, and store fresh food for you so it's available year-round—great for you readers who live in parts of the country where winter significantly limits your options. Many industrious new moms have started these programs in their cities, towns, or rural areas. Why not look into it beforehand? See http://www.localharvest.org or www.foodroutes.org for more information. Many CSAs have the ability to accommodate members who need financial assistance.

- There are many relatively inexpensive gadgets that make food preparation a breeze. A few examples of time-saving gadgets include salad spinners (to quickly rinse and dry salad greens), a few really good knives, a stainless-steel vegetable steamer basket, a cheese grater, food storage containers that are microwave- and freezer-safe, more than one cutting board, a nonstick pan, a wok, a gravy separator (a special pitcher that separates fat from broth), a handheld immersion blender (great for smoothies and pureed soups with hardly any clean-up), and an electric kitchen timer with a loud continuous ring (until you turn it off). As you probably know, appliances such as food processors, microwaves, and dishwashers also make for less work in the kitchen and are often worth the investment.

- Try to cook when you have a little extra time, and cook more food than you need for that particular meal. Immediately portion what you do not need into small, shallow containers and place them in the refrigerator or freezer for later use. This has two benefits. First, it saves you from overeating at mealtime, because you have already stored away seconds. Second, the extras can be heated and eaten as is at another meal or you can easily incorporate some of the leftovers into a totally new meal. For example, leftover baked chicken can be added to a fresh salad or sandwich one or two days later.

- In our busy world, never feel guilty if you and your partner do not have the time to make all your meals from scratch. Your grocery store carries many convenience items. It's just fine to buy a frozen lasagna or enchilada casserole to pop in the microwave or oven and add a salad from a bag of prewashed lettuce or spinach leaves (although we do advise another quick rinse). To up your seafood intake open a can of tuna for sandwiches, and add a unique salad of pre-washed, already grated broccoli slaw mixed with your favorite salad dressing. Or buy precut turkey breast tenders ready to toss into a wok with precut vegetables, minced ginger and garlic, and canned pineapple, and serve over instant rice. Or how about canned minestrone soup with extra frozen veggies added prior to warming, plus grilled cheese sandwiches using presliced cheddar cheese on whole-wheat bread? All of these are fast, convenient, and most of all healthy meals.
- If you avoid buying fresh vegetables or fruits because they often go to waste before you find the time to wash and prepare them, try keeping frozen ones on hand. Freezing does not mean that nutrient value is lost. In fact, these foods often retain very high amounts of their original nutrient composition because they are frozen soon after harvesting. And keep in mind that microwaving frozen items is a healthy and fast way to defrost and heat the items for eating. The same goes for dried culinary spices and herbs. They are less expensive overall than fresh, and they do not lose appreciable amounts of health-promoting phytonutrients when dried and stored.
- Fast foods and restaurant meals can also be a convenient part of a healthy preconception diet—when consumed in moderation. But remember that dining out often means that fatty ingredients and even sugar are added more liberally than you might at home. This is not a problem if the portion sizes are moderate or you eat out only occasionally. However, you may be accustomed to eating out regularly as part of your workday or in the evenings. More often than not, eating establishments exaggerate the concept of what is considered a normal portion and exploit customers' temptation to want more bang for their buck. Although eating out can be relaxing and fun, if done to excess it is generally not the best investment in your preconception health.

If you do eat out on a regular basis, there are several ways to keep your preconception meal habits on course. First, try ordering foods à la carte, and never hesitate to make special requests. For example, order a deli sandwich that incorporates lean meat (heated to steaming before assembly), cheese, and veggies, but no sides of potato salad or chips. At a Mexican restaurant, order fajitas or a beef and bean burrito with extra tomato, lettuce, and salsa. Try to find a Mexican restaurant that goes light on the cooking oil and doesn't use lard. Forgo the sides of rice and refried beans and do not indulge in more than a few tortilla chips.

Also, be inquisitive. Ask how food items are prepared or request printed information on nutrient composition if available (as they are with most fast-food chains and many restaurants). In most sit-down restaurants, you can request substitutions that are not written on the menu—for instance, replacing fried potatoes with steamed veggies or fresh fruit.

- Try carrying a cooler or small insulated lunch bag with an ice pack to hold extra food that requires no preparation time, such as fruits, precut and washed veggies, milk/yogurt, or high-fiber cereal. These coolers are ideal for people who cannot spare the time to find healthy meal items during the workweek and for those who travel frequently. That way, when you do eat out by necessity, you have healthy backup items to fulfill your preconception requirements over the course of the day.

- When you can eat at home, do. This is a convenience in itself, and you can get comfortable and be yourself. Where else can you put on your sweatsuit or shorts, crank up your favorite music, and dance around barefoot while preparing an enjoyable meal?

Affordability

- Premade foods and fast foods are generally more expensive. So the more you prepare foods from scratch (or close to it), the more money you save. It is up to you to decide how often the time/money trade-off is worthwhile. When you regularly prepare foods at home, you learn ways to simplify meal preparation and maximize taste. Usually breakfasts, lunches, and snacks are the easiest places to begin replacing fast foods and beverages with homemade ones. After trying that, proceed to eating out less often at dinnertime. There is a bonus: if you start preparing more food from scratch, you'll have an easier time maintaining your weight because you'll have more direct control over both preparation methods and serving sizes.

- Stick to a shopping list to avoid costly impulse buying.

- Foods that are highly processed, precut or grated, precooked, or individually packaged are generally more costly to produce. The manufacturers pass this cost on to you. Therefore, try to buy those items that you can cut, wash, flavor, or portion out at home (e.g., blocks of cheese instead of already grated; old-fashioned oats instead of prepackaged and flavored; frozen 100 percent fruit juice concentrate instead of individually bottled juices). Eliminating high-priced junk foods, soft drinks, and designer beverages will save a considerable amount of money, leaving more for you to spend on more nutritious foods. As a bonus, you can feel good because any of these actions take you one step closer to living a greener lifestyle.

- Use coupons or take advantage of store specials only if the food is something you can really use. Don't buy just because you have a coupon or it is on sale. Also, generic and store-brand items may still be more affordable than buying the national brand with a coupon. Always compare prices.

- Compare different-size food items for their price per unit to see what is really the best buy (see Figure 13-3). Don't buy the largest economy-size items to get the best buy unless you can really use that amount and still optimize variety and minimize food waste. If you do buy more food such as meats and breads than you need in order to get the better buy, you can freeze the extra for another meal. This way you aren't eating the same thing day after day just to use it up.

FIGURE 13-3
LABEL COMPARISON

Here are two sizes (15 oz vs. 20 oz) of the same brand cereal. The one on the right is the better deal because the price per ounce is less.

Total Price	$3.49	Total Price	$4.55
Net weight, ounces	15 oz	Net weight, ounces	20 oz
Price per ounce	23.3 cents/oz	Price per ounce	22.8 cents/oz

- Look for items such as nutritious legumes (dried beans, lentils, split peas), grains, and dried fruit sold in bulk bins. These are usually less expensive, and you can measure exactly the amount you want.
- Several government-funded food assistance programs such as the Special Supplemental Nutrition Program for Women, Infants, and Children (WIC) provide food assistance and other resources for women and their offspring who are at risk for hunger and in need of health care guidance.
- If you are interested in gardening, try growing some of your own vegetables and fruits. This takes time and attention, but it can be gratifying as well as economical. Gardening is also considered therapeutic by many avid gardeners. And the taste of homegrown foods is out of this world!

FOOD SAFETY: A CONSERVATIVE APPROACH

By now you are well versed in food grouping and portioning for your pre-pregnancy dietary plan. Yet within the food groups are some foods—even nutritious ones—that warrant further precautions. Here we review what foods and beverages you need to prepare differently, eat more moderately, or flat-out avoid. Don't worry, there will be plenty to eat, and we have lots of tricks to get around many of the restrictions. Some of the foods mentioned should be viewed with caution at all times, but particularly anytime conception is possible. You should be especially vigilant during your pregnancy as well. Of equal importance are safe food-handling practices, which include safe food purchasing, storage, and preparation before the foods reach your mouth.

Some foodborne illnesses or "food poisonings" that cause vague flu-like symptoms—stomachache, diarrhea, nausea, vomiting, and/or fever—can at best make you feel lousy and at worst be risky to your future fetus. Most foodborne illnesses present symptoms within several hours; others take up to six weeks to manifest, by which time some women will have crossed the threshold from preconception to pregnant. Foodborne illnesses can persist for days or even several weeks.

Before you recognize that you are pregnant, your body will already have begun tremendous hormonal changes. It used to be thought that the hormonal changes of pregnancy partially lowered a mother's immunity, making her more susceptible to certain illnesses, foodborne and otherwise. But as you may recall from Chapter 7, the maternal immune system is most certainly *not* depressed during pregnancy. It needs to be quite strong, and you are not more vulnerable to illness unless you have unresolved medical conditions or are extremely run-down. Regardless, it's simply best not to unnecessarily activate your immune system to fight off an infection that could have been prevented in the first place. You and the baby (and placenta) will all be better off that way. So both you and your partner can exercise your vocal cords while singing "Happy Birthday" twice (or whatever it takes to remind you to wash your hands for a full twenty seconds), because that's where much of germ safety begins and ends.

The pre-pregnancy months are therefore the ideal time for you and your partner to step up efforts to prevent risk of these illnesses. Pay close attention to the following to help make your body a safe haven from the moment your baby is conceived.

According to Alice Henneman, MS, RD, LMNT, extension educator at the University of Nebraska Cooperative Extension, you can be sick with a foodborne illness for as little as a few hours or as long as several months. She suggests ten food-safety practices that take thirty seconds or less, and we have extrapolated on these.

1. **Wash your hands!** The Centers for Disease Control and Prevention cite hand washing as the single most important way to prevent the spread of disease. Wash hands—front, back, in between fingers, and under nails—with regular soap and warm water for about twenty seconds before and after handling food. This is especially important when handling raw meat, poultry, or seafood; same goes for washing away the juices that accompany luncheon meats or hot dogs, even though they are precooked. (Hand sanitizing gels or wipes should be used only when you don't have access to soap and clean water.) Also wash hand towels and dish towels frequently, especially if you already have a little one who indiscriminately uses the towels!

2. **Avoid cross-contamination when using a cutting board.** Don't cut other foods on the same cutting board used to cut raw meat, poultry, or seafood. Reach for a clean cutting board and knife, or wash both with hot soapy water followed by hot rinse water before cutting the next food. According to the Agriculture Research Service, to further avoid cross-contamination, sponges and scrub brushes should be regularly replaced or sanitized by putting them through the dishwasher with a dry cycle or placing damp sponges in the microwave for one minute. Soaking in a solution of 1 teaspoon chlorine bleach to 1 quart water is less effective for sponges and brushes than the former two methods. (Do you have an extra squirt bottle, like the kind you use to mist plants? They work well for a weak bleach solution for use on the kitchen sink and counters.)

3. **Refrigerate perishable food promptly in shallow pans.** Did you know that just one bacterium can grow to 2,097,152 bacteria in seven hours if not kept under control? Never leave perishable food at room temperature more than two hours—one hour if the weather is hot. (The two-hour limit includes preparation time as well as serving time.) Perishable foods include raw *and cooked* meat, poultry, seafood, eggs, and dairy products. Once fruits and vegetables are cut, it's safest to limit their time at room temperature, too. Avoid storing foods (especially leftovers) in large, deep containers because these make it difficult for the cool refrigerator temperature to penetrate to the center of the item in a timely manner. Use shallow storage containers instead.

4. **Test food with a thermometer before serving.** Use an instant-read food thermometer to ensure that cooked food has reached a safe (high enough) temperature and to avoid overcooking. Not only will your food be safer, but it will taste better, too! (See Table 13-4.)

5. **Plan ahead when thawing food.** Take a little time today to plan tomorrow's meals so you can thaw food safely in the refrigerator, rather than at room temperature. Small items will thaw overnight in the refrigerator. Larger foods may take longer: allow approximately one day for every five pounds.

6. **Buy appliance thermometers if you don't have built-in ones.** The next time you're out shopping, purchase an appliance thermometer for both your refrigerator and your freezer. They're available at grocery, discount, hardware, and specialty stores that feature kitchen tools. Keep your refrigerator at just below 40°F and your freezer at 0°F. (Check the door seals! If your refrigerator or freezer opens too easily or you see a little mold growing, that's a sign that a seal needs replacing, which usually solves temperature inconsistencies.)

TABLE 13-4
SAFE TEMPERATURE CHART

Internal Cooking Temperatures

Product	°F
Egg & Egg Dishes	
Eggs	Cook until yolk & white are firm.
Egg dishes	160
Egg sauces, custards	160
Ground Meat & Meat Mixtures	
Turkey, Chicken	165
Beef, Veal, Lamb, Pork	160
Fresh Beef, Veal, Lamb	
Medium Rare	145
Medium	160
Well Done	170
Fresh Pork	
Medium	160
Well Done	170
Ham	
Fresh (raw)	160
Fully cooked (to reheat)	140
Roast Beef	
Cooked commercially, vacuum sealed, and ready-to-eat	140

Product	°F
Poultry*	
All products	165
Stuffing	
Cooked alone or in bird	165
Sauces, Soups, Gravies, Marinades	
Used with raw meat, poultry, or fish	Bring to a boil.
Seafood	145
Fin Fish	Cook until opaque and flakes easily with a fork.
Shrimp, lobster, crab	Should turn red and flesh should become pearly opaque.
Scallops	Should turn milky white or opaque and firm.
Clams, mussels, oysters	Cook until shells open.
Leftovers	165

Note: These temperatures are recommended for consumer cooking. They are not intended for processing, institutional, or food-service preparation. Food-service workers should consult their state or local food code, or health department.

*safe minimum internal temperature

Source: USDA-FSIS, *Cooking for Groups: A Volunteer's Guide to Food Safety (updated July 2007)*

7. **Purchase perishable foods last.** When you're in the supermarket, buy foods such as meat, poultry, seafood, eggs, and dairy products last. Then, after checkout, go straight home. When the weather's warm, carry your groceries home in the air-conditioned passenger compartment of the car rather than the hot trunk; if you don't have air-conditioning, a rolled-down window keeps the car interior cooler than the trunk.

8. **Remember: When in doubt, throw it out!**

9. **Internet help.**
Bookmark and visit these websites when you have a food-safety question:
- Fight BAC!, www.fightbac.org
- Gateway to Government Food Safety Information, www.foodsafety.gov
- www.fsis.usda.gov/Food_Safety_Education/Ask_Karen/index.asp

And here's an old-fashioned phone number to call with your questions:

- Food and Drug Administration (FDA), Center for Food Safety and Applied Nutrition Outreach and Information Center (toll free) (888) 723-3366

10. **Share this information with family and friends.** (Bookmark Alice Henneman's website, too: http://lancaster.unl.edu/food. She offers a wealth of information, everything from tips on food storage to controlling kitchen pests and cooking bison meat!)

Practical Application

Make a photocopy of the ten food safety practices, including the chart that lists all internal cooking temperatures (Table 13-4), and tape it to the inside of a kitchen cabinet for quick reference. Also, if you don't yet own an instant-read food thermometer, put it on your grocery list for the next time you go shopping.

Food and Beverage Choices

The rest of this chapter categorizes food safety issues by specific food types: dairy, meats and poultry, eggs, fresh produce, and fish. We suggest reviewing each section to see if anything conflicts with your current eating habits. Later, when confronted with the question of whether to eat, not eat, or just modify a food or beverage, you can refer back to that section and come away with a straightforward solution. You may ask yourself if all the precautions are really necessary, considering that the safety odds are definitely on your side. And sometimes the thought of making a special request at a restaurant (e.g., reheating lunch meat that's already precooked and ready-to-eat) or "insulting" the hosts of a dinner party when you choose not to eat something can be a powerful deterrent to following these guidelines. The truth is that taking chances some or all of the time won't likely affect your conception or pregnancy; then again, it could, seriously. Our goal is to offer you a plethora of tactics and food substitutes so that it will be nearly as easy to err on the side of caution.

Microwave Ovens: Tips on Safely Cooking and Reheating

Microwaves save energy and help foods retain more vitamins and minerals than most stovetop or oven cooking methods. However, the potential for uneven heating can occur in all types of foods cooked in microwaves. Where there is uneven heating, there can be "hot spots" that burn the mouth and "cold spots" that may foster bacterial growth in certain foods such as meats, chicken, eggs, casseroles, and leftovers. So for microwave-cooked foods, a few extra tips should be followed. According to the USDA's Food Safety and Inspection Service (FSIS):

- Foods should be arranged evenly covered in a dish labeled "microwave safe," potentially with a small amount of liquid added to create moist, even heating. The cover must fit loosely to allow steam to escape. Glass or ceramic containers, such as Pyrex or Corningware, work well in these cases.
- If the cover is a microwave-safe plastic wrap, it should not touch the food.
- If the food is a stirable type (like a casserole or stuffing), interrupt the heating process to stir it periodically. If your microwave doesn't have a carousel that rotates the food automatically, manually rotate the dish midway through.
- Use your food thermometer to check the finished temperature of any food mentioned by USDA/FSIS in Table 13-4. For example, leftovers should be reheated to 165°F throughout. For casseroles and other large items, test in a few places to detect uneven heating.
- Chinese take-out containers, small Styrofoam take-out boxes, and margarine tubs are safe only for food storage, not for microwave reheating. The FSIS emphasizes that these containers can get overheated and soften or melt, potentially allowing harmful chemicals to migrate into the food.

Dairy

Amrah: "I really love soft cheeses such as blue cheese and Brie and don't want to give them up. There's got to be a way to safely keep eating them." Yes, there are several. Let's look at what's off-limits first, then ideas for outsmarting some of them.

Of greatest concern in the dairy food group are raw or unpasteurized dairy products. To diminish the risk of foodborne illness from dairy products, follow these guidelines beginning three months prior to conception:

- Do not drink unpasteurized or raw milk.
- Always store milk in the regular part of the refrigerator, not in the door compartment (too warm).

Listeriosis: Foodborne Illness

Do you eat—or not wash hands off after handling—any of the following foods: raw or unpasteurized dairy products, ready-to-eat foods such as hot dogs (store-bought and sidewalk vendor sources alike), deli meats, meat spreads, store-made salads (such as ham salad, seafood salad, or chicken salad) or smoked fish (e.g., lox that is sold in the refrigerated section of the store and therefore not shelf stable), or unwashed raw vegetables? These foods may contain *Listeria monocytogenes* bacteria, to which pregnant women are particularly susceptible. Healthy nonpregnant individuals are much less susceptible but can contract a listeriosis infection if a food is highly contaminated, though tastes perfectly fine. Some of the same foods that potentially harbor listeria may carry other bacteria (such as salmonella), which can make you sick but are not as great a threat during preconception and pregnancy as listeria. Listeriosis infection can manifest up to six weeks after the food is eaten, but most life-threatening cases manifest within three weeks; this is why we add it to your preconception radar screen. The symptoms of an average case are often so mildly flu-like it frequently goes undetected and the CDC doesn't recommend testing or treatment unless more serious fever or illness occurs. The illness itself may last for a day or several weeks. Although listeriosis is less common during the first trimester of pregnancy than later, it often results in miscarriage, premature delivery, or death of the fetus or newborn.

Listeriosis can be most accurately diagnosed through testing blood or cerebrospinal fluid. Antibiotics are successfully used as treatment.

If you go a little out of your way, you can follow safety precautions that will eliminate the potential risk (more creative solutions like the ones on this and the next few pages help ease the hassle).

- Avoid eating soft cheeses such as Brie, feta, blue cheese, Camembert, and Mexican-style cheeses (queso blanco, queso panela, queso fresco, queso de hoja, queso de crema, and asadero) unless they have been melted and brought to a boil first. Why? Because most of these are made from unpasteurized milk and are at greater risk for contamination during the packaging process.[3] Remember, most blue cheese salad dressings made from scratch count, too. You don't have to avoid store-bought processed blue cheese salad dressings, but just for peace of mind, you may want to reconfirm that their processing entails pasteurization. And as already mentioned, you can eat all of these soft cheeses if they have been cooked first. Here are some ideas: baked figs stuffed with blue cheese; casseroles or enchiladas baked with Mexican-style cheeses; an appetizer of bubbly-hot baked Brie drizzled with honey and slivered almonds. But what if you love these cheeses on a salad or other cold dish? No problem. As long

---

3. If you are able to find any of the aforementioned cheeses made from *pasteurized* milk, they are safe to eat (e.g., pasteurized feta and blue cheeses are available at some markets). The ingredient label must say "pasteurized milk" first; if you're not sure, call the manufacturer.

as you heat any of them to the point of bubbling, just cool them down in a clean bowl until they harden again. They're safe and ready to recrumble or spread.

In fact, if you want to feel pampered or if you have a friend over for dinner who's pregnant and you want *her* to feel pampered, here's a recipe that gets requested over and over. It's extremely simple and has no listeria risk.

BEST PREGNANCY-FRIENDLY VINAIGRETTE SALAD DRESSING

Hint: The secret is the proportion of oil to vinegar. Regardless of how much you want to make, use 4 parts oil to 1 part vinegar (you can even do 5:1 for a less tangy taste). A common mistake is using way too much vinegar or not enough oil. Make it a few times and you'll get to the point where you can whip it up in seconds without measuring.

In a bowl, vigorously mix the following with a fork or small whisk:

¼ cup extra-virgin olive oil (or other healthy oil from Chapter 10)
1 tbsp vinegar (red wine, rice wine, balsamic, raspberry, etc.)
1 tsp Dijon mustard
½ tsp honey or fig jam
Dash of salt
Pepper to taste

Optional: fresh or dried chopped parsley or chives; chunks of that blue cheese that you brought to bubbling and cooled to eliminate risk of listeriosis.

Variation: Use a squeeze of lemon and a little less vinegar.

Nutrition info: One tablespoon of this salad dressing without added herbs or cheese is roughly 2½ tsp of oil on MyPyramid (~100 calories). It's a little higher in calories than store-bought dressings because those use more vinegar (zero calories) and less oil and add starchy thickeners (minimal calories, but thick texture). This recipe makes close to 5 tablespoons, more with cheese and herbs.

• Yogurt, cottage cheese, and cream cheese are not at risk for listeria contamination and are safe to eat.

- Don't buy dairy products that are past their sell-by date, as they likely won't stay fresh enough for the time you intend to have them on hand. Do not consume any after the use-by date.
- You may choose to drink organic or rbST-free[4] milks because you prefer these methods of raising cows, but if their price tag is prohibitive, don't fret. Fortunately, all milks should be wholesome, whether labeled organic, rbST-free, or conventionally produced. They all—yes, even organic—contain comparable levels of steroid hormones such as estradiol and progesterone from the cow, and to maintain perspective, these levels are minuscule in comparison to the amounts our own bodies produce daily. And you can breathe a sigh of relief to know that all milk that arrives in bulk tankers is tested for antibiotic residues; any that test positive are rejected before their contents can be pooled and sold (at huge financial loss to the company—another good incentive to prevent it from happening, we hope). The one area we would like to see more independent research on is milk's insulin-like growth factor 1 (IGF-1) content, a naturally occurring compound in milk. Of the three labels of milk, organic has been shown to be either the same as the other two or slightly lower, but this could be due to the fact that organic milk more often is ultrapasteurized (a method that denatures the IGF-1); it's been proposed, but far from proven, that higher IGF-1 in women could factor into a greater chance of conceiving twins.
- Heed all media reports of food recalls.

Meats and Poultry

Sandra: "The lunch meats I buy are labeled 'fully cooked, ready to eat,' as are the deli meats in my favorite sandwiches, so why should I need to reheat them again?"

Refrigerated processed meats and poultry products also have a small chance of being contaminated with *Listeria monocytogenes* bacteria during processing and packaging; canned or shelf-stable pâtés and meat spreads do not (they are pasteurized). Furthermore, raw or undercooked meats (and unwashed vegetables and refrigerated smoked seafood) can be a source of listeria as well as the parasite *Toxoplasma gondii* (see Chapter 3 for more information) and other sources of food contamination. Please note that although freezing does take care of toxoplasmosis infection, it does little or nothing to kill listeria bacteria.

---

4. Bovine somatotropin (bST) is a protein produced in all cows, regardless of how they are raised, that regulates milk production. According to 2007 statistics from the USDA, conventional milk producers treat about 17 percent of their cows with recombinant bovine somatotropin (rbST) to increase milk production. Milk labeled rbST-free is free of this supplement, whereas conventional producers pool their milk, leaving roughly 83% of the conventionally labeled cow milk rbST-free.

We advise the following preconception and pregnancy precautions to prevent all food-borne illnesses associated with certain forms of meats and poultry:

- When buying raw meats and poultry, place the wrapped item in another plastic bag right away so meat juices cannot drip on other items in the grocery cart. Keep them bagged or on a clean plate in your refrigerator at home. Never rinse raw meats or poultry; it isn't helpful, and the rinse water spreads the raw meat bacteria all over your sink.
- If meat or poultry juice gets on your kitchen counter or refrigerator shelf, wash it away immediately with soap, hot water, and disposable paper towels—not a sponge, which can hold the bacteria.
- Cook meats and poultry to the safe internal temperatures advocated in Table 13-4; check by using a meat thermometer. You may need to specifically request more thorough cooking when ordering hamburgers or other items from a restaurant menu. Stuffing and casseroles that contain these items also should be cooked (or reheated) to the recommended internal temperature.
- Hand washing before and after handling raw foods is a must.
- If you prefer to partially cook chicken or meat prior to barbecuing on the grill, do so within an hour of barbecuing to minimize bacterial growth in the interim.
- Anything (platter, utensils, cutting board) that touches raw food should be thoroughly washed before it comes in contact with the finished, cooked product.
- Leftover marinades and sauces in the marinating bowl or pan must be heated to a full boil if they are to be used again at the table. This is easy. Give it a try!
- All refrigerated, ready-to-eat deli or lunch meats, cured meats, paté and meat spreads, hot dogs, sausage, or cold cuts must be reheated until they are steaming hot before consuming them; this kills anything that contaminated the meat after it underwent cooking at the processing plant (for example, slicing machines shouldn't be, but could be, contaminated). Remember to make this request if ordering a deli sandwich—the person assembling the sandwich needs to heat only the lunch meat slices, not the whole sandwich. If you are making a sandwich at home to store until mealtime, heat the pre-sliced lunch meat—being sure to wash hands before touching it again—and cool it before assembling the sandwich, and then pop it into an insulated lunch bag that contains cold packs. A hot panini sandwich is an easier alternative.
- Make a point of eating these ready-to-eat products by the use-by date noted on the packaging.
- Reheat meat and poultry leftovers only once.
- Another hot topic is the concern over antibiotics and hormones in livestock. Many advances have been made in veterinary medicine to care for sick livestock by responsibly withdrawing

Sodium Nitrite

Regardless of whether you are planning to become pregnant, it is wise to limit your intake of sodium nitrite, a preservative intended for protection against botulism food poisoning. Nitrites can convert into nitrosamines, which have been implicated as cancer-causing agents in animals. Sodium nitrite is added to many cured luncheon meats, hot dogs, sausages, and smoked meats and fish. Fortunately, there are nitrite-free products available from local producers or in the freezer section of the store. Alternatively, some producers of cured or smoked meats add ingredients that inhibit conversion of nitrites to nitrosamines. These inhibitors are indicated on the ingredient labels as sodium ascorbate (vitamin C compound), sodium erythorbate, or vitamin E.

Don't worry about the natural sources of nitrites (and nitrates)—many veggies and fruits. They appear to have a different physiological effect and are likely healthy.

the animal from the herd and administering antibiotics when a bacterial (not viral) infection is present. Providing uncrowded living conditions is a way to prevent many infections in the first place, but this gets expensive. The bigger public health concern is the overuse and abuse of antibiotics for purposes of speeding up growth on less feed. Another issue revolves around artificial means to enhance growth, too; that of adding hormones (the term "adding" is used because animals and humans naturally produce some of the same hormones).[5] The European Union has put a ban on the use of hormone treatments as a precautionary measure; to date the United States has not done this for beef. This is an area of research that needs considerably more attention so that everyone can assess the issues more accurately. If you can afford it, buy from producers who oppose artificial means of enhancing growth of their animals; the labels will state either "no growth hormones added," "no antibiotics added," or both. Buying organic meats and poultry will cover both of those bases, though it may or may not cover what the animal is fed; for that you'll need to look specifically for terms such as "grass-fed" (slightly better) instead of "grain-fed." And if you cannot always be this specific with your purchases, tried-and-true nutrition advice prevails: eat a diet full of variety, including more modest portion sizes of meats and meat alternatives, and if you choose to live a vegetarian lifestyle, just make sure to reread that section back in Chapter 12.

- For more detailed information on topics such as safe summer barbecuing, camping, and cooking a holiday turkey, contact the U.S. Department of Agriculture, Food Safety and

5. According to the USDA, hormones are not allowed to be added to pork or poultry. Therefore, you will not see labeling on these products that say "no hormones added" unless it is followed by "Federal regulations prohibit the use of hormones."

Inspection Service Meat and Poultry Hot Line, (800) 535-4555. Burgeoning research on phytonutrients suggests that marinades or rubs containing culinary herbs and spices play a protective role against the effects of high-heat cooking (e.g., on a hot grill).

Eggs

Salmonella bacteria can be transferred from the chicken coop to the eggshell surface and into the egg carton. Unless the egg is pasteurized (very few are), these bacteria can then make their way into the egg's interior through microscopic cracks in the egg surface. To protect yourself from potential foodborne illness from unpasteurized eggs, do the following:

- Eggs should be kept refrigerated (below 40°F) at all times, because temperatures below 45°F hinder growth of salmonella bacteria.
- Cook eggs all the way through, until both the white and the yolk are firm, to kill bacteria. Healthy alternatives: scrambled eggs, omelets, frittatas and quiches, or hard-boiled eggs eaten alone, in a homemade egg salad sandwich, or as a deviled egg. With the invention of omega-3-rich eggs and the newfound importance of choline found in the yolk, these are just two more reasons to explore safe ways to get your eggs, up to seven per week. Egg drop soup, anyone?
- Batters that contain uncooked eggs should be avoided, so forgo testing the homemade cake or brownie batter and cookie dough before baking. You can get your fix of cookie dough from commercial cookie doughs and cookie dough ice cream, which typically use pasteurized eggs (read label to be sure).
- Other food items that may contain raw eggs include some Caesar salad dressings made from scratch, the Italian dessert tiramisu, and homemade chocolate mousse, ice cream, and eggnog. Ask how they're made before consuming them.
- If a recipe calls for raw eggs, as above, substitute pasteurized shell eggs (e.g., Davidsons Safest Choice) or pasteurized egg whites (e.g., Egg Beaters), which should be safe for this type of food preparation. There are also pasteurized whole-egg powders and meringue powders available in some specialty stores.
- Always wash hands thoroughly immediately after handling eggs.

Vegetables and Fruits

Laurie: "Avoid alfalfa sprouts? You're kidding. I thought they were so healthy for me."

Deidre: "The other day I noticed that my bagged spinach said 'Pre-washed.' When I looked at the fine print on the back, the asterisk was explained as 'final rinse recommended.' Is this really necessary?"*

A preconception diet with plenty of fresh produce is protective in its own right. But there's still opportunity to make it even healthier. Fresh produce that is not handled, stored, and prepared properly can be a potential source of bacterial, viral, and parasitic contamination. And although health experts consider pesticide, herbicide, or fungicide residues to be less of a concern relative to the first three, they should receive the same cautious treatment. The following tips can ensure that you reap all the benefits of these wholesome foods with the assurance of safety.

- Thoroughly rinse or scrub all vegetables and fruits under cool running water—without soap or detergent—before eating, cutting, or peeling. This is especially imperative for those that will be eaten raw or that have had contact with the ground (melons, strawberries, carrots, potatoes, greens). This washing technique should sufficiently wash away stubborn dirt, wax, and pesticide residues on the surface.[6] Certified organic produce should be washed also, if only to clean away dirt.
- For leafy vegetables such as lettuce and cabbage, discard outer leaves before washing.
- Once the vegetable or fruit is cleaned and cut, refrigerate any leftovers in a clean container as promptly as possible, certainly within the two-hour safety limit.
- Be sure to rewash any veggies that have been precut and washed (e.g., bagged salad greens, pre-cut cabbage and baby carrots) if you're going to eat them raw. If rewashing is too much trouble, try the vegetable in a different way. For example, if you have never tried fresh steamed spinach, this is a must for the novice. Add a couple tablespoons of water to a pan stuffed full of clean bagged spinach, sprinkle lightly with of salt, garlic, and/or oil, and cook covered over medium heat—delicious, worry-free, and a whopping serving or two of veggies.
- Avoid both raw and minimally cooked sprouts, homegrown or commercially grown. Al-

---

6. Currently, there is insufficient evidence to warrant the use of commercial produce washes unless they are approved by the EPA. Even if they are, the expense is considerable compared to already proven methods.

though foodborne illnesses from sprouts (mainly alfalfa, as well as bean, clover, and radish) are not particularly common, sprouts have been implicated in several outbreaks of *E. coli* as well as salmonella. The culprit appears to be the seeds themselves, so you cannot tell just by looking at the sprouts whether they are contaminated. Thorough cooking eliminates the risk, as in hot stir-fried veggies.

- Avoid drinking unpasteurized juice or cider from roadside stands or markets. Steaming-hot cider is safe. If you have a home juicer, properly clean the juicer and all fruits and vegetables before juicing.
- By attending your local farmers' market or joining a CSA (community-supported agriculture) group you can learn more about which farms are using more sustainable farming practices, such as organic methods and integrated pest management techniques, if these concerns rank high on your list. See our earlier discussion, page 398.

Fish/Seafood

A variety of fish, especially ocean fish, and other seafood can and should be included in your diet. If you are at all skeptical about following that recommendation, it's understandable. There are, in fact, some fish that are not appropriate for women who could become pregnant, and the government and media have been almost too good at getting that message across. And the fact that some—mind you, not all—in the fishing industry have done themselves no favors by indiscriminately overfishing has public sentiment even more skeptical of the news that fish could benefit them. However, much as the lowly egg was blacklisted for several years because of gaps in knowledge about its nutrient profile, seafood is in the same predicament. We'll try to walk you through this intelligently so that you will look forward to those fish meals instead of questioning if you're doing the right thing.

Before addressing the issues of mercury or PCBs, let's first address what has firmly been advised for years now:

- The FDA advises women who could become pregnant to avoid refrigerated smoked seafood, due to the risk of listeria bacterial contamination. Terms such as "lox," "nova style," "kippered," "smoked," or "jerky" on the label should cue you to skip it, unless you're planning to incorporate the item into a cooked dish such as a frittata or chowder. Canned or shelf-stable seafoods *don't* carry the risk of listeria and can be eaten just as they are, provided they are freshly opened and served soon thereafter.
- Avoid raw fish and shellfish to prevent foodborne illnesses related to raw or undercooked seafood, such as salmonella and hepatitis A, especially once there is a possibility that you could become pregnant. There is no clear evidence that ceviche is any safer than raw fish, so it's probably best not to chance it.

It's hard to surrender to this recommendation if you're a big fan of sashimi or raw sushi rolls, so try this tip given to us by a reader: "I kept a list from my favorite restaurant with the cooked sushi rolls highlighted for my quick reference."

As you know, researchers are very enthusiastic about the two long-chain omega-3 fatty acids DHA and EPA that are so abundantly found in oily ocean fish; recall that these can be found together in fish oil supplements (and DHA alone can be obtained from marine algae oil). Yet to date the research is thin on whether supplements help as much as eating the real thing: oily fish. Omega-3s aren't the only nutrients from fish that optimize your preconception health as well as your future baby's neurodevelopment. There are several more standouts, such as protein, selenium (go back and reread that section, pages 346–347), iodine, and vitamin D, to name a few. And the benefits extend beyond pregnancy. A prominent study conducted in the United Kingdom found the lowest prevalence of postpartum depression in women who ate more than 12 ounces of seafood per week during pregnancy, and their offspring were healthy as well.

To offer you more specific insight on how eating fish is beneficial, let's consider two well-known ongoing studies that have been collecting and analyzing reproductive outcome data for more than twenty years on populations who eat substantially more seafood than most people (about nine to twelve seafood meals every week): Seychelles Islanders and Faroe Islanders, who live almost halfway around the globe from each other. Both populations eat roughly the same amount of seafood. The Seychelles research clearly shows that their offspring are thriving, not just during pregnancy and infancy but into childhood and the teen years. What has had researchers scratching their heads until very recently is the fact that the Faroe Islanders were not faring as well. Offspring of these women were showing signs of subtle neurodevelopmental delays. But weren't their diets virtually the same? Well, yes and no. Both populations were consuming comparable amounts of seafood; it's just that the main seafood consumed by many Faroese was pilot whale meat and blubber (these whales are not your typical krill eaters, but predators of ocean mammals and large fish). Some women were eating more whale than others, and the others ate more ocean fish. When the researchers analyzed those differences, they found their "smoking gun." Although researchers had no direct analysis comparing the PCB content of pilot whale (especially the blubber) to the PCB content in the Faroese women's fish choices, the message became clearer.

The vast majority of ocean fish (as opposed to pilot whales) don't seem to be causing trouble. In fact, something from fish appears to be helping mom and baby (in effect, protecting against what should have been the effects of too much mercury consumption); taking fish oil alone does not yield this effect. One plausible explanation is that pilot whale meat is one of the few seafoods that contains more mercury than the antioxidant selenium, so as you'll recall from Chapter 11, when the bad guys (mercury) outnumber the good guys (antioxidants) for

What Is Methylmercury and Where Is It Found?

Mercury is released into the atmosphere through natural events such as volcanic eruptions (past and present, including active vents under the sea) or, in our more modern era, through pollution from electrical power plants and industrial waste. It vaporizes into the air and eventually rains back to earth and gathers in areas where water accumulates. On earth, bacteria transform mercury into methylmercury, a form of mercury easily absorbed by humans. Methylmercury has an affinity for fish muscle tissue, so older, bigger fish (and animals) that prey on other fish tend to accumulate the highest concentrations of methylmercury over time. These fish thrive, despite current levels of methylmercury in their tissues (notable changes haven't been detected in commercial fish for decades by current testing methods, and fortunately, monitoring is ongoing). Interestingly, fish, animals, and humans have had to evolve in an environment that naturally contains mercury (and many other potentially harmful substances), so to a certain degree, mechanisms for peaceful coexistence are built into our systems. The present concern is with how we humans can ease the global burden of man-made contributions to the mercury in our soils and oceans. In addition, in lakes where the selenium content of soil is low, fish tend to be higher in mercury; this is an area of ongoing research.

too long, things start to go wrong. Even though participants in both studies consumed far more mercury than our FDA or EPA guidelines would consider safe, it appears more important that the variety of *ocean fish* that these two populations eat (rather than whale meat) contain more than enough selenium, vitamin D, iodine, long-chain omega-3s, and other baby-friendly nutrients to protect from harm and confer additional pregnancy benefits. That, and the elimination of eating sea mammals such as whale. Even the nervous system of a developing fetus, which is perhaps five to ten times more vulnerable to mercury than that of an adult, reaps the benefits. That's profound!

Not all fish have been sufficiently analyzed for their selenium content. But we know that, like pilot whales, a few fish species don't contain enough selenium to offset mercury levels. The two main ones are large shark and swordfish (neither king mackerel nor tilefish has been well tested yet for their selenium content); an inland variety of pike is also poor. The question "What about tuna?" often comes up, and the answer is that all canned tuna species have very favorable amounts of protective selenium in comparison to their mercury content, so this is a big relief for those of you who don't have access to a year-round variety of fresh fish.

Your dietary goal should be 12 ounces of fish and shellfish (mostly marine sources, as op-

What About Farm-Raised Versus Wild Fish?

Our recommendations focus on the best fish sources of nutrients regardless of where or how the fish were harvested—ocean or farm-raised (aquaculture). That said, you may find more and more fish options labeled as "farm-raised" as the U.S. aquaculture industry expands. Several state and federal agencies regulate the aquaculture industry; thus farm-raised fish may be an excellent choice from both a sustainability and a safety perspective. On a global scale, not all countries adhere to high standards in fish farming, so you will need an additional resource that is regularly updated. The Monterey Bay Aquarium near San Francisco produces an excellent wallet-sized regional reference that lists fish harvested in ocean-friendly ways that are good for the fish and good for the environment. Download it as well as the link to pocket guide updates at montereybayaquarium.org/cr/cr_seafoodwatch/download.aspx. (Note they are also on social networking sites such as Twitter and Facebook.)

posed to freshwater fish) each week. The research trends suggest that this could be relaxed to accept more than 12 ounces within responsible parameters, as, for example, many Asian cultures as well as the Seychelles Islanders do.[7] The most important message now is to figure out how to get an average of 12 ounces of seafood into your weekly menu. Which fish and seafoods are recommended as healthy components of your preconception diet and which ones are off-limits?

- **Safest.** In general, the most popular seafoods as well as most of the smaller panfish all contain very low levels of mercury (or moderate mercury and very high selenium). As a rule of thumb, a wide variety of ocean/saltwater (S) fish and shellfish from this group should account for more than half of your choices. Examples:

7. One large coalition of respected health care experts in the United States, the National Healthy Mothers, Healthy Babies Coalition, advocated such a move in the year 2007, but this was a first in the United States and was met with more skepticism than praise. This seminal recommendation has at least paved the way for a multifaceted approach to assessing fish safety and highlighting the fact that when the right kinds of seafood are consumed, a strict 12-ounce-per-week limit for pregnant or pre-pregnant women may be unnecessary and potentially shortsighted.

Salmon (especially Alaskan) *S, F*
   (*meaning, from either salt water or fresh water*)
Shrimp *PS*
Pollock *S*
Cod *S*
Catfish (preferably farm-raised) *PF*
Clams *S*
Flatfish (e.g., flounder, halibut) *S*
Crabs *S*
Scallops *S*
Anchovies *S*
Sardines *S*
Small mackerel *S*
Herring *S, F*
Haddock *S*
Tilapia *S*
Mahi-mahi *S*
Tuna, light (mostly skipjack and yellowfin) *S*
Tuna, albacore (white)[8] *S*—you may safely consume up to six ounces per week

> Know the source of your fish and shellfish: When you buy, seek as much information as possible, from the person who is selling it or from the label on the package. You can usually obtain information such as country of origin and whether it was from a marine or freshwater source (or both). Use this key for starters.
> Key:
>   *S* = Saltwater (ocean/marine)—these (and *PS*) should predominate
>   *PS* = Primarily saltwater
>   *F* = Freshwater
>   *PF* = Primarily freshwater

- **Moderate.** Fish that may contain greater than 0.5 ppm mercury (but also have ample selenium) include the following. Eat these when you want to add more variety to your safest choices, and see the highlighted box on page 417 to answer your questions regarding sustainability. Examples:

Wahoo *S*
Bigeye *S*
Opah *S*
Striped and blue marlin *S*
Escolar *S* (be warned, eat only a small amount; this delicious oily fish may cause harmless but uncomfortable gastrointestinal symptoms after eating)
Orange roughy *S*

---

8. If you don't have fresh fatty fish available, it's a good idea to eat frozen fresh fish or canned seafood such as canned salmon, tuna, anchovies, or clams (canned albacore tuna can serve for up to 6 of your 12 ounces, but add variety for the other 6 ounces).

- **Caution.** The mercury (and selenium) content of inland-water fish will vary more. Several have been tested, but the composition varies regionally, so it's harder to be certain. Examples include:

Large pike *F*
Large perch *S, F*
Larger bass species *S, F*
Potentially any fish in selenium-poor lakes or streams
Tuna, largest *S* (the type usually prepared as tuna steaks or sushi), as many have similarly high amounts of methylmercury, though the very high selenium content from the ocean makes it more attractive than the freshwater fish in this same category.

- **Avoid or restrict.** Fish caught from contaminated inland lakes or rivers should be restricted or avoided depending on the degree of the water contamination. Examples include some trout and channel catfish. The same varieties of fish from fish farms are generally safe and need not be avoided. Oysters from contaminated waters (e.g., Gulf of Mexico, many coastal waters on the East Coast) should be avoided or restricted as well. Check your state and local public health departments for the latest fishing advisories. If you have trouble locating this information, the EPA has a listing of federal, state, and tribal contacts for up-to-date fish advisories; call (202) 260-1305 or see its Web page at www.epa.gov/waterscience/fish. If you go to this site, you can click on the state in which you are interested, then click again on "water bodies with fish advisories" for detailed reports (often with three levels of safety ratings). This resource is updated regularly and particularly important for freshwater fish species.

- **Avoid.** The FDA and the EPA make it very clear that women who could become pregnant should avoid consumption of a few fish species that consistently contain too-high levels of methylmercury or other environmental contaminants. Shark and swordfish meat are also known to be proportionately lower in selenium than other varieties of ocean fish (though their brains and other "priority" tissues such as pituitary, adrenals, and reproductive organs have evolved to contain more selenium than mercury, therefore coexisting without evident harm). Though it may be prudent to extend this recommendation to prospective fathers as well, we are unaware of evidence to mandate doing so, and male testes are even better equipped to protect themselves from mercury than the brain (there's a good joke in here somewhere, for sure). Fish species that have the highest methylmercury content are typically higher up in the aquatic food chain, meaning they eat smaller fish. Completely avoid the following:

Shark *S*
Swordfish *S*
King mackerel *S*
Tilefish *S*

Note: It goes without saying that consumption of marine mammal meat or blubber is off-limits, too.

FIGURE 13-4
HOW TO CLEAN A FISH TO GET RID OF MOST PCBs

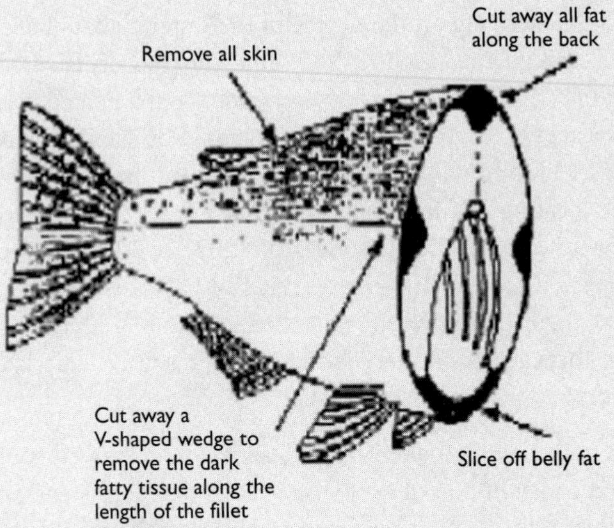

Remove all skin

Cut away all fat along the back

Cut away a V-shaped wedge to remove the dark fatty tissue along the length of the fillet

Slice off belly fat

The guidelines we've discussed should also protect you from PCBs (polychlorinated biphenyls),* as they, too, are most commonly found in large predatory sea mammals, fish species, and fish from PCB-contaminated waters (e.g., Great Lakes). Trimming fat before cooking may reduce the amount of potential contaminants such as PCBs, but the methylmercury content is not notably affected by removing the fatty skin layer.

*PCBs have not been manufactured since 1977 but remain a persistent environmental contaminant (e.g., especially in contaminated waters).

Food Irradiation

Irradiation of spices and certain foods such as beef, poultry, pork, grains, vegetables, and fruits have FDA approval for human consumption. There is no residual radiation in the food, and the nutrient composition remains healthy and essentially devoid of bacterial and parasitic contamination. The process of treating foods with gamma rays or electron beams does slightly alter or diminish certain nutrients in the process, but it's important to understand that this also happens when foods are cooked or canned. That doesn't make them harmful. Still, leeriness on the part of consumers has diminished demand for these, so they're hard to find in the grocery store.

Rest assured that these foods are considered safe as part of a varied diet for prospective parents and may prevent serious foodborne infections. These foods must be clearly labeled with the words "treated by irradiation" or "cold pasteurized" and feature the internationally recognized "radura" symbol (Figure 13-5) so people can make informed purchases.

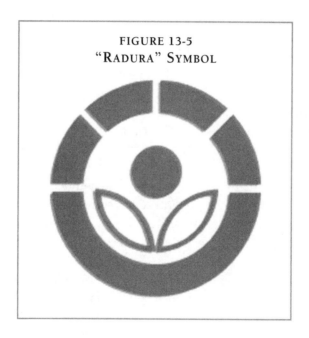

FIGURE 13-5
"RADURA" SYMBOL

CHAPTER 14

Body Weight, Body Image

*I*f ever there was a time to have a constructive relationship with food, exercise, and body weight, it is now, before you conceive. But our society is wrestling with weight-related issues. We resort to restrictive eating and/or overexercising in an effort to attain a model-skinny physique. There's also the difficulty of fitting in exercise and good nutrition while juggling the often exhausting demands of modern life. Ironically, an obsession with the scale and food actually diminishes health for some of us, distracting us from focusing where we should: on a healthy lifestyle that meets the body's most basic of needs.

Being consistently healthy sets up a "trust" relationship between your mind and body—sending a clear message that you're fit to conceive and will likely be similarly reliable once pregnant. In this chapter we'll give you the information and perspective to embrace a paradigm shift about body weight—in the words of author and social worker Kathy Kater, LICSW, we hope you will begin to "connect with health as a value in its own right, and align your actions accordingly." This approach influences a person's overall health, of which weight is only one component.

Because the weight at which you *enter* pregnancy carries with it so many short- and long-term benefits (for both you and baby), this topic simply can't be shelved until after conception, regardless of your current shape and size. What you may not realize is that in most cases, your weight (and related behaviors) when you conceive has a stronger influence on predicting pregnancy outcome than what happens to your weight *during* pregnancy. Proper pregnancy weight gain still has an important role, though. And both have a distinct impact on what will become important to you later on: an improved likelihood of a successful breastfeeding experience, a healthier infant and school-age child, healthier weight in between pregnancies should you hope to have another baby, and better health odds for you and your child(ren) later in life.

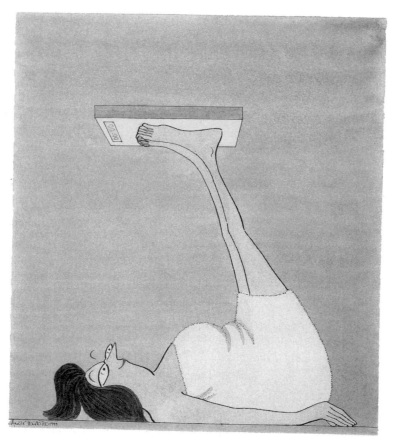

The Female Character—The ability to see facts from whatever angle suits them best . . .

Copyright © by Anne Tempest at The O'Shea Gallery, London. www.tottering.com

This chapter's layout allows you to focus on the sections that pertain to your personal situation and skim others. You might even have a few "aha" moments in these pages. After focusing on getting pregnant, we'll highlight the different role of pregnancy weight gain. Depending on your pre-pregnancy weight, your "best pace" weight gain will need to be individualized for optimizing the health of you and your baby. Of course, any discussion of weight should include what happens when eating becomes clinically disordered, an issue we address at the very end of this chapter.

When you meet your body's pre-pregnancy needs for nourishment and activity, your body weight falls in line with where it's healthiest for you. This healthy mind-set and lifestyle help you maximize your body's likelihood of ovulating predictably and conceiving more easily. Even if you had hoped to put it on the back burner, try channeling your enthusiasm for conceiving into absorbing this information to your immediate benefit. Having this mind-set in place before conception makes it easier to maintain throughout pregnancy and after delivery, when it's equally important not to trigger (or exacerbate) an obsession about the scale.

Once you understand what your body weight reveals about your preconception health, you can set realistic expectations. If there are adjustments to make—physical or mental—they're done in time to make a difference in your fertility and the baby's health. The following two anecdotes exemplify these points from very different angles:

Corrine, age thirty-one, was a full-figured, athletic woman, 5 feet 7 inches tall and 170 pounds (body mass index, or, BMI, of about 27), and had been since her late teens. Almost everyone in her family was similarly built. She had always been active, wholesomely nourished, and in otherwise good medical and gynecologic health. It was evident that Corrine was at her personal best above the "normal" BMI range. Both she and her ob-gyn were careful to acknowledge the importance of staying within the recommended range for weight gain among women categorized as "overweight" once she became pregnant (more on this later).

Natalie, age twenty-eight, was 5 feet 6 inches tall and more than 250 pounds (BMI of more than 40), and had steadily gained more than 100 pounds since being married and having a child. Her partner, Brendon, had put on close to that amount, too. They both had sedentary jobs and relaxed after work with their son and extended family and friends. In their eyes, eating healthy foods and exercising took all the fun out of life. They had no interest in it. It wasn't until Natalie's annual gynecology appointment that the nurse-practitioner expressed concern over her upwardly spiraling weight and preconception lab-work results. The nurse-practitioner firmly recommended that before trying to conceive again, Natalie (and Brendon) focus on changing their lifestyle . . . responsibly. If Natalie's weight gain was related more to lifestyle than genetic predisposition, she could expect weight loss to be a likely outcome of improved eating and exercise habits. Even if such weight loss were not the outcome, her improved overall health would go a long way toward supporting the healthiest pregnancy possible. But there was no sugar coating the risks of a BMI over 40, and this led to Natalie's decision to embrace the gift of time before trying to conceive. It was a real struggle, but she persevered, establishing sustainable routines for wholesome eating and physical activity. Her example soon set the tone for the rest of her family as well.

Our goal is to help you enter pregnancy as close as possible to your lowest-risk weight range. We also hope to capture the attention of women who may already be there but have destructive eating and exercise habits. So don't think you're off the nutrition and fitness hook based on a scale number alone. The truth is that all women need the benefit of healthy habits, independent of weight, before they go about the business of baby making. Lauren's story illustrates this point:

Lauren was 5 feet 5 inches tall and weighed 123 pounds (a BMI at the lower end of normal), worked long, intense hours as an emergency room doctor, and lived on a steady diet of soft drinks, vending machine snacks, and other fast food. She and her husband never cooked at home, and the contents of their refrigerator consisted of a few beverages, butter, random condiments, and take-out containers. Despite her medical knowledge, Lauren thought to herself, "I don't have a weight problem, so why should I worry about what I eat or whether I exercise?" Her ob-gyn assumed she was healthy, too, because of her outward appearance and low-risk weight categorization. She did conceive, but whether or not her habits played a role in her daughter's rocky start to life (born six weeks early) is a question with which she still wrestles. Lauren slowly improved her health habits during her postpartum leave as total body wellness assumed a new, more important meaning for her.

If you're behaving as if there's no tomorrow to fit into those jeans today, what's needed for true preconception readiness is a mental switch to being in it for the long haul, even for those with loudly ticking biological clocks. Obsessing over one's weight or trying to achieve a cookie-cutter appearance that doesn't respect your biological predisposition only amplifies dissatisfaction. Harsh denial of internal hunger cues and methods of changing appearance may follow. The problem lies in the focus of one's attention. What's my weight today? Why can't I look like her? These are barriers to behaviors with long-term benefit, but how does one make that mental switch to "connect with health as a value in its own right"?

Since so much of our adult body image takes root at a young age, it made sense to seek input from Kathy Kater, whom we introduced earlier. She's an expert on childhood and teen body image, and her keen insights helped us keep a constructive focus in this chapter. According to Ms. Kater, it's helpful to think back to our own childhood and adolescent experience. In particular, how much did peer, family, and media-driven influences affect how we saw ourselves? And what do we want to model for our kids? What influences will we allow to shape them? Now, more than ever, we need to be taught from an early age to be objective about societal pressures that focus on the superficial, body weight being just one example. Fortunately, if we didn't develop healthy body image attitudes when we were young, it's not too late for us now.

A young person develops a healthy perspective with an identity anchored in "substantial *inner* qualities," Kater says. It's no different for adults. We need only to look as far as our own conversations and actions to gauge where we are on this continuum. So as the topic of body weight comes up, as it does in just about every pre-pregnancy doctor visit, here are three suggestions for placing those numbers on the scale in the proper context. These same three points will help you see others from a healthier perspective too.

- First, weight is not the complete picture. We, as clinicians, (and you) cannot fully assess your health and lifestyle solely by observing your weight. Well-fed, fit people come in all sizes and shapes. We aim to weave scientific findings about weight categories with what's reasonable for you.

- Second, many complex factors beyond our control influence weight. It is therefore important to shift the primary goal from weight control to taking charge of health-enhancing behaviors that are in our power to choose, such as regular, balanced, and wholesome eating and activities that promote physical fitness. This paradigm shift in turn promotes *intrinsic* regulation of weight.

- Third, the healthy weight that's right for you can be best determined by nourishing your body well and engaging in physical activity day after day, month after month, and year after year. Sustaining this lifestyle shows your body that it will always get the food and energy it needs and should freely use it to nourish and expend through movement. But it needs that predictability and structure. If your BMI still falls in the underweight, over-weight, or obese categories, despite good eating and exercise habits, that's the weight that reflects your individuality. Attempts to alter this weight may cue your body to mount major resistance, and should always be factored into any health assessment.

As you can see, weight is often confounded by other factors, but then again, all of the sub-jects in *Before Your Pregnancy* are influenced by a number of factors. It's still important to look at what is known after those influences are peeled away. When pre-pregnancy body weight (expressed as one's body mass index, or BMI) is the lone focus, it's an independent predictor—in certain cases a very powerful indicator—of who might experience weight-related pregnancy complications. For example, folic acid supplementation doesn't offer any extra protection against neural tube defects to babies born to obese moms (those with a BMI greater than 30). That's just one example of many. So we do need to talk about basic weight information, such as what the numbers on the scale mean in relation to BMI charts.

BODY WEIGHT BASICS

The body mass index (BMI), also called the Quetelet (Q) index, is calculated as your weight in kilograms divided by your height in meters squared (see Figure 14-1). The BMI is the inter-national standard for determining body weight relative to height. Because they are not age- or gender-specific, BMI charts can be used by researchers around the globe to compare apples with apples—or maybe we should say "pears with pears," for those of us with good child-bearing hips! The "healthiest" weight ranges—those with the lowest risk for pregnancy complications—as defined by BMI are broad and take into account that women of various sizes and shapes can be ideally suited for a healthy conception.

FIGURE 14-1
BODY MASS INDEX (BMI) TABLE

Body Mass Index Table

	Normal						Overweight					Obese										Extreme Obesity														
BMI	19	20	21	22	23	24	25	26	27	28	29	30	31	32	33	34	35	36	37	38	39	40	41	42	43	44	45	46	47	48	49	50	51	52	53	54
Height (inches)																Body Weight (pounds)																				
58	91	96	100	105	110	115	119	124	129	134	138	143	148	153	158	162	167	172	177	181	186	191	196	201	205	210	215	220	224	229	234	239	244	248	253	258
59	94	99	104	109	114	119	124	128	133	138	143	148	153	158	163	168	173	178	183	188	193	198	203	208	212	217	222	227	232	237	242	247	252	257	262	267
60	97	102	107	112	118	123	128	133	138	143	148	153	158	163	168	174	179	184	189	194	199	204	209	215	220	225	230	235	240	245	250	255	261	266	271	276
61	100	106	111	116	122	127	132	137	143	148	153	158	164	169	174	180	185	190	195	201	206	211	217	222	227	232	238	243	248	254	259	264	269	275	280	285
62	104	109	115	120	126	131	136	142	147	153	158	164	169	175	180	186	191	196	202	207	213	218	224	229	235	240	246	251	256	262	267	273	278	284	289	295
63	107	113	118	124	130	135	141	146	152	158	163	169	175	180	186	191	197	203	208	214	220	225	231	237	242	248	254	259	265	270	278	282	287	293	299	304
64	110	116	122	128	134	140	145	151	157	163	169	174	180	186	192	197	204	209	215	221	227	232	238	244	250	256	262	267	273	279	285	291	296	302	308	314
65	114	120	126	132	138	144	150	156	162	168	174	180	186	192	198	204	210	216	222	228	234	240	246	252	258	264	270	276	282	288	294	300	306	312	318	324
66	118	124	130	136	142	148	155	161	167	173	179	186	192	198	204	210	216	223	229	235	241	247	253	260	266	272	278	284	291	297	303	309	315	322	328	334
67	121	127	134	140	146	153	159	166	172	178	185	191	198	204	211	217	223	230	236	242	249	255	261	268	274	280	287	293	299	306	312	319	325	331	338	344
68	125	131	138	144	151	158	164	171	177	184	190	197	203	210	216	223	230	236	243	249	256	262	269	276	282	289	295	302	308	315	322	328	335	341	348	354
69	128	135	142	149	155	162	169	176	182	189	196	203	209	216	223	230	236	243	250	257	263	270	277	284	291	297	304	311	318	324	331	338	345	351	358	365
70	132	139	146	153	160	167	174	181	188	195	202	209	216	222	229	236	243	250	257	264	271	278	285	292	299	306	313	320	327	334	341	348	355	362	369	376
71	136	143	150	157	165	172	179	186	193	200	208	215	222	229	236	243	250	257	265	272	279	286	293	301	308	315	322	329	338	343	351	358	365	372	379	386
72	140	147	154	162	169	177	184	191	199	206	213	221	228	235	242	250	258	265	272	279	287	294	302	309	316	324	331	338	346	353	361	368	375	383	390	397
73	144	151	159	166	174	182	189	197	204	212	219	227	235	242	250	257	265	272	280	288	295	302	310	318	325	333	340	348	355	363	371	378	386	393	401	408
74	148	155	163	171	179	186	194	202	210	218	225	233	241	249	256	264	272	280	287	295	303	311	319	326	334	342	350	358	365	373	381	389	396	404	412	420
75	152	160	168	176	184	192	200	208	216	224	232	240	248	256	264	272	279	287	295	303	311	319	327	335	343	351	359	367	375	383	391	399	407	415	423	431
76	156	164	172	180	189	197	205	213	221	230	238	246	254	263	271	279	287	295	304	312	320	328	336	344	353	361	369	377	385	394	402	410	418	426	435	443

Source: Adapted from *Clinical Guidelines on the Identification, Evaluation, and Treatment of Overweight and Obesity in Adults: The Evidence Report,* National Heart, Lung, and Blood Institute, 1998

Your BMI number is not the same as your percentage of body fat. You can certainly go out of your way to have your percentage of body fat measured via one of three measurement techniques: professional skin-fold measurement, an underwater immersion test called hydrostatic weighing, or dual-energy X-ray absorptiometry (DXA, formerly DEXA). However, unlike BMI, knowing your body fat percentage isn't an essential piece of information and is more subject to testing error.[1] In our opinion, a conceptual understanding is enough. The most interesting point is that muscle is 20 percent heavier than fat. Therefore, many lean, athletic women weigh more than you might suspect. And underweight women who have little muscle tone can still have near-normal body fat because it's expressed as a percentage of their weight. (You can see how undue focus on one measurement could fuel an eating disorder instead of reveal-

---

1. Bear in mind that these tests wouldn't be appropriate or accurate for pregnant women or recently pregnant women (new moms as well as women with recent miscarriage).

ing its lethal impact!) Although more often the case with men, occasionally a very muscular woman will have a BMI in the overweight category and still fall within the healthiest body fat percentage range for women of childbearing age (18 to 25 percent body fat). Physical assessment in these cases is more indicative of good health than the BMI, as was probably the case of Corrine, about whom you read at the beginning of this chapter.

Practical Application

Figuring out your BMI is very simple (flip back one page to Figure 14-1). Follow these steps:

1. Find your current height in inches along the left margin of the chart. Circle the height. (Note: 60 inches is equal to 5 feet.)
2. From this point, look to the right and find your current weight. Circle it.
3. From this point, draw an arrow straight up to the bar of BMI numbers across the top of the chart. This number is your BMI.
4. What is your BMI? _____ What range does this put you in: underweight (not shown, but less than 18.5), normal, overweight, obese, or extremely obese? _____

Take a closer look across the top of the BMI chart at the weight categorizations. With regard to preconception readiness, women with pre-pregnancy BMIs anywhere in the normal range have the most favorable odds of conceiving and having a healthy full-term baby. Women with pre-pregnancy BMIs above or below the normal range, especially those who are obese (BMI above 30), extremely obese (BMI above 40), or underweight (BMI below 18.5), increase their risk of problems associated with conception, pregnancy, and their offspring's lifelong health. Women in the overweight category (BMI 25.0–29.9) have increased risks as well, though BMIs over 30 most consistently diminish Mother Nature's ability to fully protect mom and baby. As the BMI tops 35 and 40, optimizing maternal and fetal health becomes progressively more challenging.

Let's look at a situation that many women face. Suppose you have drifted away from health-enhancing behaviors that support your healthiest BMI, and your BMI has dramatically shifted. You may not have the luxury of time to slowly and carefully lose or gain the number of pounds it would take to be comfortably within the healthiest weight range. Weighing the pros and cons of when to start trying to get pregnant at your given BMI will therefore require some personal judgment. If your BMI is outside the normal range, at a minimum consider putting on hold your date to start trying for three months—a relatively short time in the scheme of things. During that time, see whether healthier lifestyle habits will gradually improve your BMI by two to three units (e.g., increasing from 17 to 19 or decreasing from 31 to 28). The wait and wholesome efforts are well worth it, as you will likely conceive more easily and have less chance of miscarriage. If you have been trying to get (or stay) pregnant for some time now—with or without reproductive assistance—the upside to improving your BMI by a few units is all the more rewarding. Of all the things you've tried thus far, this may be what you have needed all along.

Practical Application

If you identify with the scenario of having a preconception BMI outside the normal (lowest-risk) BMI due more to unhealthy habits than true genetic predisposition, we hope you'll avoid the quick fix and instead adopt sustainable lifestyle changes (elaborated on later in this chapter). Should your weight respond by shifting toward a lower-risk BMI, here's how to figure out the tipping point at which you'll cross into a more pregnancy-friendly zone.

First, make sure that the height line you drew on the BMI chart in Figure 14-1 extends horizontally across the entire chart, and notice where it crosses through each of the weight ranges. From the points where it crosses the lower and upper ends of the normal BMI range (18.5–24.9), recall that any weight along that continuum carries with it the least statistical risk. There's also value in identifying the weight threshold below which an extremely obese woman lowers her risk to that of an obese woman, or an obese woman lowers her risk to that of someone who is overweight. Ultimately, if your BMI category does change, be prepared to alter your plan accordingly for the "best pace" weight gain once you conceive.

HAVE A HEALTHY MIND-SET ABOUT YOUR FUTURE PREGNANCY WEIGHT GAIN

Eva, a stay-at-home mom, was worried that she hadn't taken off some of her prior pregnancy weight (she was 5 feet 8 inches tall and weighed 160 pounds, with a BMI of about 24, at the high end of normal). She was equally concerned about gaining too much during her next pregnancy, having put on almost fifty pounds with her first. Eva had always gauged how she would eat with how she was feeling about her body weight. But after a couple of nutrition consultations, she exclaimed, "For the first time in my life, I'm eating for health!" She noticed that her body weight naturally started to reduce, evidence that she was improving her health. And this made it more appealing to do other things for health, such as moving more, making stroller dates with other moms, and not avoiding stairs. Eva found that her new approach made her feel less anxious, and her second pregnancy weight gain was much more evenly paced and within the recommended guidelines.

On the topic of body weight, these months prior to conception are ideal for discussing what to anticipate regarding pregnancy weight gain. Being mentally prepared for proper weight gain during pregnancy is important so that you are not caught off guard by the changes that your body needs to go through to sustain a healthy pregnancy. Pregnancy is not a license to eat, eat, eat—or worse, an opportunity to lose. Rather, it is a time to gain a type of weight that is a privilege and a gift (see Table 14-1 on the next page).

Your energy needs will increase during pregnancy, primarily in the second and third trimesters. The Dietary Reference Intake charts reflect this by advising an additional 340 and 452 calories per day in the second and third trimesters, respectively, for those who are in the normal weight category from the start. The main point here is to not gain much at first; then when support tissues and the baby grow more substantially, the scale reflects it. These are only guidelines, and many patterns of weight gain can result in good outcomes as long as the general pattern is slow and steady in the right direction. Personally speaking, it may be more comfortable to spread it out fairly evenly, so you get accustomed to the pregnancy mode of moderation and balance but aren't having to eat the highest number of calories toward the end, when your stomach has less and less room as it's crowded by the baby! Usually an extra bowl of cereal with milk and berries or a small bean and cheese burrito would suffice to give you the extra energy and balance you need. Either way you choose, begin to work on how you think of pregnancy and weight gain now.

FOR FUTURE REFERENCE: During Pregnancy/After Delivery

The website www.MyPyramid.gov has a "MyPyramid for Moms" feature. Once you are pregnant, log in to the profile that you set up a chapter or two ago, and go to the Edit Profile tab. It will prompt you to enter your estimated due date and will adjust your energy needs by trimester (so you'll see no change at first). This is a really nice way to continue tracking your intake with special attention to the nutritional value of food. If your weight gain is going more quickly or slowly than you want, work to figure out if it's the program that has misjudged your energy needs (it *does* tend to overestimate) or if you need to be more scrupulous at recording everything. Mention it to your health care practitioner if things really don't add up.

TABLE 14-1
NEW RECOMMENDED WEIGHT GAIN IN PREGNANCY

At conception, if your pre-pregnant BMI is:		You should gain this much during pregnancy:[a]
<18.5	Underweight	28–40 lb
18.5–24.9	Normal weight	25–35 lb
25.0–29.9	Overweight	15–25 lb
>30	Obese	11–20 lb

Source: Institute of Medicine, *Weight Gain During Pregnancy: Reexamining the Guidelines*, 2009.

a. Rate of weight gain varies depending on pre-pregnant weight but is very slow for the first twelve weeks (the first trimester) and largely independent of calorie intake, as discussed next. After the twelfth week, weight gain should begin averaging ½ to just over 1 pound per week based on pre-pregnant weight.

Note about multiples: Women with a normal pre-pregnancy BMI carrying twins should gain 37–54 pounds, preferably closer to 45 pounds, with 24 of the pounds gained by the twenty-fourth week. Insufficient data exist for different recommendations for underweight women carrying twins, so at a minimum, follow the goals laid out for normal-weight women. Overweight women should gain 31–50 pounds and obese women should aim for 25–42 pounds. Women carrying triplets will have higher total weight gain goals, as specified by their doctor, and should begin by aiming for 36 pounds by 24 weeks for the best outcome. For a good lay reference, see Dr. Barbara Luke and Tamara Eberlein, *When You're Expecting Twins, Triplets, or Quads* (New York: Harper Paperbacks, 2004).

So What Is the Rule of Thumb on How Fast You Should Gain Weight Once Pregnant?

It's all about what works best to achieve a healthy, full-term pregnancy. A steady weight gain of approximately four and a half pounds overall is recommended during the entirety of the first trimester, provided you're only carrying one baby in your womb (see the "note about multiples" in Table 14-1 for a preview of the different recommendations). Even if you are not increasing your calorie intake yet, most of this early weight increase reflects fluid gain (e.g., early expansion of blood volume), which is largely independent of calorie intake. Try *very* hard not to lose any weight during those critical first three months, even if you are overweight or obese from the start (in that case, do all that you can to stay at a stable weight until you begin gaining). For the second and third trimesters, those who started at a normal weight should gain approximately one pound per week, and those who conceived while underweight should gain slightly over one pound per week; those who started overweight or obese should gain approximately half a pound per week, adjusting accordingly to stay within target goals. Note: It's probably prudent to aim solely for the low end of the recommended gain (11 pounds) if you enter pregnancy at a BMI greater than 35 or 40.

Practical Application

This exercise is intended to give you an idea of where you are headed. Based on your BMI right now, if you happened to get pregnant in the next few weeks (planned or unplanned), how much total weight should you gain during the whole pregnancy, according to Table 14-1? Please make sure to base your estimate on what your weight is, not what you would like it to be, because should conception occur this soon, this is what you would need to gain to keep the baby and you healthiest. Your answer: Between _____ and _____ pounds (assume a pregnancy for a single baby). Recall the fine print below Table 14-1 to see what you would need with multiples.

The Institute of Medicine weight-gain guidelines don't specifically address the common side effect of pre-pregnancy weight gain from medications used in IVF. Most patients who undergo IVF can anticipate a gain of ten to fifteen pounds due to water retention and hormonal changes. Most often a steady pace that targets the lower end of the patient's pretreatment weight range is recommended by the attending clinician, and can be further individualized for healthiest outcome.

To some degree, most women get a bit anxious about the prospect of gaining the ideal amount of weight for pregnancy, but when they realize how different this weight is from just "getting fat," they can accept it. Occasionally, though, we counsel women who find the thought of pregnancy weight gain overwhelming, even terrifying. This is most common in women with weight preoccupation, teenagers, and especially women who have just gone the extra mile to take weight off. Feelings of anxiety are nothing to be ashamed of, but should be addressed prior to conception.

If the thought of gaining pregnancy weight is unbearable, delay conception until you are more at peace with this. Serenity of this sort doesn't usually happen spontaneously, so consider asking your obstetrician for a referral to a therapist who specializes in weight issues. Often these therapists have working relationships with registered dietitians, so while you work through emotional barriers with the therapist, the dietitian can work with you on making confident, wholesome food choices.

TAKING CONTROL OF YOUR HEALTH: IS WEIGHT LOSS OR GAIN RIGHT FOR YOUR PRECONCEPTION PLAN?

Recall how extremes in body weight exacerbate many gynecological and obstetric risks. These risks are important to understand but are not cause for sacrificing the goal of having a child. Instead, being over- or underweight is something that should be addressed on an individual basis with your health care professional.

Pregnancy: Where Does All the Weight Go?

Maternal		*Fetal*	
Uterus	2 lb	Baby	7½ lb
Breasts	1 lb	Placenta	1½ lb
Blood	2¾ lb	Amniotic fluid	2 lb
Water	3¾ lb		
Fat	7 lb (range 4–14 lb, corresponds to 25–35 lb gain)		

Adapted from F. E. Hytten and I. Leitch, eds., *The Physiology of Human Pregnancy,* 2d ed. (Oxford: Blackwell Scientific Publications, 1971).

As you know, there are occasional exceptions to the norm—women who are biologically wired to be heavier or thinner than what's normal on the BMI charts. Their low or high BMI persists despite a lifestyle of daily physical activity and faithful adherence to the "Foolproof Tips for a Preconception-Friendly Diet" in Chapter 13. If otherwise healthy, they'd be unlikely candidates for further weight loss or gain, because they're at their personal best, and to mount a lasting battle against one's genes often requires interventions that pose a whole host of other potential risks. For example, for those with a genetic predisposition to obesity to be approved for weight-loss surgery, it would be because the benefits dramatically outweighed the risks of her remaining at her gene-coded weight.

If factors other than Mother Nature are burdening your weight and health, the time has come to take control of those external influences. Give yourself at least three months' time, but don't be tempted to force a year's worth of change into those few months. Do what's responsible in the time you allow, and realize it's time well spent. Certainly, if you are fortunate to be in no rush, allow a more open-ended timeline for behavior changes to sync with your most natural size and shape.

This philosophy of allowing internal cues the opportunity to reestablish their influence is quite liberating. To give this the best chance to work, first focus on behavior strategies, and pay closer attention to calories only if weight change is occurring too fast or slow (that is, we generally recommend a pre-pregnancy weight loss or gain of about a half to one pound per week, never greater than two pounds, even for those early weeks).

For the remainder of this chapter, let's delve into practical advice to remedy, or at least minimize, weight issues that you have power to control before trying to conceive (between pregnancies, too). Skip to the preconceptional weight topic that pertains to you.

FOR FUTURE REFERENCE: During Pregnancy

*What to Do if You Gain Faster than Expected or
Have Trouble Putting on Pregnancy Weight*

The recommendations have evolved since our moms delivered us, in order to improve the odds of delivering a healthy, full-term baby. We now know that gaining more or less weight than recommended carries both short-term and long-term risks for mom and baby. Yet more than half of pregnant women don't stay within the guidelines (most are gaining too much). Even if you presently have no difficulties with body weight, at some point in your pregnancy you may find that the pounds are coming on surprisingly fast or that you need some advice on how to gain adequate weight, perhaps after a difficult first trimester. If you are having trouble staying within the recommended ranges, what you absorb from this chapter will help. (Consult your doctor if the gain seems more like swelling of ankles, hands, etc.) Some of our weight-loss tips can be adjusted to slow (though not reverse) an excessive rate of gain—an increasingly common problem, which sets you up for too much weight gain by the time you deliver. Gaining more than what's recommended (shown in the right-hand column of Table 14-1) means you'll also be more likely retain much of the excess by your baby's first birthday. Conversely, our weight-gain tips can be applied to anyone struggling to put on or keep on enough weight once pregnant.

After your baby is born, give yourself at least four to six weeks' time to settle into new motherhood and establish a good breastmilk supply (if you choose this feeding method) before devoting much attention to the remaining pregnancy pounds. Then refer back to the "Tips for Weight Loss and Maintenance Before Pregnancy" that begin on page 436 if you want guidance in shedding the postpartum pounds in a way that they're most likely to stay off.

Overweight (BMI of 25.0 to 29.9) and Obesity (BMI of 30 or More)

Kris, age thirty-five, is 5 feet 6 inches tall and weighs 189 pounds; her BMI is 30.5. Kris' weight has always been both a constant battle and a sensitive subject for her. She has yo-yoed from one quick weight-loss diet to the next, frustratingly regaining more than she lost, and keeps promising herself that she'll do more than sporadic exercise. One of the first things she said to her ob-gyn at her pre-conception appointment was, "We really had our hearts set on starting to try next month. Couldn't I just make sure to not gain any weight once I'm pregnant?"

The answer to this question is *no*. The weight you gain during pregnancy is not interchangeable with your regular body weight. Not gaining enough during your pregnancy may compromise your nutritional intake and put your baby at risk for being born before it's really ready. There's even the concern that zero net gain could program the fetal brain to develop a thrifty adaptation to hoard calories and quickly put on weight once the calories are available, an adaptation that probaby served cavemen well. On the other hand, overweight women who gain more than recommended are more likely to deliver a large baby, increasing their odds of a riskier delivery. Thus, women who do conceive at a BMI in the overweight or obese category have lower overall weight gain goals to minimize the known risks of maternal overweight as much as possible. For these women, it's just as important to gain weight gradually and consistently throughout the pregnancy as it is to not exceed the BMI-specific weight-gain goals.

If you're a little or a lot like Kris, we'd like to encourage you to stay in the preconception mode a bit longer. If you've already begun trying, perhaps even with assisted reproductive technology, put your plans on hold for a minimum of ninety days. Too many women bypass this recommendation because either they've already started trying and think they cannot turn back (viewed as a setback), or they trivialize the good that even a modest weight reduction would yield.

Ironically, the consequences of bypassing an opportunity to improve one's BMI can further delay the time to conception, even if menstrual periods seem normal. The delays are most often related to hormone levels that are thrown off. However, many overweight women do get pregnant, often as an unplanned pregnancy because birth control methods don't work as reliably. Pregnancy is sometimes achieved with medications that artificially stimulate ovulation at a time when Mother Nature had put the brakes on spontaneous ovulation, but regardless of whether the fertility hurdle is overcome, these drugs are not without their own set of risks, and they don't fix the underlying BMI risks.

Once you're pregnant, a high BMI increases one's risk of mild to moderate complications or, worse, future heartache. The higher BMI at conception might only cause long-term urinary leakage (incontinence) or increased likelihood of retaining more postpartum weight. Most often, however, the possible problems affecting both mom and baby include the following: increased susceptibility to maternal infections (a huge factor in births that occur eight or more weeks early), development of vulnerable placentas, high blood pressure, and preeclampsia. There's an increased risk of developing gestational diabetes and larger-than-normal newborns (leading to fetal injury and vaginal trauma), and Cesarean section. Some studies among women with a BMI over 30 revealed that these women had a higher likelihood of delivering a child with birth defects, particularly neural tube defects and cardiac anomalies. Unfortunately, the explanation for this is that *obesity diminishes a number of preventive measures*—folic acid supplementation, for instance—for reasons not entirely understood. Lastly, obese moms tend to discontinue breastfeeding sooner than normal-weight mothers; sadly, shorter breastfeeding duration increases the baby's future risk of childhood obesity.

Many successful studies permitted their participants to keep trying to get pregnant naturally throughout the behavior change and weight-loss process, but ideally we recommend that you first reach your healthier weight, maintain it for one month or longer, and then begin trying to conceive. After all, a baby wants a womb environment that is primed for "building," not "breakdown" mode. But it could easily be argued that our suggested pace of weight reduction (approximately half to one pound per week) is gentle enough on your body that further weight loss could safely be continued beyond the initial ninety-day waiting period. The long-term benefits dwarf the concern over a couple of pounds of weight loss at the start of pregnancy. So if you don't want to delay trying to conceive any longer than three months and choose this alternative approach, first okay it with your doctor, then test for pregnancy the minute you suspect it. When you become pregnant, maintain a steady weight through the first trimester and refer to Table 14-1 for more guidance on pacing pregnancy weight gain.

Tips for Weight Loss and Maintenance Before Pregnancy

- Do not be tempted by fad and detoxification diets, diet pills, or potions! This includes "natural" weight-loss programs that promise a weight loss of greater than two pounds per week. Drinks, pills, and powders that are touted as weight-loss products, internal cleansers, or metabolism boosters can also be extra dangerous during this preconception time period. We can't emphasize this enough!

- Listen to your body and get back in touch with moderate, balanced eating, similar to how you would feed a school-age child or elderly parent or grandparent in need of satisfying balanced meals and snacks. Avoid grazing, or you'll never develop normal hunger cues! Give the same type of thoughtful attention to what your body needs. It can be a wonderfully motivating approach to natural weight reduction and weight maintenance.

- For the first week or more, use MyPyramid to set up a baseline, or try writing down everything you eat and drink. Include the amounts, and take note of your mood. By doing this you may be able to identify what food groups you overeat or undereat. Emotional triggers that you accommodate by eating can also be uncovered this way.

  Note that when you sign up for MyPyramid's Menu Planner and enter your current height and weight, it will recognize that you are "above the healthy range for height," and then will ask if you want it to design a food plan "to gradually move toward a healthier weight." Click "yes," and continue with that plan for one to two weeks. If you see no weight change, switch to what we assume will be a lower energy intake—the minimum number of food servings in Table 13-1 (equal to 1,600 calories per day). If you have to further adjust, never dip below 1,200 calories per day, and keep your physician posted on your progress.

- Choose a variety of healthy foods and beverages from all the food groups in portion sizes that are appropriate for your body's calorie needs. You may lament that you have an appreciation for too many different foods, but this is never a curse as long as you learn to favor an assortment of leaner, less-processed foods over the high-fat, high-sugar foods. A diet with healthy variety is a very important determinant of long-term satisfaction, and your taste buds will thank you over and over. If you are a picky eater, make a pact with yourself to try one new nutritious food or a new preparation of an old favorite every few days. You'll be amazed at how many new things you can learn to like when you change your attitude.

- No skipping meals! This means eat breakfast, lunch, and dinner. If you normally skip breakfast because of lack of appetite or time, make sure you have several food groups' worth of food with you wherever you go later on in the morning, such as a small cup of precut fresh fruit, a plastic container with a generous handful of your favorite whole-grain cereal, and a yogurt or two tablespoons of nuts. Then eat all three of these separately or together by 10:30 a.m.

- Mild hunger pangs before mealtimes are not unusual for people of all sizes and shapes. In fact, consider it a sign that you are not overeating to the point where you never feel hungry. As long as you are not losing weight at a pace faster than one or two pounds per week, welcome a stomach growl now and then. To minimize this discomfort, distribute your best sources of protein evenly throughout the day, since protein helps you feel fuller longer than carbs or fats. Some feel that eating a low-glycemic-index diet works similarly for them.

- Make regular exercise a top priority (physician approval recommended), in addition to being more mobile during your daily routines. You need both, along with good nutrition, for true, long-term success.[2] Remember that the amount of physical activity you do right now depends on how active you've been all along. If you do not exercise regularly, you must be patient with your body and work slowly to a reasonable goal; your body will perceive this as a friendly new habit and gradually want more. Incorporate both aerobic (calorie-burning) exercise and strength training (muscle building) into your routine to whittle away fat and keep your metabolism revved. Studies show that believing in your ability to exercise is incredibly important, so regularly tell yourself, "I can do this!"

- Does it bug you when you are advised to "just take up a walking program"? To some it sounds hardly worthwhile. It is, but you have to figure out what will get you out that

---

2. Certain reports on people who have successfully lost weight and kept it off indicate that an expenditure of 1,500 to 2,800 calories per week from physical activity is necessary. A lower expenditure of 1,000 calories per week through exercise improves overall health but may not be quite enough to seriously influence weight.

door. If a pedometer would help inspire you (think of how a little kid loves checking how many steps he or she has gone every few paces), get one at your local sports store or order one on the Internet. For weight reduction, you will eventually work up to 12,000–15,000 steps per day. This is a lot, but you will get there, and you'll learn how to do more than the bare minimum in the course of daily activities. So push yourself to move more, but not to the point where you lack stamina for the rest of the day (watch for this, as it's a common downfall).

- Commit to a healthy pace: losing around half a pound to one pound per week, rarely two, and never more than two. This slow pace of weight loss combined with exercise will mean that you maintain adequate vitamin and mineral stores while losing mostly fat, not muscle. If you lose more than two pounds per week, you are losing a substantial amount of muscle mass (and water); this is very counterproductive, because muscle mass and muscle use are largely what keep your metabolism high. Faster weight loss may interfere with your hormonal balance and make it harder to conceive.

  This gradual pace of loss has an added bonus after pregnancy: once you have delivered your baby and have given yourself four to six weeks to ease into motherhood, take this same pace to the lose the excess postpartum pounds. It's a gentle enough pace that neither breastmilk quality nor quantity is affected.

- You do not need to set a strict weight goal on the scale, but do be aware of the nearest healthier weight ranges. A gradual decrease of ten to sixteen pounds, or two BMI units, is sometimes enough to reveal evidence that internal health is improving.

- Weigh yourself no more than once a day in the morning, and preferably only one to two times per week, so you can accurately gauge your pace of weight loss. For additional feedback, pay attention to the way your clothes fit.

- Slow down and enjoy your food. Nutrition experts from the University of Rhode Island have found that slow eaters (those who chew more and put down their fork several times during a meal) get fuller faster and consume fewer calories than speed eaters.

- If you experience a food craving shortly after eating, wait until your next meal (or snack) time. The interest often fades. If it doesn't, indulge in moderation: eat enough to satisfy, and don't feel guilty. It helps to incorporate modest portions of sweet or fatty treats during this process of behavior change, because you're really training yourself to handle similar situations in the future without triggering a binge. If you find it too tempting to have these things around your home, reserve having the treat for when you are out. Because you will be eating some of these favorite foods as part of your healthier way of eating, there is no need to have one last food fling.

- Drink approximately eight cups (8 ounces each) of water daily, and go easy on beverages with alcohol or "empty calories": regular sodas, bottled or canned flavored teas, fruit-flavored drinks, vitamin waters, or sports beverages. These sugary beverages do not fill

You Can Win!

Helpful resources from WIN (Weight-control Information Network) address the special exercise needs of larger people (featuring real people, no stick-thin waifs in their publications). Another resource from WIN is Sisters Together, specifically designed to motivate African American women to be active and eat healthfully. See www.win.niddk.nih.gov/publications/active.html or call toll-free (877) 946-4627.

you up and add a tremendous number of calories. Wine, beer, and spirits are even more calorie laden.

- Make sure you eat enough fiber every day for assistance with digestion and overall health. (See Table 10-1.)
- Take a daily multivitamin with minerals or a prenatal supplement (not both). It is much harder to get everything from whole foods when you are decreasing your food intake below maintenance needs. See Chapter 11 for help in choosing an appropriate supplement.
- Scan health-oriented cookbooks and magazines for recipe ideas. These make great gift suggestions, too, for the next time someone asks, "What would you like for your birthday?" Also a quick Google search for "healthy eating" apps or recipes will deliver tips directly to your computer screen or smartphone.
- Consider home grocery delivery as a way to avoid unhealthy impulse buys.
- Understand that sometimes you will reach a weight plateau for a week or more; this is a perfectly normal part of weight loss. If the plateau lasts it may be a cue that your portion sizes have gradually grown larger or that your level of physical activity has diminished. Consider these possibilities before assuming that you have reached your best weight.
- Develop a supportive network of people that you can be open with. You have a number of options here, including family and friends. For further nutrition assistance, seek the advice of a registered dietitian (RD). For emotional support, seek individual or group psychological counseling. Your physician should be able to make a referral to one or both. If you want to participate in a supervised weight-loss program, we advise you to consult an RD about reputable options. Internet-based programs such as the reputable VTrim online program may work well for women with schedule limitations. Your local YMCA/YWCA or church, synagogue, or mosque may even be open to starting a health-based program for like-minded women seeking more support for weight management.

- Take a good look back at Chapter 1 on how to increase willpower and reduce stress. Your brain is a powerful tool, and you need to be strong-minded to embrace behavior changes. Learn how to pamper your mind and motivate yourself.
- Get a good night's sleep. According to a study from the University of Chicago Clinical Research Center, insufficient sleep appears to negatively impact the hormones ghrelin and leptin, making you hungrier and less apt to feel full once you do eat. If you're having trouble sleeping, a great resource is the National Sleep Foundation. With the exception of shift workers who alter their eating habits out of necessity, if you are troubled by overeating at night or get up during the night to eat, talk to your doctor about ruling out a sleep disorder.

Reminder: Once you reach your goal, ideally wait one to two months before you start trying to get pregnant (the exception being gastric bypass patients, who should wait at least a year). This not only allows time for your body to recover any depleted nutrient stores but also serves as time to more fully grasp what your new body needs for weight maintenance[3] You will then get a better feel for your metabolic needs and be able to gauge how much to add, calorically, once pregnant (primarily during the second and third trimesters).

FOR FUTURE REFERENCE: During Pregnancy

When you've gone to the effort of losing weight during preconception, it can be scary to think that you will be gaining weight back during pregnancy. To ward off these negative thoughts, praise yourself for your foresight and success and acknowledge that your fears are normal. Just keep in mind the fact that pregnancy weight gain is a totally different type of body adjustment from what you just lost. And remember: it is fine to strive for the minimum amount of weight gain on Table 14-1 instead of the midrange or high end.

---

3. For those of you who have more time, the American Health Foundation's Expert Panel on Healthy Weight recommends gradually losing weight in increments of ten to sixteen pounds, followed by six months' maintenance to ensure that "the new weight becomes the usual weight." This approach can be repeated until you successfully reach a healthy BMI.

BARIATRIC SURGERY: PLANNING AND RECOVERY

Weight-loss surgery, also known as bariatric surgery (described in Chapter 7), has become a successful method of weight reduction for severely obese women. It is not something that women enter into lightly; it's considered only after less invasive nonsurgical methods of weight reduction have been exhausted, and it will succeed only if it's matched by intensive behavioral weight-loss programs with long-term follow-up, according to Dr. D. S. Bond of the Weight Control and Diabetes Research Center in Providence, Rhode Island. But the nonsurgical route can be easier said than done. We recommend that you discuss with your health care provider how much weight is essential to lose before conception to provide the greatest safety for both mom and fetus, then see if bariatric surgery should be part of your plan. Below are eleven tips if you are considering or have had weight-loss surgery (bariatric surgery) in anticipation of a future pregnancy:

1. Wait twelve to eighteen months after your bariatric surgery before trying to conceive to allow improvements in nutritional absorption and fine-tuning of other medical issues related to weight such as hypertension or diabetes.[a] This also gives enough time to avoid postsurgical issues such as leaking intestine (perforations) and hernias.

2. Meet with your bariatric surgeon, ob-gyn, internist, and/or maternal-fetal medicine (MFM) specialist to get the green light for trying to conceive. Continue to work with a registered dietitian (RD) to ensure healthy eating practices to maintain weight goals.

3. Resist the temptation not to use a birth control method when you are in the rapid-weight-loss phase after surgery (less than twelve months after surgery), thinking you are infertile. You may have been before, but fertility almost always improves with weight reduction (nonsurgical or surgical). Some methods of birth control won't work as well after surgery, so talk to your ob-gyn about what's best for you.

4. If you had your surgery a few years ago and are experiencing new complications (trouble digesting solid foods, regurgitating, abdominal pain), don't put off a checkup. Most new symptoms indicate something that can be fixed.

5. Keep a food journal during the most restrictive nutritional phase and beyond (the first six months are usually the toughest, but there are further adaptations beyond that). Get to know how your gastrointestinal tract tolerates various foods, portion sizes, and preparation methods.

6. In addition to nourishment from high-quality protein, carbs, and healthy fats, take your individually tailored vitamin-mineral supplements as prescribed by your doctor and work with your RD to emphasize food sources of folate, calcium, vitamin D, iron,

a. This is the Institute of Medicine's recommendation as of 2009; other studies recommend waiting eighteen to twenty-four months.

zinc, vitamin B$_{12}$, and vitamin K.[b] Others to keep an eye on are choline, the remaining B complex vitamins, vitamin C, and vitamin A.

7. Usually some form of behavior modification program is part of pre- and postsurgical education; you might have recognized many of those success tactics from earlier in this chapter. Embrace your ability to identify situations or feelings that trigger eating. Practice the healthy responses to triggers that you want to make into habits, and eventually they will be.

8. Studies show that regular physical activity helps patients get through surgery better and may speed weight loss afterward. If you weren't active before the surgery, you may not be confident in your ability or comfort level in being more active, but to prevent weight regain, more activity is imperative. A regular walking routine might sound challenging, but as long as your doctor approves, just get those walking shoes on, get outside, and begin walking around the block once, the next day twice, and so on.

9. Be at peace with the things you cannot control (inherited predispositions). Then actively seek out supportive influences in your social, cultural, family, and workplace environments; they are integral to your success, but acknowledge that these same influences can contribute to backsliding. Beginning with your husband or partner, make sure the two of you are working on lifestyle habits—eating, exercise, time and stress management. This will help you now and eventually offer your children an easier time with any inherited tendencies toward weight gain.

10. Get to the point where you can mentally and physically commit to *not* losing any weight once pregnant; this favorably influences fetal metabolism, as should following Table 14-1.

11. You might be well served to visit with a lactation consultant if you have any reservations about future breastfeeding. (Breastfeeding may help your weight and reduce your baby's chances of childhood obesity.) This is especially important if you have concerns about post-weight-loss sagging breasts, a history of breast reduction, or reconstruction (which is best reserved for *after* pregnancy).

b. See Chapters 7 and 11 for more information on anemias, as iron deficiency is not always the primary cause.

FOR FUTURE REFERENCE

Pregnancy and Postpartum Care for Women Who Have Had Bariatric Surgery

Once you're pregnant after bariatric surgery, fetal growth will be monitored closely with exams and ultrasounds, paying particular attention to ruling out birth defects, such as neural tube defects. Active weight loss while pregnant would be discouraged. Minimal weight gain can maintain good fetal growth if nutrition deficiencies are avoided. For example, if your BMI was in the extremely obese category (over 40) and you lost seventy-five pounds to achieve a preconception BMI of 30, notice that Table 14-1 recommends a gain of eleven to twenty pounds; it is fine for you to aim for an eleven-pound pregnancy gain. Careful vitamin and mineral supplementation is particularly important, as those nutrients are the most easily lost after bariatric surgery and are essential for healthy fetal development. Continuing the team effort between your bariatric surgeon and obstetrician throughout the pregnancy can be helpful. Clinical care for women who have had bariatric surgery prior to pregnancy is still evolving to ensure that the mother's abdominal organs remain healthy and functional despite the cramped space. When you are postpartum, continued nutrient supplementation remains very important, as is working closely with the baby's pediatrician to make sure your baby is thriving.

Underweight

Lucy is a healthy thirty-five-year-old. She is 5 feet 5 inches tall and weighs only 114 pounds (a BMI of 19, on the lowest end of normal). She has a petite build and has been thin all her life. She never skips a meal, snacks regularly, and has seen a dietitian to make sure her diet is well rounded. Her doctor and dietitian concur that there's no problem with her pre-pregnancy weight.

Lynda, a twenty-nine-year-old patient seeing her doctor for her annual gynecologic exam, notes that she went off the pill four months earlier in anticipation of trying to get pregnant. She has a high-pressure job, watches her weight strictly, sometimes skips meals, and exercises vigorously at the end of her workday. She takes pride in her "slender" figure of 5 feet 10 inches and 125 pounds (a BMI of 18). Lynda notes that she has had only one period since being off birth control pills. Her doctor expresses concern over her nutritional well-being and suggests that she gain seven to ten pounds over the next few months, and then begin trying to conceive. Although the idea of gaining this amount of weight before conception is not appealing, Lynda wants to do what is right for her future baby. She certainly doesn't want to be labeled a "pregorexic" down the road.

Is being underweight prior to conception really a big deal? The answer is a qualified yes. Most worrisome is a low BMI accompanied by suboptimal nutritional status, a combination many women resist acknowledging. After all, our culture encourages ultrathinness in women. However, undernourished women with a pre-pregnancy BMI below 18.5, as well as women who do not gain enough weight during pregnancy, are at a higher risk for a premature or low-birth-weight baby. (An underweight future father poses no risk to conception unless he is clinically malnourished.)

There is some evidence that underweight women can reduce or cancel their risks by gaining the recommended twenty-eight to forty pounds during pregnancy (the range for underweight women), but this is not a certainty, and there is no guarantee that you will find this greater-than-normal gain easy. Healthy eating habits plus gaining enough weight to bring your BMI to 18.5 or higher prior to conception may make a difference in the health of your future child.

If you are chronically underweight or if your body weight has dropped suddenly for no apparent reason, it is prudent to visit your physician to rule out other causes for low body weight. Your doctor will look for contributing factors such as a medical condition, extraordinary life stresses, an eating disorder, depression, smoking, or substance abuse. All of these should be resolved prior to trying to get pregnant. If you already eat like a horse and are simply thin due to a delicate body frame and high metabolism, you should look at whether you are overexercising and need to ease up a little to free up energy for reproduction. Work at getting up to the minimum normal BMI if your basic body build is quite slight.

Whether you have intentionally or unintentionally fostered a body weight that is too low, now is the time to prepare your body to be at its healthiest weight for supporting a pregnancy. Most women cannot fathom actually having to work to put on weight! However, as you may already know, gaining weight healthfully can be challenging, so here are a few pointers to help you. Remember these same tips during pregnancy in case you find it equally daunting to meet the calorie needs for two!

Healthy Weight Gain Before Pregnancy: Tips for Success

- Aim for a reasonable amount of weight gain per week, between half a pound and one pound, occasionally two pounds, until you reach a BMI of 19 for your height. It takes about 500 additional calories per day to add a pound of body weight per week. Adding 500 calories can be as simple as drinking a cup of milk and another of fruit juice (for 250 calories) and eating two halves of an English muffin with peanut butter (for the remaining 250 calories).

- As with any healthy diet, choose a variety of foods from all food groups. If you consider yourself a picky eater, choose your comfort foods and also be willing to incorporate new nutrient-dense foods to add flair. For example, add pesto sauce and pine nuts to a pasta meal, or grated mozzarella cheese, walnuts, kidney beans, and avocado slices to a salad. Just try and try again. You'll be amazed at how many new things you can learn to like when you change your mind-set.

- Put an end to both intentional and unintentional meal skipping. This necessitates planning ahead so that you never miss a meal even if you aren't particularly hungry. If you are notorious for skipping meals due to a busy schedule, it is okay to include fast foods, frozen items, or leftovers as part of your well-rounded diet. You can do this at home or work and even while traveling. Examples of convenient meals include microwavable entrées, fast-food submarine or bagel sandwiches, burgers, burritos, and slices of pizza. Some grocery stores carry ready-to-eat entrées such as roasted half and whole chickens and side dishes, deli sandwiches, salads, and hot Chinese foods.

Foods that you pack in an insulated lunch bag or cooler may be a more practical and economical solution. You just have to remember to freeze the individual ice packs overnight and have nutritious foods on hand to pack in the carrier. These insulated containers can hold an entire day's worth of meals, snacks, and beverages. Just as easily, they can accommodate simple side dishes, such as fresh fruits and veggies, to round out a meal that you buy. For example, you could buy a hot chicken sandwich and milk shake at a fast-food restaurant and bring fresh baby carrots, hummus dip, and slices of watermelon from home stored in your cooler; this rounds out the meal (all five major food groups) and is less expensive than buying the restaurant's choice of vegetable and fruit, if they even offer such items.

- Three balanced meals per day usually are not enough to gain weight. In fact, we can't think of a single underweight client who gained weight by eating only three times a day. This means that you'll need to make a conscious effort to snack in addition to meals. Some easy snack choices are nuts, dried fruits, crackers, pretzels, string cheese, yogurt, fresh fruit, granola bars, bagels, muffins, popcorn, and 100 percent fruit juices.

   Occasionally, supplemental beverages (e.g., Carnation Instant Breakfast, Boost, Ensure, Sustical) or bars (e.g., Lärabar, Clif Bar, PowerBar) may be eaten in place of a snack or small meal; most provide around 250 calories, so they cannot be considered a full meal.

- Eat more foods that are concentrated sources of fat and calories as part of your well-rounded diet, such as nuts, seeds, oils, fatty fish, and avocado. Unsaturated fats are preferable to saturated or partially hydrogenated fats for the baby's neurological development and for your own physical and mental health, as discussed in Chapters 10 and 12. You may also incorporate a few more sweet indulgences such as milk shakes, fruit pies, and puddings, as long as these don't take the place of balanced meals.

- Include food sources that are high in fiber (25 to 35 grams per day, not more, as discussed in Chapter 10) and drink plenty of liquids, including water. A high-fiber diet without enough liquid will make you feel full and constipated. Beverages such as 100 percent fruit juices, milk, and very modest amounts of flavored beverages and regular soft drinks are convenient liquid sources of calories at meal or snack times (no energy drinks, though).

- Keep in mind that there are no rules saying that you must have breakfast foods for breakfast and dinner foods for dinner; cereal or pancakes with milk, fruit, and chopped nuts make a perfectly nice dinner, as does a sandwich or cold pizza for breakfast.

- Take a daily multivitamin with minerals or a prenatal supplement, not both. See Chapter 11 for help in choosing an appropriate supplement.
- Although women of all sizes and shapes should quit smoking well before conception, this is imperative for underweight women. Quitting smoking may make it a little easier to gain a small amount of weight. Babies born to underweight smokers are likely to suffer greater negative effects on fetal growth and health.
- Physical activity is excellent for your mind and body in preparation for pregnancy. As much as five hours per week of moderate-level activity is what is recommended for best overall health. But until you find that you can gain weight (and make sure your periods are regular) by following these rigorous guidelines, it may be best to limit your exercise to twenty to thirty minutes per day (or 150 minutes per week) for basic good health. If you succeed in gaining weight appropriately while expending more energy through additional exercise, fine. But cut back if you find it difficult to achieve gradual weight gain.
- After you've achieved your goal, keep tabs on yourself by weighing in one or two times per week, or if you prefer to not have a scale around, pay attention to the way your clothes fit. If you start to lose the weight that you've gained, go back to eating as we've described above to maintain your weight gain.
- For further assistance about what to eat, seek the advice of a registered dietitian. For emotional support, seek a referral for psychological counseling; this may be the key factor in helping you deal with emotional issues related to being underweight.

Once a BMI of 18.5 or more is achieved, it is fine to start trying to get pregnant. After conception occurs, make sure not to lose any of the weight you have worked so hard to put on. Focus on a gradual weight gain in the range of twenty-five to thirty-five pounds over the course of your forty-week pregnancy.

EATING DISORDERS DEFINED

- **Anorexia nervosa** is an irrational fear of losing control over one's weight and getting fat, accompanied by severe calorie restriction (and often excessive exercise) in an impassioned quest for thinness. Anorexics often see themselves as fat when, in fact, they are emaciated.
- **Bulimia** is defined as secretive and cyclic behaviors of out-of-control overeating, or bingeing, followed by purges of self-induced vomiting, excessive exercising, laxative abuse, enemas, or diuretics. Temporary severe food restriction may also be intermingled with binge-purge episodes. Weight may be normal, low, or high, but fluctuates.

- **Compulsive overeating** is defined as periods of continuous eating to the point of feeling gorged, although no form of purging follows. Frequent dieting may be common. Weight may be normal to obese.

These three forms of disordered eating can be not only emotionally defeating but also physically destructive, even lethal.

WHEN WEIGHT BECOMES AN OBSESSION: EATING DISORDERS AND PRE-PREGNANCY

Our bodies are sometimes very clever. They can make it difficult to get pregnant when we abuse them. Anorexia, bulimia, and other variations of eating disorders tend to make women (and men) less fertile. Recovery improves fertility. Eating disorders also create emotional barriers that diminish intimacy and the sexual relations that lead to pregnancy. "A lot of emotional energy and time is lost in an eating disorder," says Karen Freeman, MS, RD, a nutritionist who specializes in treatment for eating disorders. "You really cannot communicate all of you if all of you isn't there."

Still, women with eating disorders can, and do, get pregnant. There are even cases of anorexic women who get pregnant although they are not menstruating. Clinical psychologist Marianne Engle, PhD, notes that women with active eating disorders often conceive successfully and have fantasies that exaggerate what being able to get pregnant says about their body's health. These women often say, "I must be healthy enough if I was able to get pregnant"; "The baby will get whatever it needs from me." They think, "The baby will get everything first," or "If I gain only the baby weight and not any of the extra, then the baby will be fine, and I'll not have any extra weight after delivery." Yet none of these fantasies are true. In fact, the mother's body will naturally give preferential treatment to the mom first. Although the fetus is able to freely withdraw a few nutrients (such as calcium) at the mother's expense, most of the time the fetus is left with the predicament of having to make do with a less-than-ideal nutrient supply. Or, in the case of eating-disordered women who exercise to the point of exhaustion to burn off calories (and water weight), the fetus is exposed to periods of oxygen restriction and dehydration. That is why it is so important to enter pregnancy healthy and able to pamper yourself and your baby at the same time.

Many women with active eating disorders who conceive change their habits once they find out they are pregnant. But this still means that the fetus's first weeks or months have been spent in a womb environment where nourishment is poor or, at best, unpredict-

A Historical Perspective on Women and Severe Nutritional Deprivation

Toward the end of World War II, western Holland was under blockade by occupying Nazi troops. Residents struggled under famine conditions from September 1944 to May 1945. These eight months were aptly termed the "Dutch Hunger Winter." Maternal and fetal adaptations were evident. Of all childbearing-age women, only about 30 percent had normal menstrual periods. More than half experienced "war amenorrhea," completely stopping ovulation and menstruation. The babies who were conceived in the midst of the famine were more likely to be miscarried, stillborn, or malformed. Those who survived pregnancy were at higher risk of dying within a week after birth. Defects of the central nervous system such as spina bifida and hydrocephalus ("water on the brain") were also more common. Later, a greater incidence of adulthood health problems, such as obesity, high cholesterol, high blood pressure, schizophrenia, and type 2 diabetes, also appeared to be linked to the timing and duration of fetal exposure to famine conditions. Ongoing research examining these relationships is discussed using terms such as "metabolic programming," "fetal origins," and "developmental origins of health and disease" (DOHaD).

Nutrition is only one factor that affected mothers, fathers, and babies during this time period. In addition to the harsh environmental and physical conditions during the Dutch Hunger Winter, it was a frightening and psychologically stressful time. It is a wonder that new lives were created in the midst of it all!

able.[4] Under these circumstances, the fetus is capable of developing adaptive mechanisms for coping with a less-than-optimal womb environment. If the child survives the pregnancy and infancy, those same adaptations may also predispose him or her to health risks early and later in life.

Eating-disordered women who suddenly mend their ways on discovering that they're pregnant often attribute their healthier behaviors to "only doing it for the baby." This attitude may land them back into their old destructive habits after the baby is born. Further, these mothers then end up modeling distorted food attitudes and behaviors for their children, despite thinking they can be concealed.

This is a cycle that can be broken—with you. If your goal is to become pregnant in the near future and you are struggling with an eating disorder, now is the time to seek professional help. When you see a doctor or nurse for a preconception visit (or if you're seeing a fertility expert), he or she may not ask you whether you have disordered eating behaviors. You will

---

4. It's not uncommon for a woman with an active eating disorder to not recognize that she is pregnant for many months. After all, signs of pregnancy such as missed periods or feelings of abdominal bloating can be just as easily misjudged as par for the course for her body as she knows it.

Practical Application

Take the following quiz if you are unsure whether your eating habits are normal. If any of these questions elicit an emphatic yes, it may be an indication that you should seek further help.

Yes / No   Do you spend more than half of your day thinking about food or planning your next meal?

Yes / No   Has anyone (family, friend, spouse) expressed concern over your eating behaviors, body weight, or unhealthy appearance?

Yes / No   Do you feel that if your weight is under control, everything else (mood, relationships, appearance) will be okay?

Yes / No   Do you eat or not eat in order to numb yourself from daily pressures or to feel less alone?

Yes / No   Do you wait too many hours between eating meals, and then feel out of control once you start eating?

Yes / No   Do you feel that for everything you eat there must be a way to compensate for it or burn it off?

Yes / No   Do you fear that everything you eat will make you fat?

Yes / No   Do you intentionally eat by yourself so no one will see you?

Yes / No   Are you often disgusted with the way your body looks and feels, to the point where you can't stop obsessing over it?

likely have to bring this up yourself and ask for help. Believe it or not, you will probably end up saying, "It's such a relief to finally be able to talk about this!" See if it's possible to get a recovery team together that includes a physician, a registered dietitian, and a qualified therapist (preferably one with experience in cognitive-behavioral therapy or interpersonal psychotherapy).[5] Ideally, you should also have a complete dental evaluation to identify and treat any underlying dental infections. Each of these specialists will help you work toward getting well for pregnancy and beyond. In addition to your health care team, see the list of available resources at the end of this chapter. Don't be afraid to reveal yourself or to ask for help.

According to Karen Freeman, MS, RD, although the willingness to tackle an eating disorder is often instigated by a very specific, sometimes traumatic emotional or physical event (e.g., death of or abandonment by a loved one; failing health), full recovery takes a long time.

5. According to Denise E. Wilfley, PhD, professor of psychiatry, medicine, pediatrics, and psychology at Washington University School of Medicine in St. Louis, Missouri, cognitive-behavior therapy appears to be very effective in the treatment of bulimia and binge eating disorder. Approximately twenty sessions are standard for most successful recoveries.

Ideally, recovery should be complete before pregnancy, but this may be asking too much considering that achieving full recovery may take years. Try to be realistic and focus on significant, sustained progress rather than perfection in getting to a point where you can physically and emotionally nourish yourself and your baby. Treatment should then continue through pregnancy and into the postpartum period to support you through the multitude of changes you will be experiencing.

"An excellent predictor of who will recover has to do with the woman's mental health prior to the eating disorder," says Marianne Engle, PhD. "If she was basically emotionally stable and had a decent support system prior to this, she will likely be able to put the disorder in its place and move on. If she has always struggled with severe emotional problems, the eating disorder will be more challenging to defeat; it may be more important here to honestly acknowledge that lifelong support may be necessary." When asked about the importance of spousal support and successful recovery, Engle notes, "What's most important is that the woman isn't being undermined, overtly or covertly." Husbands may need to take a serious look at their attitudes and preferences about their wife's appearance. Excessive praise over appearance when she is at her thinnest or frequent ogling of other thin women subtly sends the message ". . . but, please, stay [or get] skinny."

If you have an extreme preoccupation with your body weight that has developed into an eating disorder, the prospect of wanting to have a baby may well be the motivation you need to seek help. It is a very good sign if you find yourself thinking that now is the time to rescue yourself from the burden of an eating disorder. Getting professional help is the first step toward conquering the overwhelming fears associated with pregnancy weight gain and body image.

CASE COMPARISON: ANDREA AND GWEN

Andrea, twenty-two, a newlywed recovering bulimic patient, viewed her recovery as a spiritual journey. She saw the change in her eating habits as "nurturing myself just as I would if I were pregnant and another life depended on me." She wanted to consider pregnancy when she turned twenty-four, but the life depending on her at that time was her own.

This young woman obviously had a very strong spirit, but she did not come to this conclusion without outside support. She confided in a trusted family member, who helped her obtain counseling in both individual and group settings for the duration of her yearlong recovery. Also, she and her husband attended several counseling sessions together, so he could learn what was and was not helpful in facilitating her recovery. By the time Andrea was twenty-five, she was six months pregnant with their first child.

Gwen, twenty-nine, a very bright, driven woman, had battled anorexia nervosa for ten years. She had halfheartedly tried outpatient treatment for her eating disorder throughout the years but had never achieved recovery. She teetered on the border of being functional enough to hold down a full-time career as a lawyer and sick enough to focus on little else than her obsession for thinness. Gwen's husband and high-powered family felt unable to help her and had become worn down by witnessing her self-destructive behaviors. It was clear that the onus for recovery was squarely on Gwen's shoulders.

Gwen and her husband voiced a desire to have a baby, but she had not had a period in several years, and the two were seldom intimate. A fertility specialist refused to assist her until she had gained twenty-five pounds (to a BMI of 19). Once again, she attempted to tackle her eating disorder. She went through the motions of attending her dietitian appointments, mostly to appease her doctor and family, but refused to see a mental health professional because she felt she "didn't need to." Sadly, fearing loss of control, she clung to the familiar "comfort" of her disease state instead of committing to treatment from all angles. She was not capable of overcoming it alone, and has not, to our knowledge, been able to fulfill her dream of being a mother.

BODY IMAGE AND THE ELITE FEMALE ATHLETE

Some women athletes who train at very high to elite levels may consciously or unconsciously have body image anxieties that, if not handled thoughtfully, can impact fertility and pregnancy health. The following chapter addresses the unique aspects of achieving peak sports performance and preconception health through the eyes of the elite female athlete.

Resources for Body Weight, Body Image

Overeaters Anonymous; see your phone book for free local meetings
WIN—The Weight-Control Information Network, (877) 946-4627
Gürze Books, (800) 756-7533
Eating Disorders Awareness & Prevention, Inc., www.edapinc.com
Anorexia Nervosa and Related Eating Disorders, www.anred.com
National Association of Anorexia Nervosa and Associated Disorders, (630) 577-1330
American Anorexia/Bulimia Association, (212) 575-6200

Now you have a better idea of where you stand with regard to body weight and image in preparation for pregnancy. If you happen to be within your healthiest body weight range and are mentally prepared to gain the recommended weight of pregnancy, you are well on your way to having a healthy pregnancy. If, on the other hand, you've determined that you need to tackle a weight issue before conception, allow yourself the time it takes to experience success, along with normal setbacks, as you move forward. If you stick with it, you'll gain the confidence necessary to achieve your goal of being healthy for conception. Take it from new moms who have been in your shoes: in general, the hardest part for them was to refocus their energies on overcoming body weight problems (while using a reliable form of birth control) at a time when all they wanted was to become pregnant. However, they now see it as one of the wisest moves they ever made.

CHAPTER 15

Getting in Shape Before You Conceive

$\mathcal{P}$re-pregnancy fitness levels set the stage for how active you can safely be during pregnancy. So now is the time to get in shape. Below are three descriptions of women at very different fitness levels. Yet despite their differences, each of them will reap the benefits of fitness (Table 15-1) and enhance the possibility of a healthier conception. See which description best fits you.

The beginner exerciser: "I kept saying that I was going to start exercising, but everything else seemed to take precedence. I would even buy aerobics tapes, only to go home and sit on the couch and watch them! I'd joke about it with friends, but the truth was, I felt overwhelmed by my out-of-shape body. I finally admitted that if trying to get pregnant wasn't enough of a motivator to get in shape, nothing ever would be. So last week I started to walk with a friend four mornings a week before work. It's going fine, but I realize I need a backup plan for when the weather changes or she cannot make it. The other major change I'm committing to is to never sit for more than an hour or two during waking hours—for example, at work I now purposely walk upstairs to use the restroom, and at home, I get up and walk around during TV commercials."

The all-around active lifestyle: "I've always enjoyed a pretty active lifestyle—occasional doubles tennis or volleyball on the beach, and biking on a nearby bike path. If I'm inactive for a day or two, I begin to miss it. Since my husband and I had our first child two years ago (and we'd like another), I've successfully incorporated many active things into our 'mommy-and-me' days together. Sometimes that includes literally 'running errands' with my son in the jogger stroller. I've found that I love to move under my own power for fun and fitness."

The serious athlete: "I'm an aerobics instructor and competitive triathlete. I enjoy pushing myself to be my fittest. Now that my husband and I want to have a baby, we want to make sure that my exercise routine isn't going to jeopardize our ability to get pregnant and have a healthy baby. But I don't want to get out of shape, because it's taken a long time to get to this point in my athletic career. With a little coaxing from my obstetrician, I've agreed to put all-out-effort competitive events aside until after we have a baby, but my doctor is willing to allow me to continue instructing and training as long as I follow a few additional precautions."

Whatever your level, good overall pre-pregnancy fitness can be the difference that makes a woman who is anxious to conceive able to relieve stress and feel good about herself during this vital time. Take our word for it: the advantages of being fit before conception will be further accentuated during pregnancy. Good physical conditioning can be the key to making a pregnant women feel great instead of just good, or okay instead of absolutely lousy. There is no way of knowing how your body will tolerate the hormonal and physical changes that occur with pregnancy, so you want exercise and/or an active lifestyle on your side. Table 15-1 lists the benefits of exercise before and during pregnancy.

Many of the positive effects of physical activity listed in Table 15-1 are more or less immediate; they accrue from the cellular level with each muscle contraction. This is unlike most things that are "good for you" but take time to reveal their ultimate benefits. To experience this rewarding entry into pre-pregnancy fitness, you must not overdo it. In fact, as a general rule, it's best to initially set out to do about half of what you think you can do. Literally slow yourself down or cut the workout short even if you're on a roll. You'll gradually be able to add time and challenges, and you won't burn out or injure yourself along the way.

PRECONCEPTION FITNESS EVALUATION

Whether you are new or returning to fitness or a competitive athlete, it is wise to talk to your health care provider about exercise several months before getting pregnant. He will want to know your current level of fitness as well as past medical history. This information helps him anticipate whether you will require more specific exercise limitations than what is typically recommended for pregnant women. This information will also be helpful to you in the next chapter, when you individualize your own preconception fitness program.

Most inactive women can safely begin exercising in the months prior to conception. If you are already physically fit, you will likely be able to continue doing what you're doing within reason. As you read on, you may recognize that some of the activities you currently engage in are not "within reason" for pregnancy. In such cases, we recommend that you modify your activity at least two weeks before you predict conception to be possible in case you get pregnant sooner.

TABLE 15-1
THE BENEFITS OF MODERATE EXERCISE BEFORE AND DURING PREGNANCY

- Reduced stress and a bolstered sense of emotional well-being and optimism.
- Better management of pre-pregnancy weight.
- Better control over weight gain during pregnancy, but still within the desirable range; a smaller amount of maternal fat stored in the second and third trimesters.
- Greater reliance on fat as a fuel source for working muscles than in the untrained state (independent of exercise intensity).
- Greater likelihood for maintenance of pre-pregnancy fitness level. Some (not all) well-trained women who remain relatively active during pregnancy report feeling even more fit postpartum.
- Improved tolerance of pregnancy discomforts.
- Decrease in backaches. Stronger abdominal and back muscles make it easier to accommodate your pregnant tummy and facilitate better balance and coordination.
- Improved circulation. Better circulation makes it easier to dissipate heat and also alleviates swelling, varicose veins, and hemorrhoids.
- Decreased constipation (as long as good hydration and adequate fiber intake are maintained).
- More overall energy and stamina—something you'll be happy to have during pregnancy and for recovery after delivery. Most studies have found that good fitness does not make delivery any faster or easier, but fit women generally get back to feeling like their normal selves much more quickly.[a]
- Enhanced sleep.
- Better insulin sensitivity, which confers powerful risk reduction for gestational diabetes.
- Decrease in low-grade systemic inflammation; helps immune system.
- Probably protective against preeclampsia and premature delivery.
- Plenty of weight-bearing exercise, such as walking (within *all* safety limits), throughout pregnancy may even increase the odds of an on-time arrival (i.e., baby is not late for the big day!) compared to women who switch to much lower levels of exercise and/or non-weight-bearing modes (e.g., swimming) as the due date nears.
- Stronger bone density.
- Long-term risk reduction for cardiovascular disease, diabetes, and certain cancers.
- For women with preexisting medical conditions—asthma, diabetes, high blood pressure, or polycystic ovary syndrome (PCOS)—regular physical activity can offer additional benefits (as discussed in Chapters 5 and 7).
- Better brainpower: improved memory, ability to think efficiently, improved self-control.

a. If there is indeed a beneficial effect of fitness during delivery, it is probably better tolerance of the pushing stage of labor. A few studies have shown shorter labor. Athletic endurance combined with knowing when and how to simultaneously contract abdominal muscles and relax pelvic floor muscles plays a role.

Practical Application

When you visit your doctor for your preconception medical appointment, ask her to review the Preconception Fitness Evaluation that follows. Some of the information that you included earlier on your Women's Preconception Medical Checklist in Chapter 4 will assist in this fitness evaluation, too.

PRECONCEPTION FITNESS EVALUATION

Fill out the following questionnaire and take it to your preconception medical checkup along with the Women's Preconception Medical Checklist (see page 91).

- How would you rate your current level of fitness?
  Completely inactive   Just beginning   Intermediate   High   Elite

- Frequency
  For the past two months, how many times per week have you purposely done some sort of physical activity?
  Answer: _____ (average number of days per week)

- Intensity
  Your most common level(s) of intensity of exercise:
  No effort (nonexerciser)   Low   Moderate   Intense

  Do you include a slow warm-up and cool-down when you exercise?
  Never   Sometimes   Most of the time   Always

- Time (Duration)
  How much time do you spend each time you engage in physical activity?
  I spend anywhere from _____ to _____ minutes.

- Type (Mode)
  What types of activities do you typically do? Be sure to include planned exercise as well as activities that are a part of your everyday routine (e.g., walking several blocks to catch a bus or subway; frequent stair climbing at home or work; yard work/gardening):

  _____

  _____

If you have experienced any of the following, please circle and discuss with your physician:
Prior procedure that opened or cut your cervix (e.g., a D&C; LEEP, page 528)
Irregular or absent periods   High blood pressure
Complications with prior pregnancies/miscarriages
Thyroid problems   Lung disease   Heart disease   Diabetes
Previous injuries (e.g., knee injuries, back pain)

➜ *For physician to fill out:* The physical activity recommendations in this book comply with the American College of Obstetricians and Gynecologists exercise guidelines for pregnancy. Does this patient require any additional exercise precautions while conception is a possibility for her (and during pregnancy)?   Yes   No
If yes, please specify: _____
_____

WHERE THERE'S A WILL, THERE'S A WAY: MAKE EXERCISE FIT YOUR LIFESTYLE

Change is soon going to be more the norm than the exception for you. With that in mind, try to anticipate things that could disturb your good intentions to exercise. If you find yourself giving in to your own excuses, think of simple creative solutions. Tell yourself, "If X activity isn't going to work today, then Y activity is a viable alternative." Preconception fitness planning may also necessitate a change in the way you define your personal fitness satisfaction. If you are accustomed to expecting a serious level of performance from yourself in specific sports, add a few sports to your repertoire that you can enjoy for sheer pleasure. Take pride in exercise solutions that are more creative and less physically demanding. Doing something is better than doing nothing at all (unless, of course, you are told specifically not to exercise). As you adapt to your changing needs, this attitude will help you avoid quitting out of frustration if you cannot do something as well as you used to.

Furthermore, adapting now makes it easier to remain active once you are pregnant and after the baby comes. According to a study by Kathryn Schmitz, PhD, once the baby arrives, first-time moms (but not dads) typically decrease their overall physical activity level—Caucasian women by 14 percent and African American women by 9 percent. "There wasn't any additional change in physical activity when going from one to two children," adds Schmitz. It may be that the demands of motherhood require so much untapped emotional and physical energy that women feel they have no time or energy left to develop a new habit. Could this trend be reversed if more women established enjoyable exercise routines prior to and during pregnancy, ones that could be easily adapted once the baby is born?

FOR FUTURE REFERENCE: During Pregnancy/Family Life

We personally advise all parents-to-be to take up walking before they start a family so it becomes a cherished habit. Why? It can be relaxing and enjoyable and is probably one of the exercises most accommodating to new parenthood. The baby can be with you—day or night, outdoors or indoors (e.g., shopping mall, fitness club)—in a stroller, jogger stroller, front pack, or backpack, depending on his or her age. These accoutrements need not be expensive; the baby will be equally comfortable in a new jogger stroller as in one purchased on Craigslist or loaned to you by a friend. If the baby needs you, you can take a break and comfort or feed her. It's an activity that parents can do together after a busy day to nurture their companionship. The family dog, feeling outranked and desperate for attention, can come, too, and will be eternally grateful. And, as you'll discover soon enough, you'll be glad to have a fallback activity that is ideal when it's four in the afternoon, you've not showered or exercised, and you want a breath of fresh air.

One of many great resources for you is Lisa Druxman's *Lean Mommy: Bond with Your Baby and Get Fit with the Stroller Strides Program.*

Also, begin thinking about how you can overcome physical discomforts, changes in weather, daylight hours, time conflicts with work or family, travel, and holidays. Let's look at how other women have made physical activity work for them.

Jackie: "Autumn is one of my busiest times of year at work. There is always more to get done than hours in the day. In the past, everything else got put on hold, but this year I'm preparing to get pregnant, and I don't want to give up my new exercise program. I'm committing to three days of activity each week. Normally, I prefer to exercise after work, but during this time I plan to work out for an hour beforehand so that if I need to stay at the office longer, I can work with the knowledge that I've already spent time for me. As an extra incentive, I got an iPod for my birthday to listen to favorite NPR podcasts or audiobooks that I download from our local public library."

Liz: "The winters in Minnesota are often too cold and icy to run like I usually do, so if possible, I cross-country ski or snowshoe for exercise. If it's too miserable outside for that or if I simply am limited on time, I stop by the gym on my way home from work and run on the treadmill for thirty minutes or take a swim in the indoor heated pool. It's easy to just do nothing during this time of year, but getting out and exercising helps me keep my sanity."

Maria: "We've got three kids under the age of seven and want one more, so I usually go to my gym at six in the morning to walk and run on the treadmill or take "boot camp" class while my husband is at home getting ready for work. We also do active family outings on the weekends. However, during the holiday season, we visit my folks out of town, so my usual routine goes out the window. To get around this, I have my husband or other relatives watch the kids while a few of us go out after breakfast for a long walk. Or the kids come along—babies in strollers or backpacks, kids on bikes. This way I can still spend time with my family and accomplish my exercise goals at the same time. The hardest part for me was suggesting this sort of outing. I didn't want to sound selfish. However, it has now become a tradition that we all enjoy!"

Allison: "Both my husband and I work long hours. We usually exercise at home on our stationary bike or at the gym a few days a week, but what we particularly enjoy doing is walking our dog at night after the dinner dishes are done. Not only does our dog love it, but it also gives us time together. It gets us away from munching mindlessly on snacks—and from the phone and computer, too. Maybe in a year or so we'll be lucky enough to have a baby to accompany us."

Susan: "It always seems that cold and flu season fouls up my good intentions to exercise! It's usually because my three-year-old daughter gets sick, and I'm the one who has to drop everything, including my exercise class at the YMCA, and take care of her. The more workouts I miss, the harder it is to resume going. This year my husband and I sat down and coordinated a plan so that I am not always the one 'on call.' However, I also have Pilates workouts on DVD and a few old Jazzercise tapes at home as my backup."

Camille: "I had an early miscarriage three weeks ago, and last week my doctor finally gave me the green light to begin low-level exercise as long as I have no sign of problems. He has also advised us to wait for at least three months before we start trying again. I now make it a point to walk at a leisurely pace or bike almost daily, and my husband often comes with me. It has been good for us to get out and focus on enjoying life a little more. Even though in my mind I'm ready to start trying to get pregnant right away, my body is still readjusting. Being able to exercise again offers me a sense of normalcy because I'm actively doing something that will make me feel more like my old self again, ready for a future pregnancy."

Kimberly: "I travel occasionally for business, so I've had to come up with other ways to exercise while on the road. When I'm at an airport, I make a point of never taking the elevators or the moving sidewalks. If I have time between flights, I walk around the airport—walking helps to prevent my feet from swelling, too. I've also found that many hotels have swimming pools and workout rooms with treadmills, bikes, stair steppers, and weights; this is a great way to either start or end the day. If no exercise facilities are available, I make a point of using the stairs and exploring my surroundings on foot instead of taking cabs (within reason, of course)."

Lindsay: "I felt too self-conscious about my body to join a fitness club, and now that the intense summer heat is here, it's too hot to go outside for a walk. It even seems too hot inside during the day! Until recently, that was all the excuse I needed to skip exercising. It probably doesn't help that I've never been one to *really* enjoy exercise. We bought a treadmill and pulled out our old stair stepper from storage and put them both in front of the TV. I prop a floor fan up on a chair right in front of me to keep me cool while I walk or pedal. It works well, and the time goes by fast with the news or my favorite TV shows (recorded on DVR) on to keep my attention. Now I don't mind exercising so much."

Diana: "We have one toddler already and are preparing to conceive a second child. My biggest concern with fitness was making sure that I could supervise our daughter while I exercised. I have found that I can do water aerobics in the shallow end of our pool (instead of swimming with my head immersed) or use Zumba videos at home and still be able to keep my eye on her while she plays close by. I can also push her in the stroller while I walk with friends in our neighborhood. When I have more time, I take her with me to my fitness club. They have an inexpensive nursery/day care for members' children, which I use while I take a yoga class and then do light weights."

Erica: "I know that people often say that they don't have time for exercise when they really do. However, there are times in my life when things are so hectic that there literally is no time for a thirty-minute walk. When this is the case, knowing that something is better than nothing, I try to park a little farther away from my destination, take the stairs instead of elevators (or get off a couple of floors early and take the stairs the rest of the way), walk my grocery cart back to the store instead of leaving it in the parking lot, or, if possible, walk around the house or office when I'm on my cell or portable phone."

Sophia: "Six months after giving birth to our son two years ago, I found myself still thirty pounds overweight (I had gained fifty pounds during the pregnancy). I hadn't been in very good shape when I got pregnant, and I didn't exercise during the pregnancy, either. I swore that the same thing wouldn't happen again. So I began walking for exercise. At first I could barely walk a few blocks without feeling winded, but I've gradually worked up to about two to three miles per day, Sundays off. To keep myself motivated I sign up for nearby 5K and 10K races throughout the year. I walk-jog them for fun. My dresser drawer is beginning to pile up with commemorative T-shirts, and I'm back in shape. We're going to start trying to get pregnant in the fall."

DO IT NOW

Remember: if you intend to be regularly active during a normal, uncomplicated pregnancy, it is best to establish your desired level of fitness now during the months prior to conception. If you plan on trying a new mode of activity, such as walking/jogging instead of in-line skating, or cross-country skiing instead of downhill skiing, begin that now, too. You need to allow your body the time to adapt to the physical demands of a new exercise before you introduce it to the monumental demands of pregnancy. If you end up waiting until after you are pregnant to get active, first clear it with your physician and then limit yourself to low-intensity activities that require very little coordination (coordinated movements will be more difficult during pregnancy because your center of gravity changes).

#1 RULE OF EXERCISE: SAFETY FIRST

Whether you are already fit and just trying out a completely new sport, are resuming an active lifestyle after a long hiatus, or are making exercise a priority for the first time, it is good to be informed about the milestones of exercise progression.

Consider yourself de-trained if you have taken a break from exercise for longer than three weeks, according to American Heart Association spokesperson Dr. Gerald Fletcher of the Mayo Clinic Medical School. The average person takes only twelve to sixteen weeks to achieve a healthy level of fitness when starting from scratch. Improvements become more subtle after that point. From the start, it takes approximately two to three weeks for neuromuscular (nerve to muscle) adaptations to take place and improvements in strength to be noticed. These early adaptive weeks in an exercise program are also when you are most vulnerable to muscle strains; they become less of a risk when the body accustoms itself to the extra stress of exercise. The heart, lungs, and vascular systems adapt to the new exercise within about four weeks. Fit individuals have the advantage of already having some of these adaptations as a result of their prior conditioning. Finally, measurable changes in bone mineralization take at least six to eight weeks to occur. Notice that the rest of the body feels prepared to push ahead before the skeletal system is readied; injuries such as stress fractures take place most often between weeks four and six, from overdoing it too early. That is all the more reason to progress slowly and steadily. The saying "No pain, no gain" is less true than you might think.

To prevent injury from physical activity, follow these safety tips. If you adhere to them before pregnancy, the same advice applies during a normal, uncomplicated pregnancy.

1. Always include a short (five- to ten-minute) low-intensity warm-up before cardiovascular workouts (those involving continuous, repetitive motion of major muscle groups) as well as strength-training workouts. This warms you up from the inside out, and prepares the joints and cardiovascular system for the work ahead. Walking at a slow, comfortable pace is an ideal warm-up. End your workouts with a similar five-minute cool-down to ease your body back into the nonexercising state.

2. Avoid or tone down high-impact sports and aerobics. Beginners especially should keep them to a minimum.

3. Progress gradually. Do not be overenthusiastic or you may injure yourself and not be able to work out at all. Remember, too, that you want enough energy and stamina left over to carry on other daily activities.

4. Wear appropriate footwear that provides support and is specific to your activity.

5. Wear appropriate clothing: a support bra, breathable under- and outerwear, and hat and gloves when warranted.

6. Drink plenty of fluids, but not too much. See Table 15-2.

7. Be aware of environmental hazards that should steer you toward a different mode, place, or time to exercise, such as ice, loose gravel, traffic hazards if you'll be exercising near a road, and days (or times of day) when air pollution warnings are highest.

8. Listen to your body: know when to challenge it and also when to ease up.

9. Include flexibility training (stretching) after your initial warm-up or, better yet, at the conclusion of your workout.

FOR FUTURE REFERENCE: During Pregnancy

Over the course of pregnancy, hormonal changes begin relaxing the pelvic region (the pubic bone is actually a junction where the two pelvic bones join together) so it can expand to accommodate childbirth. These hormonal changes affect ligaments throughout your body, so your knees and other joints become slightly more lax, too, increasing your vulnerability to injury. Add to this the gradual change in your center of gravity, offsetting your balance as your womb and breasts grow. Non-weight-bearing activities such as pool aerobics, where balance isn't a prerequisite and injury risk is low, may become more appealing than weight-bearing activities such as jogging. Pregnant women who experience discomfort or pressure in the pelvic region during weight-bearing activities may find relief with non-weight-bearing exercise. Sometimes wearing a lower abdominal support belt (sold in maternity stores) can do the trick, although core strengthening exercises such as those in Chapter 16 may help delay or completely prevent the low-back stress and strain so common in the late stages of pregnancy. Women with recurrent knee, hip, back, or ankle injuries as well as anyone with a stubborn tendency to overtrain should also give serious consideration to gentler forms of exercise.

At moderate to high altitudes (above 8,000 to 10,000 feet) exercise is discouraged during pregnancy, especially during the first few days of altitude exposure while the body gets used to the thin air (decrease in oxygen availability). All-out, maximal effort exercise is ill-advised in all stages of pregnancy but is particularly risky at altitudes as low as 6,000 feet, even after acclimatization.

It is important to discontinue exercise and consult your physician if any of the following occurs during pregnancy:

- Vaginal bleeding or amniotic fluid leakage
- Unusual abdominal or back pain
- Shortness of breath, light-headedness
- Severe headache
- Irregular heartbeat or chest pain
- Persistent uterine contractions
- Onset of swelling or persistent pain in hands, feet, calves, or face
- Fever
- Weight loss or inability to put on weight during pregnancy

Body Temperature Safety

It's a fact: women who become fit before pregnancy are better at regulating their core body temperature and automatically keep from overheating better than unfit women.

The process of creating energy for exercise generates extra heat inside you. Recent studies have shown that the modest increases in body temperature that normally accompany sensible exercise do not harm one's chances of conception, nor do they harm the fetus. Internal temperatures will not reach anywhere near the potentially dangerous fetal threshold of 102.5°F. But this is because the body has ways of ridding itself of the heat almost as fast as it is produced.

How does the body protect itself from the heat generated by exercise? Primarily by sweating. When the sweat evaporates, the resultant cooling means you don't overheat. But sweat must vaporize—not be wiped away—to cool the body most effectively. So, aside from toweling sweat from your forehead before it drips into your eyes, leave the rest alone while you exercise.

The human body is very efficient at dissipating heat, but it has a much harder time during very high-intensity exercise and in hot, humid conditions when sweat cannot evaporate as well. This is why pregnant women should also avoid Bikram yoga and lounging in hot tubs or saunas. (Hot showers are harmless because enough of your body surface is exposed to relatively cooler ambient air.) Exercising in very dry, scorching climates and higher altitudes also makes it difficult to maintain body temperature and hydration because so much water is lost through sweating and breathing. In these extreme environmental conditions we suggest you exercise conservatively, particularly when you are trying to conceive and during the first three months of pregnancy.

Further, a woman who is dehydrated will heat up faster internally than a person who keeps well hydrated. Therefore, of greatest concern is the woman who chronically subsists in a semidehydrated state whether she knows it or not. If this practice continues, it may impair her ability to sustain a new pregnancy and make it more difficult to carry a baby to term. She may also experience greater incidence of painful muscle cramping (e.g., in the calves) at rest or during exercise. These women need to become accustomed to drinking more liquids prior to becoming pregnant, because once pregnant, water requirements increase even more. It can be challenging to keep up! As discussed in Chapter 10, thirst is not a reliable indicator of hydration status, but maintaining a pale yellow urine color is.

TABLE 15-2
HOW TO MAINTAIN GOOD HYDRATION WHEN YOU EXERCISE

1. Drink about 16 ounces of a beverage or water within the two hours before exercise, preferably closer to two hours beforehand, to permit time for the excess water to be excreted before you begin exercising.
2. Drink four to eight ounces of cool fluid every fifteen to twenty minutes during exercise. This guideline applies regardless of the sport (swimming, walking, etc). So, allow for brief water breaks during your workout; keep a water bottle handy or strategically map your exercise route past a drinking fountain. There's no need for a sports beverage unless you're a competitive athlete exercising for longer than 60 minutes (or longer than 30 minutes, if all-out effort) and you are striving for optimal performance.
3. After exercising, drink 16 ounces of fluid for every pound of water weight lost through sweating during exercise. To accurately determine sweat loss, weigh yourself before and after exercise to gauge how well you're compensating for losses. There is no need to overcompensate by drinking too much water. In fact, drinking too much water before, during, or after prolonged exercise (or profuse sweating) can lead to a dangerous health condition where your blood sodium levels get too dilute.
4. If you exercise moderately for under an hour in temperate climates, you may monitor your urine color and volume for hydration status feedback instead of the pre- and postexercise weighing. Refer back to page 284 if you need a refresher course.

FEMALE ATHLETES: GAUGING OPTIMAL FITNESS AND FERTILITY

If you are a serious athlete and have regular, predictable menstrual periods and no known fertility problems, you may be interested in reading this section, but it is primarily for the hardcore distance runner, dancer, or elite athlete who is ultra-lean and may or may not have predictable menstrual periods. If you recognize yourself in the latter description, don't worry—we're not going to put the kibosh on your entire training routine, so stay with us long enough to make sure your training is fertility-friendly.

The "female athlete triad" is a syndrome first spotlighted at an American College of Sports Medicine conference in 1992. Women involved in such activities as distance running, gymnastics, and ballet are most vulnerable to developing the triad, which is characterized by three conditions:

- Disordered eating (severe food restriction or binge-purge), as described in Chapter 14
- Absence of menstrual period (amenorrhea); we count irregular periods here, too, though it isn't mentioned in the formal definition
- Subsequent bone loss (osteoporosis)

Most often, it is the parents, coaches, or health care professionals of teenage or college-age female athletes who are most concerned about these symptoms. The athletes themselves are frequently in denial of their problem and oblivious to the long-term consequences. Many adult women in their childbearing years also have this syndrome, and it can be an underlying cause of infertility. Perhaps of even more concern, according to Wendi Buchi, MD, an obstetrician and specialist in this area, many women mistakenly believe that absent or infrequent menstrual periods serve as adequate contraception and stop taking precautions to prevent pregnancy. They resist suggestions to use effective contraception and end up with an unplanned pregnancy.

It used to be generally accepted that there was a threshold for percentage of body fat below which women would cease to have their periods. This was called the "fat loss theory," and has since been disproved. Some women have reproductive systems that are able to function perfectly well at very low percentages of body fat; others with the same body-fat percentage cease to have normal periods. Therefore, the loss of monthly menstrual flow in childbearing-age women is not directly tied to the actual amount of energy stored as body fat. It appears to be a problem of chronic imbalance of "energy in" versus "energy out": too little is coming in to the body to cover energy expenditure. Even an overweight woman can be affected in this manner if she experiences a voluntary or involuntary extreme restriction in her calorie intake, as in the case of crash diets or war blockades where food supply is shut off.

Hormones that play a critical role in regulating menstruation are disrupted by low available energy as a result of insufficient dietary calories. The energy demands of excessive physical training can then further compete with the available energy necessary to sustain normal menstrual periods. But physical activity per se has been shown to have no detrimental effect on the hormones regulating menstruation other than exacerbating this deficit in available energy. The calories just need to be replenished. If not, the cumulative drain on the body's energy reserves will disrupt important hormonal functions. The female athlete's menstrual periods will become infrequent or absent altogether.

There are more subtle consequences of the female athlete triad in addition to fertility difficulties. There is accelerated bone loss and the long-term emotional difficulties of having to unlearn disordered eating habits. Many factors, such as age and duration of the condition, determine how much damage is reversible and how much is permanent. Early intervention is certainly advantageous. Quite often, however, there is resistance on the athlete's part to heed advice involving changes in training, eating, and body weight. The athlete usually fears that her athletic performance could be hindered, although evidence points to the contrary. Athletes also tend to be acutely tuned into their bodies and may resent the perception of being second guessed.

If you feel you have some signs along the continuum of the female athlete triad, the following strategies will help you achieve your dual goals: to maintain a competitive edge and get healthier for pregnancy.

- First and foremost, train smarter, not harder, by cutting training by 10 to 20 percent. Competitive athletes are encouraged to discuss this with their coaches so that an individualized plan can be designed. If you do not have all three of the characteristic conditions associated with the syndrome (meaning you only have irregular periods and don't fit the profile of being eating disordered—this resembles Gabrielle's story on the next page), this may be all it takes to completely restore your fertility and normal periods. Give this "smarter training" intervention a chance for three to six months before any type of pharmaceutical intervention to promote ovulation and fertility.
- Gradually increase food intake to increase your body weight by 2 to 3 percent. Help from an experienced sports nutritionist or good sports nutrition book (e.g., *Nancy Clark's Sports Nutrition Guidebook* by Nancy Clark, MS, RD) is recommended. A good place to find experts who regularly see women with the female athlete triad is a university with a strong athletic program, because they often have full- or part-time health care professionals on staff to monitor and counsel their athletes and are often well connected with other clinicians outside of their immediate geographic area.
- Consume 1,500 mg calcium daily along with adequate vitamin D from food sources and the sun. (See Chapter 11 for food sources and supplements.) With physician approval, moderate strength training is encouraged to promote bone strength.

- Make sure to have at least one full day off from exercise and training each week.
- In some instances, hormone therapy is recommended to deter serious health problems.[1] Oral contraceptives, or the Pill, can be a temporary solution to prevent or slow further bone loss until you resume your normal periods naturally, an indication that your hormones are balanced and bones are protected. On the other hand, medications to enhance fertility or stimulate ovulation are *not* recommended until the athlete has first cut back on her training and addressed body weight and food issues.

LUTEAL PHASE DEFECTS: JUST SHY OF THE FEMALE ATHLETE TRIAD?

One of our readers, Gabrielle, half jokingly shared the following story with us. She writes, "Maybe I just have the 'type A triad!'" Gabrielle was a multisport endurance-trained athlete, had irregular periods, and was admittedly preoccupied with her weight. These three factors had led her to believe she had a luteal phase defect, when in fact, her training had induced the same symptoms. She didn't require medical treatment once she took a few actions on her own.

It's tempting to jump straight to ovulation induction if the luteal phase of your menstrual cycle is too short for the endometrium to support implantation of an embryo. Many female athletes experience symptoms of luteal phase defects (LPDs), where progesterone is cleared more quickly than normal, leading to shortened luteal phase and longer follicular phase. However, many of these cases of inadequate progesterone are due to a hypometabolic state (your body hasn't enough energy to reproduce). Most likely it's your body's way of cueing you to burn just a few less calories (or eat a little more). See Chapter 18 for more.

- Assuming that a physician has ruled out other possible causes of amenorrhea, normal periods should resume after there is no longer an energy deficiency. The lag time between restoring proper energy balance and restarting regular monthly periods is usually several months, sometimes longer.

Contrary to what the athlete may think, sports performance is most likely to improve with these strategies rather than decline. These strategies have been exceptionally successful in elite athletes and are meant to be permanent changes, not temporary ones. Improved sports performance often occurs in the early months of intervention and is inherently motivating.

---

1. Hormone therapy usually must be accompanied by healthy weight restoration to protect bone mass.

CHAPTER 16

Your Preconception Exercise Prescription

*I*n this chapter, we provide a two-part framework for a basic, healthy pre-pregnancy fitness routine to improve your endurance, strength, and flexibility. All three fitness components play an integral role in preparing you for perhaps the biggest forty-week physical challenge you'll ever experience. The basic exercise program is designed to be implemented now but can be continued all through pregnancy, with only a few modifications along the way. We offer tips on how to individualize the guidelines to match your desire for challenge, and you'll have a chance to consolidate the advice into a personal fitness prescription.

PHASE I: AEROBIC (CARDIOVASCULAR) CONDITIONING

There are three categories of exercises that are safe for you to do, depending on your current fitness level. Look over these lists of aerobic activities and check off all that interest you, even if you've never tried them before. Remember that variety is important to sustain your interest, so pick some that you're already comfortable with as well as some that may be refreshingly new. Make several choices from the "Safest Now and Throughout Pregnancy" category, so you'll have familiar alternatives once you do become pregnant. Also note the exercise no-nos if you are planning an active vacation that could coincide with when you are trying to get pregnant or already may be pregnant.

In the not-yet-pregnant state, your body will usually tell you if you're overdoing it—either by having irregular or nonexistent periods or by getting diminishing returns on sports performance, even when training harder. In the pregnant state, your body will again give you signals that mean you need to ease up—either by quickly fatiguing or by cramping. Pay attention and respect those signals. It usually means to *slow down,* not to stop. Discomforts related to overexertion or jerky movements should disappear almost immediately simply by toning down the intensity and/or slowing down the pace.

FOR FUTURE REFERENCE: During Pregnancy

Funny little aches and pains are more common during pregnancy and will probably occur during exercise from time to time. This is normal. However, exercise discomforts that persist are not always normal. Should this happen to you, stop the activity and call your health care provider just to be on the safe side.

Activities That Are Safest Now and Throughout Pregnancy

The following activities are among the easiest on your body, but you can still get a great workout. Although these exercises carry the least risk, please do consult your health care provider if you have reservations about participating in any of them.

_____ Walking/treadmill

_____ Stair stepping/stair climbing

_____ Stationary cycling, self-paced

_____ Swimming

_____ Snorkeling

_____ Water aerobics/pool jogging

_____ Hiking on even, steady terrain/trekking

_____ Nordic walking (ski walking)

_____ Low-impact aerobics

_____ Golf (walking the course)

_____ Light work, such as raking leaves, light snow shoveling, washing and waxing the car or floors

_____ Other _____ (verify with health care provider)

Activities That Are Safe for Preconception, but *Require Additional Safety Precautions During Pregnancy*

The following activities are ones that you should have at least some experience with prior to conception so you're not dealing with the rookie learning curve after conception. These can usually be continued through the early months of pregnancy but may require modification (or stopping) later on. For instance, you may be able to jog during your entire pregnancy, but at a gradually slower pace, whereas you may choose to give up beach volleyball if you become less nimble on your feet. Environmental factors (as discussed in the safety tips on pages 461–464 in Chapter 15) as well as your level of experience and that of those participating with you should always be taken into consideration.

Many of the activities listed below require more balance than you may retain as pregnancy progresses, increasing your risk of falls or sprains. Some women feel less coordinated right from the start of pregnancy. It may also become progressively more difficult to maintain proper technique as your belly grows more cumbersome. Remember, compensating for your new body by using improper form can also increase risk of injury. If your sport involves deep squatting or stretching movements and during pregnancy you notice that this bothers your pubic bone (really a joint) or any other joints, absolutely scale back on your range of motion or ask about an alternative exercise that does not provoke pain. Sports that require agile side-to-side motions, especially quick moves, should be tempered or stopped altogether. If you participate in an exercise class where the instructor sets the pace, choose one in which you can keep up with the beat of the music and not be pushed beyond your comfort zone. Unless you're the overzealous type, none of the sports in the following list involve aggressive physical contact or extremely ballistic movement, but if your version of them does, stop them prior to trying to conceive.

____ Rowing

____ Jogging/running

____ Dance exercise (e.g., ballroom dancing, salsa dancing, hip-hop, square dancing)

____ Step aerobics on two or fewer platforms (medium-high impact)

____ Ballet

____ Ice-skating

____ In-line skating

____ Tennis

____ Racquetball/squash

____ Badminton

___ Kayaking/canoeing/paddling

___ Stand-up paddleboarding (SUP) in calm water

___ Outdoor cycling/mountain biking

___ Studio cycling, instructor-led spinning classes

___ Volleyball

___ Cross-country skiing/snowshoeing (according to altitude guidelines)

___ Yoga (most types, such as hatha, Iyengar, vinyasa, and ashtanga); see next category for Bikram

___ Tai chi

___ Pilates

___ Martial arts/kickboxing, solo

___ Skipping rope

___ Plyometrics

___ Video-based exer-games such as Dancetown and Wii Sports (typically the ones that allow more freedom of movement are the better workout; most are not close to matching the real thing, though)

No-Nos: Activities That Must Be Discontinued Two Weeks Before Starting to Try and for the Entire Pregnancy

One could argue that basically any sport carries inherent risks, yet there are a few particularly dangerous ones that women nearing pregnancy should avoid. The reason for stopping two weeks before conception is in case you conceive earlier than anticipated.

___ Downhill skiing/snowboarding: sudden ski falls can cause abdominal trauma. Even if you are a great skier, the out-of-control novice behind you poses too much collision risk. All experienced skiers can recall a time when their ski bindings were too loose, causing their ski boot to pop out and triggering a hard fall.

___ Waterskiing: a hard fall could result in abdominal trauma; an unintentional squat-position skid on the water surface could cause water to be forced up into the vagina (and rectum), causing trauma to the cervical area.

___ Scuba diving: there is severe decompression risk to a fetus regardless of how good you may feel.

___ Diving: risk of abdominal trauma from belly-flop landing; your center of gravity changes too dramatically as pregnancy progresses.

___ Surfing: risk of hard fall is too high.

___ Horseback riding: risk of jarring is too high, as is the potential for a hard fall.

___ Rock climbing: risk of jarring is too high; potential for hard fall; too physically cumbersome as abdomen grows.

___ High-altitude exercise such as hiking or snowshoeing above 10,000 feet.

___ Soccer: potential for traumatic contact is too high.

___ Ice hockey and field hockey: potential for traumatic contact is too high.

___ Basketball: potential for traumatic contact is too high.

___ Gymnastics (especially at sophisticated levels): risk of abdominal trauma from a fall is too high; certain apparatuses are too jarring.

___ Bikram yoga: risk of overheating is too great when sweat cannot evaporate and cool the body.

Exercise for Health Benefits: Not-Too-Demanding Workouts Are All It Takes

Not too long ago women and men were advised to do thirty minutes or more of moderate-intensity physical activity on most (preferably all), days of the week. Not much has changed; however, the recommendation was thought to be too specific. A new recommendation, this one from the U.S. Department of Health and Human Services, has received broad approval and allows people to design their own way of meeting the guidelines. The new *2008 Physical Activity Guidelines for Americans* (*PA Guidelines*) basic recommendation states:

- Adults should get a minimum of 2 hours and 30 minutes (150 minutes) a week of moderate-intensity aerobic physical activity (a brisk walk, for instance).[1]
- Already-fit individuals can save time and get the same benefits by doing 1 hour and 15 minutes (75 minutes) a week of high-intensity exercise, if they prefer.

---

1. Researchers from San Diego State University School of Exercise and Nutritional Sciences have come up with a way to translate the "moderate-intensity walking" recommendation to something you can monitor with a pedometer. They found that 1,000 steps in ten minutes, or 3,000 steps in thirty minutes, meets the level of exertion that will lead to the health benefits that you want. *Consumer Reports* (2009) rates the Omron brand pedometer most favorably. Another reputable and affordable pedometer is the Yamax Digi-Walker SW-200.

Though you can customize how you work these minutes into your weekly schedule, bouts should be at least ten minutes long to count in the tally. This level of activity expends roughly 1,000 calories per week. You gain substantial health benefits from meeting this basic *PA Guidelines* goal, including all the benefits you read about for preconception and pregnancy (see Chapter 15, Table 15-1).

If you are just beginning to exercise, it's best not to embark on anything more challenging than this until completing at least three months of moderate training. Also, higher levels of exercise do not definitively confer greater benefits once you become pregnant, and the risks can be significant (e.g., higher injury rates, more difficulty replenishing calories for adequate weight gain). But if after three consecutive months of following the above guidelines you want more of a challenge, go ahead, and continue to do so, but once pregnant, monitor your RPE (Rating of Perceived Exertion; see Table 16-1), hydration level, and calorie goals even more closely because these will change as pregnancy progresses.

Taking It to the Next Level: More Intensive Workouts for Greater Health Impact

If you're a regular exerciser already, you are probably most interested in improving total fitness and health. To reap greater health benefits and high-level cardiorespiratory fitness requires exercise expenditures of approximately 2,000 calories of energy per week, 1,000 more than that recommended for health benefits alone.

- Adults should aim for five hours (300 minutes) or more a week of moderate-intensity aerobic activity or two hours and thirty minutes (150 minutes) or more a week of vigorous physical activity; adults who are trying to lose weight (or maintain a weight loss) should work up to this goal for better long-term success.

• A combination of moderate- and high-intensity aerobic activity works quite nicely, too; in fact, we highly recommend this mix for optimal fitness.

This can be broken down into multiple ten-minute sessions accumulated throughout the week. The time frame excludes the time spent warming up and cooling down.

The appropriate duration of a workout depends on how strenuous an activity feels. There is an inverse relationship between the two (see Figure 16-1). If you constantly find yourself pinched for time, you may be most successful at working up to a point where you can exercise vigorously for a shorter time. But if you prefer to walk at an easier pace, aim for the longer duration. You are free to alternate heavy and light workouts on different days. And there is no rule that says you need to exercise almost every day, though if you don't it makes it harder to reach the energy expenditure necessary for greater fitness gains. Try not to bunch your workout minutes into one or two days back to back unless there's no alternative. Exercise at regular intervals is better for you.

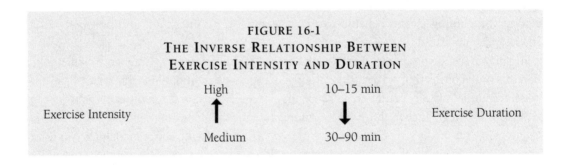

FIGURE 16-1
THE INVERSE RELATIONSHIP BETWEEN
EXERCISE INTENSITY AND DURATION

You may do more than this recommendation when in good health, but if you do vigorous exercise regularly, be sure to take at least one rest day per week. By participating in a variety of different activities, as suggested (cross-training), you may naturally have easier or harder workouts based on your prior experience and proficiency at the sport.

The more demanding the fitness routine, the more challenging it can be to meet your food and water needs, and the more diligent you must be to replenish calories and liquids. If you avidly exercise and are underweight (or normal weight) prior to pregnancy and have irregular or absent menstrual periods, this could be a telltale sign that your energy needs are not being met (see "Female Athletes: Gauging Optimal Fitness and Fertility" in Chapter 15 for more on this). It may be wise to scale back exercise until your body weight and menstrual function normalize. During pregnancy, poor weight gain is another sign that exercise should be cut back until you can get your weight to where it should be for your stage of pregnancy.

Monitoring Exercise Intensity

The American College of Obstetricians and Gynecologists has issued physical activity guidelines for both pregnant and planning-to-be-pregnant women using a Rating of Perceived Exertion (RPE) scale to estimate exercise intensity. The RPE is a reliable measure that takes into account individual differences and requires no monitors or measuring tools. All you need to do is rate your level of exertion on a scale of 1 to 10 for a particular activity, 1 being lowest, 10 highest. Be mindful of how your *whole* body feels—your legs, arms, heart, breathing—and rate what you feel.

TABLE 16-1
EXERCISE INTENSITY BASED ON RATING OF
PERCEIVED EXERTION (RPE) SCALE

0	No effort at all: "couch potato" level
0.5	Very, very weak
1	Very weak
2	Weak
3	Moderate
4	Somewhat strong
5	Strong
6	
7	Very strong
8	
9	
10	Very, very strong
*	Maximal—unable to continue. Never, ever exercise to the point of exhaustion during this pre-pregnancy time or during pregnancy.

Adapted from G. A. Borg, "Psychophysical Bases of Perceived Exertion," *Medicine and Science in Sports and Exercise* 14, no. 5 (1982): 377–81.

We suggest the following routine for a workout. Follow along using the RPE chart in Table 16-1.

- Begin with an easy five- to ten-minute warm-up at an RPE of 1 to 2.
- Next, aim for a workout intensity between 3 and 7 on the RPE scale. Where exactly should you be in this range? Your workout should not be so exhausting that you have to quit before your allotted workout time is up. It should be challenging enough so that you can carry on a conversation, but not quite sing.
- If you're a beginner and working on moderate-intensity activity, strive for several short and long workouts at an RPE of 3 to 4. Once you are past the novice stage, intersperse a few one- to two-minute intervals of higher intensity for challenge; this will improve your endurance, and you'll begin to see more definition to your waistline and whole body.
- If you're a trained athlete, you've built up endurance and, from experience, you know your body's capabilities and limitations better. You can safely exercise in the higher workout RPE range of 4 to 7—or incorporate intervals of both—without tiring out too early.
- Always slow down to a lower RPE or stop if you begin to feel too fatigued.
- End your workout with another easy five-minute cool-down at an RPE of 1 to 2.

No two people rate the same activity exactly the same unless their athletic abilities are identical. As an example, consider an exercise such as swimming eight laps in a pool. If you asked two women of different fitness levels to do this exercise in fifteen minutes and then to rate their perceived exertions, you'd probably hear completely different answers. The woman who swims regularly might give this a 1 or 2 on the RPE scale, a good warm-up pace, after which she could speed up for her workout pace. For the woman who is out of shape and hasn't swum in fifteen years, this is an RPE of 7, too intense to sustain for a full workout, but if she allowed herself thirty minutes to complete the eight laps at a slower pace, she'd rate it as a 3 or 4 on the RPE scale and be able to achieve her goal of thirty minutes of moderate-intensity exercise that day.

Whatever exercise intensity rating you become accustomed to now can be continued during a normal, uncomplicated pregnancy, without overheating or jeopardizing your baby's oxygen.[2] But keep in mind that your perception of an exercise workload will go through a few normal transitions from pre-pregnancy through late pregnancy. For example, right now you may rate a brisk walk of forty-five minutes as a 5 on the RPE scale. When you become pregnant, you'll still aim for a workout RPE of 5, because your body is accustomed to that intensity. But, as you will discover (especially in the third trimester), your RPE of 5 may occur when

---

2. If you've previously had preterm labor (or are at risk for it) or delivered a baby small for his or her gestational age, you should automatically decrease your activity level in the second and third trimester, regardless of how fit you are.

you're going at a slower pace. Stick with that slower pace, because maintaining your former workload would mean exceeding your pre-pregnancy level of exertion.

If you don't become active now but decide you want to begin exercising after you've conceived, you should first get physician approval to begin low-level activity. Then maintain a workout RPE of 2 to 4—no higher—with activities such as leisurely swimming, walking at an easy pace on flat ground, stationary cycling, or very low-impact aerobics (with only modest use of your arms). (Remember, overexerting when unconditioned jeopardizes the baby's safety.)

Practical Application

Design your preconception "F.I.T.T.ness" (Frequency, Intensity, Type, Time) routine for promoting overall health and cardiovascular (aerobic) fitness by filling in the blanks below. Remember: you can always revise as needed. The next section focuses on adding strength and flexibility, so allow a bit of leeway in your time commitment for these as well.

F = Frequency: I intend to be physically active _____ days per week.

I = Intensity: I intend to exercise at an RPE between _____ and _____ after an easy warm-up.

T = Type (mode) of activity: I would like to do the following physical activities prior to pregnancy:_____

_____.

As I get closer to conception, I'll consider adjustments to my exercise routine accordingly.

T = Time (duration): I intend to devote _____ minutes of time to each workout. I may/may not (circle one) break the exercise sessions down into several shorter time periods.

Notes to self on success and rate of progression (or if you have been advised to cut back, note how you intend to reduce your mileage, intensity, range of motion, or duration):

_____

PHASE II: STRENGTH AND FLEXIBILITY

In preparation for your pregnancy, it is important to target strength as well as aerobic conditioning. The new *PA Guidelines* send a clear message that strength training, also called resistance training or weight training, should be done at least two days per week and provides additional health benefits. Strength training is different from aerobic conditioning. Aerobic exercises such as walking will greatly improve the endurance of your heart, lungs, and blood vessels, but they play a minor role in building lean muscle mass. This is why you see female and male athletes (tennis players, skiers, gymnasts) doing weight training as well as practicing their given sport.

To strike a balance between muscles that are strong but not too tight, flexibility training is also essential. Flexibility not only lessens the risk of muscle and tendon injury but also enhances the muscles' response to strength training. Therefore, to complete your preconception fitness program, the remainder of this chapter focuses on muscular strength, stamina, and flexibility. This final fitness component may have particular relevance if you already have children and are feeling untoned or are experiencing muscle imbalances (from actions such as lifting the heavy car seat or carrying and resting the child on one of your arms or hips).

Strength training prior to conception focuses on strengthening the muscles of five areas: those of the upper and lower back, abdomen, pelvic floor, and lower body. The muscles in these areas will be called on to support the extra weight of pregnancy. Back and abdominal muscles are also the most important muscles for good posture. Once pregnant, women who have strong abdominal and back muscles find that they still have the strength and stability to maintain good posture throughout pregnancy. Toning the muscles of the upper back also discourages the tendency for the back muscles to get overstretched when the gravitational pull of enlarging breasts tugs the shoulders forward and shortens the chest (pectoral) muscles. The eventual cradling and carrying of your child will strengthen your chest but also further promotes the slouched position if the opposing back muscles aren't strengthened, too. The most common consequence of neglecting these muscle groups is back pain, which more than half of all pregnant women experience during some part of their pregnancy. Fit women experience back pain to a much lesser degree.

There are more benefits to resistance training. It used to be thought that drawing in your abdomen to target the deepest of the four abdominal muscles, the transverse abdominis, would reduce or prevent a separation (diastasis) of the most superficial abdominal muscle, the rectus abdominis, as it stretches during pregnancy. A diastasis recti is a separation of the vertical connective tissue that joins together the two halves of the rectus abdominis muscle, which runs from your pubic bone to the rib cage. Such separation weakens the pregnant abdomen and secondarily provides less support for the back. (It doesn't, however, harm the baby.) This happens in the majority of healthy pregnancies to some extent, and some women have an unhealed diastasis recti from a prior pregnancy. (Look ahead to Figures 16-3A and 16-3B.)

But Stuart McGill, PhD, a professor of spine biomechanics and author of the textbook *Low Back Disorders*, debunks the concept of focusing only on the transverse ab muscles. The best way to build core stability and repair and restore full strength to the abdominal wall muscles is to contract the entire abdominal wall. Think of how you might tense up your entire abdomen, instead of sucking in the belly button, to deflect a mild stomach punch (feel the difference?); it's called abdominal bracing.

Strength in the pelvic floor, or genital area, is another plus. Good tone in these muscles prevents the gradual weakening that may occur *during* the pregnancy, not just from delivery. More specifically, this could make *the* difference in averting urine leakage during exertion (such as during high-impact exercise, coughing, or sneezing) late in pregnancy and postpartum. Yet another benefit of resistance training includes greater muscle stamina for labor itself. You'll have more power for pushing the baby out, and you'll also have trained yourself to relax specific muscles in between pushes. Should you choose to assume a deep squat position to deliver the baby, strong leg and hip muscles will give you greater stamina as well.

GOOD POSTURE = STRONGER CORE

Unlike formal strength training, *subtle* strength training can be done over and over throughout the day simply by maintaining proper posture (see Figure 16-2).

FIGURE 16-2
NEUTRAL SPINE POSITION: POSTURE FOR STANDING AND SITTING

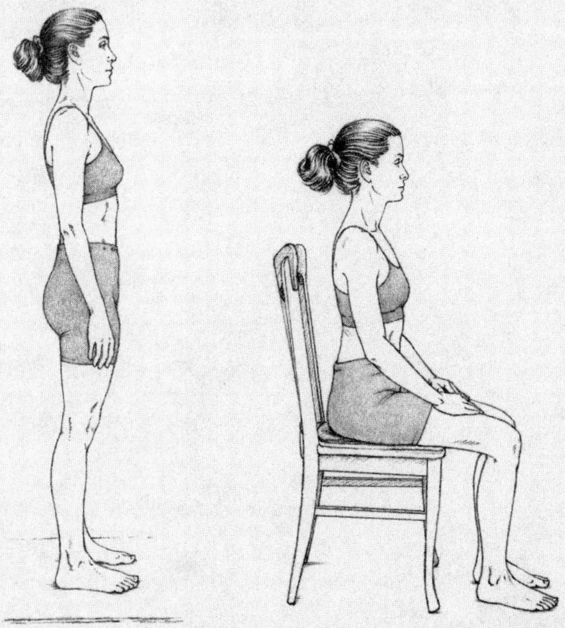

Notice how the spine looks when good posture is maintained in this neutral spine position. It has natural curvatures. The tendency during pregnancy is for the normally subtle curve in the lower back to become exaggerated. A well-designed strength workout can prevent that.

So get in the habit of maintaining good postural alignment not only during exercise but also when you stand, sit, get dressed, or lean over to pick up something. It will soon become automatic. Don't underestimate the effectiveness of numerous small efforts toward improving the stamina of the postural muscles, including the abdominal muscles pictured below. Attention to postural alignment could be the single most important defense against developing back pain.

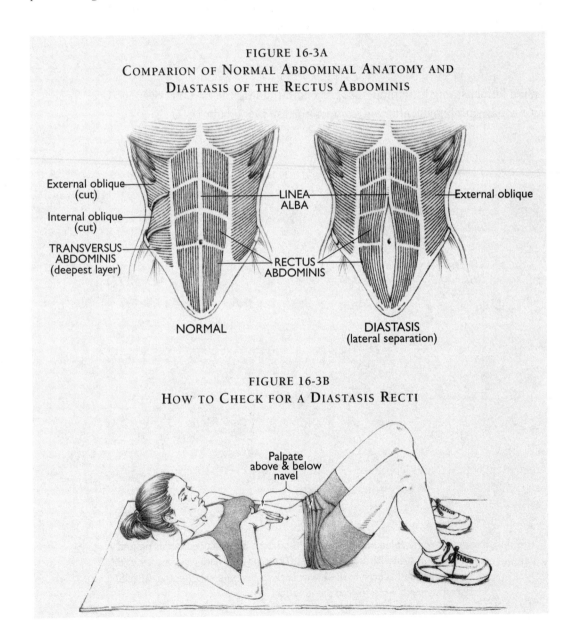

FIGURE 16-3A

COMPARION OF NORMAL ABDOMINAL ANATOMY AND DIASTASIS OF THE RECTUS ABDOMINIS

External oblique (cut)

Internal oblique (cut)

TRANSVERSUS ABDOMINIS (deepest layer)

LINEA ALBA

External oblique

RECTUS ABDOMINIS

NORMAL

DIASTASIS (lateral separation)

FIGURE 16-3B

HOW TO CHECK FOR A DIASTASIS RECTI

Palpate above & below navel

Lie on your back with knees bent and feet on the floor as if you were going to do an abdominal crunch exercise. Instead of putting your hands behind your head, rest one hand down along your side and the other on your abdomen. Place your index fingertip and middle fingertip together on your belly button so that both fingertips point in the direction of the pubic bone. Now lift your head a couple of inches off the floor to produce a minor ab contraction and hold it. Press your fingertips firmly above and then below the navel to check for a separation of the connective tissue in the midline of the rectus abdominis muscle. If you've never been very overweight and you've never been pregnant, there is probably no separation. If there is a separation, you'll feel the firm edge of the connective tissue on the sides of the fingertip(s) as it fits into the gap. The separation may be one or two fingertips wide; sometimes it's greater. Neither is painful. At your normally scheduled medical appointment, notify your physician of a separation wider than three fingertips so it can be monitored. The exercises in this preconception program are safe to do when there is a diastasis recti present.

FOR FUTURE REFERENCE: During Pregnancy

It's safe to lie on your back long enough to check for a diastasis recti in all trimesters of pregnancy. It's just not advisable to lie on your back for much longer than that after the second trimester. This is to prevent a drop in blood pressure caused by the enlarging uterus pressing on the vein that carries blood back to the heart. It doesn't happen to all pregnant women when they lie on their back, but if you suddenly feel nauseous, dizzy, and short of breath, don't worry. You don't need to call the doctor; just roll onto your side! These symptoms should disappear quickly thereafter. (Rolling on your side and then tightening your ab and back muscles when you're ready to push up to a seated position will also have a back-sparing effect. Use this when you get out of bed, too.)

The flexibility component of this preconception fitness program aims to relieve muscle and tendon tightness in areas of the body that normally get even tighter over the course of pregnancy. The stretches should be performed at least two to three times per week. The lower back, chest, and hip flexor regions need special attention. For example, hip flexor muscles are tightened by the forward tilting of the pelvis as the pregnant tummy grows, and this is further exacerbated by long durations of sitting at work or home.

Flexibility training, like strength training, is best accomplished after the body has been warmed up. Do a five- to ten-minute warm-up, with particular attention to the areas you will be conditioning. Stretching at the end of a full aerobic workout is even better, because it may take the muscles as long as fifteen to thirty minutes to warm to optimal levels.

Props, Tips, and Breathing Technique for Your Strength and Flexibility Workout

Strength training can be performed using a variety of props. Weight-training machines, free weights, elastic tubing or bands, stability balls, or buoyant devices (for pool exercise) all are wonderful tools. However, when you get down to the basics, all you really need is a chair, a soft mat or carpet, and the force of your own body weight against gravity. You can strength-train in the privacy of your own home or home-away-from-home with no specialized equipment at all (think playground!).

The following fourteen-step pre-pregnancy strength- and flexibility-training program is best done two to three times per week, in about thirty minutes. The first two times you do this workout, we suggest that someone be present (your husband or a friend) who can guide you through the poses to make sure you maintain proper form throughout each movement. After you have read through the workout on your own, have your partner read through the prompts as you do the exercises, and allow him to adjust your posture so that your technique matches the picture. He can remind you to breathe, too, in case you forget and hold your breath. (This is more common than you think!) A full-length mirror can be a substitute here, but a partner can spare you from having to crane your neck to read the prompts or look in the mirror.

Remember: once you have successfully conceived, all of these preconception exercises are appropriate to continue throughout pregnancy, provided you have no discomfort or medical reasons that preclude resistance training.

STRENGTH-TRAINING TIPS

Posture
Maintain proper posture in the neutral spine position (see Figure 16-2).

Warm-up
Remember to warm up for at least five to ten minutes before you strengthen or stretch. Examples of warm-up activities include walking, *slow* stair stepping, and gentle arm circles.

Repetitions, Sets, and Pace
Unless stated otherwise, aim for a set of twelve repetitions of each exercise at a slow, controlled pace: each repetition can last three to seven seconds. When training at the very slowest pace (the seven second speed per repetition), eight repetitions is sufficient for one set. Do *one* set of *each* exercise; if you have the time and the inclination, you may do two or three sets per exercise. The exercises should be a challenge, *not* a strain. An exercise is

too difficult if you cannot do eight to twelve repetitions in each set while maintaining excellent technique. (Proper breathing is discussed below.)

Rest Periods
Rest between sets for about thirty seconds to two minutes. You can increase the length of the rest period during pregnancy as desired.

How Often?
Perform resistance-training exercises two to three days per week. Allow at least one day between sessions. After you've completed several months of strength training, you can *periodically* get away with as little as one day per week without significantly losing strength.

FOR FUTURE REFERENCE: During Pregnancy

During pregnancy, some of these exercises will inevitably become more difficult to execute. It doesn't mean you're turning into a wimp; after all, you're living with the extra physical challenges of pregnancy twenty-four hours a day! Please take our suggestions for making the moves easier or even stop if necessary.

FOCUS ON BREATHING

Proper breathing technique is important anytime strenuous physical exertion comes into play, even outside the realm of strength training. But it takes practice. For starters, try the following: put one hand on your belly and the other in the middle of your chest. Now take a deep breath. Did your chest and shoulders elevate, causing your top hand to move? Or did your belly expand—shoulders and chest staying relatively stationary—causing your lower hand to move outward? If you answer yes to the latter, you already know how to perform a deep, full *diaphragmatic breath* (more fondly termed a "belly breath"). However, if you're like most people, you probably are used to taking the shallower breath that expands only the upper part of the lungs, and your abdominal muscles, or "abs," may actually pooch out as you forcefully blow out. This is the opposite of what you want.

Try it again the right way a few times. This time, let your abdomen *expand* when you inhale, and allow your abdomen to firm up on exhalation. Now try this correct breathing technique the next time you vigorously exert yourself, even during a task other than your workout. Good opportunities for practice include taking a heavy shopping bag out of your car, straining during a bowel movement, coughing or sneezing, and going from a lying to a sitting position, such as when you're rolling out of bed. Before you exert, inhale with a belly breath. As you exert, breathe out and firm your torso. You'll actually cue your abs to protect the rectus abdominis from separating too much during pregnancy. Good breathing technique also protects against blood pressure spikes and light-headedness on exertion.

With the fundamental preconception exercises you see on the next pages, there is debate over whether you need to train your breath to the phases of movement. In fact, Dr. McGill, the spine mechanics expert mentioned earlier in this chapter, recommends that in all but the most strenuous exertions, it's better to breathe freely during resistance training while bracing the abdominals (contracting abs firmly throughout the movement); this is particularly pertinent for superslow training. But as long as you aren't holding your breath, you will find that your natural breathing rhythm flows through the exertion and relaxation phases of an exercise. As a precaution for those of you who simply forget to breathe while you're strength training or want to progress to harder exercises, we have included breathing prompts, but take it in stride that these shouldn't be strenuous enough to necessitate entrained breathing.

FOR FUTURE REFERENCE: During Pregnancy (Labor and Delivery)

The "Focus on Breathing" vignette (above) concentrated on proper form and breathing cues during physical exertion—even through something as basic as a difficult bowel movement. And during pregnancy, it is important to preserve oxygen flow to the womb; breathing during exertion achieves that end. However, you may be advised differently during the pushing phase of labor when short periods of breath-holding while bearing down is typical (called Valsalva-type pushing). Practitioners usually try to avoid *prolonged* Valsalva bearing down, but if needed, they have fetal monitors that keep tabs, too. Your practitioner will guide your pushing technique to maximal effect during delivery!

The 14-Step Preconception Strength and Flexibility Workout (After Warm-up)

Step 1: One-Arm Bent-over Row

This strengthens the back muscles as well as the upper arms and back part of the shoulders. It requires the use of a chair or bench. This is the only exercise in which you are advised to hold a weight or a weighted object such as a hardcover book or full water bottle.

PROMPTS.

Begin by placing your right hand on the far front corner of the chair and your right knee on the closest front corner, as pictured in Figure 16-4. If the chair is too narrow, causing your body to feel bunched up, slip the knee back off the chair, allowing the right foot to rest on the floor. Your back and head should be in the same plane parallel to the ground, torso stabilized by slight contraction in the abdominal area. Without any weight in your left hand (palm in), allow your left arm to hang directly below the shoulder. Inhale and on exhalation retract your shoulder blades, especially the left one (as you'd do with a backward shoulder roll to create "cleavage" between your shoulder blades). Without pausing, bend the elbow toward the ceiling and slowly raise your fist to your waist, keeping the elbow close to the body the whole time. Slowly lower the arm to the starting position as you inhale. The full motion is similar to sawing wood slowly. Repeat twelve times per set. Then alter your position on the chair and do the same for the right side. After you've practiced once, do the exercise holding a weight.

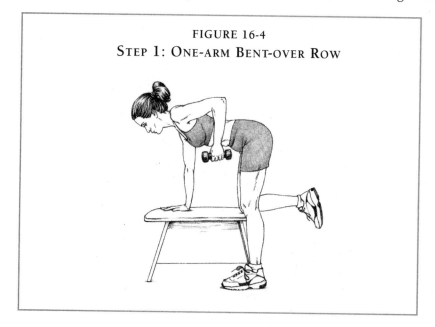

FIGURE 16-4
STEP 1: ONE-ARM BENT-OVER ROW

COMMON MISTAKES.

Forgetting to retract the shoulder blade makes this an exercise for the arm's biceps muscle rather than the back strengthener it is intended to be.

Step 2: Desk or Kitchen Counter Push-ups

Although the upper-body portion of your preconception workout targets the back muscles, a balanced workout design never neglects the opposing chest musculature. A simple push-up will strengthen the chest area as well as the shoulders and triceps (back of upper arm).

PROMPTS.

Stand at least three feet away from a counter or sturdy desktop with your feet slightly apart (see Figure 16-5). Place hands slightly wider than shoulder-width apart on the counter's edge, arms straight. Your head and body should make a straight line—a slight contraction in the abs helps stabilize this rigid posture. Breathe in while slowly bending the elbows. Lower the chest to within an inch or two of the surface. Your heels should lift from the floor. Slowly breathe out while pushing back up to the start position. After the first push-up, you may find that you need to adjust your feet backward or forward to allow the chest (not the waist or the neck) to be even with your hands in the down position. Repeat twelve times per set.

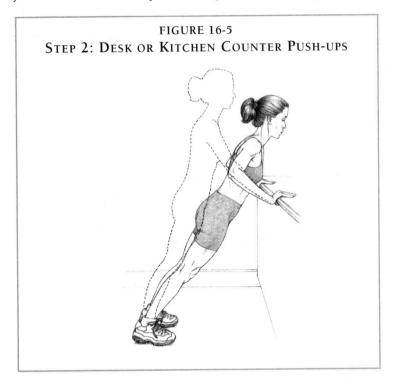

FIGURE 16-5
STEP 2: DESK OR KITCHEN COUNTER PUSH-UPS

If you find these push-ups too strenuous, try doing them against a wall, starting with your feet approximately two feet from the wall. To make the push-ups more difficult you can do them on the floor, with or without your knees touching the floor. Some women find it more comfortable to keep the *wrists taut* and place their fists against the wall or floor instead of open palms.

COMMON MISTAKES.

Allowing the buttocks to arch upward or the hips to sway down. Don't lose your abdominal contraction.

Step 3: Chest and Shoulder Stretch

Not only does this stretch the chest and front of the shoulder area, but it also helps pull the shoulder blades together to aid in good posture.

PROMPTS.

Stand tall, abs contracted, with your feet hip-width apart, and clasp your hands together behind your back near your buttocks (see Figure 16-6). Keep your head from jutting forward by tucking in your chin. Now focus on gently squeezing your shoulder blades together *and* down at the same time. Elbows will automatically face the back of the room when you do this. Hold this position for an out-loud count of ten to thirty seconds (as recommended by the American College of Sports Medicine) for effective stretching. Repeat up to four times.

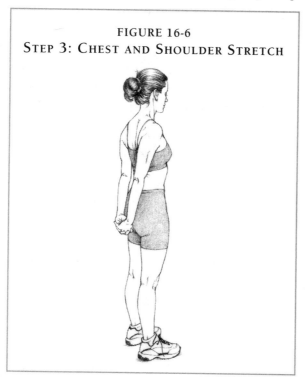

FIGURE 16-6
STEP 3: CHEST AND SHOULDER STRETCH

Step 4: Standing Pelvic Tilt Abdominal Exercise

The pelvic tilt primarily strengthens the rectus abdominis muscle (recall Figure 16-3A) to aid in postural alignment. Although traditional abdominal crunches strengthen the same muscle, the pelvic tilt challenges the muscle fibers in a more functional manner, making this the better choice as you prepare to conceive. Pelvic tilts can be continued throughout pregnancy, whereas back-lying exercises like stomach crunches are not advised after the first trimester.

PROMPTS.

Begin in a standing position with a neutral spine, feet hip-width apart, knees slightly bent (see Figure 16-7). Envision a rocking chair—how the seat and back tilt backward and forward as it rocks. Now picture your pelvis as that rocking chair. Place your hands on your hips as if you were grasping the back (sides) of the rocking chair and had to help it rock by twisting your wrists back and forth. Now, without moving your legs or upper body, slowly tilt your pelvis backward and then forward and backward again. When you stop in between those two extremes your spine is in neutral position. From here, do only backward tilts. Your spine will temporarily flatten. Then rock back to neutral, rock backward again, and then again to neutral. Repeat this *slowly* twelve times per set.

Keep in mind that pregnancy tends to tilt the pelvis excessively forward, causing more than the normal inward curve of the lower back. We work on the backward pelvic tilt to strengthen the pull toward neutral, effectively preventing the strain of improper posture.

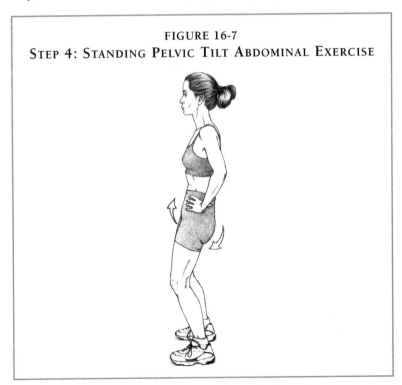

FIGURE 16-7
STEP 4: STANDING PELVIC TILT ABDOMINAL EXERCISE

COMMON MISTAKES.

When you tilt the pelvis backward, your belly button is drawn in and your tailbone will slightly tuck under, but your gluteal (buttocks) muscles should not tighten. By taking the gluteal muscles out of the action, the rectus abdominis muscle must do all of the work.

Step 5: Opposite Arm and Leg Raises (also called Bird Dog)

This exercise strengthens the muscles of the lower back, abdomen, and lower body. It also develops balance and coordination.

PROMPTS.

First, place a chair seat just beyond arm's reach in front of you to aid in balance. On your hands and knees on a soft mat or carpet, begin with wrists directly below shoulders, knees directly under hips. Your back is in the neutral position (with a slight normal curvature); head is in the same plane as the spine. Activate your abdominal muscles so your tummy doesn't sag. In a slow, controlled manner, simultaneously extend one arm forward and the opposite leg backward so that they are both parallel to the floor (see Figure 16-8), though full extension isn't necessary. Lengthen the spine and keep hips stationary. You should feel this strengthening through your torso as well as feel your limb muscles tightening as they assist in stabilizing your balance.

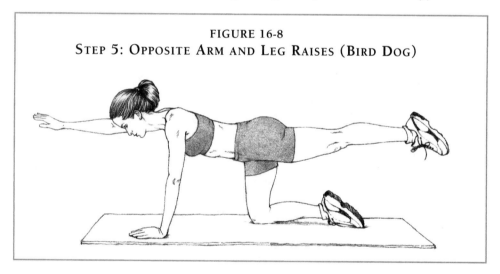

FIGURE 16-8
STEP 5: OPPOSITE ARM AND LEG RAISES (BIRD DOG)

Hold the stretch for three to five seconds, then fluidly switch to the other arm and opposite leg. Build up to about six or seven repetitions on each side (not necessarily twelve, in this case). Breathe normally while keeping core muscles activated.

If the hand position bothers your wrists, you can make a fist instead of an open palm. If you find it too difficult to maintain your balance by working arms and legs together, decrease your range of motion or split it into two separate exercises, alternating arms first while both knees remain stationary, and then switch to alternating legs while both hands remain on the floor.

COMMON MISTAKES.

There is a tendency to lift the straight leg too high. Although you can safely raise your leg past parallel to the ground to create an angle of 10 degrees above the ground, raising your leg higher causes strain in your lower spine.

Step 6: Plank Pose (also called Elbow Plank or Front Bridge)

This exercise will help develop your core muscles, particularly the ab region.

PROMPTS.

While still on your hands and knees, walk your hands out in front of you until you can rest your forearms on the mat with your elbows directly in line with your shoulders. Then anchor your toes to the ground and lift your knees off the floor so that your entire body is hovering parallel to the ground (see Figure 16-9). With particular emphasis on tightening your abdominal muscles, make your body stable like a board from your head to toes. Watch that you don't strain your neck backward; keep it level. Straighten hips by using a pelvic tilt to help, and hold the pose for ten to twenty seconds, over time building up to one minute (it can be quite challenging). Breathe! And keep reminding yourself to breathe freely the entire time.

This exercise is one that might need the following modification during pregnancy (or if you are unconditioned now, this may be a good place to start). You can make plank pose more comfortable by starting in a standing position facing a wall, feet planted hip-width apart about two to three feet from the wall. Walk your hands up the wall so that the elbows land at shoulder level on the wall, forearms and hands resting vertically on the wall. Now you are looking like a human lean-to, and your muscles, especially those of the abdomen, contract and stabilize the body. Add extra challenge by shuffling feet backward by one foot. Breathe freely and hold up to one minute.

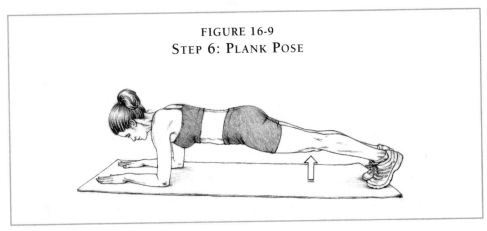

FIGURE 16-9
STEP 6: PLANK POSE

Common Mistakes.

Watch out for the sway-back potential or the opposite, bottom sticking out again. This is where your partner can give you feedback. Is your bottom popping up? The goal is to be rigid like a plank.

Step 7: Tail Wag

This exercise stretches and relieves tension in your hip and side muscles while tightening the abdomen.

Prompts.

The tail wag is a nice way to lightly stretch and strengthen while still on all fours. Your back is in the neutral position with a slight normal curve; abs are lightly contracted to stabilize the torso; head is in the same plane as the spine. Take a belly breath, and then for a count of two to three seconds slowly breathe out as you turn your head to the right in an attempt to look in the direction of your right foot. Move the right hip simultaneously slightly to the right, too (see Figure 16-10). You will feel a nice stretch along the left side of your torso and hip. Return to neutral in a controlled manner as you breathe in. Alternate by simultaneously looking left and turning your left hip out. Repeat eight to twelve times per set.

If the hand position bothers your wrists, you can make a fist instead of an open palm.

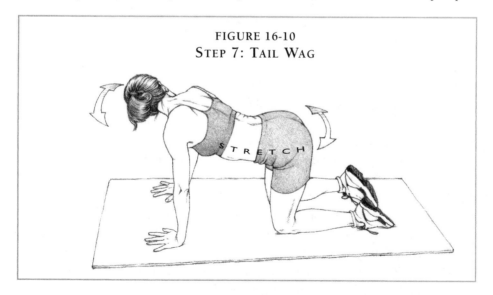

FIGURE 16-10
STEP 7: TAIL WAG

Common Mistakes.

If the head is lifted up to look back, this tends to cause the lower back to sway out of the neutral zone. Make sure your head remains at the same level as your shoulder when you peer around it.

Step 8: Side-lying Leg Raises for Outer Thigh

This exercise should be felt in your upper hip region, and some of the gluteal muscles will be at work, too.

PROMPTS.

Lie straight on your left side on a soft mat or carpet. Allow the bottom leg to bend at the knee and bring your right hand in front of you for support at the waist or chest level. The left arm extends directly overhead, bent at the elbow to cradle the head. Abdominals are tightened to support the pelvis and back. Now slowly raise your top leg about 1½ feet from the floor (see Figure 16-11). Lower the leg at the same pace and repeat twelve times for one set. You may vary the pace by pausing at the top for two to three seconds and then slowly lowering. Roll over and repeat on the other side.

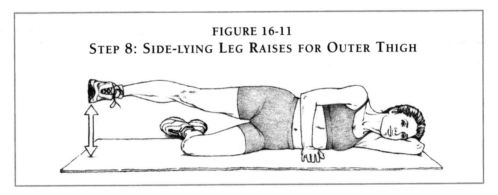

FIGURE 16-11
STEP 8: SIDE-LYING LEG RAISES FOR OUTER THIGH

COMMON MISTAKES.

Allowing the working leg to drift forward or backward.

Step 9: Side-lying Leg Raises for Inner Thigh

With this variation, you should feel most of the contraction in your inner thigh region.

PROMPTS.

Lie straight on your left side on a soft mat or carpet. Keep the bottom leg straight while bending the top leg at the hip and knee, creating a right angle, with the tip of your toe touching the floor for support (you may prop a pillow under the knee and foot for added comfort; see Figure 16-12). Bring your right hand in front of you for support at the waist or chest level. The left arm extends directly overhead, bent at the elbow to cradle the head. Tighten your abdominals to support the pelvis and back. Now slowly raise the bottom leg straight up toward the ceiling, about six to twelve inches from the floor. Lower the leg at the same slow pace and repeat twelve times for one set. You may vary the pace by pausing at the top for two to three seconds and then slowly lowering. Roll over and repeat on the other side.

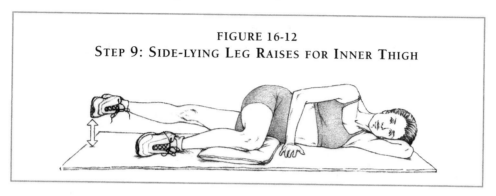

FIGURE 16-12
STEP 9: SIDE-LYING LEG RAISES FOR INNER THIGH

COMMON MISTAKES.

Allowing the hips to drift forward or backward out of alignment.

Step 10: Squats

This exercise strengthens the front and back of the thighs and the buttock muscles. Your torso muscles also help stabilize posture and balance during the exercise.

PROMPTS.

Do this exercise on a hard surface and not a cushy mat. Try it near a doorjamb or back of a chair where you can take hold for balance if needed. Stand with feet shoulder-width apart, toes pointing either forward or turned slightly outward. Hold both arms out in front of you for balance (like a sleepwalker) as you begin bending into the squat position (see Figure 16-13). The key to doing this exercise correctly is to make sure the knees track in the same direction as your middle to little toes, and that they never go forward enough to hover over or beyond the toes. For this to happen, you need to keep most of your weight on your heels and allow the buttocks to jut backward, with your chest lifted, abs engaged, and back straight. Depending on your strength, you may squat low enough to where the thighs are parallel with the floor, but no lower, as this is too stressful on the knees. Now slowly stand back up. Repeat twelve times for one set.

To make this exercise easier, do not dip quite as low, or do wall squats (find a slick vertical surface, or put a stability ball between your back and the wall for ease of movement). The same principles apply, but your back remains up against the wall the whole time. Make sure your feet begin far enough from the wall so that if we saw a side view of you in the down position, your knees would be over your ankles, not your toes. To add challenge to the original exercise, you may hold light hand weights at your sides. During pregnancy, if this is still too much or you experience pain anywhere, ease up on the range of motion and stop if that doesn't help.

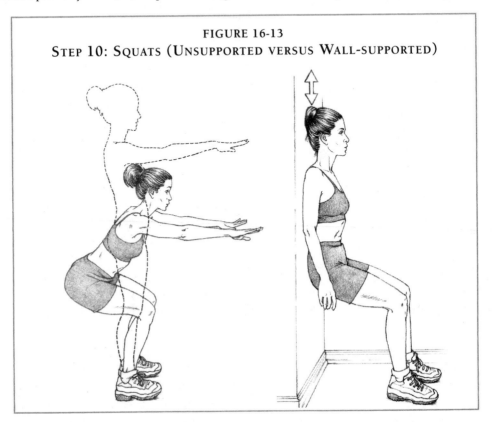

FIGURE 16-13
STEP 10: SQUATS (UNSUPPORTED VERSUS WALL-SUPPORTED)

COMMON MISTAKES.
Knees hovering over your toes or farther, knees turning in or out, and squatting too deep.

Step 11: Standing Calf Stretch

PROMPTS.
Lean with palms or forearms at chest level against a wall or at waist level on the edge of a countertop. Place your right toe an inch from the baseboard, your knee over your ankle. Take a large stride backward with the left foot. Now look down and make sure both feet point straight toward the wall. You may need to move the back heel slightly outward to straighten the foot alignment. Maintain neutral postural alignment. Keep hips squared toward the wall; your partner may need to adjust your hips so that one is not more forward than the other. Now press

that back heel slowly and firmly down toward the floor until you feel a good stretch in the calf muscle (see Figure 16-14). If you don't feel much of a stretch, move the back leg farther away.

Hold the stretch for ten to thirty seconds to the point of mild discomfort. Do not bounce. Then switch to the other leg. Repeat up to four times.

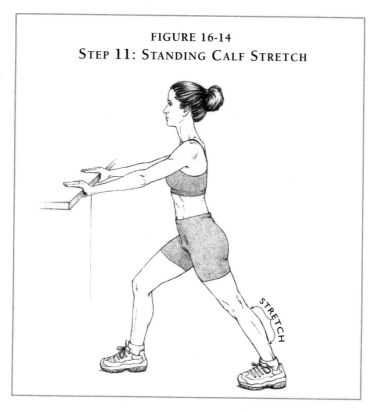

FIGURE 16-14
STEP 11: STANDING CALF STRETCH

COMMON MISTAKES.

Forgetting to maintain body alignment—torso, hips, toes, and heels—toward the wall.

FOR FUTURE REFERENCE: During Pregnancy

Do you ever experience painful calf cramps at night while lying in bed? If you cannot move quickly enough to get up and do this standing calf stretch, remember the phrase "Toes to the nose." Don't worry, we're not referring to a Rockettes-style kick! To alleviate the cramp while still lying in bed, simply straighten the leg and flex the foot in the direction of the nose, as opposed to the foot of the bed. (If you mistakenly point your toe, the cramp will worsen.) Also, remember the importance of keeping well hydrated, *not* strictly limiting sodium intake, and eating a good balance of foods from Chapter 11 containing calcium, potassium, and magnesium. All of these potentially aid in cramp prevention.

Step 12: Standing Quadriceps Stretch (Front of the Thigh)
PROMPTS.

Standing near a countertop or chair for balance, grab your right toe (or heel, if you prefer) with your right hand, and pull it slowly toward the buttocks. Knees should be fairly close together. Posture is erect, not bent forward (see Figure 16-15). You will feel a good stretch on the front of the thigh. For a little extra challenge and a better stretch where the hip flexes, add a backward pelvic tilt so the buttocks tuck slightly under. Hold the stretch for ten to thirty seconds to the point of mild discomfort. Do not bounce. Then switch to the other leg. Repeat up to four times.

You may find this stretch easier to negotiate in a side-lying position, as shown in steps 8 and 9.

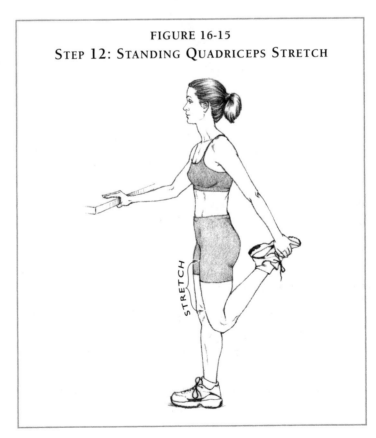

FIGURE 16-15
STEP 12: STANDING QUADRICEPS STRETCH

COMMON MISTAKES.

Bending forward and not standing tall.

Step 13: Standing Hamstring Stretch (Back of the Thigh)

PROMPTS.

The leg that you're stretching stays straight, heel on the floor (or on a low step) and toe up. The other foot is planted firmly below the body and the leg is bent. Both hands rest on the thigh of the bent leg. Then lean forward from the hip joint, keeping a straight back, not rounded (see Figure 16-16). Feel the stretch all along the back of the straight leg. Hold the stretch for ten to thirty seconds to the point of mild discomfort. Do not bounce. Then switch to the other leg. Repeat up to four times.

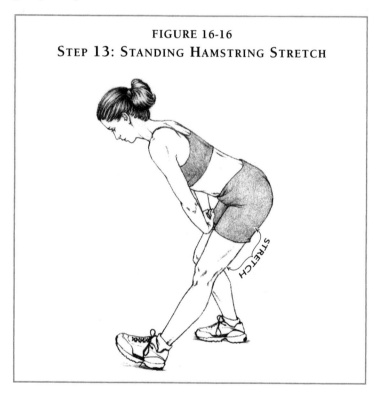

FIGURE 16-16
STEP 13: STANDING HAMSTRING STRETCH

COMMON MISTAKES

Insufficient flexion at the hip joint. To really feel this stretch, be sure the buttocks stick out and up.

Step 14: Kegels

These strengthen the muscles of the pelvic floor, and they can be done discreetly anytime, anywhere, and especially if you are between pregnancies and have less control of your bladder (stress incontinence). Kegel exercises should actually be continued into old age to maintain bladder control and healthy vaginal tone. Maintaining a healthy body weight is also important because according to the Nurses' Health Study, women who gain weight are much more likely to develop problems with controlling urination.

PROMPTS.

Take a belly breath, and then forcefully exhale as you tighten and "pull up" the muscles of the pelvic floor as if you were trying to halt the flow of urine and tighten the anal area at the same time. You might initially try this in the bathroom while urinating to determine if you're doing it correctly, but normally it is best *not* to intentionally stop the flow of urine because this could promote a urinary tract infection. Hold each contraction for five seconds, and eventually work up to holding it for ten seconds. Maintain normal breathing rhythm. Repeat five times for one set. You may do as many as fifty Kegels (ten sets) during the course of a day.

COMMON MISTAKES.

Not holding contractions for long enough; forgetting to breathe. (Counting aloud helps.)

These fourteen exercises constitute a basic, thorough preconception strength, and flexibility-training workout. If you consistently stick with it, you'll be in great shape for pregnancy. If you have any history of significant back pain or really problematic bladder control, your doctor may even recommend consultation with a physical therapist to assist you with customized muscle-strengthening exercises. For future reference, there are entire books devoted to pregnancy fitness. One of our personal favorites is physical therapist Elizabeth Noble's *Essential Exercises for the Childbearing Year.* Another is *Expecting Fitness* by Birgitta Gallo and Sheryl Ross, MD.

CHAPTER 17

Romancing the Egg

$\mathcal{Y}$ou and your partner have spent the past three months or so doing everything in your power to prepare for pregnancy. You've eaten right, taken vitamins, addressed unhealthy habits, and, we hope, replaced them with more beneficial new ones, such as exercising regularly. Perhaps you've also taken steps to improve certain aspects of your physical environment. Now that you're both prepared for the healthiest possible conception, you can actually start trying to have a baby. It will take timing, persistence, and luck, but also a little bit of fun and romance!

HOW DO YOU GET PREGNANT? IT'S JUST THE BIRDS AND BEES, RIGHT?

Every couple considering conception has their own timeline, which depends on maternal age, previous obstetrical history, personal timing needs, and medical issues. To help you decide what your time horizon is, and your "fertility personality," please complete the following brief questionnaire. It is not a scientifically tested survey, but it will help personalize this chapter while you get a feel for your desired pregnancy timing, or how relaxed or rushed you are. Those of you who desire a more leisurely approach to conception (the "Zen" group) may wish to skip the more detailed sections geared to those in a hurry to get pregnant (the "Zoom" group). For our Zoom readers, we note sections with details, tools, or strategies specifically geared to you by a . Some of our Zoom readers may be more apprehensive about the pregnancy pursuit than necessary. This chapter will refine your fertility awareness and help you relax and enjoy the process a bit more.

FERTILITY "PERSONALITY" PROFILE

This short questionnaire will help focus your reading from here on. It may also help you manage expectations about how long it will take to conceive. By circling your responses to these questions, you'll see at a glance where along the conception quest you most realistically fall. Those with

higher scores will naturally prefer to cut to the chase, paying particular attention to the information, which is scaled to your needs, and you can "zoom" right to it.

Circle your score (or "red flag" symbol) for each question and record in column to right.

					POINTS	SCORE
Time spent trying to conceive:	Haven't started yet **0 pts**	1–6 months **5 pts**	7–12 months **10 pts**	>12 months **20 pts**		
Unprotected sex for:	Haven't started yet **0 pts**	1–6 months **5 pts**	7–12 months **10 pts**	>12 months **15 pts**		
Age	<30 years **0 pts**	30–34 years **2 pts**	35–39 years **10 pts**	≥40 years **20 pts**		
Previous successful pregnancy?	none **5 pts**	1 **2 pts**	2 **1 pt**	>2 **0 pts**		
Previous miscarriage?	none **0 pts**	1 **0 pts**	2 🚩	>2 🚩🚩		
Timing to desired conception	Now **10 pts**	Within 3 months **5 pts**	Within 6 months **2 pts**	Within a year **1 pt**		
Body mass index (BMI) (See Fig. 14-1)	<18.5 🚩	18.5–24.9 —	25–29.9 🚩	≥30 🚩🚩		
Medical condition requiring daily medication?	Yes 🚩	No —				

TOTAL POINTS: _____

Key

 "Zen" = <25 points

 "Zoom" = ≥25 points

Any red flags? _____ (refer to following notes)

 If your weight or a medical condition is flagged, use a little extra time to incorporate recommendations from earlier chapters and work toward your best preconception health. Otherwise, there's the potential to be hindered by an uncontrolled medical condition or weight that's too low or high. We also recommend paying close attention to the zoom points so that you are savvy about your fertility signs once you're ready

 Those in the Zoom group are preconception-healthy and want to do everything in their power to improve the odds of quickly conceiving by predicting ovulation and pinpointing possible fertility issues right away (Chapter 18). We know you'll pay careful attention to the text and Zoom-designated features.

 Those who are not predominantly Zen-minded are preconception-healthy, but at peace *not* knowing all the details of their body's fertility signals. They'll likely toss out birth control and let nature take its course, skimming or skipping over the Zoom features. (Yes, we know this is the populist interpretation of the Zen state, not true Zen, which is a highly focused state achieved by meditation.)

Here is how a couple of our readers used this guide:

Score 1 + . Lani is twenty-six and Jai is twenty-eight. They married recently and dream of having a large family, but they are not in a rush. They both have careers and have not yet decided how they will balance work and family. Lani's health and weight are good and she is active. She does have asthma but it is under control with daily medication, and they have both been following the preconception-friendly lifestyle outlined in this book for three months. If anyone is asking, they are "not trying" but would be happy if they conceived within a year.

What happened? After four months of unprotected intercourse, Lani and Jai conceived their first child!

Score 37. Jill, age thirty-three, and Jerod, age thirty-eight, would like to have a baby as soon as possible (now!) but have not conceived after seven months of trying. Jill enjoys being physically fit and is an avid runner. She is lean, with a BMI of 19. She has been charting her fertility signs, but her cycle seems to be irregular. Her friends recommended that she quit running, and her doctor gave her a prescription for Clomid to promote ovulation.

What happened? Jill wanted to avoid the potential risks and side effects that accompany medication, so with the support of her physician, she put off filling her prescription to see whether a change in her running habits might help enough. She didn't quit running, but she did cut back her weekly mileage. She also monitored all her fertility signs, which became more predictable once she understood exactly what to look for. Three months later their baby was conceived!

Score 55+ 🚩 🚩 Kendra, age thirty-six, and her husband, Cody, age forty, have been trying to conceive without success for a year. Fertility signs are more than admittedly a bit of a mystery to her, even now. Kendra's weight has been an issue all her life, and her BMI is 33; otherwise, she is relatively healthy.

What happened? Even though Kendra's score indicated she might fall into the category of a Zoom fertility personality, she paid attention to the red flags that cautioned her to refocus her energy on healthier eating and exercise to give her BMI a fighting chance (Chapter 14). Five months later her BMI had dropped below 30 (a lower risk category and her best effort) and she was in tune with her fertility signals, ready to conceive! She maintained her new lifestyle habits and healthier weight, and conceived within four months.

Practical Application

Predicting Your Period

In order to figure out when the best baby-making time is for you, you'll need to know your cycle. In the menstrual chart shown in Figure 17-1, pencil in the first day you begin menstruating and the last. If you can remember the dates when your periods started for the past two to three months, you can record that, too. Soon you'll observe a pattern, or perhaps notice a lack of pattern, either of which will help you understand fertility signs. If you take note of how long your cycles are, you can be almost certain that you are most likely to conceive 14 to 17 days before you begin to bleed. And if your periods are predictable, you can begin to see when you'll be most fertile for the months to come. You should notice changes in your cervical mucus just before ovulation—it will become stretchy instead of sticky. We provide more detail on this in the next section.

For Zens, this may be all you need to take note of for now, but if you are a Zoom or have irregular periods, you should also focus on additional fertility signals (see "Signs That Ovulation Is Imminent," pages 505–508). Keep these records until you conceive. If you keep track of your menstrual period, it will also be much easier for you and your doctor to identify any fertility issues as well as determine your due date when you conceive.

FIGURE 17-1
MENSTRUAL DIARY CHART WITH SAMPLE FIRST MONTH MARKED

Menstrual Chart
Record your menstrual blood flow and cervical mucus changes to detect ovulatory patterns each month.

Date	1	2	3	4	5	6	7	8	9	10	11	12	13	14	15	16	17	18	19	20	21	22	23	24	25	26	27	28	29	30	31	Length of cycle (no. of days from start of period to beginning of next period)	Breast self-exam done (✓)
(Sample)																																	
Jan																																	
Feb																																	
Mar																																	
Apr																																	
May																																	
June																																	
July																																	
Aug																																	
Sept																																	
Oct																																	
Nov																																	
Dec																																	

My notes: _____
_____

The first day of the cycle, called "DOC1," is the first day of normal bleeding (January 26 in the sample above).
During your period: L = light blood flow and X = normal blood flow
Near ovulation: cm = white/sticky cervical mucus, CM = clear egg-white cervical mucus, * = mittelschmerz

For your convenience, there is another full-page version of this chart in Appendix D that you can either tear out or photocopy.

OVULATION 411: THE BASICS OF HOW TO GET PREGNANT

Each month during our reproductive years the female reproductive system releases one (or two) eggs that can be fertilized by spermatozoa. The entire goal of a woman's menstrual cycle is to make it possible for her to conceive but, ironically, some of us spend most of our lives impeding fertility.

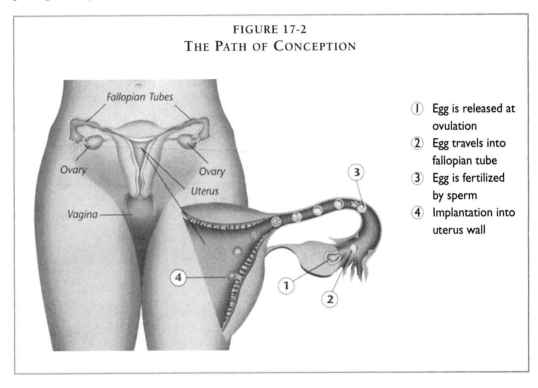

FIGURE 17-2
THE PATH OF CONCEPTION

① Egg is released at ovulation
② Egg travels into fallopian tube
③ Egg is fertilized by sperm
④ Implantation into uterus wall

The average couple has a 20 to 25 percent chance of conceiving each month if they make love on or around ovulation. This means about 84 percent of couples will conceive naturally within a year of trying. It is a fallacy that you are only fertile on the day you ovulate. After a symphony of hormonal changes, fifteen to twenty eggs per month are prepared but usually only one egg is released. These "chosen ones" survive approximately twenty-four hours as they travel through the fallopian tubes—hoping to encounter sperm—to the uterus. The good news is that sperm can survive from twenty-four to ninety-six hours in the female reproductive tract, where they lie in wait for the egg. (See Figure 17-2.) This results in a three-to-four-day fertile period or "prime time" for conception each month. That is, the two days before you ovulate and the day of ovulation are the most likely to lead to success. With this timing in mind, if you are making love every other day of the week you expect to ovulate, it's a good bet that you won't miss the time that the egg is released. But you don't have to be militant about the every-other-day guideline—a Saturday/Sunday/Wednesday schedule would work, too, for those with no suspicion of a low sperm count (otherwise go with Friday/Sunday/Wednesday). Just be sure to hit one of your peak fertile days, and remember, lovemaking should still be fun!

Though it is commonly believed that every woman ovulates on the fourteenth day of the cycle, there is great variation in normal menstrual cycles and you'll be best able to predict ovulation if you learn to read your body's signs. A normal menstrual cycle can vary from twenty-four to thirty-five days, which means ovulation can occur any time between ten and twenty-one days after the last menstrual period started.

There are a number of reasons why ovulation may not be occurring to provide an egg for fertilization. Extremes in body weight can have a negative impact on ovulation. If you're underweight, there is a dearth of estrogen available to help release mature eggs. Likewise, when you're overweight, the hormones available to control ovulation can be unbalanced. In men and women, the use of tobacco, alcohol, and recreational drugs can reduce the viability of sperm and the likelihood of healthy ovulation. The use of certain herbal supplements may also disrupt your hormonal milieu and potentially damage egg or sperm DNA, possibly leading to birth defects or miscarriage. Studies are now suggesting that extreme mental and emotional stress may have a negative effect on ovulation as well. All of these risk factors are discussed in detail in previous chapters. The next chapter focuses on how to diagnose a fertility problem.

Signs That Ovulation Is Imminent

Although you know the basics of getting pregnant, it's more efficient if you know your body well enough to predict when you're ovulating. As we discussed in Chapter 5, ovulation is triggered by a surge of luteinizing hormone, or LH, that tells the ovary to release the egg. Some women feel a lower abdominal cramp or achy feeling for up to a day or two when the egg is released; however, this midcycle discomfort, known as *mittelschmerz,* doesn't affect all women and is not the only sign that ovulation is occurring.

When you are about to ovulate, your cervical mucus becomes wetter, slippery, and stretchier, similar in appearance to uncooked egg whites. Some women produce enough of this cervical mucus as a vaginal discharge that it can be seen on the underwear or when wiping after urinating. For others it may be most noticeable after a bowel movement. Knowing your body's usual signs helps discriminate between a natural change in vaginal discharge, such as with ovulation, and signs of a vaginal infection, which would require medical treatment. (For instance, a vaginal discharge accompanied by vaginal itching, burning, and odor change would be most likely due to a vaginal infection.)

Changes in cervical mucus reflect an increase in the estrogen level, preparing your body for ovulation. Since these cervical mucus changes are not always obvious, you can see if you are about to ovulate by placing your index finger gently into the vagina and bringing a little of the discharge out. Usually you want to start checking for these changes as early as a few days after your period has stopped. Then place your thumb against your index finger with the discharge already on it and see if you can stretch the mucus between them. The further you can stretch the discharge (the maximum will be about two inches), the closer you are to ovulation. You can also feel your cervix, which becomes softer at this time, by gently inserting a clean finger into your vagina and pressing up and forward. The cervix is the only firm object in the area and feels a little like the tip of your nose. (Don't be alarmed if you feel something hard back toward your buttocks; it's probably stool in your rectum.)

If you don't notice any of these physical signs of ovulation but are having a regular menstrual cycle, do not be concerned. You are probably still releasing an egg each month. If you are a Zen

reader, 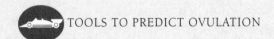, you may want to give it a couple of months and see if you conceive before exploring your fertility signs further. However, it is possible to have a period without ovulation, and conversely, you can ovulate when you don't have menstrual bleeding. If you are a Zoom person, you may want to try one or two more technical means of determining when and if you ovulate (see "Tools to Predict Ovulation" below). You may also wish to consult Toni Weschler's definitive guide, *Taking Charge of Your Fertility* (Collins Living, 2006). Her comprehensive book is an excellent reference regarding fertility and ovulation.

TOOLS TO PREDICT OVULATION

Basal body temperature (BBT) charts keep track of the changes in your body temperature that occur throughout the month and that reflect the changes in your hormonal milieu as you ovulate. This means that if a rise in temperature is seen, ovulation already occurred during the past twenty-four to thirty-six hours, so optimal timing for conception would have been in the days just before your temperature began rising (a modest dip in temperature may or may not be detected before the main rise); some women are still fertile during the twenty-four hours that span the temperature rise as charted. With a few months of active charting under your belt, you'll be better able to predict when the rise is about to happen. This progesterone supports the growth of the next endometrium (womb lining) that will be needed to welcome an embryo. After you are done menstruating, you can begin to chart a BBT trend. Take your temperature immediately upon awakening and *while still in bed* each morning. Whatever device you use to check your temperature, be consistent and use the same device daily. If your temperature remains elevated for fourteen days after your most likely day of ovulation, you may be pregnant! (See Figure 17.3.)

By maintaining a BBT chart for a few months, you can spot the temperature change that occurs at ovulation. Usually if you count fourteen days back from the first day of your period, you can confirm that ovulation occurred when your BBT predicted it would. You can then use this information to predict your *next* ovulation for the purpose of conception. If your body temperature seems to rise and fall haphazardly, this may indicate that you are ill (e.g., a cold or flu), that you are not ovulating, or that your sleep patterns are too unpredictable for this method to work correctly.

See Appendix D for a blank BBT chart that you can use for your own cycle.

FIGURE 17-3
SAMPLE BASAL BODY TEMPERATURE CHART—PREGNANCY DETECTED

Below is a sample BBT chart of a woman who achieved pregnancy during the recorded cycle. The intersection of the horizontal and vertical lines indicates the day of ovulation. Note that egg-white cervical mucus was recorded for three days prior to ovulation ("E" noted in the "CM" rows in the chart) and the BBT rose within twenty-four hours after ovulation, an indicator that ovulation has occurred. Pregnancy is likely when the BBT remains elevated after ovulation, as seen in this cycle. A blank BBT chart is provided in Appendix D for your use—either tear out or photocopy. Additional copies can be printed at the website address noted below the chart.

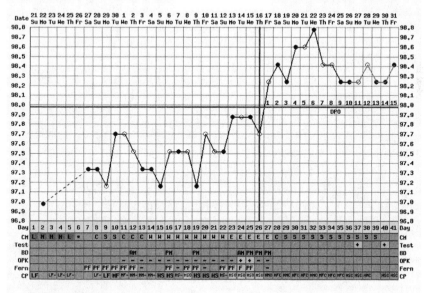

CM (row)—cervical mucus
www.FertilityFriend.com
E—Raw egg white consistency (slippery and clear)

Used with permission (www.FertilityFriend.com)

OVULATION PREDICTOR KITS

These kits measure the level of luteinizing hormone in your urine (or saliva), which surges for two to three days prior to ovulation. When the kit indicates the hormone surge has occurred, ovulation is *about* to happen, twelve to thirty-six hours later. The kits can be purchased at any drugstore for about $30–$50 per cycle, and each kit will provide five to nine days of testing. Many women, especially those whose bodies don't overtly signal ovulation or whose cycles are somewhat irregular, have found them to be very helpful. On the other hand, some women are frustrated by readings that say that they *are* ovulating when they actually are *not* (false positives), or vice versa (false negatives). This can happen if your hormone levels fluctuate more than average, which is especially common over the age of forty. Many other factors can influence the validity of the ovulation predictor kits. To improve the likelihood of an accurate reading, we recommend consistently testing at the same time of the day and around the time ovulation should occur; testing the first (concentrated) urine of the day, which may contain a higher hormone level; and using kits before the expiration date so the reagents are fresh. Don't use the kits if you are taking hormonal medications (Menopur, Repromix, or any human gonadotropin or HCG-containing injections). A positive result late in your cycle may even mean the possibility that you are already pregnant! We therefore recommend that you observe as many of the natural signs of ovulation—cervical mucus changes, middle-cycle discomfort, and temperature fluctuation—that are pertinent to *your* body for a successful understanding of your reproductive cycle.

Saliva Ovulation Testing
Examining your saliva with a special mini-microscope allows you to detect imminent ovulation up to three days in advance. The rising estrogen level prior to ovulation causes changes to your cervical mucus and your saliva. Two devices can detect these changes in saliva—a saliva microscope (about $50) and an electrolyte-measuring device (about $250; OvaCue). For the microscope (we tested the Fertile-Focus model), a drop of saliva is placed on the slide and allowed to dry. When observed at 50X magnification through the microscope, you look for evidence of "ferning"—which looks like frost on a windowpane. The testing should be done first thing in the morning, before eating, drinking, or brushing your teeth. While some women are frustrated by trying to discern the difference between "not fertile," "transitional," and "fertile," other women swear by the convenience, portability, and early detection. Another advantage for both devices is that there is a one-time expense rather than a monthly expense to resupply test strips. These mini-microscopes are the size of a lipstick case. Imagine your friends' reaction when you pull one of these out of your purse at the next girls' night out!

Angie and Dan are in their early thirties and have been married for three years. They both have fairly demanding jobs that require frequent travel. When they decided that they were ready to start trying to get pregnant, Angie began reading books to find out how to improve their chances by trying to tell when ovulation occurs. She wanted to do this before buying expensive ovulation predictor kits. Much to her frustration, it was very difficult to decipher her body's signals. Angie worried that this, coupled with travel schedules that kept her and Dan apart several days each month, would make it difficult for them to conceive a baby. To her credit, Angie persisted with monitoring her fertility signs and began to recognize that the signs were there—just too subtle to recognize when it was all new. Now she and Dan just needed to work on the logistics of being to-gether at the right time.

If, like Angie and Dan, you are one of the many couples who travel often on business, or who work on opposite shifts, you may have difficulty getting together when ovulation is most likely to occur. Sometimes it requires creative solutions and even tough decisions in order to routinely spend time with your partner. Interestingly enough, though, it's also possible to get *too* focused on spending time together. Some of our patients have spontaneously conceived after one or the other (or both) has had some time to themselves, such as a fishing trip with the guys or a weekend visit to a best girlfriend. Returning to each other mentally refreshed and glad to see each other could be all you need.

Common Questions When You're Trying to Conceive

My partner says having sex on demand takes the fun out of our lovemaking. What should I do?

For some couples, lovemaking for the sake of conception can have an enhancing effect on the libido. For others it can have a dampening effect. Most couples tell us that they experience both at different times. Certainly, if your cervical mucus, basal body temperature, or ovulation predictor kit tells you that an egg is on its way, you will probably feel some degree of urgency about having sex, regardless of whether you or your partner is actually in the mood. But stress can inhibit arousal and performance, making conception that much more difficult to achieve. So try to avoid rolling over in bed on the day you ovulate and saying to your partner, "Honey, it's now or never!" Remember that sexual desire is very individualized and that whatever feels right to you *as a couple* is right. If you find that lovemaking three to four times a week (roughly every other day) puts too much pressure on you, stick with your usual sexual activity for a few months and see what happens.

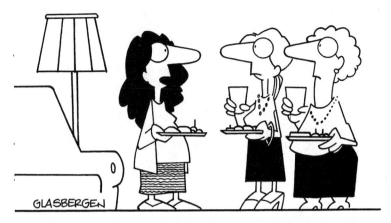

"My husband and I had to try 70 times before I got pregnant—that was one weekend I'll never forget!"

Copyright © 1998 by Randy Glasbergen. www.glasbergen.com

Will a lubricant prevent conception?

Most women are naturally more lubricated during midcycle, but if you wish to use an additional lubricant, read the label to make sure that it contains no spermicide or alcohol. A Committee Opinion of the American Society for Reproductive Medicine (2008) reported no negative effects on sperm function if canola oil, mineral oil, or hydroxycellulose-based lubricants such as Pre-Seed were used; other lubricants such as K-Y Jelly, Astroglide, and saliva all may negatively affect sperm motility. Avoid using highly perfumed soaps or lotions, as they may irritate your vagina and vulva. Douching is also not advisable when trying to conceive because it changes the normal acidity in the vaginal environment and can result in vaginal dryness and/or yeast and bacterial infections. If you must douche for any reason, speak to your doctor first. (Once you are pregnant, *never* douche.)

When I stand up after making love, a great deal of discharge comes out of my vagina. Am I losing too much of my husband's sperm?

The fluid that is discharged after lovemaking is a combination of your natural vaginal fluids, lubricants (either natural or synthetic), and semen, approximately 90 percent of which remain at the cervix as a reservoir and the other 10 percent of motile sperm entering the uterus less than sixty to ninety seconds after ejaculation. Those sperm present in discharge released from the vagina would not have made it all the way to the egg anyway.

Is there a recipe for blue or pink?

Although the first wish of most prospective parents is for a healthy baby, regardless of gender, many couples are interested in trying to influence nature's preference for the sex of their baby. You may have heard the old wives' tales that specify foods to eat, various lovemaking positions to use, and allowing the phases of the moon to determine when to make love so that you can conceive a boy or a girl. Although some of these suggestions have been studied by researchers and might be fun to try, they have little effect on gender determination. However, there are ways to "stack the deck," so to speak, in favor of one sex or the other. It all has to do with the sperm.

All eggs carry an X chromosome, while sperm cells carry either an X or a Y chromosome. An XX combination will produce a girl, while an XY combination will result in a boy. The X-carrying sperm are larger, hardier, and longer-lived, making them better able to tolerate higher vaginal acidity levels. The Y-carrying sperm are smaller and faster but are more fragile and thrive in alkaline vaginal conditions.

Most "natural" gender selection techniques manipulate the female reproductive environment to favor one or the other type of sperm. None, however, is foolproof. Research shows that under normal circumstances a slight majority of the embryos conceived are male, but for a variety of reasons male fetuses are the ones more likely to be spontaneously miscarried.

To date, the only method that can almost guarantee gender selection is preimplantation genetic diagnosis (PGD) via IVF, offering 95 to 100 percent success rates, with an embryo tested for its gender re-implanted into the uterus. Sperm sorting, with 65 to 70 percent accuracy for gender selection, choose a girl-bound X-carrying sperm or a boy-bound Y-carrying sperm that can be isolated by weight and speed. Once a specific type of sperm is isolated, it can then be implanted into the egg for fertilization, with one specific male- or female-producing sperm injected into an egg, known as intracellular sperm injection (ICSI). Both PGD and ICSI require IVF, which is quite expensive and is usually reserved for those couples with infertility or hereditary concerns (see Chapter 6). In the end, most couples wishing to have a choice in the sex of their baby have to accept a wide margin of uncertainty. The mystery remains.

AM I PREGNANT?

Once you've made love at the time that you believed you were most fertile, you will probably spend the rest of your cycle wondering whether or not you've conceived. If your period doesn't start when it should, you should take a home urine pregnancy test or call your doctor's office to schedule a test. Most women first use a home pregnancy test because they are fast and inexpensive. More importantly, if used properly, the urine pregnancy test is between 91 and 97 percent accurate as soon as seven to ten days after conception has occurred. We still recom-

Strategy for Gender Selection: The Shettles Method

In the early 1970s, Dr. Landrum Shettles developed a method of timed lovemaking based on the different characteristics of X- and Y-carrying sperm that has been 75 percent effective in selecting a particular gender, and similar success rates for both natural intercourse and artificial insemination were reported.

This method can be confusing to remember, especially in the moment, and it requires an acute body awareness to predict your ovulation accurately. While we are not recommending you go to these lengths, we'll try to help clarify his recommendations.

Remember the tale of the tortoise and the hare? Think of the X-sperm as the tortoise (slow, but with a lot of stamina) and the Y-sperm as the hare (faster, and easily fatigued). Keep this metaphor in mind as you review the Shettles method.

TO IMPROVE YOUR CHANCES OF HAVING A BOY

- You want the faster Y-sperm (the hares) to reach the egg first, when the environment in the vagina is more alkaline than usual due to increased cervical mucus production.
- Lovemaking should occur exclusively during the day before and the day of ovulation (and if your timing is precise enough, aim for the twelve hours before ovulation).
- Avoid vaginal lubricants and jellies, as they increase the acidity of the vaginal fluid.

TO IMPROVE YOUR CHANCES OF HAVING A GIRL

- You want the slower X-sperm (the tortoises) to reach the egg first, so give them a head start by having intercourse frequently (even daily) from near the end of menstrual flow up to two to three days before ovulation. Abstain from normal sexual activity for a few days until ovulation has passed.
- The X-sperm can handle the more acidic vaginal environment prior to ovulation and can wait patiently for the egg's debut. The Y-sperm competitors have less staying power in these race conditions. The end result is more X-sperm waiting around at the "finish line," effectively stacking the deck in favor of a girl being conceived.
- Though Shettles theoretically says you could conceive a girl if you wait until after ovulation (when cervical mucus dries and pH reverts back to acidic), the chances are much lower because the egg may no longer be viable.

The Shettles method also recommends mapping your cycle at least two to three months in advance using cervical mucus testing (confirming stretchy, egg-white-like mucus for two days), BBT charts, or ovulation predictor kits to determine your specific pattern of ovulation. His method also works best if abstinence or a condom is used during the nonoptimal days to increase the odds that the desired gender-specific sperm are available for fertilization.

mend waiting until your usual menstrual time has passed before checking a urine pregnancy test. Always keep track of the date of your menstrual periods because your doctor will use your last menstrual period (or LMP) to determine your due date. The expected date of delivery is usually 284 days after your LMP, or 270 days after conception.

To get the most accurate reading of your pregnancy test:

- Use the first urine of the day, when the concentration of the pregnancy hormone human chorionic gonadotropin (HCG) is highest and can be most readily detected by the test.
- Follow the instructions carefully.
- Recheck the test results the next morning and, if you have not had a menstrual cycle, repeat it again in a week.

If you continue to get negative test results but your period still hasn't started, call your doctor to schedule a blood test, which is more sensitive and can detect a pregnancy five to seven days after conception. False negative results from home urine tests are usually due to an error in carrying out the test and are quite common. False positives, that is, a positive urine pregnancy test when a pregnancy doesn't exist, are rare and may be the result of a previous pregnancy loss that is not yet completely resolved, test error, or an error in reading the test.

Even if the pregnancy test hasn't confirmed a pregnancy yet, it's important to continue the baby-friendly habits you've been practicing up to this point. Remember, what you might think is a light period could instead be spotting caused by the embryo burrowing into the uterine lining during implantation, a normal occurrence for some women.

If you are pregnant, you can skip to the Epilogue to whet your appetite for the next stage in this wonderful journey.

I'm Not Pregnant Yet—Should I Be Concerned?

Once you start trying to conceive, every month you are not pregnant may raise doubts about your fertility. Remember, only a minority of couples become pregnant right off the bat, and it's totally normal for it to take more time.

When is the right time to be concerned about your ability to conceive? For women under thirty-five years of age, the usual recommendation is to try to conceive for twelve months before evaulation or fertility treatment is even considered, because success is likely. If you are over thirty-five years of age, an evaluation of your fertility is reasonable after six months of trying. If you are over forty, seek evaluation after three to four months of trying because the need to optimize each cycle becomes more crucial. However, for some couples who have a specific concern, medical condition, or firm timeline, some fertility evaluation can be performed after six months of trying to conceive (especially for those who have been meticulously tracking fertility signs for those six months).

Based on your individual circumstances, you may want to read more about diagnosing infertility in the next chapter. However, if you began in Zen mode and see that your timeline is narrowing, first read the Zoom information carefully for a few menstrual cycles before becoming concerned about your fertility.

CHAPTER 18

Understanding Infertility

*N*o matter what your timeline was to begin with, not conceiving as quickly as you had hoped can be a disappointing blow. Every menstrual cycle can lead to greater desperation in attempting pregnancy and a heavier strain on one's relationship. Be reassured that getting pregnant, no matter your age or your issues, will take time and patience. Contrary to how you might feel, each month actually brings you one step closer to pregnancy. But don't despair— if you can't get pregnant the "old-fashioned" way, the medical community can help you. And you can help yourself by staying positive, by keeping the lines of communication open between you and your partner, and by engaging in moments of intimacy without a conception goal.

At the end of the last chapter we discussed when to be concerned about your ability to conceive (see summary on page 516). If these guidelines indicate that you or your spouse may need a fertility evaluation, try not to think of it as a disease. Some fertility issues are readily resolved. After all, our bodies were designed to create new life! If that's so, you may be wondering, "Why, then, are women in the most developed countries having such trouble?" Beyond spending more time pursuing education and careers, which often means we put more energy into fewer children at a later age, the advances of the last century inadvertently created barriers to fertility. Some are environmental, such as increased exposure to chemicals in our daily lives. Others are lifestyle-related, such as extremes in weight and tobacco use. The industrial revolution modernized everything from sewing clothes to harvesting grain. We simply don't have to work as hard at just living our lives, we are more sedentary, and we tend to overeat but undernourish, becoming overweight or obese as a result. Some women strive for the other end of the continuum and overexercise or undereat. Because many fertility issues are unexplained, trying to find a balance between exertion and consumption will help improve health overall, and potentially fertility, too.

When to Seek a Fertility Evaluation

- Over forty years: after three to four months of trying.
- Thirty-five to forty years: after six months of trying.
- Less than thirty-five years: after twelve months of trying. Sometimes an evaluation is reasonable after six months of trying if there is a specific concern, medical condition, or firm timeline. However treatment for unexplained infertility is typically discouraged until after a total of twelve months of trying because success is likely without medical intervention.
- Any age: if irregular cycles, or regular cycles longer than forty days, are noted.
- If you have had two or more miscarriages (see Chapter 5 for more details about recurrent losses).

Let's redouble our effort to strive for a balance in exercise, work/life stresses, and weight to help you conceive. Other conditions can be treated with medical interventions, such as medication to induce ovulation or even surgery to address endometriosis. Your body is not your enemy, and you are not at war with your ovaries. Try to relax, because our experience is that in many cases, less is more: less thinking, less stress, less analyzing, less testing . . . To that end, we'll review some things you can do to become healthy first, fertile second. We'll start with the basics, then step you through the most common fertility issues and medical workups so you know what to expect.

ARE THERE THINGS I CAN DO NOW TO IMPROVE FERTILITY?

Yes! This is a good time to reflect on the preceding chapters, consider areas that you may still need to address, and revisit priorities that might need some adjustment. For instance, our athletic readers may need to reflect on their training intensity by asking "Am I *really* willing to reduce my running mileage?" Slight adjustments may be all it takes to improve your chances of conceiving. We're not saying to stop running; we're saying to seek balance.

That being said, there are only so many things that *are* under your control. Identifying and coming to peace with factors beyond your control is essential. The following round-up of previous chapters may help you identify things you *can* do to further promote fertility.

- Maybe you hoped to escape tackling a weight issue. Often just a *small* amount of weight loss or gain can rebalance the hormones to favor fertility. See Chapter 14.
- Or maybe you skipped over some of the gynecological information because you aren't

entirely comfortable knowing more about your genitalia or vaginal secretions. This takes some getting used to but is incredibly empowering! See Chapters 5 and 17 for help predicting your fertile window.

- Maybe you see restrictions on your or your partner's drinking, smoking, or drug use as strictly moralizing instead of considering the solid scientific data to back it. These data often come from countries where such practices are more socially acceptable. See Chapter 2.
- Maybe you feel like you have no good options for exercise (due to lack of time, bad weather, discomfort) so you skipped over the anecdotes about how people just like you made it work. See Chapter 15. Pair this with Chapter 13's "Preconception Meal Makeovers."
- Maybe you or your partner have been avoiding dealing with something—a miscarriage or abortion, or even a history of abuse as a child—and this is placing additional strain on your relationship. See Chapter 1.
- Maybe you tend to be more naturally pessimistic than optimistic, which has a definite impact on fertility. Or maybe you are depressed. Now is the time to reach out and seek some help. This is important to resolve before pregnancy, as it has an impact on your postpartum adjustment as well. See Chapters 1 and 7.
- Maybe a career change is needed to facilitate being less stressed or being in a more environmentally suitable conditions. See Chapter 1, including financial readiness, and Chapter 3.

Perhaps the toughest part of needing to tackle any remaining issues is knowing that many people can get pregnant without having to go this far. It seems so unfair. Although this work can be a tremendous challenge, you *will* be better off in the end, and all these changes will benefit you as a parent. Keep in mind your focus: the body favors reproduction when the physical, mental, emotional, and environmental conditions are conducive to sustaining life. You and your partner *can* make a difference.

Complementary Approaches

In addition to a healthy diet and exercise, coupled with traditional medical interventions, many women are also turning to complementary approaches to encourage ovulation and fertility. They often express a sense of having greater control over their bodies, a feeling that is particularly appealing when it may seem as if you're completely out of synch with your own body. Yoga and meditation to achieve relaxation and emotional balance may be helpful in improving fertility rates. Recent studies of mind-body programs demonstrated improvements in women who underwent IVF, with success rates increasing from 17 percent up to 40 percent when yoga and meditation were used in addition to traditional therapies.

Although herbal products are recommended by alternative medicine, they have not been proven to assist in fertility and in some cases are harmful to a developing fetus. See Chapter 8 for more information about herbal safety before and after conception.

One of the most popular natural therapies for improving fertility is acupuncture. Studies show that blood flow to female reproductive organs increases after acupuncture is performed. Acupuncture has been proven to be helpful in a number of medical circumstances such as the treatment of asthma, nausea, and vomiting as a result of chemotherapy, fibromyalgia, and chronic pain syndromes. Many small studies have looked at the potential benefits of acupuncture to the fertility patient, but the findings have been inconsistent. However, all agree that acupuncture can lead to greater relaxation, which can assist in overall fertility in both men and women who were studied.

The hope is that acupuncture can also increase blood flow to the uterus (increasing its ability to receive an embryo after fertilization), increase blood flow to the ovaries, and change the hormonal milieu by increasing beta-endorphins to allow more consistent ovulation. One recent study from Hong Kong found that IVF patients who undergo egg retrieval and who received auricular (outer ear) acupuncture achieved a slightly improved pregnancy outcome compared to those who did not receive acupuncture. Other studies in men have shown an improved semen quality and sperm count after acupuncture sessions twice a week for five weeks. But a recent British meta-analysis (compiling all of the randomized trials looking at fertility and acupuncture) showed no improvement in the live birthrate among women who received acupuncture as part of their IVF protocol.

While the evidence is mixed, it is fair to say that acupuncture may increase blood flow to the female and male reproductive organs. And although the usefulness remains unproven, there is little harm in trying. Side effects of acupuncture include needle site infection and rare reports of internal bleeding after deep acupuncture by the unskilled or overenthusiastic. Researchers will undoubtedly focus on determining if and how acupuncture can facilitate pregnancy achievement and how many sessions of acupuncture are required to get the desired result. For now, it is safe to say that acupuncture will not discourage fertility.

DIAGNOSING INFERTILITY

Marjorie, thirty-four, a recently married lawyer, said, "I know I will have trouble getting pregnant because all of my friends have had to get help to get pregnant."

Sandra and John, both thirty-seven years of age, have had unprotected intercourse since they got married two years ago and have not conceived during that time. Even though they were not trying to get pregnant then, they are both worried about their fertility now that they want to try to conceive.

If no pregnancy results from spontaneous or timed intercourse, that is, intercourse during ovulation confirmed by BBT (basal body temperature) or ovulation predictor kits for the number of months mentioned earlier in this chapter, a workup for infertility should be considered. A couple may suffer from infertility caused by one or a combination of the following factors (illustrated graphically in Figure 18-1):

- 25 to 30 percent of couples have male factor infertility—this is a reduced sperm count or other sperm abnormalities that make conception more difficult.
- 25 to 30 percent of women have difficulty ovulating—this is a reflection of hormonal imbalances in estrogen and luteinizing hormones (LH), which affect egg release and development, as well as progesterone levels, which can lead to luteal phase defects. This also includes diminished ovarian reserve.
- 18 percent of women have a blockage in the fallopian tubes.
- 2 to 5 percent of women have a cervical factor that prevents the sperm from getting into the uterus.
- 20 to 30 percent of couples have no known reason for their infertility.

Your initial evaluation will begin with a thorough history in which you will be asked to describe:

- Your menstrual cycle history
- The timing and frequency of intercourse
- Medications and supplements you and your spouse may be using
- Your behavioral habits such as tobacco, alcohol, or illicit substance use
- Any previous history of pelvic pain, pelvic inflammatory disease (PID), previous abdominal or pelvic surgeries, or spontaneous losses in the first trimester
- Signs and symptoms of vaginal and sexually transmitted infections
- Use of lubricants, spermicides, perfumes, or scented oils that might be detrimental to your fertility

Female Athletes and Pseudo–Luteal Phase Defects

As introduced in Chapter 15 (pages 465–467), runners and other endurance athletes may need to rebalance their energy demands by eating more or exercising less in order to induce ovulation. Studies of female runners, for instance, have shown that the metabolic clearance of progesterone is significantly higher after exercise.

Progesterone is required to sustain the blastocyst implanted in the uterine lining, so even if you are ovulating and have a regular cycle, you may be jeopardizing the viability of your womb by clearing too much progesterone from your system.

Low progesterone is certainly not an issue for all female athletes, but if it is, it's probably only mimicking a true luteal phase defect. Those who have progesterone levels less than 10 ng/mL (tested on DOC [day of cycle] 22–24 in a 28- to 30-day cycle) may want to seriously consider toning down their workouts or liberalizing their calorie intake, or both, for at least ninety days to see if this tips the energy balance to favor both fitness and fertility. Remember how this worked for Jill in the last chapter (pages 501–502)? A true luteal phase defect involves more "players" on the reproductive playing field, an issue discussed next.

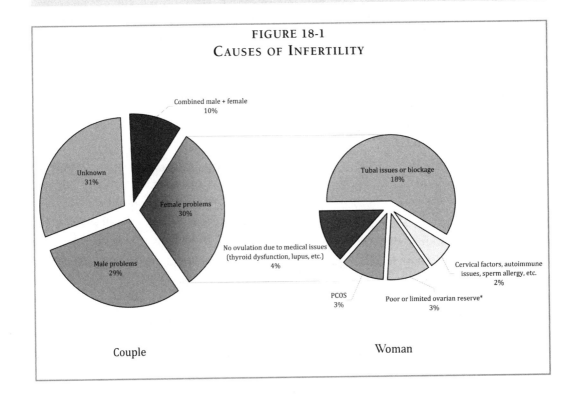

FIGURE 18-1
CAUSES OF INFERTILITY

Combined male + female
10%

Unknown
31%

Female problems
30%

Male problems
29%

No ovulation due to medical issues
(thyroid dysfunction, lupus, etc.)
4%

Tubal issues or blockage
18%

Cervical factors, autoimmune
issues, sperm allergy, etc.
2%

PCOS
3%

Poor or limited ovarian reserve*
3%

Couple

Woman

After a thorough history and physical examination, your infertility workup may begin with a month of testing to see if a cause can be found for the lack of fertility. Typically, a semen analysis is best performed at least forty-eight hours after the last ejaculation (via masturbation or intercourse) to determine if the movement and anatomy of the sperm are likely to result in fertilization. The semen analysis is usually done at an andrology laboratory or fertility clinic, where a semen sample is obtained after the man masturbates to ejaculation into a sterile cup. If the semen analysis identifies a problem, further evaluation of the male genitalia by a urologist can be helpful. (See Chapter 9 for more information on evaluation of the male reproductive system.)

Identifying and Treating Ovulatory Problems

The most common fertility issues for women are related to reduced ovarian reserve and/or difficulty with ovulation. The suspicion of ovulatory problems usually begins with a history of irregular or absent menstrual cycles, reinforced by disappointing trends in basal body temperatures (BBT) and ovulation predictor kit results. To further evaluate whether you may have ovulatory problems, several blood tests can be run over the course of a month to trace the hormonal signals from the brain to the ovaries. On the second to fifth day of your cycle, a blood test for thyroid hormone, follicle stimulating hormone (FSH), estrogen, and prolactin can identify gaps in the complex hormonal signaling pathway that may be preventing the ovaries from functioning properly. Around the twenty-first day of your cycle, a test for progesterone may be conducted to determine if ovulation did occur. One of the newest tools that determine *your* egg availability for ovulation is a simple blood test that measures your Anti-Müllerian hormone or AMH.

If your progesterone levels are low, you may have what is called a *luteal phase defect* or LPD, which is the inability to develop a mature endometrium, which would serve as a nest for the embryo. Diagnosis requires interpretation of menstrual cycle history and progesterone blood levels, but a definitive diagnosis is more elusive due to a wide range of normal variation in cycle length and hormone levels between women. LPDs may account for a small but significant percentage of infertility cases, but most experts still feel it is uncommon for an LPD to be the sole source of a couple's infertility. If a true LPD is suspected, treatment with supplemental timed progesterone is a relatively easy and safe way to correct the problem.

If ovulation does not appear to be occurring, there are a number of treatments available to stimulate ovulation. Each option has different side effects, risks, and pregnancy success rates; you, your partner, and your doctor have to choose a path comfortable for both of you to follow in your pursuit of fertility. The three most common methods used today include:

- **Clomid.** Also known as clomiphene citrate, this oral medication has been used for many years to stimulate ovulation among women whose ovarian systems are believed to have the potential to function if given some assistance. The cost of the medication is between $100 and $200 per cycle, and is usually not covered by insurance. The cost for Clomid cycling increases with various lab tests, possible intrauterine insemination, and ultrasounds to manage your cycle. (The ultrasounds are done to adjust the Clomid dosage to maximally encourage ovulation, but not so much that you are creating too many follicles.) If the appropriate follicle production occurs with Clomid therapy, it's usually advised to try three to six cycles stimulated by Clomid before going on to another form of induced ovulation, known as "superovulation." Before Clomid is tried, or if it fails to induce ovulation, your medical team may recommend an assessment of tubal patency to see if there is a blockage. A hysterosalpingogram uses a radioopaque dye to trace your tubes and see if an egg could travel from the ovaries to the uterus (see Figure 18-2). Using Clomid will not be appropriate if your tubes are blocked. Fertility rates, which range based on maternal age, can improve about 5 to 10 percent with Clomid. Common side effects can include mood changes, headaches, visual changes, significant abdominal bloating, and thickening of the cervical mucus, which can make it harder for the sperm to travel. (The cervical mucus can be thinned by taking 1 teaspoon of Robitussin CF two times per day from DOC 11 to DOC 18.) The increased likelihood of twins as a result of Clomid is approximately 5 to 10 percent, and 2 percent for triplets. There is no increased risk of early miscarriage or birth defects using this medication.

Laura, a thirty-four-year-old lawyer, and her husband, Doug, a thirty-six-year-old high school teacher, had tried to conceive for six months and were frustrated because Laura's menstrual cycle came every forty-five days. Otherwise she was healthy. Although ovulation predictor kits and medical evaluation confirmed Laura was not ovulating, she was reluctant to try any artificial technology to conceive. After three more months, she underwent one cycle of Clomid superovulation and is now six months pregnant.

- **Injectables (FSH related: Follistim, Gonadil-f; HMG related: Menopur, Repronex).** These are synthetic forms of follicle stimulating hormone (FSH) with or without LH, followed by an injection that "triggers" ovulation. Injectables are considered if ovulation doesn't occur with the use of Clomid. Ovulation with these medications can improve fertility 15 to 25 percent, when compared with a natural cycle (i.e., dependent on maternal age), with the exception of those women who are not ovulating due to polycystic ovary syndrome (see PCOS section in Chapter 5). The cost can range from $1,000 to $3,000 a cycle depending on how much medication is used and how much surveillance is needed to monitor your cycle. There is a 15 percent higher risk of multiple gestations such as twins or triplets if this form of medication-induced ovulation is used.

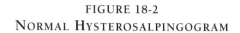

FIGURE 18-2
NORMAL HYSTEROSALPINGOGRAM

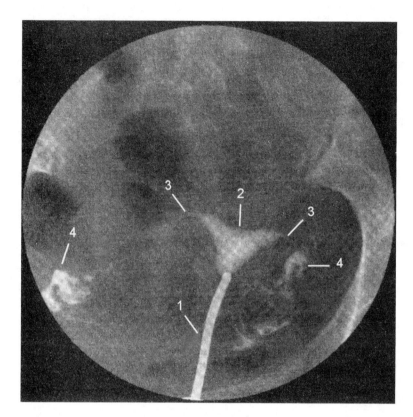

1. Catheter delivers dye into the uterus.
2. Normal uterine cavity is outlined by dye.
3. Fallopian tubes are faintly visible.
4. Dye spills from open fallopian tubes into the abdomen.

- **In vitro fertilization (IVF).** For women with ovulatory and/or tubal problems or men with very low sperm counts, IVF can be an effective treatment because mature eggs are harvested from dominant follicles in the ovaries, then combined with sperm outside of the potential mother, which allows a fertilized embryo to be replaced within her uterus, bypassing the fallopian tubes. IVF may be the right choice for you if your fallopian tubes are blocked (see "tubal factor infertility" on the next page) or a limited number of eggs are available, such as among women with limited ovarian reserve (fewer eggs) or premature ovarian failure and those over age forty. During one cycle of IVF, more embryos may be made than can or should be reimplanted in a woman. More is not always better, as the greater the number of embryos implanted in a potential mother, the higher the likelihood she may have a multiple gestation with twins, triplets, and so on. Extra unused embryos can be frozen for future implantation in your next pregnancy. Prior to 2007, the success rate of implantation with a frozen embryo was not as good as a fresh embryo (up to 10 to 20 percent less effective at implantation), and a slightly higher risk of miscarriage and failure of implantation were noted. New freezing techniques used since 2007 have resulted in pregnancy rates that are almost equivalent to fresh transfer cycles. Reproductive specialists are often asked if *unfertilized* eggs can be frozen. Improvements have been made in egg cryopreservation, but eggs are still more fragile than embryos. Continued improvements are being made to the technology of egg cryopreservation, particularly for women who are undergoing cancer treatment and want to try to save their eggs for future use, but the birth-rates and successful IVF rates when egg preservation is done are definitely less than when a fresh or frozen embryo is used.

Diagnosing and Treating Tubal-Factor Infertility

A blockage of the fallopian tubes is the second most common reason for women to be infertile. This is where fertilization actually occurs—it is essential to check and see if your fallopian tubes are open if standard medication strategies haven't led to pregnancy or if you are at increased risk for tubal blockage, such as with the following (introduced in Chapter 5):

- History of a sexually transmitted infection or pelvic inflammatory disease
- Endometriosis
- Adhesions due to previous surgery in your abdomen or pelvis
- Diverticulitis, an inflammation in the intestines causing pockets to develop that can cause scarring around the tubes.
- Previous ectopic pregnancy
- History of synthetic estrogen (diethylstilbestrol or DES) exposure while you were in utero (in other words, your mother took DES while you were in the womb)
- Fibroids in the sides of the uterus, which may obstruct the fallopian tube opening.

To confirm that your fallopian tubes are open and can act as a conduit for the egg to get to the waiting sperm, a hysterosalpingogram is performed between days seven and nine of your menstrual cycle. In this test, radioopaque dye is inserted through your cervix, outlines your uterine cavity, and spills out of your fallopian tubes if they are open (see Figure 18-2). This procedure carries a less than 1 percent risk of infection, which if found must be treated promptly to minimize the possibility of tubal damage from the test itself. It is also commonly thought that there is a slight increase in pregnancy rates in the month that follows a hysterosalpingogram, but these reports are mostly anecdotal. An ultrasound (sonohysterogram) may also prove helpful in evaluating the shape and normalcy of your tubal anatomy.

A more invasive technique to evaluate the fallopian tubes is done with laparoscopy via chromopertubation. In this case, a small telescope, called a laparoscope, is inserted into a tiny incision just below your navel that allows your doctor to see the inside of your abdomen. Blue dye is then injected into the uterus, and your doctor will watch to see if it travels out of your fallopian tubes.

The most common physical reasons for tubal blockage are STDs and endometriosis. Discussed earlier, STDs or pelvic inflammatory disease (or PID, which is caused by infection in the fallopian tubes) can cause scarring of the fallopian tubes, which prevents a normal passage for the egg to travel to meet the sperm. Endometriosis occurs when endometrial tissue ends up outside the uterine cavity. Almost 7 percent of reproductive-age women suffer from fertility problems and pelvic pain from endometriosis. We do not know the exact cause of endometriosis, but we think it is the result of menstrual blood that has been expelled in the wrong direction—upward through the fallopian tubes. These pieces of endometrium can then attach themselves to other abdominal organs such as the bladder, bowel, or ovaries, where they grow, shrink, and bleed in response to your usual monthly hormone cycle (see Figure 18-3).

Modern science has still not revealed why some women have endometriosis as a result of this menstrual blood retrograde travel and others do not. Researchers continue to better understand and cure this problem, which leads to chronic pelvic pain and infertility. Endometriosis carries a high physical and emotional toll due to chronic pain, costly medical therapy, such as Lupron, with the side effects of menopausal-like symptoms, or surgical removal of the ovaries if medical therapy is not helpful. The good news is that dramatic strides have been taken in medical treatments and reproductive technology to overcome the damage endometriosis does.

Many women with endometriosis will still be able to conceive and have babies. But among women who are infertile, endometriosis accounts for approximately one-third of the infertility problems. Symptoms of endometriosis include:

- **Pelvic pain.** When implanted endometrial tissue responds to hormonal stimulation of ovulation and menstrual cycling, it causes cyclic pain that occurs in midcycle or before the menstrual period. Over time the bleeding and scarring from the endometriosis can cause continuous pelvic pain as well as pain with and after intercourse.

- **Infertility.** If you have been unable to conceive after twelve cycles of trying and you have any history of pelvic pain, you may want to discuss an evaluation of endometriosis with your doctor.

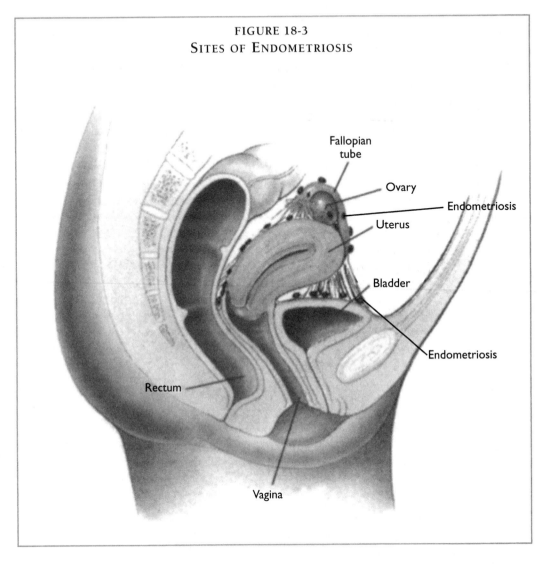

FIGURE 18-3
SITES OF ENDOMETRIOSIS

Fallopian tube

Ovary

Endometriosis

Uterus

Bladder

Endometriosis

Rectum

Vagina

A physical exam may reveal the scarring on the internal organs, but the definitive diagnosis is best made via laparoscopic surgery. Treatment for pelvic pain is available with the continuous use of oral contraceptives to reduce cyclic stimulation to the endometriosis, or a gonadotropin-releasing hormone agonist known as Lupron that mimics menopause, thereby removing hormonal stimulation and hopefully reducing scarring and pain. Combining surgical removal of the endometriosis (when it is more extensive) with medical therapy before trying to conceive seems to increase the likelihood of fertility. For milder endometriosis, surgery adds little benefit to drug treatment. If after surgery for endometriosis you are not able to conceive, IVF may be your next step, in consultation with your doctor or reproductive endocrinologist.

One final note regarding tubal issues pertains to women who have had a previous tubal ligation, or tying of the fallopian tubes, as a method of birth control. The decision to have a tubal ligation is a permanent change, but circumstances do sometimes arise that may make a woman consider a reversal. Reversal of a tubal ligation, known as "tuboplasty," is a $15,000–$20,000 procedure with less than a 20 percent success rate. Tuboplasty is the surgical procedure used to open the tubes, via laparoscopy or laparotomy, and involves general anesthesia. Risks include infection, bleeding, and nearby organ injury as well as a higher likelihood of tubal or ectopic pregnancy.

If the reason for fertility difficulties includes tubal blockage, there are two choices for resolution: tuboplasty or IVF. Currently, the standard, and much preferred treatment for tubal factor infertility is IVF, which is equally expensive but offers less surgical risk to the potential mother and a greater success rate for fertility. Since the first successful IVF in 1981, birthrates have improved. Today, up to 1 percent of all births in the United States are the result of IVF treatment; the process allows eggs to be retrieved from the ovaries, combined with sperm under carefully controlled laboratory conditions, and then the fertilized embryo is implanted in the mother's uterus. Success, measured as live birthrate, is up to 40 to 50 percent in women under thirty and 25 to 30 percent in women between thirty-five and thirty-nine years of age. After age forty, the IVF success rates drop below 10 percent; these rates drop even further among more mature women unless donor eggs are used.

The disadvantages of IVF include cost, increased incidence of twins and triplets, and increased pregnancy risks (almost twofold in one study) of preterm labor, gestational hypertension, and gestational diabetes. These medical concerns in pregnancy may be more prevalent in IVF patients who are also more mature, that is, more than thirty-five years old. The safety of IVF has been enhanced by implanting a limited number of embryos to reduce the likelihood of multiples. Ultimately, IVF can be the difference between the dream of conceiving a child and the reality of having one.

Evaluation and Treatment of Cervical Factors

Cervical factors come into play when the cervical mucus is unfriendly or hostile to the sperm or there is a cervical stenosis, or narrowing, that does not allow the sperm to enter the uterine cavity. Cervical problems account for about 5 percent of fertility problems. You may be at increased risk for this issue if you have any of these:

- Increasing maternal age narrows the fertile window, meaning the cervical mucus is less runny and hospitable to sperm and may not last as many days.
- History of synthetic estrogen (diethylstilbestrol or DES) exposure while in your mother's womb, which can change the cervical canal and uterine shape (see Chapter 5 for details).

- Previous cervical surgery, which can cause stenosis, or narrowing of the cervix, the opening of the uterus, making it difficult for sperm to penetrate. Examples of cervical surgery include cryotherapy, a freezing of the cervical tissue, or loop electrosurgical excision procedure, known as LEEP, a cone-shaped biopsy of the cervix. These techniques would be performed if abnormal Pap smears and cervical dysplasia were a problem for you (see Chapter 5 for details). If you have had only one LEEP procedure in your life time, studies have shown no change in your fertility or pregnancy risks. If you have had more than one LEEP procedure, there is a slightly higher risk for cervical incompetence or compromise, which is when the cervix opens in pregnancy much earlier than safe for delivery of a healthy baby (usually between fourteen and twenty-two weeks; see Chapter 5).

Treatment for cervical problems may include something as simple as timing intercourse more precisely if cervical mucus (CM) is only plentiful and watery for one day. If the texture of the CM is too thick through the entire ovulatory part of your menstrual cycle then take an expectorant for a few days. As mentioned in the section on Clomid use, the expectorant Robitussin CF is used to thin the mucus and improve its ability to carry sperm. If additional evaluation shows cellularity, or too many white blood cells in the cervical mucus, an allergy or infection may be present. Bacteria known as *Mycoplasma urealyticum* often cause the increased cellularity; presence of these bacteria can be easily determined by your doctor. Your doctor may recommend intrauterine insemination (IUI), in which the sperm are directly inserted into the uterus, bypassing the cervix, or a cervical dilation that can be done in the office.

Postcoital Testing

Postcoital testing (PCT) evaluates the health of your cervical mucus and is performed four to six hours after intercourse during midmonth when you are likely to be ovulating. The PCT evaluates:

- Spinnbarkeit or cervical mucus texture. An egg-white-like quality is optimal. The normal stretchiness of the mucus is also evaluated.
- Microscopic assessment of the number of the sperm per high-powered field (hpf). More than 5 to 10 sperm per hpf are adequate.
- Ferning (see Figure 18-4). The presence of fern-like patterns in the cervical mucus midcycle, which reflects appropriate estrogen levels.

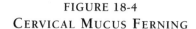

FIGURE 18-4
CERVICAL MUCUS FERNING

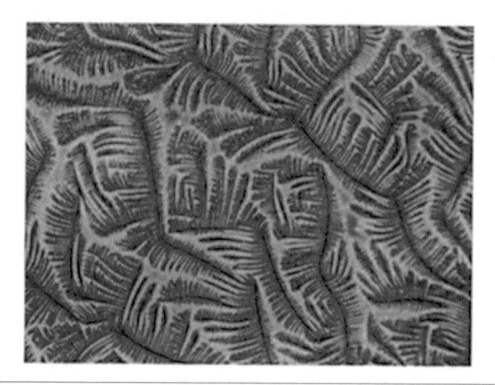

Evaluating and Treating Male Factor Infertility

Donna, a thirty-two-year-old homemaker, and her husband, Michael, had a healthy baby girl two years earlier, right before Michael was diagnosed with testicular cancer. Now they wanted to expand their family but were faced with a limited time to obtain sperm before he underwent cancer therapy and testicular surgery, which would make him sterile. With only two ejaculates to use for conception, they went through Michael's therapy with great success but then wondered how best to get pregnant. Due to the limited sperm availability, they were advised to undergo IVF to maximize the small number of sperm available. After their first cycle of IVF Donna conceived, and nine months later they welcomed a healthy baby boy into their family.

A low sperm count or abnormal sperm can account for up to 25 to 30 percent of all cases of infertility. While these issues can be emotionally devastating for a man, or at least embarrassing, they are the easiest issues to fix. The causes of male infertility can be due to:

Vasectomy Reversal

The overall success rate is 50 to 90 percent, depending on the man's age, type of vasectomy, skill of the surgeon, length of time since the vasectomy, and the health of the partner. Compared to a tubal ligation reversal (in women), vasectomy reversal is easier and less risky, and the risk of an ectopic pregnancy is not elevated. The alternative to vasectomy reversal, obtaining sperm directly from the testicle, is very difficult and not usually recommended. The cost is not usually covered by insurance and can range from $6,000 to $15,000.

- **Difficulty in growing healthy sperm due to a hormonal imbalance.** Glands in the brain may not be able to stimulate testosterone production or may produce an excess of estrogen or prolactin. Tumors or trauma to the brain can also change the hormonal messages to the male reproductive system.

- **Obstruction of the route sperm use to travel during phases of development from immaturity to mature growth.** The obstruction can be due to:
  - A birth defect, such as an absence of the vas deferens, the tube that connects the testicles to the epididymis
  - A surgical blockage, such as a vasectomy or hernia repair
  - Infections, such as *Chlamydia trachomatis,* which can scar the tubes closed (much like the effect of untreated chlamydia in women)
  - Prostate enlargement or inflammation
  - Trauma, such as in a motor vehicle accident or if a pelvic fracture occurs.

- **Inability of the sperm to move normally.** The most common reasons for this are:
  - Dilated veins around the sperm development sites in the testicles, known as a *varicocele,* which increases the ambient temperature in the testicles and damages the development of sperm
  - Partial blockage of the vas deferens (see Figure 9-1), which can occur after sexually transmitted disease and can lead to a longer than normal transit time for sperm to be ejaculated. Under these circumstances only very old, dead sperm reach the ejaculate, making them much less effective if not impotent, in fertilizing an egg
  - A congenital disorder, known as *immotile cilia syndrome,* which means the sperm lack the ability to move
  - Use of drugs such as marijuana

Varicoceles

A varicocele is the most common reason for a low sperm count. The dilated veins of the varicocele surround the testicle, which increases the testicular temperature, and makes sperm production less efficient.

A simple surgical procedure can repair the dilated veins and restore normal temperature around the testicles. Within a few months, there may be an improvement in the sperm count.

- **Sexual disturbance that doesn't allow the sperm to be released effectively,** such as ejaculation problems and erectile dysfunction (ED). (More about this can be found in Chapter 9.)

If your spouse or partner has a history of the following conditions, he may be at increased risk for male infertility:

- Testicular surgery or removal, common after testicular cancer or trauma
- Mumps in adolescence or adulthood
- Chemotherapy
- Radiation therapy in the pelvic area
- History of testicular torsion (twisting that deprives the testicles of blood supply)
- Recurrent sexually transmitted disease (particularly chlamydia)
- Exposure to the synthetic estrogen diethylstilbestrol (or DES) in his mother's uterus, if she took it during pregnancy
- History of retrograde ejaculation (as described in Chapter 9)
- History of erectile dysfunction or decreased libido
- History of medical conditions that can lead to some of the above issues, such as diabetes, obesity, high blood pressure, sedentary lifestyle, depression, or anxiety
- History of substance abuse

Additional, but less severe, influences on your partner's fertility include:

- Fever in the four months prior to trying to conceive
- History of trauma or injury to the penis or testicles
- History of inflammation of the epididymis or prostate
- Family history of infertility
- Frequent use of Jacuzzi, steam room, or hot tubs

Typically, the initial workup for suspected male infertility is a thorough sexual history, simple blood tests to evaluate the hormonal milieu, and a semen analysis, which you'll find detailed in Chapter 9. In general, the sperm have to be able to recognize their goal (the egg), be able to move toward it unencumbered (not carrying antibodies), and be able to get through to the uterus and fallopian tubes and into the egg, which is a bit of an uphill climb.

If the sperm count is found to be lower than normal or even absent, do not despair: assisted reproduction can be very successful. Intrauterine insemination (IUI) is the injection of sperm into the uterus of the prospective mother. By direct placement of the sperm into the uterus, this procedure overcomes the attrition of sperm that occurs when traveling through thick cervical mucus. (For instance, if your partner's semen contains twenty million sperm, the number that actually find the egg is only two hundred.) Bypassing these barriers with IVI maximizes the number of sperm in the vicinity of the egg waiting to be fertilized.

During IVF, another technique called intracytoplasmic sperm injection (ICSI) can isolate the most vital sperm, even only one excellent sperm, and inject it into an egg. This is a very successful process—it uses the fewest number of healthy sperm to achieve fertilization—but it is highly technical and can be fairly expensive. Simpler ways of restoring male fertility may include treating any infections that may be present, correcting anatomical disturbances (such as varicocele, for example), and stopping medications that may be disturbing sexual function. After a general medical evaluation, your spouse or partner may be referred to a urologist for further evaluation and treatment.

A Last Word on Medical Intervention

It is appropriate to consider these interventions under the following conditions: the unsuccessful trial of three to six months of ovulation medications, with or without intrauterine sperm insemination; if tubal blockage is suspect; or if severe male factor infertility is present. The chances of conception in women under the age of forty with the assistance of artificial reproduction technology (ART) are quite good, depending on the source of your fertility problem. It may sound a little harsh, but it often comes down to how much you are willing and able to spend and what you are willing to endure to achieve the pregnancy.

Today's IVF success rates (that is, IVF that results in a live birth) can vary based on maternal and paternal age, ovarian response to medication-induced ovulation, the experience of the reproductive endocrinologist assisting you, and the expertise of the embryologist. Generally speaking, you should expect that IVF can result in a 20 to 25 percent likelihood of a multiple pregnancy (that is, twin or triplet pregnancies) and a success rate (or "take-home baby rate") of 40 to 50 percent for women under age thirty-five, 25 to 30 percent if you are thirty-five to thirty-nine, and 10 percent for women age forty and older. Keep in mind that each cycle of IVF can cost between $10,000 and $15,000.

If you are looking to find a reproductive endocrinologist to assist in fertility therapies, ask your health care provider for a referral. You can evaluate fertility clinics by their successful pregnancy rates and their rates of multiple gestations. Birthrates are tracked by the Society for Assisted Reproductive Technology www.sart.com) and the Centers for Disease Control and Prevention (www.cdc.gov/ART).

Reproduction technology offers a very encouraging picture to most couples having difficulty conceiving, but occasionally you and your partner may need a break from attempting to conceive. Many infertility specialists and ob-gyns suggest taking a little "holiday" now and then. Try taking the spotlight off your urgent desire to make a baby and focus on the reason you got together in the first place. Enjoy each other and make love when the mood strikes, not just when the basal body temperature chart tells you it's time. In addition to helping you reduce stress, it is advisable to limit medication-induced ovulation to twelve lifetime cycles to reduce the risk of future ovarian cancer, so don't spend your dozen cycles all in one year! And here's an interesting fact: if you've struggled with infertility in a previous pregnancy, conception is often a little easier the next time. Maybe it's like running your first distance race—your body just knows the drill! Confidence and other positive diversions may help. So have some fun while you're trying.

SUCCESSFULLY MANAGING THE FERTILITY QUEST

Some experts consider the emotional stress of infertility and its treatment to be equal to the stress that one suffers when diagnosed with cancer or heart disease. The need for sexual intimacy on a schedule, the technical poking and prodding, and the general unfairness of infertility when you have spent the majority of your adult sexual life preventing fertility can become overwhelmingly frustrating. The stress of infertility can result in an even greater difficulty in conceiving.

Previous studies have found more fertility issues among depressed or anxious women, and it was speculated that a reduced libido, which led to less interest in intimacy and less sexual activity, resulted in reduced opportunities to conceive. One recent study, looking at women with known depression prior to trying to conceive, revealed a twofold increase in infertility. Positive imagery and thought processes seemed to result in an improved fertility rate for these couples. The mechanism explaining this change for women suffering from depression still remains unclear. Mind-body programs, in similar studies, improved fertility when relaxation techniques were employed.

As much as we like to think a positive attitude will conquer all, the truth is that the stress of trying to get pregnant can pose a serious relationship challenge for you and your spouse. You may both need to vent your frustrations, but doing so to each other may only make things worse. Don't hesitate to consider counseling. Even if you don't think of yourself as a "joiner," you might find a great deal of strength and wisdom in an infertility support group that in-

Online Information

Researching fertility information online is fast and easy. However, please keep in mind that not all of the information out there is clinical, or even factual. Look for sites that end in .edu or .gov to be safe. Some sites we have found to be reliable include:

- cdc.gov/ART/
- Fertilityfriend.com
- Fertilitylifelines.com
- resolve.org
- babycenter.com

cludes people who have been there, done that, and have the baby pictures to prove it. Check with your ob-gyn or fertility specialist for any suggestions about lectures or groups in your community. You may also find it very reassuring to explore reference material and message boards on the Internet. Just look for material that has been produced by a trustworthy source (a .gov or a .edu site is usually a good bet).

TOP 10 URBAN LEGENDS ABOUT FERTILITY

Fears are often raised by misinformation or urban legends promoted by friends, the media, and questionable Internet sites. Here are the facts to help you counter those urban legends!

1. **Pregnancy is possible every day of the month, except during my period.** Conception is most likely when intercourse occurs during the three-day interval ending on the day of ovulation,* usually the fourteenth day of your cycle if you have a twenty-eight-day menstrual cycle. (Cycle day number one is the first day of normal or heavier bleeding.)

2. **The "missionary position" increases your odds of pregnancy.** There is no proof that certain positions, such as the "missionary" position (man on top), are optimal for pregnancy. In fact, sperm get through the cervical mucus barrier within the first sixty to ninety seconds after ejaculation. (No stopwatches over the shoulder please!) So, have sex in any position preferable. Placing your hips on a pillow is not necessary, but you may want to "stay together" and relax for a few minutes anyway before you get up to void after intercourse.

---

*For example, in a twenty-eight-day menstrual cycle, ovulation usually occurs on DOC 14, so prime time would be DOC 12–15. We recommend lovemaking every other day during DOC 11–18 to account for the variety of cycle lengths.

3. **If I have a tilted uterus, I will have more trouble conceiving.** If you have been told by your gynecologist that you have a tilted or retroverted uterus, you are in good company. Almost 30 percent of women have a uterus bending toward your back (as opposed to a uterus that is anteverted, that is, tilts forward toward the bladder). To date, there is little research to support the common myth that this uterine position will make it more difficult to conceive. You may have been advised to use a rear entry or side-to-side position in order to optimize conception. Unfortunately, there is no conclusive research to substantiate those beliefs, so we recommend you enjoy your preferred position(s).

4. **Having an orgasm during intercourse will make it harder to get pregnant.** Studies have shown that female orgasm may actually assist the sperm and egg in their first introduction to each other by creating spasms of the uterine anatomy that draw the egg and sperm toward each other. There is also a favorable cervical mucus change with orgasm versus without. This doesn't make an orgasm vital, but it doesn't hurt to have one.

5. **I will never get a period if I am pregnant.** Often a woman may already be pregnant and still appear to get a menstrual flow. Usually this flow is not her normal type and consistency. If you are trying to conceive and your period is very light, late, or heavy compared to your normal cycle, we suggest that you take a pregnancy test with the first void of the morning. Also, never hesitate to inform your health care provider of these changes for further evaluation.

6. **It's best to have sex daily when you want to get pregnant.** Sexual activity with the intent of pregnancy can become cumbersome for couples. If your partner's sperm count is in the lower range of normal, taking a day off from lovemaking will increase sperm counts for the next ejaculation. In general, lovemaking during "prime time" (the three-day interval ending on the day of ovulation) should occur every other day, but can occur daily if normal sperm counts are known. Making love or masturbating too frequently (that is, more than one time per day) reduces the amount of sperm available in each ejaculation, thus reducing the likelihood of fertilization. Of course, if your opportunity to be together is limited to only two consecutive days during your fertile time, you have nothing to lose by trying two days in a row.

7. **I must not be ovulating if I don't get my menstrual flow every twenty-eight days.** Variations in women's cycles mean a "normal" cycle can be as short as twenty-four days or as long as thirty-five days. There are also women who do not get any menstrual flow at all—when breastfeeding, for example—yet they still can ovulate and conceive during this time.

8. **Just relax, or quit running, or adopt a child—then you'll get pregnant!** There are many anecdotes about couples who suffer unexplained or persistent infertility, then go on vacation, give up trying, or even adopt a child and then conceive spontaneously. There are no studies proving a link, though we often speculate that once the pressure to become pregnant is gone, pregnancy may actually be easier to achieve. And while the link is still speculative, female athletes may need to consider reducing the strenuousness of their workouts to free up more available energy or avoid clearing too much progesterone from their bodies. There may be a grain of truth to this urban legend after all.

9. **There is one test that can diagnose fertility issues.** There is no single test to determine the source of a couple's fertility problem. There are so many possible explanations, including ovulation irregularities, fallopian tube abnormalities, cervical factors, and male factors. In fact, fertility specialists are unable to pinpoint the cause for up to 30 percent of couples who do not spontaneously conceive. This is called unexplained infertility. We do not encourage fertility testing of either member of the couple *prior* to trying to conceive unless there have been extenuating circumstances in one's history where semen analysis or fallopian tube testing would be recommended (e.g., prior tubal surgery, adult male history of mumps, etc.).

10. **I want to have twins so I can get my childbearing done in one pregnancy.** Twins are a blessing, and are more common with fertility drug usage, maternal age over thirty-five, BMI over 30, or tall height (yes, really), and family history. However, twin pregnancies are not courted because they do increase the risk for preterm delivery, maternal hypertension, and gestational diabetes as well as creating a demanding postpartum adjustment above and beyond that which accompanies one newborn.

Be well, and be well informed. We hope this chapter has helped you with both. And we wish you the best in your baby quest!

After You Conceive

*I*f a positive result on a pregnancy test isn't enough evidence for you, there are normal bodily changes that begin fairly soon after conception. You may experience breast tenderness, abdominal bloating, and inexplicable fatigue. Sometimes the nausea we call morning sickness (but which can happen at any time of day) can begin very early as well. Some women describe feeling as though they have "very bad PMS" and find themselves to be unusually irritable or moody. Elation, anxiety, fear, or a combination of all of the above are some of the typical emotions experienced by newly pregnant woman. Alternatively, some women become anxious that they feel too well in the first few months of pregnancy. Every woman and each pregnancy she has is different, and so may be her symptoms.

Certainly it can take a few days for the knowledge that you are pregnant to actually sink in. It can take even longer than that for your spouse or partner, who might not experience the pregnancy as real until you start to "show." Many women wait until after the first trimester (twelve weeks) to begin really planning, sharing, and buying. Women, and couples, make a personal decision about when and with whom to share their news about pregnancy. If you tell folks that you are pregnant as soon as you know, there may be awkwardness later if a miscarriage occurs. With this in mind, we usually recommend that you share the joy of being pregnant with those in your life that you would also share the despair of miscarriage with—who could be supportive to you. Likewise, we often recommend telling work associates when you are showing, around the sixteenth week of pregnancy.

The preconception time of your life is over (at least for now), and you've embarked on the most miraculous journey of your life. The lifestyle changes you may have made before pregnancy will need to continue. Your improved eating habits, avoidance of smoking and alcoholic beverages, regular exercise habits, and careful manipulation of your home and work environment are all excellent ways to optimize your health and that of your growing fetus. You are now the master chef and caterer providing "womb service" twenty-four hours a day, seven days a week for a little guest who is receiving an optimal balance of nutrients and improved blood circulation because of the care you took before pregnancy. Preparing your body and your world for a healthy pregnancy is an act of profound love and devotion to the new life within you. Your baby is truly lucky.

A FETUS SLEEPING AT THIRTY-TWO WEEKS GESTATION

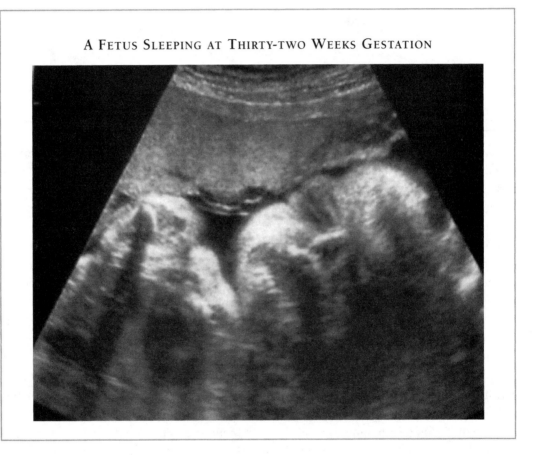

APPENDIX A: Income and Expense Worksheets

ESTIMATED CURRENT AFTER-TAX INCOME AND LIVING EXPENSES WORKSHEET

DATE: _____

	Monthly	or	Annual
Household After-Tax Income			
Income A	_____		_____
Income B	_____		_____
Other Income Sources	_____		_____
TOTAL INCOME			
House/Apartment Expenses			
Mortgage or Rent	_____		
Real Estate Property Taxes			_____
Utilities			
Electricity	_____		
Water	_____		
Cable	_____		
Trash	_____		
Telephone	_____		
Maintenance & Repairs	_____		
Lawn Care	_____		
Cleaning Help	_____		
New Household Purchases	_____		
Homeowner's Dues	_____		_____
	_____		_____
Food and Household Goods			
Groceries and Sundries	_____		_____
Work Lunches/Eating Out	_____		_____
Pet Food	_____		_____
	_____		_____
Clothing			
Purchases	_____		_____
Cleaning	_____		_____
	_____		_____

Transportation
Auto Payments/Lease _____
Gas and Oil _____
Maintenance, Repairs, and Tires
    Regular   _____
    Major   _____
License _____   _____

_____   _____   _____

Insurance Premiums
Homeowner's Insurance _____   _____
Auto Insurance _____   _____
Umbrella Policy _____   _____
Health Insurance _____   _____
Disability Insurance _____   _____
Long-Term-Care Insurance _____   _____
Life Insurance _____   _____

_____   _____

Recreation
Entertainment _____   _____
Hobbies _____   _____
Vacations _____   _____

_____   _____

Medical
Doctors and Dentist _____   _____
Medicines _____   _____

_____   _____

Personal Expenses
Subscriptions _____   _____
Education _____   _____
Allowances _____   _____
Hair Care _____   _____
Pet Care _____   _____

_____   _____

Child Care (if applicable)
Day Care/Babysitting _____ _____

Schooling _____ _____
Children Allowances _____ _____

_____ _____

Miscellaneous Expenses
Gifts _____ _____
Charitable Contributions _____ _____
Miscellaneous _____ _____

_____ _____

TOTAL EXPENSES

Source: Adapted from Creative Capital Management, Inc.

APPENDIX B: Dietary Reference Intake (DRI) Charts

On the following pages you will find two tables prepared by the Institute of Medicine of the National Academies of Sciences. The DRI charts show the Recommended Dietary Allowances (RDAs) in bold type and Adequate Intakes (AIs) in ordinary type followed by an asterisk (*) for vitamins and minerals at different life stages. The RDAs and AIs are daily goals for individual intake. Note that, unless otherwise specified, these levels refer to total intake from foods and supplements.

Dietary Reference Intakes (DRIs): Recommended Intakes for Individuals, Vitamins
Food and Nutrition Board, Institute of Medicine, National Academies

Life Stage Group	Vit A (µg/d)[a]	Vit C (mg/d)	Vit D (µg/d)[b,c]	Vit E (mg/d)[d]	Vit K (µg/d)	Thiamin (mg/d)	Riboflavin (mg/d)	Niacin (mg/d)[e]	Vit B6 (mg/d)	Folate (µg/d)[f]	Vit B12 (µg/d)	Pantothenic Acid (mg/d)	Biotin (µg/d)	Choline[g] (mg/d)
Infants														
0–6 mo	400*	40*	5*	4*	2.0*	0.2*	0.3*	2*	0.1*	65*	0.4*	1.7*	5*	125*
7–12 mo	500*	50*	5*	5*	2.5*	0.3*	0.4*	4*	0.3*	80*	0.5*	1.8*	6*	150*
Children														
1–3 y	**300**	**15**	5*	**6**	30*	**0.5**	**0.5**	**6**	**0.5**	**150**	**0.9**	2*	8*	200*
4–8 y	**400**	**25**	5*	**7**	55*	**0.6**	**0.6**	**8**	**0.6**	**200**	**1.2**	3*	12*	250*
Males														
9–13 y	**600**	**45**	5*	**11**	60*	**0.9**	**0.9**	**12**	**1.0**	**300**	**1.8**	4*	20*	375*
14–18 y	**900**	**75**	5*	**15**	75*	**1.2**	**1.3**	**16**	**1.3**	**400**	**2.4**	5*	25*	550*
19–30 y	**900**	**90**	5*	**15**	120*	**1.2**	**1.3**	**16**	**1.3**	**400**	**2.4**	5*	30*	550*
31–50 y	**900**	**90**	5*	**15**	120*	**1.2**	**1.3**	**16**	**1.3**	**400**	**2.4**	5*	30*	550*
51–70 y	**900**	**90**	10*	**15**	120*	**1.2**	**1.3**	**16**	**1.7**	**400**	**2.4**[h]	5*	30*	550*
>70 y	**900**	**90**	15*	**15**	120*	**1.2**	**1.3**	**16**	**1.7**	**400**	**2.4**[h]	5*	30*	550*
Females														
9–13 y	**600**	**45**	5*	**11**	60*	**0.9**	**0.9**	**12**	**1.0**	**300**	**1.8**	4*	20*	375*
14–18 y	**700**	**65**	5*	**15**	75*	**1.0**	**1.0**	**14**	**1.2**	**400**[i]	**2.4**	5*	25*	400*
19–30 y	**700**	**75**	5*	**15**	90*	**1.1**	**1.1**	**14**	**1.3**	**400**[i]	**2.4**	5*	30*	425*
31–50 y	**700**	**75**	5*	**15**	90*	**1.1**	**1.1**	**14**	**1.3**	**400**[i]	**2.4**	5*	30*	425*
51–70 y	**700**	**75**	10*	**15**	90*	**1.1**	**1.1**	**14**	**1.5**	**400**	**2.4**[h]	5*	30*	425*
>70 y	**700**	**75**	15*	**15**	90*	**1.1**	**1.1**	**14**	**1.5**	**400**	**2.4**[h]	5*	30*	425*
Pregnancy														
14–18 y	**750**	**80**	5*	**15**	75*	**1.4**	**1.4**	**18**	**1.9**	**600**[j]	**2.6**	6*	30*	450*
19–30 y	**770**	**85**	5*	**15**	90*	**1.4**	**1.4**	**18**	**1.9**	**600**[j]	**2.6**	6*	30*	450*
31–50 y	**770**	**85**	5*	**15**	90*	**1.4**	**1.4**	**18**	**1.9**	**600**[j]	**2.6**	6*	30*	450*
Lactation														
14–18 y	**1,200**	**115**	5*	**19**	75*	**1.4**	**1.6**	**17**	**2.0**	**500**	**2.8**	7*	35*	550*
19–30 y	**1,300**	**120**	5*	**19**	90*	**1.4**	**1.6**	**17**	**2.0**	**500**	**2.8**	7*	35*	550*
31–50 y	**1,300**	**120**	5*	**19**	90*	**1.4**	**1.6**	**17**	**2.0**	**500**	**2.8**	7*	35*	550*

NOTE: This table (taken from the DRI reports, see www.nap.edu) presents Recommended Dietary Allowances (RDAs) in **bold type** and Adequate Intakes (AIs) in ordinary type followed by an asterisk (*). RDAs and AIs may both be used as goals for individual intake. RDAs are set to meet the needs of almost all (97 to 98 percent) individuals in a group. For healthy breastfed infants, the AI is the mean intake. The AI for other life stage and gender groups is believed to cover needs of all individuals in the group, but lack of data or uncertainty in the data prevent being able to specify with confidence the percentage of individuals covered by this intake.

[a] As retinol activity equivalents (RAEs). 1 RAE = 1 µg retinol, 12 µg β-carotene, 24 µg α-carotene, or 24 µg β-cryptoxanthin. The RAE for dietary provitamin A carotenoids is twofold greater than retinol equivalents (RE), whereas the RAE for preformed vitamin A is the same as RE.

[b] As cholecalciferol. 1 µg cholecalciferol = 40 IU vitamin D.

[c] In the absence of adequate exposure to sunlight.

[d] As α-tocopherol. α-Tocopherol includes *RRR*-α-tocopherol, the only form of α-tocopherol that occurs naturally in foods, and the 2*R*-stereoisomeric forms of α-tocopherol (*RRR*-, *RSR*-, *RRS*-, and *RSS*-α-tocopherol) that occur in fortified foods and supplements. It does not include the 2*S*-stereoisomeric forms of α-tocopherol (*SRR*-, *SSR*-, *SRS*-, and *SSS*-α-tocopherol), also found in fortified foods and supplements.

[e] As niacin equivalents (NE). 1 mg of niacin = 60 mg of tryptophan; 0–6 months = preformed niacin (not NE).

[f] As dietary folate equivalents (DFE). 1 DFE = 1 µg food folate = 0.6 µg of folic acid from fortified food or as a supplement consumed with food = 0.5 µg of a supplement taken on an empty stomach.

[g] Although AIs have been set for choline, there are few data to assess whether a dietary supply of choline is needed at all stages of the life cycle, and it may be that the choline requirement can be met by endogenous synthesis at some of these stages.

[h] Because 10 to 30 percent of older people may malabsorb food-bound B₁₂, it is advisable for those older than 50 years to meet their RDA mainly by consuming foods fortified with B₁₂ or a supplement containing B₁₂.

[i] In view of evidence linking folate intake with neural tube defects in the fetus, it is recommended that all women capable of becoming pregnant consume 400 µg from supplements or fortified foods in addition to intake of food folate from a varied diet.

[j] It is assumed that women will continue consuming 400 µg from supplements or fortified food until their pregnancy is confirmed and they enter prenatal care, which ordinarily occurs after the end of the periconceptional period—the critical time for formation of the neural tube.

Dietary Reference Intakes (DRIs): Recommended Intakes for Individuals, Elements
Food and Nutrition Board, Institute of Medicine, National Academies

Life Stage Group	Calcium (mg/d)	Chromium (µg/d)	Copper (µg/d)	Fluoride (mg/d)	Iodine (µg/d)	Iron (mg/d)	Magnesium (mg/d)	Manganese (mg/d)	Molybdenum (µg/d)	Phosphorus (mg/d)	Selenium (µg/d)	Zinc (mg/d)	Potassium (g/d)	Sodium (g/d)	Chloride (g/d)
Infants															
0–6 mo	210*	0.2*	200*	0.01*	110*	0.27*	30*	0.003*	2*	100*	15*	2*	0.4*	0.12*	0.18*
7–12 mo	270*	5.5*	220*	0.5*	130*	11	75*	0.6*	3*	275*	20*	3	0.7*	0.37*	0.57*
Children															
1–3 y	500*	11*	340	0.7*	90	7	80	1.2*	17	460	20	3	3.0*	1.0*	1.5*
4–8 y	800*	15*	440	1*	90	10	130	1.5*	22	500	30	5	3.8*	1.2*	1.9*
Males															
9–13 y	1,300*	25*	700	2*	120	8	240	1.9*	34	1,250	40	8	4.5*	1.5*	2.3*
14–18 y	1,300*	35*	890	3*	150	11	410	2.2*	43	1,250	55	11	4.7*	1.5*	2.3*
19–30 y	1,000*	35*	900	4*	150	8	400	2.3*	45	700	55	11	4.7*	1.5*	2.3*
31–50 y	1,000*	35*	900	4*	150	8	420	2.3*	45	700	55	11	4.7*	1.5*	2.3*
51–70 y	1,200*	30*	900	4*	150	8	420	2.3*	45	700	55	11	4.7*	1.3*	2.0*
>70 y	1,200*	30*	900	4*	150	8	420	2.3*	45	700	55	11	4.7*	1.2*	1.8*
Females															
9–13 y	1,300*	21*	700	2*	120	8	240	1.6*	34	1,250	40	8	4.5*	1.5*	2.3*
14–18 y	1,300*	24*	890	3*	150	15	360	1.6*	43	1,250	55	9	4.7*	1.5*	2.3*
19–30 y	1,000*	25*	900	3*	150	18	310	1.8*	45	700	55	8	4.7*	1.5*	2.3*
31–50 y	1,000*	25*	900	3*	150	18	320	1.8*	45	700	55	8	4.7*	1.5*	2.3*
51–70 y	1,200*	20*	900	3*	150	8	320	1.8*	45	700	55	8	4.7*	1.3*	2.0*
>70 y	1,200*	20*	900	3*	150	8	320	1.8*	45	700	55	8	4.7*	1.2*	1.8*
Pregnancy															
14–18 y	1,300*	29*	1,000	3*	220	27	400	2.0*	50	1,250	60	12	4.7*	1.5*	2.3*
19–30 y	1,000*	30*	1,000	3*	220	27	350	2.0*	50	700	60	11	4.7*	1.5*	2.3*
31–50 y	1,000*	30*	1,000	3*	220	27	360	2.0*	50	700	60	11	4.7*	1.5*	2.3*
Lactation															
14–18 y	1,300*	44*	1,300	3*	290	10	360	2.6*	50	1,250	70	13	5.1*	1.5*	2.3*
19–30 y	1,000*	45*	1,300	3*	290	9	310	2.6*	50	700	70	12	5.1*	1.5*	2.3*
31–50 y	1,000*	45*	1,300	3*	290	9	320	2.6*	50	700	70	12	5.1*	1.5*	2.3*

NOTE: This table presents Recommended Dietary Allowances (RDAs) in **bold type** and Adequate Intakes (AIs) in ordinary type followed by an asterisk (*). RDAs and AIs may both be used as goals for individual intake. RDAs are set to meet the needs of almost all (97 to 98 percent) individuals in a group. For healthy breastfed infants, the AI is the mean intake. The AI for other life stage and gender groups is believed to cover needs of all individuals in the group, but lack of data or uncertainty in the data prevent being able to specify with confidence the percentage of individuals covered by this intake.

SOURCES: *Dietary Reference Intakes for Calcium, Phosphorous, Magnesium, Vitamin D, and Fluoride* (1997); *Dietary Reference Intakes for Thiamin, Riboflavin, Niacin, Vitamin B₆, Folate, Vitamin B₁₂, Pantothenic Acid, Biotin, and Choline* (1998); *Dietary Reference Intakes for Vitamin C, Vitamin E, Selenium, and Carotenoids* (2000); *Dietary Reference Intakes for Vitamin A, Vitamin K, Arsenic, Boron, Chromium, Copper, Iodine, Iron, Manganese, Molybdenum, Nickel, Silicon, Vanadium, and Zinc* (2001); and *Dietary Reference Intakes for Water, Potassium, Sodium, Chloride, and Sulfate* (2004). These reports may be accessed via http://www.nap.edu.

APPENDIX C: Resources for Safety Information

Resources for Lead Information

National Lead Information Center, (800) 424-5323 or www.epa.gov/lead.

Lead Listing, (888) LEADLIST (532-5478) or www.leadlisting.org, helps you locate lead service providers in your area.

Local Department of Health Services can guide you to their lead poisoning prevention programs. Also refer to your State Department of Environmental Protection.

Environmental Protection Agency (EPA) Safe Drinking Water Hotline, (800) 426-4791 or www.epa.gov/safewater. The EPA recommends two organizations that can provide information on safe water filtration products: the Water Quality Association (WQA) at (630) 505-0160, www.wqa.org, or the National Sanitation Foundation (NSF) at (800) NSF-MARK (673-6275), www.nsf.org.

Note: If you are interested in more resources, some key words to use in your phone book Yellow Pages are: *Lead Testing & Consulting, Lead Removal & Abatement,* and *Environmental Services.*

General Resources

EPA (Environmental Protection Agency) Washington, D.C. (local chapters may be present in your community)
Evaluation of potential air and water contamination, waste management, and pesticide usage
www.epa.gov

National Domestic Violence Hotline
(800) 799-SAFE (7233)
www.ndvh.org
Phone number can be accessed from a public pay phone; website can be accessed from a library computer if confidentiality is a concern.

National Institute of Occupational Safety
Guide to Chemical Hazards
(800) CDC-INFO (232-4636)
www.cdc.gov/niosh

OSHA (Occupational Safety and Health Administration), Washington, D.C.
Evaluates limits of safety in health care environments, provides teaching in health hazards disposal and safety
www.osha.gov

REPROTOX (Reproductive Toxicology Center), Columbia Hospital for Women, Washington, D.C.
Contains referenced information on three thousand physical and chemical agents
www.reprotox.org

TERIS (Teratogen Information Service). Many states have their own bureaus.
www.otispregnancy.org

APPENDIX D: Charts for Tracking Your Cycle

Menstrual Chart

Record your menstrual blood flow and cervical mucus changes to detect ovulatory patterns each month.

Date	1	2	3	4	5	6	7	8	9	10	11	12	13	14	15	16	17	18	19	20	21	22	23	24	25	26	27	28	29	30	31	Length of cycle (no. of days from start of period to beginning of next period)	Breast self-exam done (✓)
(Sample)																																	
Jan																																	
Feb																																	
Mar																																	
Apr																																	
May																																	
June																																	
July																																	
Aug																																	
Sept																																	
Oct																																	
Nov																																	
Dec																																	

My notes: _____

The first day of the cycle, called "DOC1," is the first day of normal bleeding (January 26 in the sample above).

During your period: L = light blood flow and X = normal blood flow

Near ovulation: cm = white/sticky cervical mucus, CM = clear egg-white cervical mucus, * = mittelschmerz

APPENDIX E: Shopping List

GRAINS   *pages 361–362*

(whole-grain bread, cereal, rice, and pasta)

_____

_____

_____

_____

_____

_____

_____

VEGETABLES   *page 363*

_____

_____

_____

_____

_____

_____

_____

_____

FRUITS   *pages 363–364*

_____

_____

_____

_____

_____

_____

_____

MILK   *pages 364–365*

(nonfat or low-fat milk or yogurt; cheese)

_____

_____

_____

_____

_____

MEAT and BEANS   *page 366*

(meat, poultry, fish, and shellfish; eggs; dried beans, lentils, soy products; nuts and seeds)

_____

_____

_____

_____

OILS   *page 367*

(canola and extra virgin olive oil; mayonnaise or aioli; oil-based salad dressings)

_____

_____

_____

MISCELLANEOUS

Essentials include *iodized* salt, pages 348–349.

Nonessential "discretionary extras" include solid fats and sweets, pages 368–369 and alcoholic beverages, according to preconception guidelines, pages 38–44.

APPENDIX F: Common Acronyms

BMI—body mass index

DOC—day of cycle

IVF—in vitro fertilization

A1C or HbA1C—hemoglobin A1C or glycated hemoglobin

LMP—last menstrual period

PMS—premenstrual syndrome

PCOS—polycystic ovary syndrome

STD/STI—sexually transmitted disease/infection

VBAC—vaginal birth after Cesarean section

MFM—maternal-fetal medicine specialist

ADHD—attention-deficit hyperactivity disorder

AUB—Abnormal uterine bleeding

ED—erectile dysfunction

To our delight, the impetus to revise this book the has stemmed directly from couples who have allowed us to help guide them on the path towards parenthood. We have been continually challenged and motivated by the couples who share their curiosity and their questions about preconception health and the science and technology that has been changing rapidly in the years between our first and second editions of *Before Your Pregnancy*. Thank you to patients, clients, and colleagues for continued support and willingness to learn more about the exciting advances in preconception care. We are touched and inspired to live up to your expectations and pave the way for more confident, healthy prospective moms and dads.

It would be very difficult to mention everyone who assisted in this project, but we'd like to thank a few special people. The revision of our book would have been impossible, and not nearly as enjoyable, without the editing and writing talents of Allison Krug, MPH. She expressed endless patience, resilience, professionalism, and intelligence with each challenge we faced in revising the second edition to be the most up to date and accurate book it could be. In the first edition of *Before Your Pregnancy,* without the writing expertise and assistance of Andrea Stein, Linda Gross Kahn, Jill Gagnon, and Ramona Segreti, the original book would never have been completed. Under the grace and guidance of our literary agent, Angela Rinaldi, and the appreciated editorial guidance of Christina Duffy, Rebecca Shapiro, Tracy Bernstein, Elisabeth Dyssegaard, Patricia Peters, Maureen O'Neal, the Ballantine staff (Judith Hoover, Helene Berinsky, Nancy Delia, Jie Yang, Elizabeth Cochrane, Stacey Witcraft), and Leslie Meredith, we were able to create a book from a dream that would allow all couples to have healthier pregnancies from the moment of conception and make healthier babies. To Judith Cummins, our thanks for her beautifully rendered anatomical and exercise illustrations.

We deeply appreciate the time and knowledge shared with us by many experts, who are committed to the betterment of reproductive health for men and women, that has enabled this book to be as accurate and thorough as possible, including Jeanne Blankenship, MS, RD (bariatric nutrition), Robert Brannigan, MD (urology), Wendi Buchi, MD (ob-gyn/eating disorders), A. Correa, M.D. (endocrinologist), Jean Cox, MS, RD, LN (nutrition), Mary D'Alton, MD (maternal-fetal medicine), Marianne Engle, PhD (psychology), Cathy Fagan (reproductive nutrition), Karen Freeman, MS, RD (nutrition/eating disorders), Angela Grassi, MS, RD, LDN (PCOS/nutrition/disordered eating), Peter Hurst, DDS (dental), Kathy Kater, LICSW (healthy body image/psychotherapy), Ralph Kazer, MD (reproductive endocrinology), Carl Keen, PhD (reproductive nutrition), Diane Machcinski, MEd, RD (nutrition), Carrie McMahon, MS, GC (genetic counseling), Patti Tveit Milligan, MS, RD (nutrition/herbs), Gil Mor, MD (immunology), Eugene Pergament, MD (genetics), Richard Phelps, MD (endocrinology), Lois Platt-Koch, RN, MSW (psychology), Nick Ralston, PhD (selenium physiology), Cherie Roussos, RD, CDE (nutrition/diabetes), Arthur Segreti, PhD (psychology), Ramona Segreti, MSW (psychology), Lee Shulman, M.D. (genetics), Judy Simon, MS, RD, CD, CHES (reproductive nutrition), Christopher Sipe, MD (reproductive endocrinology), Cindy Swann, MS, RD (nutrition), the late Varro Tyler, PhD, ScD (herbal medicine), Nicki Ward, RN, IBCLC (lactation), Sheila Watkins, MS (perinatal fitness), Chris Westbrook, MD (pediatrics), Denise Wilfley, PhD (eating disorders/psychology), and Sheri Zidenberg-Cherr, PhD (reproductive nutrition). Additional thanks to Ross Afsahi and Kerri Sullivan, CFP, for their input on the intricacies of preconceptional medical insurance and financial planning, respectively. To Janice Janecki for her vision of what the original video edition of *Before Your Pregnancy* could become, and to Cheryl Gill and Holly Retz for their candid feedback on the flow and intelligibility of this revised edition, as well as to Linn Bekins, Merri Metcalfe, Chaela Pastori, Briana and Bill Ruff, and Hope Roel for their thoughtful attention and feedback on various versions of the manuscript or related works.

We continue to be humbled and awed by the support, saintly patience, and good humor of our dear families, friends, partners, and colleagues. We are grateful for the individual ways that they have enriched our writing experience—not just once, but twice now—and our everyday lives.

ABOUT THE AUTHORS

AMY OGLE, MS, RD, is a registered dietitian, exercise physiologist, and ACE-certified personal trainer in private practice in San Diego, California. She has produced a popular video, which has been used in medical practices, university courses, and corporate wellness programs, on which this book is based.

LISA MAZZULLO, MD, is a practicing ob-gyn and assistant professor of obstetrics and gynecology at Northwestern University Medical School.